P9-DDN-740

THE WILLS EYE MANUAL

Office and Emergency Room
Diagnosis and Treatment of Eye Disease

Fourth Edition

THE WILLS EYE MANUAL

Office and Emergency Room
Diagnosis and Treatment of Eye Disease

Fourth Edition

Derek Y. Kunimoto, M.D.
Kunal D. Kanitkar, M.D.
Mary S. Makar, M.D.
Editors for the Fourth Edition

Mark A. Friedberg, M.D.
Christopher J. Rapuano, M.D.
Founding Editors

LIPPINCOTT WILLIAMS & WILKINS
A **Wolters Kluwer** Company
Philadelphia • Baltimore • New York • London
Buenos Aires • Hong Kong • Sydney • Tokyo

Acquisitions Editor: Jonathan Pine
Developmental Editor: Stacey L. Baze
Production Editor: Jonathan Geffner
Manufacturing Manager: Colin Warnock
Cover Designer: Brian Crede
Compositor: Lippincott Williams & Wilkins Desktop Division
Printer: R. R. Donnelley–Crawfordville

© 2004 by LIPPINCOTT WILLIAMS & WILKINS
530 Walnut Street
Philadelphia, PA 19106 USA
LWW.com

All rights reserved. This book is protected by copyright. No part of this book may be reproduced in any form or by any means, including photocopying, or utilized by any information storage and retrieval system without written permission from the copyright owner, except for brief quotations embodied in critical articles and reviews. Materials appearing in this book prepared by individuals as part of their official duties as U.S. government employees are not covered by the above-mentioned copyright.

Printed in the USA

Library of Congress Cataloging-in-Publication Data

The Wills eye manual: office and emergency room diagnosis and treatment of eye disease.— 4th ed. / Derek Y. Kunimoto, Kunal D. Kanitkar, Mary S. Makar, editors ; Mark A. Friedberg, Christopher J. Rapuano, founding editors.
    p. ; cm.
  Includes bibliographical references and index.
  ISBN: 0-7817-4207-2
    1. Eye—Diseases—Handbooks, manuals, etc. 2. Ophthalmologic emergencies—Handbooks, manuals, etc. I. Kunimoto, Derek Y. II. Kanitkar, Kunal D. III. Makar, Mary S. IV. Wills Eye Hospital (Philadelphia, Pa.)
  [DNLM: 1. Eye Diseases—diagnosis—Outlines. 2. Eye Diseases—therapy—Outlines. 3. Emergencies—Outlines. WW 18.2 W741 2004]
  RE48.9 W54 2004
  617.7—dc22   2003065975

Care has been taken to confirm the accuracy of the information presented and to describe generally accepted practices. However, the authors, editors, and publisher are not responsible for errors or omissions or for any consequences from application of the information in this book and make no warranty, expressed or implied, with respect to the currency, completeness, or accuracy of the contents of the publication. Application of this information in a particular situation remains the professional responsibility of the practitioner.

    The authors, editors, and publisher have exerted every effort to ensure that drug selection and dosage set forth in this text are in accordance with current recommendations and practice at the time of publication. However, in view of ongoing research, changes in government regulations, and the constant flow of information relating to drug therapy and drug reactions, the reader is urged to check the package insert for each drug for any change in indications and dosage and for added warnings and precautions. This is particularly important when the recommended agent is a new or infrequently employed drug.

    Some drugs and medical devices presented in this publication have Food and Drug Administration (FDA) clearance for limited use in restricted research settings. It is the responsibility of the health care provider to ascertain the FDA status of each drug or device planned for use in their clinical practice.

10 9 8 7 6 5 4 3

CONTENTS

CHAPTER 6: EYELID 111

CHAPTER 7: ORBIT 126

CHAPTER 8: PEDIATRICS 141

CHAPTER 9: GLAUCOMA 164

CHAPTER 10: NEURO-OPHTHALMOLOGY 198

CORNEA

Major Consultants
Elisabeth J. Cohen, M.D.
Christopher J. Rapuano, M.D.

Consultants
Sadeer B. Hannush, M.D.
Peter R. Laibson, M.D.
Irving M. Raber, M.D.

GLAUCOMA

Consultants
L. Jay Katz, M.D.
Marlene R. Moster, M.D.
Jonathan S. Myers, M.D.
Douglas J. Rhee, M.D.
Louis W. Schwartz, M.D.
George L. Spaeth, M.D.
Richard P. Wilson, M.D.

NEURO-OPHTHALMOLOGY

Consultants
Peter J. Savino, M.D.
Robert C. Sergott, M.D.

OCULOPLASTICS

Consultants
Jurij R. Bilyk, M.D.
Joseph C. Flanagan, M.D.
Marlon Maus, M.D.
Robert Penne, M.D.
Mary A. Stefanyszyn, M.D.

ONCOLOGY

Consultants
Carol L. Shields, M.D.
Jerry A. Shields, M.D.

PEDIATRICS

Consultants
Joseph H. Calhoun, M.D.
Leonard B. Nelson, M.D.
Bruce M. Schnall, M.D.

RETINA

Major Consultants
William E. Benson, M.D.
David H. Fischer, M.D.
William Tasman, M.D.

Consultants
Jonathan B. Belmont, M.D.
Gary C. Brown, M.D.
Allen C. Ho, M.D.
Joseph I. Maguire, M.D.
Carl D. Regillo, M.D.
Arunan Sivalingam, M.D.
James F. Vander, M.D.
Tamara R. Vrabec, M.D.

GENERAL

Consultants
Elizabeth L. Affel, M.S., R.D.M.S.
Michael DellaVecchia, M.D.
Edward A. Jaeger, M.D.
John B. Jeffers, M.D.
Robert D. Reinecke, M.D.
Richard Tipperman, M.D.

CONTRIBUTORS TO THE FOURTH EDITION

Seema Aggarwal, M.D.
Brian C. Bigler, M.D.
Vatinee Y. Bunya, M.D.
Christine Buono, M.D.
Jacqueline R. Carrasco, M.D.
Sandra Y. Cho, M.D.
Carolyn A. Cutney, M.D.
Brian D. Dudenhoefer, M.D.
John A. Epstein, M.D.
Colleen P. Halfpenny, M.D.
Stephen S. Hwang, M.D.
ThucAnh T. Ho, M.D.
Kunal D. Kantikar, M.D.
Derek Y. Kunimoto, M.D.

R. Gary Lane, M.D.
Henry C. Lee, M.D.
Mimi Liu, M.D.
Mary S. Makar, M.D.
Anson T. Miedel, M.D.
Parveen K. Nagra, M.D.
Michael A. Negrey, M.D.
Heather A. Nesti, M.D.
Vasudha A. Panday, M.D.
Nicholas A. Pefkaros, M.D.
Robert Sambursky, M.D.
Daniel E. Shapiro, M.D.
Derrick W. Shindler, M.D.

CONTRIBUTORS TO THE THIRD EDITION

Christine W. Chung, M.D.
Brian P. Connolly, M.D.
Vincent A. Deramo, M.D.
Kammi B. Gunton, M.D.
Mark R. Miller, M.D.
Ralph E. Oursler III, M.D.
Mark F. Pyfer, M.D.

Douglas J. Rhee, M.D.
Jay C. Rudd, M.D.
Brian M. Sucheski, M.D.

Medical Illustrator
Marlon Maus, M.D.

CONTRIBUTORS TO THE SECOND EDITION

Mark C. Austin, M.D.
Jerry R. Blair, M.D.
Benjamin Chang, M.D.
Mary Ellen Cullom, M.D.
R. Douglas Cullom, Jr., M.D.
Jack Dugan, M.D.
Forest J. Ellis, M.D.
C. Byron Faulkner, M.D.
Mary Elizabeth Gallivan, M.D.
J. William Harbour, M.D.
Paul M. Herring, M.D.
Allen Ho, M.D.
Carol J. Hoffman, M.D.
Thomas I. Margolis, M.D.
Mark L. Mayo, M.D.

Michele A. Miano, M.D.
Wynne A. Morley, M.D.
Timothy J. O'Brien, M.D.
Florentino E. Palmon, M.D.
William B. Phillips, M.D.
Tony Pruthi, M.D.
Carl D. Regillo, M.D.
Scott H. Smith, M.D.
Mark R. Stokes, M.D.
Janine G. Tabas, M.D.
John R. Trible, M.D.
Christopher Williams, M.D.

Medical Illustrator
Neal H. Atebara, M.D.

CONTRIBUTORS TO THE FIRST EDITION

Melissa M. Brown, M.D.
Catharine J. Crockett, M.D.
Bret L. Fisher, M.D.
Patrick M. Flaharty, M.D.
Mark A. Friedberg, M.D.
James T. Handa, M.D.
Victor A. Holmes, M.D.
Bruce J. Keyser, M.D.

Ronald L. McKey, M.D.
Christopher J. Rapuano, M.D.
Paul A. Raskauskas, M.D.
Eric P. Suan, M.D.

Medical Illustrator
Marlon Maus, M.D.

It has been 14 years since the first edition of *The Wills Eye Manual* was published. Over that period of time, each edition has been well received and the third edition has been translated into Japanese, Spanish, Portuguese, and Czechoslovakian.

The fourth edition features many changes. The uveitis section has been completely redone, as well as the section on hyphema. Of particular importance is the addition of new diagnostic techniques such as ultrasound biomicroscopy, ocular computerized tomography, and confocal biomicroscopy. Another very important new highlight is the updated material relating to clinical trials. For example, since the last edition, the Ocular Hypertension Study (OHTS),

Treatment of Age-Related Macular Degeneration with Photodynamic Therapy (TAP) study, and Age-Related Eye Disease Study (AREDS) have been added, to mention a few. And, finally, this edition has been prepared in a more reader-friendly format.

The editors for the fourth edition are Derek Y. Kunimoto, M.D., Kunal D. Kanitkar, M.D., and Mary S. Makar, M.D. As did their predecessors, they have worked diligently to make this volume a success. However, nothing could have been achieved had it not been for all three resident classes who volunteered their time and effort to bring this project to fruition.

William Tasman, M.D.

We are pleased to present the Fourth Edition of *The Wills Eye Manual*, the most widely used text of office and emergency room-based ophthalmic management.

As with previous editions, *The Wills Eye Manual* should continue to appeal to residents, comprehensive ophthalmologists, optometrists, emergency room physicians, primary care practitioners, medical students, and other health care professionals delivering eye care. In this new edition, our goals are to provide a timely, comprehensive manual and to present the information in an easy-to-use format. We have updated all sections with current concepts of diagnosis and management and have included pertinent recommendations from recent major clinical trials, including among others, the Age-Related Eye Disease Study (AREDS), the Ocular Hypertension Treatment Study (OHTS), and the Controlled High-Risk Subjects Avonex Multiple Sclerosis Prevention Trial (CHAMPS).

Major revisions have been made to sections on Hyphema, Ocular Hypertension, Optic Neuritis, Anterior Uveitis, Intermediate Uveitis, Posterior Uveitis, Acute Retinal Necrosis, Vogt–Koyanagi–Harada Syndrome, Pregnancy, Vitamin A Deficiency, and Neurofibromatosis. New sections have been added on Ocular Vaccinia, Chronic Angle-Closure Glaucoma, Commonly Used Ophthalmic Drugs, Ultrasound Biomicroscopy, Optical Coherence Tomography, Confocal Scanning Laser Ophthalmoscopy, and Confocal Biomicroscopy.

We also have created a new look for this latest edition of *The Wills Eye Manual*, so that it is easier and quicker to use, is streamlined in size, and is therefore a more portable companion. The wealth of wisdom from leading clinicians at Wills Eye Hospital is apparent throughout the manual.

It is our hope that the fourth edition of *The Wills Eye Manual* will continue to be a comprehensive handy resource for managing the ophthalmic problems of your patients.

Derek Y. Kunimoto, M.D.

Kunal D. Kanitkar, M.D.

Mary S. Makar, M.D.

Our goal has been to produce a concise book, providing essential diagnostic tips and specific therapeutic information pertaining to eye disease. We realized the need for this book while managing emergency room patients at one of the largest and busiest eye hospitals in the country. Until now, reliable information could only be obtained in unwieldy textbooks or inaccessible journals.

As residents at Wills Eye Hospital we have benefited from the input of some of the world-renowned ophthalmic experts in writing this book. More importantly, we are aware of the questions that the ophthalmology resident, the attending ophthalmologist, and the emergency room physician (not trained in ophthalmology) want answered immediately.

The book is written for the eye care provider who, in the midst of evaluating an eye problem, needs quick access to additional information. We try to be as specific as possible, describing the therapeutic modalities used at our institution. Many of these recommendations are, therefore, not the only manner in which to treat a particular disorder, but indicate personal preference. They are guidelines, not rules.

Because of the forever changing wealth of ophthalmic knowledge, omissions and errors are possible, particularly with regard to management. Drug dosages have been checked carefully, but the physician is urged to check the *Physicians Desk Reference* or *Facts and Comparisons* when prescribing unfamiliar medications. Not all contraindications and side effects are described.

We feel this book will make a welcome companion to the many physicians involved with treating eye problems. It is everything you wanted to know and nothing more.

Christopher J. Rapuano, M.D.

Mark A. Friedberg, M.D.

ACKNOWLEDGMENTS

We thank the growing generations of Wills residents who have contributed to this manual over the last 15 years. Their hard work has created a text that has fundamentally impacted the ophthalmic care of patients across the country and, indeed, throughout the world. We are grateful to the many Wills attending ophthalmologists who have shared their knowledge and experience, always dedicated to resident education. Lastly, a special acknowledgment must be made to Dr. William Tasman, Dr. Edward Jaeger, and Dr. Christopher Rapuano for their unwavering support of this endeavor.

CHAPTER 1

DIFFERENTIAL DIAGNOSIS OF OCULAR SYMPTOMS

BURNING

More common. Blepharitis, meibomianitis, dry-eye syndrome, conjunctivitis (infectious, allergic, mechanical, chemical).

Less common. Corneal problem (fluorescein staining of the cornea, usually), inflamed pterygium/pinguecula, episcleritis, superior limbic keratoconjunctivitis, ocular toxicity (medication, makeup, contact lens fluid).

CROSSED EYES IN CHILDREN

See 8.3, Esodeviations in Children (eyes turned in), or 8.4, Exodeviations in Children (eyes turned out).

DECREASED VISION

1. **Transient visual loss** (vision returns to normal within 24 hours, usually within 1 hour).

   More common. Few seconds (usually bilateral): Papilledema. Few minutes: Amaurosis fugax (transient ischemic attack; unilateral), vertebrobasilar artery insufficiency (bilateral). 10 to 60 minutes: Migraine (with or without a subsequent headache).

   Less common. Impending central retinal vein occlusion, ischemic optic neuropathy, ocular ischemic syndrome (carotid occlusive disease), glaucoma, sudden change in blood pressure, central nervous system (CNS) lesion, optic disc drusen, giant cell arteritis.

2. **Visual loss lasting longer than 24 hours**

   —**Sudden, painless loss**

   More common. Retinal artery or vein occlusion, ischemic optic neuropathy, vitreous hemorrhage, retinal detachment, optic neuritis (usually pain with eye movements), sudden discovery of preexisting unilateral visual loss.

   Less common. Other retinal or CNS disease (e.g., stroke), methanol poisoning.

   —**Gradual, painless loss** (over weeks, months, or years).

   More common. Cataract, refractive error, open-angle glaucoma, chronic retinal disease [e.g., age-related macular degeneration (ARMD), diabetic retinopathy].

   Less common. Chronic corneal disease (e.g., corneal dystrophy), optic neuropathy/atrophy (e.g., CNS tumor).

   —**Painful loss:** Acute angle-closure glaucoma, optic neuritis (pain with eye movements), uveitis, endophthalmitis, corneal hydrops (keratoconus).

3. **Posttraumatic visual loss:** Eyelid swelling, corneal irregularity, hyphema, ruptured globe, traumatic cataract, lens dislocation, commotio retinae, retinal detachment, reti-

nal/vitreous hemorrhage, traumatic optic neuropathy, CNS injury.

Note: Always remember nonphysiologic visual loss.

DISCHARGE

See Red Eye in this chapter.

DISTORTION OF VISION

More common. Refractive error [including presbyopia, acquired myopia (from cataract, diabetes, ciliary spasm, retinal detachment surgery), acquired astigmatism (from anterior segment surgery, chalazion)], macular disease (e.g., central serous chorioretinopathy, macular edema, or ARMD), corneal irregularity, intoxication (ethanol, methanol), pharmacologic (e.g., scopolamine patch).

Less common. Keratoconus, topical eye drops (miotics, cycloplegics), retinal detachment, migraine (transient), hypotony, CNS abnormality (including papilledema), nonphysiologic.

DOUBLE VISION (DIPLOPIA)

1. **Monocular** (The double vision remains when the uninvolved eye is occluded.).

   More common. Refractive error, incorrect spectacle alignment, corneal opacity or irregularity (including corneal/refractive surgery), cataract.

   Less common. Dislocated natural lens or lens implant, extra pupillary openings, macular disease, retinal detachment, CNS causes (rare), nonphysiologic.

2. **Binocular** (The double vision is eliminated when either eye is occluded.).

   —**Typically intermittent:** Myasthenia gravis, intermittent decompensation of an existing phoria.

   —**Constant:** Isolated sixth, third, or fourth nerve palsy; orbital disease (e.g., thyroid eye disease, orbital inflammatory pseudotumor, tumor); cavernous sinus/superior orbital fissure syndrome; status postocular surgery (e.g., residual anesthesia, displaced muscle, undercorrection/overcorrection after muscle surgery); status posttrauma (e.g., orbital wall fracture with extraocular muscle entrapment, orbital edema); internuclear ophthalmoplegia, vertebrobasilar artery insufficiency, other CNS lesions; spectacle problem.

DRY EYES

See 4.3, Dry-Eye Syndrome.

EYELASH LOSS

Trauma, thyroid disease, Vogt–Koyanagi–Harada syndrome, eyelid infection/inflammation, radiation, chronic skin disease (e.g., alopecia areata), cutaneous neoplasm.

EYELID CRUSTING

More common. Blepharitis, meibomianitis, conjunctivitis.

Less common. Canaliculitis, nasolacrimal duct obstruction, dacryocystitis.

EYELIDS DROOPING (PTOSIS)

See Ptosis and Pseudoptosis in Chapter 2, Differential Diagnosis of Ocular Signs.

EYELID SWELLING

1. **Associated with inflammation** (usually erythematous).

   More common. Hordeolum, blepharitis, conjunctivitis, preseptal or orbital cellulitis, trauma, contact dermatitis, herpes simplex/zoster dermatitis.

   Less common. Ectropion, corneal abnormality, urticaria/angioedema, blepharochalasis, insect bite, dacryoadenitis, erysipelas, eyelid or lacrimal gland mass.

2. **Noninflammatory:** Chalazion; dermatochalasis; prolapse of orbital fat (retropulsion of the globe increases the prolapse); laxity of the eyelid skin; cardiac, renal, or thyroid disease; superior vena cava syndrome; eyelid or lacrimal gland mass.

EYELID TWITCH

Fatigue, excess caffeine, habit, corneal or conjunctival irritation (especially from an eyelash, cyst, or conjunctival foreign body), dry eye, blepharospasm (bilateral), hemifacial spasm, albinism (photosensitivity), serum electrolyte abnormality, anemia (rarely).

EYELIDS UNABLE TO CLOSE (LAGOPHTHALMOS)

Severe proptosis, severe chemosis, eyelid scarring, eyelid retractor muscle scarring, cranial nerve VII palsy, status postfacial cosmetic/reconstructive surgery.

EYES "BULGING" (PROPTOSIS)

See 7.1, Orbital Disease.

EYES "JUMPING" (OSCILLOPSIA)

Acquired nystagmus, internuclear ophthalmoplegia, myasthenia gravis, vestibular function loss, opsoclonus/ocular flutter, superior oblique myokymia, various CNS disorders.

FLASHES OF LIGHT

More common. Retinal break or detachment, posterior vitreous detachment, migraine, rapid eye movements (particularly in darkness), oculodigital stimulation.

Less common. CNS (particularly occipital lobe) disorders, retinitis, entoptic phenomena.

FLOATERS

See Spots in Front of the Eyes in this chapter.

FOREIGN BODY SENSATION

Dry-eye syndrome, blepharitis, conjunctivitis, trichiasis, corneal abnormality (e.g., corneal abrasion or foreign body, recurrent erosion, superficial punctate keratitis), contact lens–related problem, episcleritis, pterygium, pinguecula.

GLARE

Cataract, corneal edema or opacity, altered pupillary structure or response, status postrefractive surgery, posterior vitreous detachment, pharmacologic (e.g., atropine).

HALLUCINATIONS (FORMED IMAGES)

Blind eyes, bilateral eye patching, Charles Bonnet syndrome, psychosis, parietotemporal area lesions, other CNS causes, various drugs.

HALOS AROUND LIGHTS

Cataract, acute angle-closure glaucoma or corneal edema from another cause (e.g., aphakic/pseudophakic bullous keratopathy, contact lens overwear), corneal dystrophies, corneal haziness or mucus, pigment dispersion syndrome, vitreous opacities, drugs (e.g., digitalis, chloroquine).

HEADACHE

See 10.24, Headache.

ITCHY EYES

Conjunctivitis (especially allergic, vernal, and viral), blepharitis, dry-eye syndrome, topical drug allergy or contact dermatitis, giant papillary conjunctivitis or another contact lens–related problem.

LIGHT SENSITIVITY (PHOTOPHOBIA)

1. **Abnormal eye examination**

   More common. Corneal abnormality (e.g., abrasion or edema), anterior uveitis.

   Less common. Conjunctivitis (mild photophobia), posterior uveitis, albinism, total color blindness, aniridia, drugs (e.g., atropine), congenital glaucoma in children.

2. **Normal eye examination:** Migraine, meningitis, retrobulbar optic neuritis, subarachnoid hemorrhage, trigeminal neuralgia, or a lightly pigmented eye.

NIGHT BLINDNESS

More common. Refractive error (especially undercorrected myopia), advanced glaucoma or optic atrophy, small pupil (especially from miotic drops), retinitis pigmentosa, congenital stationary night blindness, drugs (e.g., phenothiazines, chloroquine, quinine).

Less common. Vitamin A deficiency, gyrate atrophy, choroideremia.

PAIN

1. **Ocular**

   —**Typically mild to moderate:** Dry-eye syndrome, blepharitis, infectious conjunctivitis, episcleritis, inflamed pinguecula or pterygium, foreign body (corneal or conjunctival), corneal disorder (e.g., superficial punctate keratitis), superior limbic keratoconjunctivitis, ocular medication toxicity, contact lens–related problems, postoperative, ocular ischemic syndrome.

   —**Typically moderate to severe:** Corneal disorder (abrasion, erosion, infiltrate/ulcer, ultraviolet burn), chemical conjunctivitis, trauma, anterior uveitis, scleritis, endophthalmitis, acute angle-closure glaucoma.

2. **Periorbital:** Trauma, hordeolum, preseptal cellulitis, dacryocystitis, dermatitis (contact, chemical, herpes zoster/simplex), referred pain (dental, sinus).

3. **Orbital:** Sinusitis, trauma, orbital pseudotumor/myositis, orbital tumor/mass, optic neuritis, orbital cellulitis or abscess, acute dacryoadenitis, migraine/cluster headache, diabetic cranial nerve palsy.

4. **Asthenopia:** Uncorrected refractive error, phoria/tropia, convergence insufficiency, accommodative spasm, pharmacologic (miotics).

RED EYE

1. **Adnexal causes:** Trichiasis, distichiasis, floppy eyelid syndrome, entropion/ectropion, lagophthalmos (incomplete eyelid closure), blepharitis, meibomianitis, acne rosacea, dacryocystitis, canaliculitis.

2. **Conjunctival causes:** Ophthalmia neonatorum in infants, conjunctivitis (bacterial, viral, chemical, allergic/atopic/vernal, medication toxicity), subconjunctival hemorrhage, injected pinguecula, superior limbic keratoconjunctivitis, giant papillary conjunctivitis, conjunctival foreign body, cicatricial pemphigoid, Stevens–Johnson syndrome, conjunctival neoplasia.

3. **Corneal causes:** Infectious/inflammatory keratitis, recurrent corneal erosion, pterygium, neurotrophic keratopathy, contact lens–related problems, corneal foreign body, ultraviolet burn.

4. **Other:** Trauma, postoperative, dry-eye syndrome, endophthalmitis, anterior uveitis, episcleritis, scleritis, pharmacologic (e.g.,

prostaglandin analogs), angle-closure glaucoma, carotid–cavernous fistula (corkscrew conjunctival vessels), cluster headache.

"SPOTS" IN FRONT OF THE EYES

1. **Transient:** Migraine.

2. **Permanent or long-standing**

   More common. Posterior vitreous detachment, posterior uveitis, vitreous hemorrhage, vitreous condensations/debris.

   Less common. Retinal break/detachment, corneal opacity/foreign body.

   Note: Some patients are referring to a blind spot in their visual field caused by a retinal, optic nerve, or CNS disorder.

TEARING

1. **Adults**

   —**Pain present:** Corneal abnormality (e.g., abrasion, foreign body/rust ring, recurrent erosion, edema), anterior uveitis, eyelash or eyelid disorder (trichiasis, entropion), conjunctival foreign body, dacryocystitis, trauma.

   —**Minimal/no pain:** Dry-eye syndrome, blepharitis, nasolacrimal duct obstruction, punctal occlusion, canaliculitis, lacrimal sac mass, ectropion, conjunctivitis (especially allergic and toxic), emotional states, crocodile tears (congenital or Bell palsy).

2. **Children:** Nasolacrimal duct obstruction, congenital glaucoma, corneal/conjunctival foreign body or other irritative disorder.

CHAPTER 2

DIFFERENTIAL DIAGNOSIS OF OCULAR SIGNS

ANTERIOR CHAMBER/ANTERIOR CHAMBER ANGLE

BLOOD IN SCHLEMM CANAL ON GONIOSCOPY

Compression of episcleral vessels by a gonioprism (iatrogenic), Sturge–Weber syndrome, arteriovenous fistula (e.g., carotid–cavernous sinus fistula), superior vena cava obstruction, hypotony.

HYPHEMA

After trauma or intraocular surgery (including laser iridectomy), iris neovascularization, herpes simplex or zoster iridocyclitis, blood dyscrasia or clotting disorder (e.g., hemophilia), anticoagulation, intraocular tumor (e.g., juvenile xanthogranuloma, retinoblastoma, angioma).

HYPOPYON

Infectious corneal ulcer, endophthalmitis, severe iridocyclitis, reaction to an intraocular lens or retained lens protein after cataract surgery, intraocular tumor necrosis (e.g., pseudohypopyon from retinoblastoma), retained intraocular foreign body, tight contact lens, chronic corneal edema with ruptured bullae.

CORNEA/CONJUNCTIVAL FINDINGS

CONJUNCTIVAL SWELLING (CHEMOSIS)

Allergy, any ocular or periocular inflammation, postoperative, drugs, venous congestion, angioneurotic edema, myxedema.

CONJUNCTIVAL DRYNESS (XEROSIS)

Vitamin A deficiency, after cicatricial conjunctivitis, Stevens–Johnson syndrome, ocular cicatricial pemphigoid, exposure (e.g., lagophthalmos, absent blink reflex, proptosis), radiation, long-standing inflammation of the lacrimal gland.

CORNEAL CRYSTALS

Schnyder crystalline dystrophy, multiple myeloma, cystinosis, gout, uremia, hypergammaglobulinemia, drugs (e.g., indomethacin, chloroquine), infectious crystalline keratopathy.

CORNEAL EDEMA

1. **Congenital:** Congenital glaucoma, congenital hereditary endothelial dystrophy, posterior polymorphous dystrophy (PPMD), birth trauma (forceps injury).

2. **Acquired:** Early postoperative edema, aphakic or pseudophakic bullous keratopathy, Fuchs endothelial dystrophy, contact lens overwear, traumatic/exposure/chemical

injuries, acute angle-closure glaucoma and other causes of acute increase in intraocular pressure, corneal hydrops (acute keratoconus), herpes simplex or zoster keratitis, iritis, failed corneal graft, iridocorneal endothelial (ICE) syndrome, PPMD.

DILATED EPISCLERAL VESSELS (IN THE ABSENCE OF OCULAR IRRITATION OR PAIN)

Underlying uveal neoplasm, arteriovenous fistula (e.g., carotid–cavernous fistula), polycythemia vera, leukemia, ophthalmic vein or cavernous sinus thrombosis.

ENLARGED CORNEAL NERVES

Most important. Multiple endocrine neoplasia type IIb (medullary carcinoma of the thyroid gland, pheochromocytoma, mucosal neuromas; may have marfanoid habitus).

Others. Keratoconus, keratitis, neurofibromatosis, Fuchs endothelial dystrophy, Refsum syndrome, trauma, congenital glaucoma, failed corneal graft, leprosy, ichthyosis, idiopathic.

FOLLICLES ON THE CONJUNCTIVA

See 5.1, Acute Conjunctivitis and 5.2, Chronic Conjunctivitis.

MEMBRANOUS CONJUNCTIVITIS

(Removal of the membrane is difficult and causes bleeding.) Streptococci, pneumococci, chemical burn, ligneous conjunctivitis, *Corynebacterium diphtheriae*, adenovirus, herpes simplex virus, ocular vaccinia. See also Pseudomembranous Conjunctivitis in this chapter.

OPACIFICATION OF THE CORNEA IN INFANCY

Congenital glaucoma, birth trauma (forceps injury), congenital hereditary endothelial or stromal dystrophy (bilateral), PPMD, developmental abnormality of the anterior segment (especially Peters anomaly), metabolic abnormalities (bilateral; e.g., mucopolysaccharidoses, mucolipidoses), interstitial keratitis, herpes simplex virus, corneal ulcer, corneal dermoid, sclerocornea.

PANNUS (SUPERFICIAL VASCULAR INVASION OF THE CORNEA)

Rosacea, tight contact lens or contact lens overwear, phlyctenule, chlamydia (trachoma and inclusion conjunctivitis), superior limbic keratoconjunctivitis (micropannus only), staphylococcal hypersensitivity, vernal keratoconjunctivitis, herpes simplex virus, chemical burn, aniridia, molluscum contagiosum, leprosy.

PAPILLAE ON THE CONJUNCTIVA

See 5.1, Acute Conjunctivitis and 5.2, Chronic Conjunctivitis.

PIGMENTATION/DISCOLORATION OF THE CONJUNCTIVA

Racial pigmentation (perilimbal), nevus, primary acquired melanosis, melanoma, ocular and oculodermal melanocytosis (congenital, blue–gray, episcleral), Addison disease, pregnancy, radiation, jaundice, resolving subconjunctival hemorrhage, mascara, pharmacologic (e.g., chlorpromazine, topical epinephrine).

PSEUDOMEMBRANOUS CONJUNCTIVITIS

(Removal of the membrane is easy, and no bleeding results.) All of the causes of membranous conjunctivitis, as well as ocular cicatricial pemphigoid, Stevens–Johnson syndrome, superior limbic keratoconjunctivitis, gonococci, staphylococci, chlamydia in newborns, and others.

SYMBLEPHARON [FUSION OF THE EYELID (PALPEBRAL) CONJUNCTIVA WITH THE CONJUNCTIVA COVERING THE GLOBE (BULBAR)]

Ocular cicatricial pemphigoid, Stevens–Johnson syndrome, chemical burn, trauma, drugs, long-standing inflammation, epidemic keratoconjunctivitis, atopic conjunctivitis, radiation, congenital.

WHORL-LIKE OPACITY IN THE CORNEAL EPITHELIUM

Amiodarone, chloroquine, Fabry disease and carrier state, phenothiazines, indomethacin.

EYELID ABNORMALITIES

EYELID EDEMA

See Eyelid Swelling in Chapter 1, Differential Diagnosis of Ocular Symptoms.

EYELID LESION

See 6.11, Malignant Tumors of the Eyelid.

PSEUDOPTOSIS

Dermatochalasis (laxity of the eyelid skin from old age), brow ptosis, enophthalmos (e.g., from a traumatic blow-out fracture), phthisis bulbi, microphthalmia (small eye), chalazion or other eyelid tumor, eyelid edema, hypotropia (e.g., in double-elevator palsy) and retraction of the contralateral eyelid, blepharospasm, Duane syndrome.

PTOSIS

More common. Aging (e.g., levator dehiscence), after intraocular surgery or trauma, congenital.

Less common. Myasthenia gravis, Horner syndrome, third nerve palsy, chronic progressive external ophthalmoplegia, corneal or anterior segment disease (e.g., corneal abrasion), prolonged use of topical steroids, botulinum toxin or sub-Tenon's steroid injection.

FUNDUS FINDINGS

BONE SPICULES (WIDESPREAD PIGMENT CLUMPING)

More common. Retinitis pigmentosa and associated syndromes, disseminated chorioretinitis

(especially old syphilis), trauma, pigmentary changes of aging.

Less common. After spontaneous reattachment of a retinal detachment (e.g., toxemia of pregnancy, Harada disease), Kearns–Sayre syndrome, abetalipoproteinemia, vitamin A deficiency, viral infections (e.g., rubella), drugs (e.g., thioridazine and other phenothiazines), retinopathy of prematurity (when seen years later as an adult), cystinosis, old vascular occlusions.

BULL'S-EYE MACULAR LESION

Age-related macular degeneration (ARMD), Stargardt disease, cone dystrophy, chloroquine retinopathy, Spielmeyer–Vogt syndrome.

CHOROIDAL FOLDS

Orbital or choroidal tumor, thyroid orbitopathy, orbital inflammatory pseudotumor, posterior scleritis, hypotony, retinal detachment, marked hyperopia, scleral laceration, papilledema, postoperative.

CHOROIDAL NEOVASCULARIZATION (GRAY–GREEN MEMBRANE OR BLOOD SEEN DEEP TO THE RETINA)

More common. ARMD, ocular histoplasmosis syndrome, high myopia, angioid streaks, choroidal rupture (trauma).

Less common. Drusen of the optic nerve head, tumors, after retinal laser photocoagulation, idiopathic.

COTTON-WOOL SPOTS (WHITE, FLUFFY LESIONS WITH FEATHERED EDGES, OFTEN OBSCURING RETINAL VESSELS)

More common. Acquired immunodeficiency syndrome retinopathy, hypertension, diabetes, connective tissue disease (e.g., systemic lupus erythematosus), retinal artery/arteriole occlusion.

Less common. Retinal vein occlusion, cardiac valvular disease, carotid artery obstruction, chest trauma (Purtscher retinopathy), anemia, leukemia, lymphoma.

EMBOLUS

See 10.20, Amaurosis Fugax; 11.6, Branch Retinal Artery Occlusion; 11.5, Central Retinal Artery Occlusion.

• Platelet–fibrin [dull gray and elongated (as opposed to round)]: Carotid disease.

Note: Similar-appearing fibrin emboli also may arise from the heart.

• Cholesterol (sparkling yellow, usually at an arterial bifurcation): Carotid disease.

• Calcium (dull white, typically around or on the disc): Cardiac disease.

• Cardiac myxoma (common in young patients, particularly in the left eye; often occludes the ophthalmic or central retinal artery behind the globe and is not seen).

• Talc and cornstarch (small yellow–white glistening particles in macular arterioles; may produce peripheral retinal neovascularization): Intravenous (i.v.) drug abuse.

• Lipid or air (cotton-wool spots, not emboli, are often seen): Results from chest trauma (Purtscher retinopathy) and fracture of long bones.

• Others (tumors, parasites, other foreign bodies).

MACULAR EXUDATES

More common. Diabetes, choroidal (subretinal) neovascular membrane, hypertension.

Less common. Macroaneurysm, Coats disease (children), peripheral retinal capillary hemangioma, retinal vein occlusion, papilledema, radiation.

NORMAL FUNDUS IN THE PRESENCE OF DECREASED VISION

Retrobulbar optic neuritis, cone degeneration, Stargardt disease/fundus flavimaculatus, other optic neuropathy (e.g., tumor, alcohol/tobacco), rod monochromatism, amblyopia, nonphysiologic visual loss.

OPTOCILIARY SHUNT VESSELS ON THE DISC

Orbital or intracranial tumor (especially meningioma), status postcentral retinal vein occlusion, chronic papilledema (e.g., pseudotumor cerebri), chronic open-angle glaucoma, optic nerve glioma.

RETINAL NEOVASCULARIZATION

1. **Posterior pole:** Diabetes, after central retinal vein occlusion.

2. **Peripheral:** Sickle cell retinopathy, after branch retinal vein occlusion, diabetes, sarcoidosis, retinopathy of prematurity, embolization from i.v. drug abuse, chronic uveitis, others (e.g., leukemia, anemia, Eales disease).

ROTH SPOTS (HEMORRHAGES WITH WHITE CENTERS)

More common. Leukemia, septic chorioretinitis (e.g., secondary to subacute bacterial endocarditis), diabetes.

Less common. Pernicious anemia (and rarely other forms of anemia), sickle cell disease, scurvy, systemic lupus erythematosus, other connective tissue diseases.

SHEATHING OF RETINAL VEINS (PERIPHLEBITIS)

More common. Syphilis, sarcoidosis, pars planitis, sickle cell disease.

Less common. Tuberculosis, multiple sclerosis, Eales disease, viral retinitis (e.g., human immunodeficiency virus, herpes), Behçet disease, fungal retinitis, bacteremia.

TUMOR

See 11.32, Malignant Melanoma of the Choroid.

INTRAOCULAR PRESSURE

ACUTE INCREASE IN INTRAOCULAR PRESSURE

Acute angle-closure glaucoma, glaucomatocyclitic crisis (Posner–Schlossman syndrome), inflammatory open-angle glaucoma, malignant glaucoma, postoperative (see Postoperative Problems, this chapter), suprachoroidal hemorrhage, hyphema, carotid–cavernous fistula, retrobulbar hemorrhage, or other orbital disease.

CHRONIC INCREASE IN INTRAOCULAR PRESSURE

See 9.1, Primary Open-Angle Glaucoma.

DECREASED INTRAOCULAR PRESSURE (HYPOTONY)

Ruptured globe, phthisis bulbi, retinal/choroidal detachment, iridocyclitis, severe dehydration, cyclodialysis cleft, ocular ischemia, drugs (e.g., glaucoma medications), postoperative (see Postoperative Problems, this chapter), traumatic ciliary body shutdown.

IRIS

IRIS HETEROCHROMIA (IRIDES OF DIFFERENT COLORS)

1. **Involved iris is lighter than normal:** Congenital Horner syndrome, most cases of Fuchs heterochromic iridocyclitis, chronic uveitis, juvenile xanthogranuloma, metastatic carcinoma, Waardenburg syndrome.

2. **Involved iris is darker than normal:** Ocular melanocytosis or oculodermal melanocytosis, hemosiderosis, siderosis, retained intraocular foreign body, ocular malignant melanoma, diffuse iris nevus, retinoblastoma, leukemia, lymphoma, ICE syndrome, some cases of Fuchs heterochromic iridocyclitis.

IRIS LESION

1. **Melanotic** (brown): Nevus, melanoma, adenoma, or adenocarcinoma of the iris pigment epithelium.

   Note: Cysts, foreign bodies, neurofibromas, and other lesions may appear pigmented in heavily pigmented irides.

2. **Amelanotic** (white, yellow, or orange): Amelanotic melanoma, inflammatory nodule or granuloma (sarcoidosis, tuberculosis, leprosy, other granulomatous disease), neurofibroma, patchy hyperemia of syphilis, juvenile xanthogranuloma, foreign body, cyst, leiomyoma, seeding from a posterior segment tumor.

NEOVASCULARIZATION OF THE IRIS

Diabetic retinopathy, central retinal vein or artery occlusion, branch retinal vein occlusion, ocular ischemic syndrome (carotid occlusive disease), chronic uveitis, chronic retinal detachment, intraocular tumor (e.g., retinoblastoma), other retinal vascular disease.

LENS (SEE ALSO 13.1, ACQUIRED CATARACT)

DISLOCATED LENS (ECTOPIA LENTIS)

Trauma, Marfan syndrome (usually superior), Weill–Marchesani syndrome, homocystinuria (usually inferior), syphilis, microspherophakia.

IRIDESCENT LENS PARTICLES

Drugs, hypocalcemia, myotonic dystrophy, hypothyroidism, familial, idiopathic.

LENTICONUS

1. **Anterior** (marked convexity of the anterior lens): Alport syndrome (hereditary nephritis).

2. **Posterior** (marked concavity of the posterior lens surface): Usually idiopathic, may

be associated with persistent hyperplastic primary vitreous.

NEUROOPHTHALMIC ABNORMALITIES

AFFERENT PUPILLARY DEFECT

1. **Severe** (2 to 3+): Optic nerve disease (e.g., ischemic optic neuropathy, optic neuritis, tumor, glaucoma); central retinal artery or vein occlusion; less commonly, a lesion of the optic chiasm/tract.

2. **Mild** (1+): Any of the preceding, amblyopia, vitreous hemorrhage, macular degeneration, branch retinal vein or artery occlusion, retinal detachment or other retinal disease.

ANISOCORIA (PUPILS OF DIFFERENT SIZES)

See 10.1, Anisocoria.

LIMITATION OF OCULAR MOTILITY

1. **With exophthalmos and resistance to retropulsion:** See 7.1, Orbital Disease.

2. **Without exophthalmos and resistance to retropulsion:** Isolated third, fourth, or sixth nerve palsy; multiple ocular motor nerve palsies (see 10.9, Cavernous Sinus and Associated Syndromes), myasthenia gravis, chronic progressive external ophthalmoplegia, orbital blow-out fracture with muscle entrapment, ophthalmoplegic migraine, Duane syndrome, other central nervous system (CNS) disorders.

OPTIC DISC ATROPHY

More common. Glaucoma; after central retinal vein or artery occlusion; ischemic optic neuropathy; chronic optic neuritis; chronic papilledema; compression of the optic nerve, chiasm, or tract by a tumor or aneurysm; traumatic optic neuropathy.

Less common. Syphilis, retinal degeneration (e.g., retinitis pigmentosa), toxic/metabolic op-

tic neuropathy, Leber optic atrophy, congenital amaurosis, retinal storage disease (e.g., Tay–Sachs), radiation neuropathy, other forms of congenital or hereditary optic atrophy (nystagmus almost always present in the congenital forms).

OPTIC DISC SWELLING (EDEMA)

See 10.14, Papilledema.

OPTOCILIARY SHUNT VESSELS

See Fundus Findings in this chapter.

PARADOXICAL PUPILLARY REACTION (PUPIL DILATES IN LIGHT AND CONSTRICTS IN DARKNESS)

Congenital stationary night blindness, congenital achromatopsia, optic nerve hypoplasia, congenital amaurosis, Best disease, optic neuritis, dominant optic atrophy, albinism, retinitis pigmentosa. Rarely, amblyopia and strabismus.

ORBIT

EXTRAOCULAR MUSCLE THICKENING ON COMPUTED TOMOGRAPHY SCAN

More common. Thyroid orbitopathy, orbital inflammatory pseudotumor.

Less common. Tumor (especially lymphoma, metastasis, or spread of lacrimal gland tumor to muscle), carotid–cavernous fistula, cavernous hemangioma (usually appears in the muscle cone without muscle thickening), rhabdomyosarcoma (children).

LACRIMAL GLAND LESIONS

See 7.7, Lacrimal Gland Mass/Chronic Dacryoadenitis.

OPTIC NERVE LESION (ISOLATED)

More common. Optic nerve glioma (especially children), optic nerve meningioma (especially adults).

Less common. Metastasis, leukemia, orbital inflammatory pseudotumor, sarcoidosis, increased intracranial pressure with secondary optic nerve swelling.

ORBITAL LESIONS/PROPTOSIS

See 7.1, Orbital Disease.

PEDIATRICS

LEUKOCORIA (WHITE PUPILLARY REFLEX)

See 8.1, Leukocoria.

NYSTAGMUS IN INFANCY (SEE ALSO 10.19, NYSTAGMUS)

Congenital nystagmus, albinism, Leber congenital amaurosis, CNS (thalamic) injury, spasmus nutans, optic nerve or chiasmal glioma, optic nerve hypoplasia, congenital cataracts, aniridia, congenital corneal opacities.

POSTOPERATIVE PROBLEMS

SHALLOW ANTERIOR CHAMBER

1. **Accompanied by increased intraocular pressure:** Pupillary block glaucoma, suprachoroidal hemorrhage, malignant glaucoma.

2. **Accompanied by decreased intraocular pressure:** Wound leak, choroidal detachment.

HYPOTONY

Wound leak, choroidal detachment, cyclodialysis cleft, retinal detachment, ciliary body shutdown, pharmacologic aqueous suppression.

REFRACTIVE PROBLEMS

PROGRESSIVE HYPEROPIA

Orbital tumor pressing on the posterior surface of the eye, serous elevation of the retina (e.g.,

central serous chorioretinopathy), posterior scleritis, presbyopia, hypoglycemia, cataracts, after radical keratotomy.

PROGRESSIVE MYOPIA

High (pathologic) myopia, diabetes, cataract, staphyloma and elongation of the globe, corneal ectasia (keratoconus or after corneal refractive surgery), medications (e.g., miotic drops, sulfa drugs, tetracycline), childhood (physiologic).

VISUAL FIELD ABNORMALITIES

ALTITUDINAL FIELD DEFECT

More common. Ischemic optic neuropathy, hemibranch retinal artery or vein occlusion.

Less common. Glaucoma, optic nerve or chiasmal lesion, optic nerve coloboma.

ARCUATE SCOTOMA

More common. Glaucoma.

Less common. Ischemic optic neuropathy (especially nonarteritic), optic disc drusen, high myopia.

BINASAL FIELD DEFECT

More common. Glaucoma, bitemporal retinal disease (e.g., retinitis pigmentosa).

Rare. Bilateral occipital disease, tumor or aneurysm compressing both optic nerves or chiasm, chiasmatic arachnoiditis.

BITEMPORAL HEMIANOPSIA

More common. Chiasmal lesion (e.g., pituitary adenoma, meningioma, craniopharyngioma, aneurysm, glioma).

Less common. Tilted optic discs.

Rare. Nasal retinitis pigmentosa.

BLIND SPOT ENLARGEMENT

Papilledema, glaucoma, optic nerve drusen, optic nerve coloboma, myelinated (medullated) nerve fibers off the disc, drugs, myopic disc with a crescent.

CENTRAL SCOTOMA

Macular disease; optic neuritis; ischemic optic neuropathy (more typically produces an altitudinal field defect); optic atrophy (e.g., from tumor compressing the nerve, toxic/metabolic disease); rarely, an occipital cortex lesion.

CONSTRICTION OF THE PERIPHERAL FIELDS LEAVING A SMALL RESIDUAL CENTRAL FIELD

Glaucoma; retinitis pigmentosa or other peripheral retinal disorder; chronic papilledema; after panretinal photocoagulation; central retinal artery occlusion with cilioretinal artery sparing; bilateral occipital lobe infarction with macular sparing; nonphysiologic visual loss; carcinoma-associated retinopathy; rarely, medications.

HOMONYMOUS HEMIANOPSIA

Optic tract or lateral geniculate body lesion; temporal, parietal, or occipital lobe lesion of the brain (stroke and tumor more common; aneurysm and trauma less common). Migraine may cause a transient homonymous hemianopsia.

VITREOUS

VITREOUS OPACITIES

Asteroid hyalosis; synchysis scintillans; vitreous hemorrhage; inflammatory cells from vitritis or posterior uveitis; snowball opacities of pars planitis or sarcoidosis; normal vitreous strands from age-related vitreous degeneration; tumor cells; foreign body; hyaloid remnants; rarely, amyloidosis or Whipple disease.

CHAPTER 3

TRAUMA

3.1 CHEMICAL BURN

Treatment should be instituted IMMEDI-
ATELY, even before testing vision.

Note: This includes alkali (e.g., lye, cements, plasters), acids, solvents, detergents, and irritants (e.g., mace).

EMERGENCY TREATMENT

1. Copious irrigation of the eyes, preferably with saline or Ringer lactate solution, for at least 30 minutes. However, if nonsterile water is the only liquid available, it should be used. Do not use acidic solutions to neutralize alkalis or vice versa. It is helpful to place an eyelid speculum and topical anesthetic (e.g., proparacaine) in the eye before irrigation. Pull down the lower eyelid and evert the upper eyelid, if possible, to irrigate the fornices. Manual use of intravenous (i.v.) tubing connected to an irrigation solution facilitates the irrigation process.

2. Five to 10 minutes after ceasing irrigation (to allow equilibration), litmus paper should be touched to the inferior cul-de-sac. Irrigation should be continued until neutral pH is reached (i.e., 7.0).

3. The conjunctival fornices should be swept with a moistened cotton-tipped applicator or glass rod for crystallized particles if there is

a persistently abnormal pH. Double eversion of eyelids with a Desmarres eyelid retractor may aid in identifying and removing particles in the deep fornix.

Note: The volume of irrigation fluid required to reach neutral pH varies with the chemical and with the duration of the chemical exposure. The volume required may range from a few liters to several liters (more than 8 to 10 L). As stated earlier, irrigation should ideally be continued until neutral pH is reached.

MILD TO MODERATE BURNS

SIGNS

Critical. Corneal epithelial defects range from scattered superficial punctate keratitis (SPK) to focal epithelial loss to sloughing of the entire epithelium. No significant areas of perilimbal ischemia are seen (no sign of interrupted blood flow through the conjunctival or episcleral vessels).

Other. Focal areas of conjunctival chemosis, hyperemia, hemorrhages, or a combination of these; mild eyelid edema; mild anterior chamber (AC) reaction; first- and second-degree burns of the periocular skin.

WORKUP

1. History: Time of injury? Chemical to which the patient was exposed? Duration of the exposure until irrigation was started? Duration of the irrigation? Eye protection?

2. Slit-lamp examination with fluorescein staining: Evert the eyelids to search for foreign bodies. Check the intraocular pressure (IOP). In the presence of a distorted cornea, IOP may be most accurately measured with a Tono-Pen or pneumotonometer.

TREATMENT DURING AND AFTER IRRIGATION

1. Fornices should be thoroughly searched, including a sweep with a moistened cotton-tipped applicator or glass rod, to remove any sequestered particles of caustic material and necrotic conjunctiva, which may contain residual chemicals. Calcium hydroxide particles may be more easily removed with a cotton-tipped applicator soaked in disodium ethylenediaminetetraacetic acid (EDTA).

2. Cycloplegic (e.g., scopolamine 0.25%). Avoid phenylephrine because of its vasoconstrictive properties.

3. Topical antibiotic ointment (e.g., erythromycin) q1–2h while awake or pressure patch for 24 hours.

4. Oral pain medication (e.g., acetaminophen with or without codeine) as needed.

5. If IOP is increased, acetazolamide (e.g., Diamox) 250 mg p.o., q.i.d.; acetazolamide 500 mg sequel p.o., b.i.d.; or methazolamide (e.g., Neptazane) 25 to 50 mg p.o., b.i.d. or t.i.d., may be given. Add a topical beta-blocker (e.g., timolol 0.5%, b.i.d.) if additional IOP control is required.

6. Frequent (e.g., q1h while awake) use of preservative-free artificial tears or gel if not pressure patched.

FOLLOW-UP

Recheck and treat with antibiotic ointment, cycloplegic, and repatching (if desired) every day until the corneal defect is healed. Topical steroids may then be used to reduce significant inflammation. Watch for corneal ulceration and infection.

SEVERE BURNS

SIGNS

Critical. Pronounced chemosis and conjunctival blanching; corneal edema and opacification, sometimes with little to no view of the AC, iris, or lens; a moderate to severe AC reaction (may not be appreciated if the cornea is opaque).

Other. Increased IOP, second- and third-degree burns of the surrounding skin, and local necrotic retinopathy as a result of direct penetration of alkali through the sclera.

Note: If you suspect an epithelial defect but do not see one on fluorescein staining, repeat the fluorescein application to the eye. Sometimes the defect is slow to take up the dye. Occasionally, the whole epithelium may slough off, leaving only Bowman membrane, which may take up fluorescein poorly.

WORKUP

Same as for mild to moderate burns.

TREATMENT AFTER IRRIGATION

1. Admission to the hospital may be necessary for close monitoring of IOP and corneal healing.

2. Debride necrotic tissue containing foreign matter.

3. Cycloplegic (e.g., scopolamine 0.25% or atropine 1%, t.i.d. to q.i.d.). Avoid topical phenylephrine because it is a vasoconstrictor.

4. Topical antibiotic [e.g., trimethoprim/polymyxin (Polytrim) or fluoroquinolone drops, q.i.d.; erythromycin ointment, b.i.d. to q.i.d.].

5. Topical steroid (e.g., prednisolone acetate 1%, or dexamethasone 0.1%, four to nine times per day) if significant inflammation of the AC or cornea is present. May use a combination antibiotic–steroid such as tobramycin/dexamethasone q1–2h.

6. Consider a pressure patch between drops/ointment.

7. Antiglaucoma medications if the IOP is increased or cannot be determined. (See the earlier antiglaucoma recommendations.)

8. Lysis of conjunctival adhesions by using a glass rod or a moistened cotton-tipped applicator covered with an antibiotic ointment, sweeping the fornices b.i.d. If symblepharon begins to form despite attempted lysis, consider using a scleral shell or ring to maintain the fornices.

9. Frequent (e.g., q1h while awake) use of preservative-free artificial tears or gel.

10. Other considerations:

—Therapeutic soft contact lens, collagen shield, amniotic membrane transplant, or tarsorrhaphy (usually used if healing is delayed beyond 2 weeks).

—Intravenous ascorbate and citrate for alkali burns has been reported to speed healing time and allow better visual outcome.

—If any melting of the cornea occurs, collagenase inhibitors may be used [e.g., acetylcysteine 10% to 20% (Mucomyst) q4h].

—If the melting progresses (or the cornea perforates), consider cyanoacrylate tissue adhesive. An emergency patch graft or corneal transplantation may be necessary; however, the prognosis is better if this procedure is performed at least 12 to 18 months after the injury.

FOLLOW-UP

These patients need to be monitored closely, either in the hospital or daily as outpatients. Topical steroids must be tapered after 7 to 10 days because they can promote corneal melting. Long-term use of artificial tears and lubricating ointment (e.g., Refresh Plus, q1–6h, and Refresh PM ointment, q.d. to q.i.d.) may be required. A severely dry eye may require a tarsorrhaphy or a conjunctival flap. A conjunctival or limbal stem cell transplantation from the fellow eye may be performed in unilateral injuries that fail to heal within several weeks to several months.

SUPER GLUE (CYANOACRYLATE) INJURY TO THE EYE

Note: Rapid-setting super glues harden quickly on contact with moisture.

TREATMENT

1. If the eyelids are glued together, they can be separated with gentle traction. Lashes may need to be cut to separate the eyelids. Misdirected lashes or hardened glue mechanically rubbing the cornea, as well as glue adherent to the cornea, should be carefully removed with fine forceps.

2. Resulting epithelial defects are treated as corneal abrasions (see 3.2, Corneal Abrasion).

3. Warm compresses q.i.d. may help remove any remaining glue stuck in the lashes that did not require urgent removal.

FOLLOW-UP

Daily until corneal epithelial defects are healed.

3.2 CORNEAL ABRASION

SYMPTOMS

Sharp pain, photophobia, foreign body sensation, tearing, history of scratching the eye.

SIGNS

Critical. Epithelial defect that stains with fluorescein.

Other. Conjunctival injection, swollen eyelid, mild AC reaction.

DIFFERENTIAL DIAGNOSIS

- Recurrent erosion syndrome (see 4.2, Recurrent Corneal Erosion).

- Herpes simplex keratitis (see 4.14, Herpes Simplex Virus).

WORKUP

1. Slit-lamp examination: Use fluorescein dye, measure the size of the abrasion, diagram its location, and evaluate for an AC reaction. Evaluate for infiltrate, corneal laceration, or penetrating trauma.

2. Evert the eyelids to make certain no foreign body is present.

TREATMENT

1. Antibiotic

—Non–contact lens wearer: Antibiotic ointment (e.g., erythromycin, bacitracin, or ciprofloxacin, q2–4h) or antibiotic drops [e.g., polymyxin B/trimethoprim (Polytrim) or a fluoroquinolone, q.i.d.].

—Contact lens wearer: Must have antipseudomonal coverage. May use antibiotic ointment (e.g., tobramycin or ciprofloxacin, q2–4h) or antibiotic drops (e.g., tobramycin, levofloxacin, ofloxacin, ciprofloxacin, gatifloxacin, or moxifloxacin, q.i.d.).

Note: The decision to use drops versus ointment depends on the needs of the patient. Ointments offer better barrier function between eyelid and abrasion but tend to blur vision (not an issue if pain is so intense that the patient cannot open his or her eye). We prefer frequent ointments.

2. Cycloplegic agent (e.g., cyclopentolate 1% to 2%) for discomfort from traumatic iritis, which may develop 24 to 72 hours after trauma. Avoid steroid use for iritis because it may retard epithelial healing and increase the risk of infection. Avoid use of long-acting cycloplegics for small abrasions.

3. Consider patching for comfort, but DO NOT patch if the mechanism of injury involves vegetable matter or false fingernails, or if the patient wears contact lenses. We usually avoid patching but encourage patients to keep eyes shut.

4. Consider topical nonsteroidal antiinflammatory drug (NSAID) drops (e.g., ketorolac, q.i.d., for 3 days) for pain control. Avoid in patients with other ocular surface disease and in postoperative patients.

5. Consider debriding loose or hanging epithelium because it may inhibit healing.

6. NO contact lens wear. Some clinicians use bandage contact lenses for therapy. We do not.

FOLLOW-UP

Non–contact lens wearer

1. If patched, patient should return in 24 hours (or sooner if the symptoms worsen) for reevaluation.

2. Central or large corneal abrasion: Return the next day to determine if the epithelial defect is improving. If the abrasion is healing, may see 2 to 3 days later. Instruct the patient to return sooner if symptoms worsen. Revisit every 3 to 5 days until healed.

3. Peripheral or small abrasion: Return 2 to 5 days later. Instruct the patient to return sooner if symptoms worsen. Revisit every 3 to 5 days until healed.

Contact lens wearer

Have the patient return every day until the epithelial defect resolves, and then treat with topical tobramycin or fluoroquinolone drops for an additional 1 or 2 days. The patient may resume contact lens wear after the eye feels perfectly normal for a week without medication. Remember to examine the lens for tears, scratches, protein buildup, and other defects.

Note: *If, at any time, a corneal infiltrate is observed, appropriate smears and cultures should be obtained and more aggressive antibiotic therapy instituted (see 4.11, Bacterial Keratitis).*

3.3 CORNEAL AND CONJUNCTIVAL FOREIGN BODIES

SYMPTOMS

Foreign body sensation, tearing, history of trauma.

SIGNS

Critical. Conjunctival or corneal foreign body with or without rust ring.

Other. Conjunctival injection, eyelid edema, mild AC reaction, and SPK. A small infiltrate may surround a corneal foreign body; this infiltrate is usually sterile. Linear, vertically oriented corneal scratches may indicate a foreign body under the upper eyelid.

WORKUP

1. History: Determine the mechanism of injury. Was the patient wearing safety goggles? Did the foreign body arise from metal striking metal (which may suggest an intraocular foreign body)?

2. Document visual acuity before any procedure is performed. One or two drops of topical anesthetic may be necessary to control blepharospasm and pain.

3. Slit-lamp examination: Locate and assess the depth of the foreign body. Rule out self-sealing lacerations, iris tears, lens opacities, AC shallowing, and asymmetrically low IOP in the involved eye. If there is no evidence of perforation, evert the eyelids and inspect the fornices for additional foreign bodies. Double-everting the upper eyelid with a Desmarres eyelid retractor may be necessary.

Carefully inspect a conjunctival laceration to rule out a scleral laceration or perforation. Measure the dimensions of any infiltrate, the degree of any AC reaction, and the IOP.

4. Dilate the eye and examine the vitreous and retina for a possible intraocular foreign body.

5. Consider a B-scan ultrasound, a computed tomography (CT) scan of the orbit (axial and coronal views, 1-mm cuts), or ultrasonographic biomicroscopy (UBM) to exclude an intraocular or intraorbital foreign body. Avoid magnetic resonance imaging (MRI) if there is a history of possible metallic foreign body.

TREATMENT

Corneal foreign body

1. Apply topical anesthetic (e.g., proparacaine). Remove the corneal foreign body with a foreign body spud or fine forceps at a slit lamp. Multiple superficial foreign bodies may be more easily removed by irrigation.

2. Remove the rust ring. This may require an ophthalmic drill. It is sometimes safer to leave a deep, central rust ring to allow time for the rust to migrate to the corneal surface, at which point it can be more easily removed.

3. Measure the size of the resultant corneal epithelial defect.

4. Treat as for corneal abrasion (see 3.2, Corneal Abrasion).

Conjunctival foreign body

1. Remove foreign body under topical anesthesia.

   —Multiple or loose foreign bodies can often be removed with saline irrigation.

   —A foreign body can be removed with a cotton-tipped applicator soaked in topical anesthetic or with fine forceps. For deeply embedded foreign bodies, consider pretreatment with a cotton-tipped applicator soaked in phenylephrine (e.g., Neo-Synephrine) 2.5%, to reduce conjunctival bleeding.

   —Small, relatively inaccessible, buried subconjunctival foreign bodies may sometimes be left in the eye without harm. Occasionally, they will surface with time, at which point they may be removed more easily.

2. Sweep the conjunctival fornices with a glass rod or cotton-tipped applicator soaked with a topical anesthetic to catch any remaining pieces.

3. See 3.6, Conjunctival Laceration if there is a significant conjunctival laceration. If no laceration is noted:

   —A topical antibiotic (e.g., erythromycin or bacitracin ointment, b.i.d.; trimethoprim/polymyxin B or fluoroquinolone drops, q.i.d.) may be used.

   —Artificial tears (e.g., Refresh, q.i.d. for 2 days) may be given for a mildly irritated eye.

FOLLOW-UP

1. **Corneal foreign body:** Follow up as with corneal abrasion (see 3.2, Corneal Abrasion). If residual rust ring remains, reevaluate in 24 hours.

2. **Conjunctival foreign body:** Follow up as needed, or in 1 week if residual foreign bodies were left in the conjunctiva.

   Note: An infiltrate accompanied by a significant AC reaction, purulent discharge, or extreme redness and pain should be cultured to rule out an infection and treated with antibiotics more aggressively (see 4.11, Bacterial Keratitis).

3.4 HYPHEMA AND MICROHYPHEMA

TRAUMATIC

SYMPTOMS

Pain, blurred vision, history of blunt trauma.

SIGNS

Blood in the AC.

Hyphema. Gross layering or clot or both, usually visible without a slit lamp. A total (100%) hyphema may be black or red; when black, it is called an "8-ball" or "black ball" hyphema; when red, the circulating blood cells may settle out to become less than a 100% hyphema.

Microhyphema. Suspended red blood cells (RBCs) only, visible only with a slit lamp. Sometimes there may be enough suspended RBCs to see a haziness of the AC without a slit lamp; in these cases, the RBCs may settle out as a gross hyphema.

WORKUP

1. History: Mechanism (including force and direction) of injury; approximate time and day of injury; time of visual loss, if any use of protective goggles. Usually the visual loss occurs at the time of injury; decreasing vision over time suggests a rebleed or continued bleed. Inquire about medications with anticoagulant properties [aspirin, NSAIDs, warfarin (e.g., Coumadin)] and history or family history of sickle cell disease/trait.

2. Complete ocular examination, first ruling out a ruptured globe (see 3.14, Ruptured Globe and Penetrating Ocular Injury). External and periocular examinations should be performed, evaluating for other traumatic injuries. Quantitate (percentage) and draw the extent and location of any clot. Measure the IOP. Perform a dilated retinal evaluation, if possible. Do not perform scleral depression. Avoid gonioscopy unless intractable IOP increase develops. If gonioscopy is necessary, use a Zeiss 4 mirror lens gently. Consider a B-scan ultrasound if view to the fundus is poor. Consider UBM to evaluate anterior segment/lens if lens capsule rupture, foreign body, or other anterior segment abnormalities are suspected but are not clearly visible.

3. Consider a CT scan of the orbits and brain (axial and coronal views, with 1- to 3-mm cuts through the orbits), when indicated.

4. Black and Mediterranean patients should be screened for sickle cell trait or disease (order Sickledex screen; if necessary, may check hemoglobin electrophoresis).

FACTORS ASSOCIATED WITH POOR OUTCOME

Some studies suggest that the following are associated with a higher risk of poor outcome:

1. Poor visual acuity at presentation (worse than 20/200).

2. Sickle cell disease/trait with increased IOP.

3. Medically uncontrollable increased IOP.

4. Large initial hyphema size (at least one third of AC).

5. Recent aspirin or NSAID use, especially in large amounts.

6. Delayed presentation to the ophthalmologist. (This frequently represents delayed visual deterioration or pain, as may occur with rebleeding or increased IOP.)

TREATMENT

Many aspects remain controversial, including whether hospitalization and absolute bed rest are necessary. Most microhyphemas can be treated as outpatient cases. Consider hospitalization for noncompliant patients, patients at high risk for secondary hemorrhage, and patients with other severe ocular or orbital injuries. In addition, consider hospitalization and generally more aggressive treatment for children, especially those at risk for amblyopia or when child abuse is suspected.

Treatment for All Patients

1. Confine either to bed rest with bathroom privileges or to limited activity. Elevate head 30 degrees (use pillows if not in hospital using an adjustable bed). No strenuous activity allowed.

2. Place a shield (metal or clear plastic) over the involved eye at all times. Do not patch because this prevents recognition of sudden visual loss in the event of a rebleed.

3. Atropine 1% drops, t.i.d., for patients with hyphema; q.d. to b.i.d., for patients with microhyphema.

4. No aspirin-containing products or NSAIDs.

5. Mild analgesics only (e.g., acetaminophen). Avoid sedatives.

6. To prevent heavy, fibrinous AC reaction, or if the eye becomes photophobic, consider a topical steroid (e.g., prednisolone acetate 1%, four to eight times per day). Traumatic iritis symptoms and itching often develop 2 to 3 days after trauma.

7. For increased IOP:

   Note: Increased IOP, especially soon after trauma, may be transient, secondary to acute mechanical plugging of the trabecular meshwork. Elevating the patient's head may decrease the IOP by causing RBCs to settle inferiorly.

   Non–sickle cell disease/trait (more than 30 mm Hg):

   —Start with a beta-blocker (e.g., timolol or levobunolol 0.5%, b.i.d.).

   —If that is unsuccessful, add topical alpha-agonist (e.g., apraclonidine 0.5%, or brimonidine 0.2%, t.i.d.) or topical carbonic anhydrase inhibitor (e.g., dorzolamide 2%, or brinzolamide 1%, t.i.d.). Avoid prostaglandin analogs and miotics because they may increase inflammation.

—If still unsuccessful, add acetazolamide (500 mg p.o. q12h for adults, 20 mg/kg/day divided three times per day for children) or mannitol (1 to 2 g/kg i.v. over 45 minutes q24h). If mannitol is necessary to control the IOP, surgical evacuation may be an imminent necessity.

Sickle cell disease/trait (at least 24 mm Hg):

—Start with a beta-blocker (e.g., timolol or levobunolol 0.5%, b.i.d.). All other agents must be used with extreme caution: Topical dorzolamide and brinzolamide may reduce AC pH and induce more sickling; topical alpha-agonists (e.g., brimonidine or apraclonidine) may affect iris vasculature; miotics and epinephrine are vasoactive and may promote inflammation. Avoid prostaglandin analogs because they also may promote inflammation.

—Try to avoid systemic diuretics because they promote sickling owing to systemic acidosis and volume contraction. If a carbonic anhydrase inhibitor is necessary, use methazolamide 50 mg p.o. q8h instead of acetazolamide, although this is also controversial. If mannitol is necessary to control the IOP, surgical evacuation may be an imminent necessity.

—AC paracentesis is safe and effective if IOP cannot be safely lowered medically. See 11.5, Central Retinal Artery Occlusion. This procedure is often only a temporizing measure, when the need for surgical evacuation is anticipated.

8. If admitting patient, see the following for hospitalized patients; for outpatients, see later for nonhospitalized patients.

Treatment for Hospitalized Patients with Hyphema

All previously mentioned treatment as well as:

1. Aminocaproic acid 50 mg/kg p.o. q4h (maximum, 30 g per 24 hours). Aminocaproic acid may cause postural hypotension during the first 24 hours. It should not be used as an outpatient treatment, in pregnant patients, or in those with coagulopathies or renal disease. It should be used with caution in patients with hepatic, cardiovascular, or cerebrovascular disease. A syrup form of aminocaproic acid (250 mg/mL) may be better tolerated by children.

2. Antiemetics [e.g., prochlorperazine 10 mg intramuscularly (i.m.) q8h or 25 mg pr q12h as needed (prn); younger than 12 years of age, trimethobenzamide suppositories, 100 mg q6h prn].

3. In hospital, check visual acuity and IOP and perform a slit-lamp examination at least twice daily. Look for new bleeding, increased IOP, corneal stromal blood staining, and other intraocular lesions as the blood clears (e.g., iridodialysis; subluxated, luxated, or cataractous lens). Hemolysis, which may appear as bright red fluid, should be distinguished from a rebleed, which forms a new, bright red clot. If the IOP is increased, treat as previously described (see Treatment for All Patients), depending on the patient's age and the status of the optic nerve.

4. **If a rebleed does not occur:**

   —Posttrauma day 2: Decrease the dose of aminocaproic acid by one half. Allow gradual increase in activity level (e.g., walking).

   Note: *When the aminocaproic acid is decreased, fibrinolysis increases over the next 48 to 72 hours, which may result in increased IOP.*

   —Posttrauma day 3: Discontinue oral aminocaproic acid and discharge if stable. Continued observation may be necessary if rapid resolution of clot causes an elevated IOP.

5. If a rebleed does occur, continue the aminocaproic acid for an additional day. Check coagulation profile and aminocaproic acid dose. Patients rarely rebleed on the appropriate dose of aminocaproic acid.

6. Surgical evacuation of hyphema may be indicated for the following: corneal stromal blood staining (surgery should be done urgently), significant visual deterioration, total filling of AC with blood, persistent clot packed in the angle for 7 days, uncontrollable IOP for more than 24 hours in sickle cell–positive individuals, or IOP increase despite maximal medical therapy (IOP greater than 50 mm Hg for 5 days or greater than 35 mm Hg for 7 days).

7. On discharge, maintain patients with atropine, topical steroid, and antiglaucoma medications (if needed). Instructions regarding activity should be given (see Follow-up).

Treatment for Nonhospitalized Patients

1. **Hyphema:** The patient should return daily for 3 days after initial trauma to check visual acuity and IOP, and for a slit-lamp examination. Look for new bleeding, increased IOP, corneal blood staining, and other intraocular lesions as the blood clears. Hemolysis, which may appear as bright red fluid, should be distinguished from a rebleed, which forms a new, bright red clot. If the IOP is increased, treat as described earlier (see Treatment for All Patients), depending on the patient's age and the status of the optic nerve.

2. **Microhyphema:** The patient should return on the third day after the initial trauma and again at 2 weeks. If the IOP is greater than 25 mm Hg at presentation, the patient should be followed for 3 consecutive days for pressure monitoring, and again at 2 weeks. Patients with initial IOP of at least 24 mm Hg who are sickle cell positive should also be followed for 3 consecutive days.

3. The patient should be instructed to return immediately for reevaluation if a sudden increase in pain or decrease in vision is noted (which may be symptoms of a rebleed or secondary glaucoma).

4. If a rebleed or an intractable IOP increase occurs, the patient should be hospitalized.

5. Administer prednisolone 1%, q.i.d., if symptoms of traumatic iritis exist.

6. After the initial close follow-up period, the patient may be maintained on atropine 1% drops, one to two times per day, depending on the severity of the condition. Other instructions should be given as follows.

FOLLOW-UP (HOSPITALIZED AND NONHOSPITALIZED PATIENTS)

1. Glasses or eye shield during the day and eye shield at night for 2 weeks after trauma, after which the patient should wear protective eyewear (polycarbonate or Trivex lenses) any time the potential for an eye injury exists.

2. The patient must refrain from strenuous physical activities (including bearing down or Valsalva maneuvers) for 2 weeks after the initial injury or rebleed. The patient may resume normal activities after the initial 2 weeks from the date of injury or rebleed.

3. Outpatient examinations after discharge (or after initial daily follow-up, for outpatients):

—For hospitalized patients, 2 to 3 days after discharge; for nonhospitalized patients, several days to 1 week after initial daily follow-up period, depending on severity of condition (amount of blood, potential for IOP increase, other ocular or orbital pathologic processes).

—Two weeks after trauma for gonioscopy and dilated fundus examination with scleral depression for all patients.

—Yearly, because of the potential for development of angle-recession glaucoma.

—If any complications arise, more frequent follow-up is required.

—If filtering surgery was performed, the patient may be advised to refrain from strenuous physical activity for 4 to 8 weeks.

NONTRAUMATIC (SPONTANEOUS) AND POSTSURGICAL HYPHEMA OR MICROHYPHEMA

SYMPTOMS

May present with decreased vision or with transient visual loss (intermittent bleeding may cloud vision temporarily).

ETIOLOGY (OF SPONTANEOUS HYPHEMA OR MICROHYPHEMA)

Must exclude the possibility of occult trauma.

• Neovascularization of the iris or AC angle (e.g., from diabetes, old central retinal vein occlusion, ocular ischemic syndrome, chronic uveitis).

• Blood dyscrasia.

• Iris–intraocular lens chafing.

• Other (e.g., iris microaneurysm, leukemia, retinoblastoma, juvenile xanthogranuloma, child abuse).

WORKUP

As for traumatic hyphemas, also:

1. Gonioscopy.

2. For spontaneous hemorrhages, may consider additional studies.

—Consider checking prothrombin time/partial thromboplastin time, complete blood count with platelet count, bleeding time, proteins C and S.

—Consider i.v. fluorescein angiogram of iris.

—Consider UBM to evaluate position of intraocular lens haptic.

TREATMENT

Consider atropine 1% drops, one to three times per day; limited activity; elevation of head of bed; avoidance of aspirin or NSAIDs. Recommend protective plastic or metal shield if etiology unclear. Monitor IOP. Postsurgical hyphemas and microhyphemas are usually self-limited and often require observation only, with close attention to IOP.

3.5 TRAUMATIC IRITIS

SYMPTOMS

Dull, aching/throbbing pain, photophobia, tearing, onset of symptoms within 3 days of trauma.

SIGNS

Critical. White blood cells and flare in the AC (seen under high-power magnification by focusing into the AC with a small, bright beam from the slit lamp).

Other. Pain in the traumatized eye when light enters *either* eye; lower (although sometimes higher) IOP; smaller pupil (which dilates poorly) or larger pupil (caused by iris sphincter tears) in the traumatized eye; perilimbal conjunctival injection; occasionally, decreased vision.

DIFFERENTIAL DIAGNOSIS

• Traumatic corneal abrasion (Corneal epithelial defect that stains with fluorescein. May have an accompanying AC reaction. See 3.2, Corneal Abrasion.).

• Traumatic microhyphema (RBCs suspended in the AC. Often accompanied by iritis. See 3.4, Hyphema and Microhyphema.).

• Traumatic retinal detachment (May produce an AC reaction. May also see pigment in the anterior vitreous. A detachment is seen on dilated fundus examination. See 11.3, Retinal Detachment.).

• Nongranulomatous anterior uveitis (No history of trauma, or the degree of trauma is not consistent with the level of inflammation. See 12.1, Anterior Uveitis.).

WORKUP

Complete ophthalmic examination, including IOP measurement and dilated fundus examination.

TREATMENT

Cycloplegic agent (e.g., cyclopentolate 2%, q.i.d., or scopolamine 0.25%, t.i.d.).

Note: Some physicians also give a steroid drop (e.g., prednisolone acetate 0.125% to 1%, q.i.d.); initially, we do not. Avoid steroid use if an epithelial defect is present.

FOLLOW-UP

1. Recheck in 5 to 7 days.

2. If there is no improvement after 5 to 7 days, a steroid drop (e.g., prednisolone acetate 1%, q.i.d.) may be given in addition to the cycloplegic agent.

3. If resolved, the cycloplegic agent is discontinued.

4. One month after trauma, examine the AC angle in both eyes by gonioscopy to look for angle recession. Also, perform indirect ophthalmoscopy with scleral depression to detect retinal breaks or detachment.

3.6 CONJUNCTIVAL LACERATION

SYMPTOMS

Mild pain, red eye, foreign body sensation; usually, a history of ocular trauma.

SIGNS

Fluorescein staining of the conjunctiva. The conjunctiva may be torn and rolled up on itself. Exposed white sclera may be noted. Conjunctival and subconjunctival hemorrhages are often present.

WORKUP

1. History: Determine the nature of the trauma and whether a ruptured globe or intraocular or intraorbital foreign body may be present (e.g., metal-striking-metal or BB gun injuries).

2. Complete ocular examination, including a careful exploration of the sclera (after topical anesthesia, e.g., proparacaine) in the region of the conjunctival laceration to rule out a scleral laceration or a subconjunctival foreign body. The entire area of sclera under the conjunctival laceration must be inspected. Use a proparacaine-soaked, sterile cotton-tipped applicator to manipulate the conjunctiva to rule out underlying scleral injury. Dilated fundus examination, especially evaluating the area underlying the conjunctival injury, must be carefully performed with indirect ophthalmoscopy.

3. Consider a CT scan of the orbit (axial and coronal views, 1- to 3-mm cuts) to exclude an intraocular or intraorbital foreign body or a ruptured globe. B-scan ultrasound or UBM may be helpful.

4. Exploration of the site in the operating room under general anesthesia may be necessary when a ruptured globe is suspected.

5. Children often do not give an accurate history of trauma. They must be questioned and examined especially carefully.

TREATMENT

In case of ruptured globe or penetrating ocular injury, see 3.14, Ruptured Globe and Penetrating Ocular Injury. Otherwise:

1. Antibiotic ointment (e.g., erythromycin or bacitracin t.i.d.) for 4 to 7 days. A pressure patch may be used for the first 24 hours.

2. Large lacerations (greater than 1 to 1.5 cm) may be sutured with 8-0 polyglactin 910 (e.g., Vicryl), but most lacerations heal without surgical repair. When suturing, take care not to bury folds of conjunctiva. Do not incorporate Tenon capsule into the wound. Avoid suturing the plica semilunaris or caruncle to the conjunctiva.

FOLLOW-UP

If there is no concomitant ocular damage, patients with large conjunctival lacerations are re-examined within 1 week. Patients with small injuries are seen only as needed.

3.7   EYELID LACERATION

SYMPTOMS

Mild periorbital pain, epiphora.

SIGNS

Superficial laceration/abrasion that may mask a deep laceration.

WORKUP

1. History: Determine mechanism of injury: bite, foreign body potential, and so forth.

2. Complete ocular examination, including bilateral dilated fundus evaluation. Make sure there is no injury to the globes.

3. Determination of the depth of the laceration, which can look deceptively superficial. We recommend using toothed forceps or cotton-tipped applicators to gently pull open one edge of the wound to determine depth of penetration.

4. CT scan of brain and orbit (axial and coronal views, 1- to 3-mm cuts) should be obtained when a foreign body, ruptured globe, or severe blunt trauma is suspected. Loss of consciousness necessitates CT scan of the brain.

5. If laceration is nasal to either upper or lower eyelid punctum, even if not obviously through the canalicular system (i.e., seems very superficial), perform punctal dilation and irrigation of canalicular system to exclude canalicular involvement.

Note: Dog bites are notorious for causing canalicular lacerations. Probing should be performed in all such cases, even with lacerations that appear to be superficial.

6. With uncooperative children, conscious sedation or an examination under anesthesia may be necessary to examine fully the eyelids and globe.

TREATMENT

Consider tetanus prophylaxis (see Appendix 10 for indications).

1. Assess eyelid laceration. The following lacerations require repair in the operating room and are beyond the scope of this book:

a. Those associated with ocular trauma requiring surgery (e.g., ruptured globe or intraorbital foreign body).

b. Those involving the lacrimal drainage apparatus (i.e., punctum, canaliculus, common duct, or lacrimal sac), except when uncomplicated and near the punctum in a cooperative patient.

c. Those involving the levator aponeurosis of the upper eyelid (producing ptosis) or the superior rectus muscle; orbital fat is often exposed.

d. Those in which the medial canthal tendon is avulsed (exhibits a displaced medial canthus or abnormal laxity of the medial canthus).

e. Those that cause extensive tissue loss (especially more than one third of the eyelid) or severe distortion of anatomy.

2. Eyelid lacerations reparable in the office or emergency department.

   a. Clean the area of injury and surrounding skin [e.g., povidone–iodine (e.g., Betadine)].

   b. Give local subcutaneous anesthetic (e.g., 2% lidocaine with epinephrine).

   c. Irrigate the wound thoroughly with saline in a syringe.

   d. Search the wound carefully for foreign bodies. Remove them only if there is no evidence of globe penetration or extension into the orbit.

   Note: Lacerations resulting from human or animal bites or those otherwise with significant risk of contamination may require minimal debridement of necrotic tissue. Contaminated wounds may be left open for delayed repair, although some believe that the excellent blood supply of the eyelid allows primary repair. If electing primary repair, proceed to the subsequent steps.

   e. Isolate the surgical field with a sterile eye drape.

   f. Place a drop of topical anesthetic (e.g., proparacaine) into the eye. Place a protective eye shell over the eye before suturing.

   g. Lacerations involving the eyelid margin: Repair by using one of many methods. Figure 3.1 illustrates the method described. (Regardless of the technique used, the tarsus must be realigned with several sutures to allow for proper eyelid alignment and healing. Marginal repair alone will not provide structural integrity to the eyelid; the injured tarsus will splay apart, resulting in eyelid notching.)

      i. Place a 5-0 polyglactin 910 (e.g., Vicryl) suture on a spatulated needle through the tarsus on one side of the laceration, entering 3 to 4 mm deep to the eyelid margin; exit next to the eyelid margin. Enter the tarsus on the opposite side of the laceration next to the eyelid margin, and exit in the same vertical plane, 3 to 4 mm deep to the eyelid margin. Tie the suture. If the margin is well aligned, proceed to g iii.

      ii. If the eyelid margin is not aligned after tying the suture, place a 6-0 silk vertical mattress suture (near-to-near, far-to-far) just anterior to the gray line. Near-to-near: enter the eyelid margin 1 mm from one edge of the laceration, exiting 1 mm from the edge of the laceration. Far-to-far: reenter the eyelid margin 2 to 3 mm from one edge of the laceration, and exit through the opposite side of the laceration 2 to 3 mm from the edge. Tie the suture, leaving the ends long, and incorporate the ends into the skin suture closest to the eyelid margin (see g iv).

      iii. Use 5-0 polyglactin 910 sutures to close the subcutaneous tissues and remaining tarsus along the length of the laceration. Take a partial-thickness bite through the tarsus on one side. Enter the tarsus on the opposite side of the laceration at the corresponding point, and exit in the same horizontal plane slightly anterior to the tarsus. Tie the suture, and repeat until the laceration is closed.

      iv. Over the nonmarginal aspect of the laceration, close the skin with interrupted 6-0 plain gut suture.

   h. Lacerations of the eyelid not involving the eyelid margin. Close the skin, as in g iv. Be aware that deeper, buried subcutaneous sutures can incorporate the orbital septa, resulting in eyelid tethering.

   i. Remove the protective eye shell.

   j. Apply antibiotic ointment (e.g., bacitracin) to the wound, b.i.d.

   k. Give systemic antibiotics if contamination is suspected [e.g., dicloxacillin or

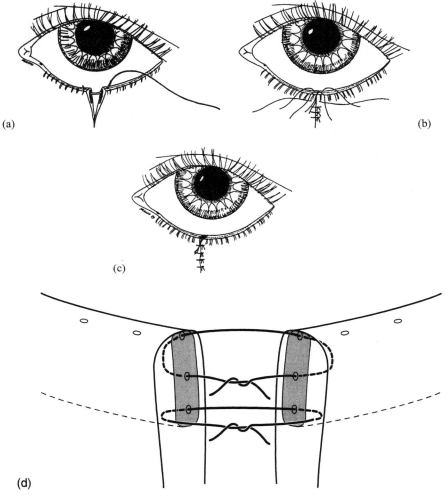

FIGURE 3.1 Eyelid margin repair. **a:** Suture 1 (see text). **b, c:** At the conclusion of the repair, the eyelid margin sutures are tied under the knot of the skin suture closest to the eyelid margin. **d:** Eyelid margin repair (preferred method). See text.

cephalexin, 250 to 500 mg p.o., q.i.d. (adults); 25 to 50 mg/kg/day divided into four doses (children); for human or animal bites, consider penicillin V (same dose as dicloxacillin)]. Continue for 2 to 5 days. For animal bites, if indicated, consider rabies prophylaxis.

Note: Do not shave the eyebrow if it has been lacerated; in some cases, the hair will not grow back or will do so irregularly.

FOLLOW-UP

The methods described use mostly absorbable sutures (except for the optional silk eyelid-margin suture described in g ii). If nonabsorbable sutures are used, eyelid-margin sutures should be left in place for 10 to 14 days, and other superficial sutures for 4 to 7 days. In an emergency department setting, it may be more prudent to use absorbable sutures because some patients may not return for follow-up.

3.8   ORBITAL BLOW-OUT FRACTURE

SYMPTOMS

Pain (especially on attempted vertical eye movement), local tenderness, binocular double vision (the double vision disappears when one eye is covered), eyelid swelling and crepitus after nose blowing, recent history of trauma.

SIGNS

Critical. Restricted eye movement (especially in upward or lateral gaze or both), subcutaneous or conjunctival emphysema, hypesthesia in the distribution of the infraorbital nerve (ipsilateral cheek and upper lip), point tenderness, enophthalmos (may initially be masked by orbital edema).

Other. Nosebleed, eyelid edema, and ecchymosis. Superior rim and orbital roof fractures may show hypesthesia in the distribution of the supratrochlear or supraorbital nerve (ipsilateral forehead) and ptosis. Trismus, malar flattening, and a palpable stepoff deformity of the inferior orbital rim are characteristic of tripod fractures.

DIFFERENTIAL DIAGNOSIS

• Orbital edema and hemorrhage without a blow-out fracture (May have limitation of ocular movement, periorbital swelling, and ecchymosis, but these resolve over 7 to 10 days.).

• Cranial nerve palsy (Limitation of ocular movement, but no restriction on forced-duction testing. Will have abnormal results on force generation testing.).

WORKUP

1. Complete ophthalmologic examination, including measurement of extraocular movements and globe displacement. Compare the sensation of the affected cheek with that on the contralateral side; palpate the eyelids for crepitus (subcutaneous emphysema); palpate the orbital rim for stepoffs; and evaluate the globe carefully for a rupture, hyphema or microhyphema, traumatic iritis, and retinal or choroidal damage. IOP should be measured. Check pupils and color vision carefully to rule out a traumatic optic neuropathy.

2. Forced-duction testing is performed if restriction of eye movement persists beyond 1 week (see Appendix 5).

3. CT scan of the orbits (axial and coronal views, 3-mm cuts) is obtained in all cases of suspected orbital fractures. If there is any history of loss of consciousness, brain imaging is also recommended.

TREATMENT

1. Nasal decongestants [e.g., pseudoephedrine (Afrin) nasal spray, b.i.d.] for 3 days.

2. Broad-spectrum oral antibiotics [e.g., cephalexin (Keflex) 250 to 500 mg p.o., q.i.d.; or erythromycin 250 to 500 mg p.o., q.i.d.] for 7 days may be used but are not mandatory.

3. Instruct the patient not to blow his or her nose.

4. Apply ice packs to the orbit for the first 24 to 48 hours.

5. Surgical repair should be considered based on the following criteria:

Immediate repair (usually within 24 hours)

—If there is evidence on CT scan of entrapped muscle or periorbital tissue in combination with diplopia and nonresolving bradycardia, heart block, nausea, vomiting, or syncope.

—In patients younger than 16 years of age with a quiet external periocular appearance and marked motility restriction (usually vertical).

Repair in 1 to 2 weeks

—Persistent, symptomatic diplopia in primary or downgaze that has not improved at

1 week, with positive forced ductions and evidence of entrapment on CT.

—Large floor fractures (more than one half of the orbital floor) that have caused or are likely to cause cosmetically unacceptable enophthalmos.

—Complex trauma involving rim or zygomatic arch with displacement.

6. Neurosurgical consultation is recommended for most orbital roof fractures and for all patients with intracranial hemorrhage.

Note: Most adult orbital fractures can initially be followed conservatively. If there is a question of entrapment, some physicians use an oral steroid to decrease the inflammatory reaction and reevaluate the patient in a few days.

FOLLOW-UP

Patients should be seen at 1 and 2 weeks after trauma and evaluated for persistent diplopia or enophthalmos after the acute orbital edema has subsided. The presence of these findings may indicate entrapment of the orbital contents or a large displaced fracture and the need for surgical repair. Patients should also be monitored for the development of associated ocular injuries (e.g., orbital cellulitis, angle-recession glaucoma, and retinal detachment). Gonioscopy of the AC angle and dilated retinal examination with scleral depression is performed 3 to 4 weeks after trauma if a hyphema or microhyphema was present. Warning symptoms of retinal detachment and orbital cellulitis are explained to the patient.

3.9 TRAUMATIC RETROBULBAR HEMORRHAGE

SYMPTOMS

Pain, decreased vision, recent history of trauma or surgery to the eye or orbit.

SIGNS

Critical. Proptosis with resistance to retropulsion, diffuse subconjunctival hemorrhage, tight eyelids, vision loss, afferent pupillary defect, dyschromatopsia.

Other. Eyelid ecchymosis, chemosis, congested conjunctival vessels, increased IOP; often, limited extraocular motility in any or all fields of gaze.

DIFFERENTIAL DIAGNOSIS

• Orbital cellulitis (Fever, proptosis, chemosis, limitation of eye movement, pain with eye movement; also may follow trauma, but usually not as acute. See 7.4, Orbital Cellulitis.).

• Orbital fracture (Blow-out, medial wall, or tripod fracture; limited extraocular motility, in-fraorbital hypesthesia, and crepitus; enophthalmos or proptosis may be present. See 3.8, Orbital Blow-out Fracture.).

• Ruptured globe [Subconjunctival edema and hemorrhage may mask a ruptured globe. A shallow or deep AC (compared with the other eye), hyphema, and limitation of ocular motility are often present. IOP is commonly low, and there is usually no proptosis. See 3.14, Ruptured Globe and Penetrating Ocular Injury.].

• Carotid–cavernous fistula (May follow trauma. Pulsating exophthalmos, ocular bruit, corkscrew-arterialized conjunctival vessels, chemosis, and increased IOP may be seen. Often, bilateral involvement because of venous communications. See 10.9, Cavernous Sinus and Associated Syndromes.).

• Varix (Increased proptosis with Valsalva maneuver. Is not usually seen acutely, and there is usually no history of trauma or surgery.).

• Lymphangioma (Usually in younger patients. May have acute proptosis, ecchymosis, and external ophthalmoplegia after minimal trauma or upper respiratory tract infection. MRI is usually diagnostic.).

WORKUP

1. Complete ophthalmic examination; check specifically for an afferent pupillary defect, loss of color vision (color plates), increased or decreased IOP, pulsations of the central retinal artery, and choroidal folds (signs that vision is threatened). Pulsations of the central retinal artery often precede a central retinal artery occlusion.

2. CT scan of the orbit (axial and coronal views). The CT scan should be delayed until definitive treatment has been instituted in cases in which vision is threatened.

TREATMENT

If IOP is increased (e.g., more than 30 mm Hg in a patient with a normal optic nerve, or more than 20 mm Hg in a patient whose optic cup is very large and who normally has a lower IOP), any or all of the following methods are used to reduce the IOP. When vision is threatened, all of them are instituted immediately.

1. Oral carbonic anhydrase inhibitor (e.g., acetazolamide, take two 250-mg pills simultaneously).

2. Topical beta-blocker (e.g., timolol or levobunolol 0.5%), alpha-agonist (e.g., brimonidine 0.2%), or topical carbonic anhydrase inhibitor (e.g., dorzolamide 2% or brinzolamide 1%). May repeat each drop once after 30 minutes.

3. Hyperosmotic agent (e.g., mannitol, 1 to 2 g/kg i.v. over 45 minutes).

Note: A 500-mL bag of mannitol 20% contains 100 g of mannitol.

4. Lateral canthotomy and cantholysis (Fig. 3.2). After local injection with lidocaine 2%, with epinephrine, a hemostat is placed horizontally over the lateral canthus and clamped for 1 minute to compress the tissues and reduce bleeding. (a) The clamp is released, and sterile scissors are used to make a horizontal incision approximately 1 cm into the tissue compressed by the hemostat. (b) The skin and conjunctiva in the area of the incision are separated, and the scissors are placed between them to cut the inferior arm of the lateral canthal tendon. The lower eyelid usually will prolapse forward and medially if the tendon is completely cut. (c) Hemostasis is usually achieved with pressure. A sterile dressing is placed over the wound.

Note: A lateral canthotomy alone or an incomplete inferior cantholysis is NOT adequate therapy.

5. Hospitalization is indicated in all cases of orbital hemorrhage affecting visual function. In cases of normal vision, the patient should be followed in the emergency department or office for 4 to 6 hours before discharge with detailed instructions.

FOLLOW-UP

In cases in which vision is threatened, monitor the patient closely until stable. After the acute episode has resolved, reexamination should be performed every few weeks at first. Fibrosis may develop later, limiting extraocular motility. Fracture repair should be delayed until the orbit has softened.

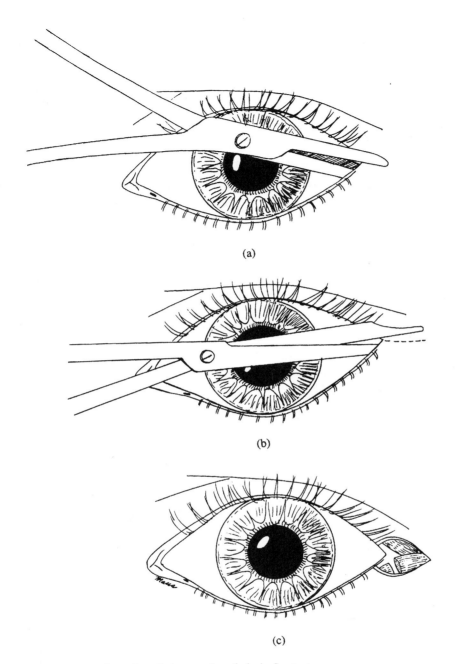

(a)

(b)

(c)

FIGURE 3.2 **a–c:** Lateral canthotomy and cantholysis. See text.

3.10 INTRAORBITAL FOREIGN BODY

SYMPTOMS

Decreased vision, pain, double vision, or may be asymptomatic; history of trauma (can be years before presentation).

SIGNS

Critical. Orbital foreign body identified by radiograph, CT scan, orbital ultrasonogram, or a combination of these.

Other. A palpable orbital mass, limitation of ocular motility, proptosis; an eyelid or conjunctival laceration; erythema, edema, or ecchymosis of eyelids. The presence of an afferent pupillary defect may indicate a traumatic optic neuropathy.

TYPES OF FOREIGN BODIES

1. Poorly tolerated (often lead to inflammation): Organic (e.g., wood and vegetable matter) and sometimes copper foreign bodies.

2. Fairly well tolerated (typically produce a chronic low-grade inflammatory reaction): Copper alloys that are less than 85% copper (e.g., brass, bronze).

3. Well tolerated (inert): Stone, glass, plastic, iron, lead, steel, aluminum, and most other metals.

   Note: BBs and shotgun pellets are typically made of 80% to 90% lead and 10% to 20% iron.

WORKUP

1. History: Determine the nature of the injury and the foreign body. Must have a high index of suspicion in all trauma.

2. Complete ocular and periorbital examination, with special attention to pupillary reaction, IOP, and retinal evaluation. Examine carefully for an entry wound. Carefully rule out occult globe rupture.

3. CT scan of the orbit and brain (axial and coronal views, 1- to 1.5-mm cuts of the orbit) is the study of choice but may miss some foreign bodies (e.g., wood may look like an air bubble on CT acutely). Rule out a ruptured globe, determine the location of the intraorbital foreign body, and rule out optic nerve or central nervous system involvement. MRI is contraindicated if a metal foreign body is suspected or cannot be excluded, but MRI may be better at demonstrating wood if suspicion of this is high and the CT is negative.

4. Conduct B-scan orbital ultrasonography if a foreign body is suspected but not detected by CT scan.

5. Culture any drainage sites.

TREATMENT

1. Surgical exploration and extraction, based on the following indications:

   —Signs of infection/inflammation (e.g., fever, proptosis, restricted motility, severe chemosis, a palpable orbital mass, an abscess on CT scan).

   —Any organic or wooden foreign body (because of the high risk for sight-threatening complications). Many copper foreign bodies need to be removed because they can incite a marked inflammatory reaction.

   —Fistula formation.

   —Signs of optic nerve compression or directional amaurosis (i.e., decreased vision in a specific gaze direction).

   —A large or sharp-edged foreign body (independent of composition) that can be easily extracted.

   Note: Posteriorly located foreign bodies are often simply observed if inert and not causing optic nerve compression. This is due to the risk of iatrogenic optic neuropathy or diplopia. Alternatively, even an inert metallic foreign body that is anterior and easily removable may be considered for surgery.

2. Tetanus toxoid prn (see Appendix 10).

3. Consider hospitalization, especially if surgery is contemplated. Management in the hospital:

—Administer systemic antibiotics promptly (e.g., cefazolin, 1 g i.v. q8h, for clean, inert objects). If the object is contaminated or organic, treat as orbital cellulitis (see 7.4, Orbital Cellulitis).

—Follow vision; assess degree (if any) of afferent pupillary defect; evaluate motility, proptosis, and eye discomfort daily.

—Surgical exploration and removal of the foreign body when indicated (as above).

—If the decision is made to leave the foreign body in place, discharge when stable with oral antibiotics (e.g., amoxicillin–clavulanate, 250 to 500 mg, p.o. q8h) to complete a 10- to 14-day course.

4. Patients with small nonorganic foreign bodies not requiring surgical intervention may be discharged without hospitalization with oral antibiotics for a 10- to 14-day course. Daily follow-up until stable.

FOLLOW-UP

After hospitalization or when stable, the patient is told to return in 1 week (or sooner if the condition worsens). See 3.14, Ruptured Globe and Penetrating Ocular Injury; 3.16, Traumatic Optic Neuropathy; and 7.4, Orbital Cellulitis.

3.11 COMMOTIO RETINAE

SYMPTOMS

Decreased vision or asymptomatic; history of recent ocular trauma.

SIGNS

Confluent area of retinal whitening.

Note: The retinal blood vessels are undisturbed in the area of retinal whitening. Other signs of ocular trauma may be noted.

DIFFERENTIAL DIAGNOSIS

• Retinal detachment (Retinal vessels can be seen to rise upward with the detached retina. A retinal break or dialysis, anterior vitreous pigment, and an AC reaction may be seen. See 11.3, Retinal Detachment.).

• Branch retinal artery occlusion (Rarely follows trauma. Whitening of the retina with edema occurs along the distribution of an artery; cotton-wool spots, narrowed arterioles, and sludging of blood in the affected vessels

may be seen. See 11.6, Branch Retinal Artery Occlusion.).

• White without pressure (A common retinal anomaly unrelated to trauma. A prominent vitreous base is seen in the peripheral retina, often bilaterally.).

WORKUP

Complete ophthalmic examination, including dilated fundus examination. Scleral depression is performed except when a hyphema, microhyphema, or iritis is present.

TREATMENT

No treatment is required because this condition usually clears without therapy.

FOLLOW-UP

Dilated fundus examination is repeated in 1 to 2 weeks. Patients are instructed to return sooner if retinal detachment symptoms are experienced (see 11.3, Retinal Detachment).

3.12 TRAUMATIC CHOROIDAL RUPTURE

SYMPTOMS

Decreased vision or asymptomatic; history of ocular trauma.

SIGNS

Critical. A yellow or white crescent-shaped subretinal streak, usually concentric to the optic disc. It may be single or multiple. Often the rupture cannot be seen until several days or weeks after trauma because it may be obscured by overlying blood.

Other. Rarely, the rupture may be radially oriented. A choroidal neovascular membrane (CNVM) may later develop. Traumatic optic neuropathy may be present.

DIFFERENTIAL DIAGNOSIS

• Lacquer cracks of high myopia (Often bilateral. A tilted disc, a scleral crescent adjacent to the disc, or a posterior staphyloma also may be seen. A CNVM also may develop in this condition. See 11.16, High Myopia.).

• Angioid streaks (Bilateral reddish-brown or gray subretinal streaks that radiate out from the optic disc, sometimes associated with a CNVM. See 11.17, Angioid Streaks.).

WORKUP

1. Complete ocular examination, including dilated fundus evaluation to rule out retinal breaks and to detect traumatic choroidal ruptures. A CNVM is best seen with slit-lamp biomicroscopy with either a fundus contact or 60- or 90-diopter lens.

2. Consider fluorescein angiography to confirm the location of a late CNVM.

TREATMENT

Laser therapy should be considered when a CNVM greater than 200 μm from the center of the fovea is detected. Treatment should be applied within 72 hours of obtaining the fluorescein angiogram. Surgical removal of the CNVM as well as photodynamic therapy may be options for subfoveal lesions, although experience with these options is limited.

FOLLOW-UP

After ocular trauma, patients with hemorrhage obscuring the underlying choroid are reevaluated every 1 to 2 weeks until the choroid can be well visualized. If a choroidal rupture is present, patients are instructed in the use of an Amsler grid and told to return if a change in the appearance of the grid is noted (see Appendix 3). Ruptures that are longer or closer to the fovea are at greater risk for development of CNVM, although, overall, CNVMs are rare. Fundus examinations may be performed every 6 to 12 months, depending on severity and risk of progression to CNVM. Patients treated for a CNVM must be followed closely after treatment to watch for a persistent or new CNVM (see 11.14, Exudative Age-Related Macular Degeneration, for further follow-up guidelines).

3.13 CORNEAL LACERATION

PARTIAL-THICKNESS LACERATION

SIGNS

The AC is not entered and, therefore, the cornea is not perforated.

WORKUP

1. Complete ocular examination; use a slit lamp carefully to exclude ocular penetration. Carefully inspect the cornea, conjunctiva, and sclera. Make sure the AC is deep and does not contain blood. Check iris for defects and lens for traumatic cataract (must have high level of suspicion with projectile objects) and, if present, see Full-Thickness Laceration, later. Measure the IOP by applanation tonometry only if the laceration site can be avoided (otherwise, use a Tono-Pen or gently assess IOP with your fingers).

2. Seidel test (see Appendix 4). If the Seidel test is positive, a full-thickness laceration is present (see Full-Thickness Laceration).

TREATMENT

1. A cycloplegic (e.g., scopolamine 0.25%) and an antibiotic [e.g., frequent polymyxin B/bacitracin ointment (e.g., Polysporin) or fluoroquinolone drops, depending on the nature of the wound].

2. When a moderate to deep corneal laceration is accompanied by wound gape, it is often best to suture the wound closed in the operating room to avoid excessive scarring and corneal irregularity, especially in the visual axis.

3. Tetanus toxoid for dirty wounds (see Appendix 10).

FOLLOW-UP

Reevaluate daily until the epithelium heals.

FULL-THICKNESS LACERATION

See 3.14, Ruptured Globe and Penetrating Ocular Injury. Note that small, self-sealing, or slow-leaking lacerations may be treated with aqueous suppressants, bandage soft contact lenses, fluoroquinolone drops q.i.d., and precautions as listed in 3.14. Alternatively, a pressure patch and twice-daily antibiotics may be used. Avoid topical steroids. If an intraocular foreign body is present, see 3.15, Intraocular Foreign Body.

3.14 RUPTURED GLOBE AND PENETRATING OCULAR INJURY

SYMPTOMS

Pain, decreased vision, history of trauma.

SIGNS

Critical

• Ruptured globe: Severe subconjunctival hemorrhage (often involves 360 degrees of bulbar conjunctiva), a deep or shallow AC compared with the contralateral eye, hyphema (often with clotted blood), peaked or irregular pupil, limitation of extraocular motility (greatest in the direction of rupture), intraocular contents may be outside of the globe.

• Penetrating injury: Full-thickness scleral or corneal laceration, with or without distortion or irregularity of the iris; traumatic cataract; accompanying signs of a ruptured globe; history of a sharp object entering the globe.

Other. Low IOP (although it may be normal or increased), iridodialysis, cyclodialysis, periorbital ecchymosis, vitreous hemorrhage, dislocated or subluxed lens, and traumatic optic neuropathy. Commotio retinae, choroidal rupture, and retinal breaks may be seen but are typically obscured by vitreous hemorrhage.

WORKUP/TREATMENT

Once the diagnosis of a ruptured globe or penetrating ocular injury is made, further examination should be deferred until the time of surgical repair in the operating room. This is to avoid placing any pressure on the globe and risking extrusion of the intraocular contents. Diagnosis is made by penlight or, if possible, by slit-lamp examination (very gentle manipulation to evaluate the status of the lens and to look for signs of infection). The following measures should be taken:

1. Protect the eye with a shield.

2. Admit patient to the hospital with no food or drink (NPO).

3. Systemic antibiotics should be administered within 6 hours of injury, if possible, unless there is a posterior rupture only, with no communication to the outside world. For adults, give cefazolin 1 g i.v., q8h or vancomycin 1 g i.v., q12h. Also give ciprofloxacin 400 mg p.o./i.v., b.i.d. (Newer fluoroquinolones, such as gatifloxacin 400 mg, q.d. or moxifloxacin 400 mg, q.d., may have better vitreous penetration.) For children younger than age 12 years, give cefazolin 25 to 50 mg/kg/day i.v. in three divided doses, and gentamicin 2 mg/kg i.v., q8h.

Note: Antibiotic doses may need to be reduced if renal function is impaired. Gentamicin peak and trough levels are obtained one-half hour before and after the fifth dose, and blood urea nitrogen and creatinine levels are evaluated every other day.

4. Administer tetanus toxoid prn (see Appendix 10).

5. Administer antiemetic [e.g., prochlorperazine (Compazine) 10 mg i.m., q8h] prn to prevent Valsalva.

6. Place patient on bed rest with bathroom privileges.

7. Determine when the patient had his or her last meal. The timing of surgical repair is often influenced by this information.

8. Obtain CT scan (axial and coronal views) of the orbits and brain. B-scan ultrasonography may be needed to localize the rupture site(s) and to rule out an intraocular or intraorbital foreign body.

9. Arrange for surgical repair to be done as soon as possible.

Note: In any severely traumatized eye in which there is no chance of restoring vision, enucleation should be considered initially or within 7 to 14 days after the trauma to prevent the rare occurrence of sympathetic ophthalmia.

Note: Infection is more likely to occur in eyes with dirty injuries, retained intraocular foreign bodies, or rupture of lens capsule, and in patients with a long delay until primary surgical repair. In patients at high risk of infection, some groups recommend intravitreal antibiotics (see 12.12, Traumatic Endophthalmitis).

3.15 INTRAOCULAR FOREIGN BODY

SYMPTOMS

Eye pain, decreased vision, or may be asymptomatic; often suggestive history (e.g., ocular foreign body after hammering metal).

SIGNS

Critical. May have a clinically detectable corneal or scleral perforation site or an intraocular foreign body. Intraocular foreign bodies are usually seen on CT scan, B-scan ultrasonography, or both.

Other. Microcystic (epithelial) edema of the peripheral cornea (a clue that a foreign body may be hidden in the AC angle in the same sector of the eye), an iris transillumination defect (see Workup), an irregular pupil, anterior or posterior segment inflammation, vitreous hemorrhage, decreased IOP. Long-standing iron-containing intraocular foreign bodies may cause siderosis, manifesting as anisocoria, heterochromia, corneal endothelial and epithelial deposits, anterior subcapsular cataracts, lens dislocation, and optic atrophy.

TYPES OF FOREIGN BODIES

1. Frequently produce severe inflammatory reactions.

   —Magnetic: Iron and steel.

   —Nonmagnetic: Copper and vegetable matter.

2. Typically produce mild inflammatory reactions when left in the eye.

   —Magnetic: Nickel.

   —Nonmagnetic: Aluminum, mercury, and zinc.

3. Inert foreign bodies: Carbon, coal, glass, lead, plaster, platinum, porcelain, rubber, silver, and stone. Note that brass is also relatively nontoxic.

   Note: *Even inert foreign bodies can be toxic to the eye because of a coating or* *chemical additive. Most BBs and gunshot pellets are made of 80% to 90% lead and 10% to 20% iron.*

WORKUP

1. History: Composition of foreign body and time of last meal.

2. Perform ocular examination, including visual acuity assessment and careful evaluation of whether the globe is intact. If there is an obvious perforation site, the remainder of the examination may be deferred until surgery. If there does not appear to be a risk of extrusion of the intraocular contents, the globe is inspected gently to localize the site of perforation and to detect the foreign body.

   —Slit-lamp examination; search the AC and iris for a foreign body and look for an iris transillumination defect (direct a small beam of light directly through the pupil and look at the iris for a red reflex penetrating through it). Examine the lens for disruption, cataract, or embedded foreign body. Check the IOP.

   —Consider gonioscopy of the AC angle if no wound leak can be detected and the globe appears intact.

   —Dilated retinal examination using indirect ophthalmoscopy.

3. Obtain a CT scan of the orbit and brain (coronal and axial views with thin, 1- to 1.5-mm cuts through the orbit); MRI is contraindicated in the presence of a metallic foreign body. It may be difficult to visualize wood, glass, or plastic on a CT scan, especially acutely. Wood may look like air.

4. Obtain B-scan ultrasonogram of the globe and orbit. (Note that intraocular air can mimic a foreign body.)

5. Culture the object from which the foreign body arose, if possible. Culture the wound site, if it appears infected.

6. Determine whether the foreign body is magnetic (e.g., examine material from which the foreign body came).

TREATMENT

1. Hospitalization.

2. No food or drink (NPO).

3. Place a protective shield over the involved eye.

4. Tetanus prophylaxis as needed (see Appendix 10).

5. Antibiotics (e.g., vancomycin 1 g i.v., q12h; and ceftazidime 1 g i.v., q12h or ciprofloxacin 750 mg p.o., q12h).

   Note: Ciprofloxacin is contraindicated in children and pregnant women.

6. Cycloplegic (e.g., atropine 1%, t.i.d.) for posterior segment foreign bodies.

7. Surgical removal of any acute intraocular foreign body, even if nontoxic, is advisable to prevent infection. For some metallic foreign bodies, a magnet may be useful during surgical extraction. Copper or contaminated foreign bodies require especially urgent removal. A long-standing intraocular foreign body may require removal if associated with severe recurrent inflammation, if in the visual axis, or if causing siderosis.

8. If endophthalmitis is present, treat as per 12.12, Traumatic Endophthalmitis.

FOLLOW-UP

Observe the patient closely in the hospital for signs of inflammation or infection. Examine both eyes. Periodic follow-up for years is required; watch for a delayed inflammatory reaction. When an intraocular foreign body is left in place, an electroretinogram (ERG) should be obtained as soon as it can be done safely. The patient should have serial ERGs to look for toxic retinal metallosis. If found, this retinal toxicity often reverses after the foreign body is removed.

3.16 TRAUMATIC OPTIC NEUROPATHY

SYMPTOMS

Decreased vision after a traumatic injury to the eye or periocular area; other trauma symptoms (e.g., pain).

SIGNS

Critical. A new afferent pupillary defect in a traumatized eye that cannot be accounted for by retinal or other ocular lesions (which would have to be severe).

Other. Decreased color vision in the affected eye, a visual field defect, and other signs of trauma. The optic disc acutely appears normal in most cases. Optic disc avulsion is obvious on funduscopic examination unless obscured by vitreous hemorrhage.

Note: Optic disc pallor usually does not appear for weeks after a traumatic optic nerve injury. If pallor is present immediately after trauma, a pre-existing optic neuropathy should be suspected.

DIFFERENTIAL DIAGNOSIS

(Other causes of a traumatic afferent pupillary defect).

• Severe retinal trauma (Retinal lesion evident on examination.).

• Traumatic vitreous hemorrhage (Obscured retinal view on dilated fundus examination. The relative afferent pupillary defect is mild.).

• Intracranial trauma with asymmetric damage to the optic chiasm.

- Functional/nonphysiologic visual loss (No afferent pupillary defect; must be a diagnosis of exclusion. See 10.23, Nonphysiologic Visual Loss.).

ETIOLOGY

- Shearing injury from blunt trauma.

- Compression of the nerve by bone, hemorrhage, or perineural edema.

- Laceration of the nerve by bone or an intraorbital foreign body (which may or may not still be present in the orbit).

WORKUP

1. Complete ocular examination. A pupillary evaluation is essential to diagnose a traumatic optic neuropathy.

2. Color vision testing in each eye (color plates).

3. Visual fields by confrontation. Formal visual field testing is helpful if available.

4. CT scan of the head and orbit (coronal and axial views) to rule out an intraorbital foreign body or an impinging fracture through the optic canal. Thin cuts through the optic canal should be obtained.

5. B-scan ultrasonography when a foreign body is suspected but not discovered by CT scan.

TREATMENT

Depends on type of traumatic optic neuropathy.

1. Compressive optic neuropathy from orbital hemorrhage: See 3.9, Traumatic Retrobulbar Hemorrhage.

2. Compressive optic neuropathy from orbital foreign body: See 3.15, Intraorbital Foreign Body.

3. Bone impingement of orbital apex or optic canal: Endoscopic optic canal/orbital apex decompression by an oculoplastic specialist.

4. Optic nerve sheath hematoma: Optic nerve sheath fenestration.

5. There is no effective treatment for optic nerve head avulsion or intraorbital optic nerve laceration.

6. Chiasmal injury: Immediate i.v. steroids because of possibility of pituitary gland injury and addisonian crisis. Immediate neurosurgical consultation and admission to neurosurgical intensive care unit.

7. Posterior indirect traumatic optic neuropathy: Treatment is controversial. There has been no clearly proven benefit of megadose corticosteroids as used in spinal cord injury. However, anecdotal reports have shown improvement in uncontrolled, nonrandomized, small series. Options at present include:

—No treatment; follow-up for repeat visual field testing at monthly intervals. Visual function may show improvement for up to 6 months.

—Megadose corticosteroids (i.v. methylprednisolone, loading dose of 30 mg/kg, then 5.4 mg/kg, q6h for 48 hours, plus histamine type 2 receptor antagonist such as ranitidine 150 mg p.o., b.i.d.). All patients must be told of lack of definitive proof of efficacy as well as the potential for severe systemic side effects. Because of the increased potential for side effects from corticosteroids, this treatment is usually not offered to young children, the elderly, and patients with brittle diabetes.

FOLLOW-UP

Daily evaluation of vision, pupillary reactions, and color vision. If vision deteriorates after discontinuing steroids, they should be reinstituted as previously described. If visual deterioration occurs despite steroids, surgery may be considered (controversial).

CHAPTER 4

CORNEA

4.1 SUPERFICIAL PUNCTATE KERATITIS

SYMPTOMS

Pain, photophobia, red eye, foreign body sensation, mildly decreased vision.

SIGNS

Critical. Pinpoint corneal epithelial defects (stain with fluorescein); may be confluent if severe. Pain is relieved by the instillation of anesthetic drops.

Note: Relief of pain with the instillation of anesthetic drops (e.g., proparacaine) strongly suggests corneal epithelial disease as the etiology of pain. Although anesthetic drop instillation is an essential part of the ocular examination, patients should never be prescribed topical anesthetic drops for use at home. When used chronically, these drops inhibit epithelial healing and predispose to corneal ulcer formation.

Other. Conjunctival injection, watery or mucoid discharge.

ETIOLOGY

Superficial punctate keratitis (SPK) is nonspecific but is most commonly seen with the following disorders:

• Dry-eye syndrome (Poor tear lake or a decreased tear break-up time. See 4.3, Dry-Eye Syndrome.).

• Blepharitis (Erythema, telangiectases, or crusting of the eyelid margins, meibomian gland dysfunction. See 5.8, Blepharitis/Meibomianitis.).

• Trauma (Can occur from relatively mild trauma, such as chronic eye rubbing.).

• Exposure keratopathy (Poor eyelid closure with failure of eyelids to cover the entire globe. See 4.5, Exposure Keratopathy.).

• Topical drug toxicity (e.g., neomycin, gentamicin, trifluridine, or any drops with preservatives, including artificial tears).

• Ultraviolet burn/photokeratopathy (Often in welders or from sun lamps. See 4.7, Thermal/Ultraviolet Keratopathy.).

• Mild chemical injury (See 3.1, Chemical Burn.).

• Contact lens–related disorder (e.g., chemical toxicity, tight lens syndrome, contact lens overwear syndrome, giant papillary conjunctivitis; see 4.19, Contact Lens–Related Problems).

• Thygeson SPK (Bilateral, recurrent SPK without conjunctival injection. See 4.8, Thygeson Superficial Punctate Keratitis.).

• Foreign body under the upper eyelid (Typically linear SPK, fine scratches arranged vertically.).

- Conjunctivitis (Discharge, conjunctival injection, eyelids stuck together on awakening. See 5.1, Acute Conjunctivitis and 5.2, Chronic Conjunctivitis.).

- Trichiasis/distichiasis (One or more eyelashes rubbing against the cornea. See 6.4, Trichiasis.).

- Entropion or ectropion (Eyelid margin turned in or out. Area of SPK is superior or inferior. See 6.2, Ectropion and 6.3, Entropion.).

- Floppy eyelid syndrome (Extremely loose upper eyelids that evert very easily. See 6.5, Floppy Eyelid Syndrome.).

WORKUP

1. History: Trauma? Contact lens wear? Eyedrops? Discharge or eyelid matting? Chemical or ultraviolet light exposure? Time of day when worse?

2. Evaluate the cornea and tear film. Evert the upper and lower eyelids and look for a foreign body. Check eyelid closure and eyelid laxity. Look for inward-growing lashes.

3. Inspect contact lenses for fit (if still in the eye) and for the presence of deposits, sharp edges, and cracks.

Note: A soft contact lens should be removed before placing fluorescein in the eye.

TREATMENT

See the appropriate section to treat the underlying disorder. SPK is often treated nonspecifically as follows:

1. Non–contact lens wearer with a small amount of SPK

—Artificial tears q.i.d., preferably nonpreserved (e.g., Refresh Plus or TheraTears) or neutral preservative (e.g., GenTeal or Refresh Tears).

—Can add a lubricating ointment q.h.s. (e.g., Refresh PM).

2. Non–contact lens wearer with a large amount of SPK

—Preservative-free artificial tears q2h.

—Antibiotic (e.g., erythromycin ointment q.i.d. for 3 to 5 days).

—Consider a cycloplegic drop (e.g., cyclopentolate 1% to 2%, or scopolamine 0.25%) for relief of pain and photophobia.

3. Contact lens wearer with a small amount of SPK

—Artificial tears four to six times per day, preferably nonpreserved (e.g., Refresh Plus or TheraTears).

—Lenses may or may not be worn, depending on the symptoms and the degree of SPK.

4. Contact lens wearer with a large amount of SPK

—Discontinue contact lens wear.

—Fluoroquinolone [e.g., ciprofloxacin (e.g., Ciloxan), levofloxacin (e.g., Quixin), ofloxacin (e.g., Ocuflox), gatifloxacin (e.g., Zymar), moxifloxacin (e.g., Vigamox)] or tobramycin drops four to six times per day, and tobramycin or ciprofloxacin ointment q.h.s.

—Consider a cycloplegic drop (e.g., cyclopentolate 1% to 2% or scopolamine 0.25%) for relief of pain and photophobia.

Note: DO NOT patch contact lens–related epithelial defects.

FOLLOW-UP

1. Non–contact lens wearers with SPK (especially traumatic SPK) are not seen again solely for the SPK unless the patient is a child or is unreliable. Reliable patients are told to return if their symptoms worsen or do not improve. When underlying ocular disease is responsible for the SPK, follow-up is in accordance with the guidelines for the underlying problem.

2. Contact lens wearers with a large amount of SPK are seen every day until significant improvement is demonstrated. Contact lenses are not to be worn until the condition clears. The antibiotic may be discontinued when the SPK resolves. The patient's contact lens

regimen (e.g., wearing time, cleaning routine) is corrected or the contact lenses are changed if either is thought to be responsible (see 4.19, Contact Lens–Related Problems). Contact lens wearers with a small amount of SPK are rechecked in several days to 1 week, depending on their symptoms and degree of SPK.

Note: In general, contact lens wearers should not wear their lenses when their eyes feel irritated.

4.2 RECURRENT CORNEAL EROSION

SYMPTOMS

Recurrent attacks of acute ocular pain, photophobia, foreign body sensation, and tearing. These often occur at the time of awakening, or during sleep when the eyelids are rubbed or opened. There is often a history of prior corneal abrasion in the involved eye. The unpredictability of recurrent corneal erosions may cause patients intense anxiety.

SIGNS

Critical. Localized roughening of the corneal epithelium (fluorescein dye may lightly outline the area) or a corneal abrasion. Epithelial changes may resolve within hours of the onset of symptoms so that an abnormality is difficult to detect when the patient is examined.

Other. Corneal epithelial dots or small cysts (microcysts), a fingerprint pattern, or maplike lines may be seen between episodes in both eyes if anterior basement membrane (map–dot–fingerprint) dystrophy is the underlying problem.

ETIOLOGY

Damage to the corneal epithelium or epithelial basement membrane from one of the following:

• Anterior corneal dystrophy [e.g., anterior basement membrane (most common), Meesmann, and Reis–Bücklers dystrophies].

• Previous traumatic corneal abrasion (occasionally, years before the current presentation).

• Stromal corneal dystrophy (e.g., lattice, granular, and macular dystrophies).

• Keratorefractive, corneal transplant, or cataract surgery.

WORKUP

1. History: Recent or remote history of a traumatic corneal abrasion? Ocular surgery? Family history (corneal dystrophy)?

2. Slit-lamp examination with fluorescein staining (visualization of abnormal basement membrane lines may be enhanced by staining the tear film thickly with fluorescein and looking for areas of rapid tear breakup, referred to as "negative staining").

TREATMENT

1. Acute episode: A cycloplegic drop (e.g., cyclopentolate 1% to 2%, or homatropine 2%) is applied, and antibiotic ointment (e.g., erythromycin) is used three to four times per day. If the defect is large, a pressure patch or bandage contact lens may be placed. Oral analgesics (e.g., acetaminophen with or without codeine) as needed.

2. Patients should never be prescribed topical anesthetic drops for use at home.

3. After epithelial healing is complete, artificial tears (e.g., Refresh Plus, TheraTears, or Celluvisc) four to eight times per day and artificial tear ointment (e.g., Refresh PM) q.h.s. for at least 3 to 6 months, or 5% sodium chloride drops four to eight times

per day and 5% sodium chloride ointment q.h.s. for at least 3 months.

4. If the corneal epithelium is loose and heaped and is not healing, consider debridement of the abnormal epithelium. Apply a topical anesthetic (e.g., proparacaine) and use a sterile cotton-tipped applicator gently to remove the loose epithelium.

5. Erosions not responsive to the preceding treatment:

—Consider an extended-wear bandage soft contact lens for several months.

—Consider anterior stromal puncture. This is usually used in extremely symptomatic, refractory cases, with erosions outside the visual axis. It can be performed with or without an intact epithelium. The patient must be very cooperative. This treatment may cause small permanent corneal scars that are usually of no visual significance.

—Epithelial debridement with diamond burr polishing of Bowman membrane. Effective for large areas of epithelial irregularity and lesions in the visual axis.

—Phototherapeutic keratectomy (PTK): Excimer laser ablation of the superficial stroma is successful in up to 90% of patients with recurrent erosions from corneal dystrophies.

FOLLOW-UP

Every 1 to 2 days until the epithelium has healed, and then every 1 to 3 months, depending on the severity and frequency of the episodes.

4.3 DRY-EYE SYNDROME

SYMPTOMS

Burning or foreign body sensation, mildly to moderately decreased vision, may have excess tearing, often exacerbated by smoke, wind, heat, low humidity, or prolonged use of the eye (commonly when working on a computer, and worse later in the day). Usually bilateral and chronic (although patients sometimes are seen with recent onset in one eye). Often causes more discomfort than the clinical signs would suggest.

SIGNS

Critical (either or both may be present)

• Scanty tear meniscus seen at the inferior eyelid margin: The normal meniscus should be at least 1 mm in height and have a convex shape.

• Decreased tear breakup time (measured from a blink to the appearance of a tear film defect, by using fluorescein stain): Normally should be longer than 10 seconds.

Other. Punctate corneal or conjunctival fluorescein, rose bengal, or lissamine green staining; usually inferiorly or in the interpalpebral area. Excess mucus or debris in the tear film and filaments on the cornea may be found.

DIFFERENTIAL DIAGNOSIS

See 4.1, Superficial Punctate Keratitis.

ETIOLOGY

• Idiopathic (Commonly found in menopausal and postmenopausal women.).

• Connective tissue diseases (e.g., Sjögren syndrome, rheumatoid arthritis, Wegener granulomatosis, systemic lupus erythematosus).

• Conjunctival scarring (e.g., ocular cicatricial pemphigoid, Stevens–Johnson syndrome, trachoma, chemical burn).

- Drugs (e.g., oral contraceptives, antihistamines, beta-blockers, phenothiazines, atropine).

- Infiltration of the lacrimal glands (e.g., sarcoidosis, tumor).

- Postradiation fibrosis of the lacrimal glands.

- Vitamin A deficiency (Usually from malnutrition or intestinal malabsorption. See 13.11, Vitamin A Deficiency.).

- After laser in situ keratomileusis (LASIK) (Likely secondary to disruption of corneal nerves and interference with normal reflex tearing.).

WORKUP

1. History and external examination to detect underlying etiology.

2. Slit-lamp examination with fluorescein stain to examine the tear meniscus and tear breakup time. Can use rose bengal or lissamine green stain to examine the cornea and conjunctiva.

3. Schirmer test. Technique: After drying the eye of excess tears, Schirmer filter paper is placed at the junction of the middle and lateral one third of the lower eyelid in each eye for 5 minutes.

   —Unanesthetized: Measures basal and reflex tearing. Normal is wetting of at least 15 mm in 5 minutes.

   —Anesthetized: Topical anesthetic (e.g., proparacaine) is applied before drying the eye and placing filter paper. Measures basal tearing only. Abnormal is wetting of less than 5 mm in 5 minutes. We prefer the anesthetized method, which is less irritating to the patient.

TREATMENT

Mild Dry-Eye

Artificial tears q.i.d. (e.g., Refresh Tears, GenTeal, HypoTears, Systane, Tears Naturale II).

Moderate Dry-Eye

1. Increase frequency of artificial tear application up to q1–2h; use preservative-free artificial tears (e.g., Refresh Plus, TheraTears, Bion tears, Celluvisc).

2. Add a lubricating ointment or gel q.h.s. (e.g., Refresh PM, Lacri-Lube, GenTeal gel).

3. If these measures are inadequate or impractical, consider punctal occlusion. Use collagen inserts (temporary) or silicone or acrylic plugs (reversible), occasionally followed by thermal punctal cautery (permanent) after a successful trial of plugs.

4. Cyclosporine 0.05% (e.g., Restasis, b.i.d.) has recently been approved for patients with chronic dry eye in whom tear production is thought to be suppressed because of ocular inflammation. Although promising, we have not yet had significant clinical experience with this medication. Note that the medication takes 1 to 3 months for most patients to experience clinical improvement.

Severe Dry-Eye

1. Punctal occlusion, as described earlier (both lower and upper puncta if necessary), with preservative-free artificial tears up to q1–2h as needed.

2. Cyclosporine 0.05% (e.g., Restasis), as described earlier.

3. Add lubricating ointment or gel (e.g., Refresh PM, GenTeal gel) two to four times during the daytime if needed.

4. Patch or moist chamber (plastic film sealed at orbital rim) with lubrication at night. May need to patch during the day pending more definitive treatment.

5. If mucus strands or filaments are present, remove with forceps and consider 10% acetylcysteine (e.g., Mucomyst) q.i.d.

6. Consider a lateral tarsorrhaphy if all of the previous measures fail. A temporary adhesive tape tarsorrhaphy (to tape the lateral one third of the eyelid closed) can also be used, pending a surgical tarsorrhaphy.

1. *In addition to treating the dry eye, treatment for contributing disorders (e.g., blepharitis, exposure keratopathy) should be instituted if these conditions are present.*

2. *Always use preservative-free artificial tears if using them more frequently than q4h to prevent preservative toxicity.*

3. *If the history suggests the presence of a previously undiagnosed connective tissue disease (e.g., history of arthritic pain), referral should be made to an internist or rheumatologist for further evaluation.*

FOLLOW-UP

In days to months, depending on the severity of the drying changes and the symptoms. Anyone with severe dry eyes caused by an underlying chronic systemic disease (e.g., rheumatoid arthritis, sarcoidosis, ocular pemphigoid) may need to be monitored more closely.

Note: Patients with significant dry eye should be discouraged from contact lens wear as well as LASIK surgery. Patients with Sjögren syndrome have an increased incidence of lymphoma and mucous membrane problems and may require internal medicine, rheumatologic, dental, and gynecologic follow-up.

4.4 FILAMENTARY KERATOPATHY

SYMPTOMS

Moderate to severe pain, red eye, foreign body sensation, photophobia.

SIGNS

Critical. Short strands of epithelial cells and mucus attached to the anterior surface of the cornea at one end of the strand. The strands stain with fluorescein.

Other. Conjunctival injection, poor tear film, punctate epithelial defects.

ETIOLOGY

• Dry-eye syndrome (Most common cause. Can be associated with an autoimmune connective tissue disease such as Sjögren syndrome. See 4.3, Dry-Eye Syndrome.).

• Superior limbic keratoconjunctivitis (Filaments are located in the superior cornea, in association with superior conjunctival injection and fluorescein staining, and with superior corneal pannus. See 5.4, Superior Limbic Keratoconjunctivitis.).

• Recurrent corneal erosions (Recurrent spontaneous corneal abrasions often occurring upon awakening. See 4.2, Recurrent Corneal Erosion.).

• Patching (e.g., postoperative, after corneal abrasions).

• Neurotrophic keratopathy (see 4.6, Neurotrophic Keratopathy).

• Chronic bullous keratopathy (see 4.26, Aphakic Bullous Keratopathy/Pseudophakic Bullous Keratopathy).

• Adjacent to irregular corneal surface (e.g., postoperative, near a surgical wound).

WORKUP

1. History, especially for the previously mentioned conditions.

2. Slit-lamp examination with fluorescein staining.

TREATMENT

1. Treat the underlying condition.

2. Consider debridement of the filaments. After applying topical anesthesia (e.g., proparacaine), gently remove filaments at their base with fine forceps or a cotton-tipped ap-

plicator. This gives temporary relief, but the filaments will recur if the underlying etiology is not treated.

3. Lubrication with one of the following regimens

—Preservative-free artificial tears four to eight times per day (e.g., Refresh Plus, TheraTears, Bion tears) and lubricating ointment q.h.s. (e.g., Refresh PM).

—Punctal occlusion as described earlier.

—Acetylcysteine 10% (e.g., Mucomyst) q.i.d. (Not commercially available as a drop but can be made by a compounding pharmacy.).

4. If the symptoms are severe or treatment fails, then consider a bandage soft contact lens (unless the patient has severe dry eyes). Extended-wear bandage soft contact lenses may need to be worn for weeks to months.

FOLLOW-UP

In 1 to 4 weeks, if the condition is not improved, consider repeating the filament removal or applying a bandage soft contact lens. Lubrication must be maintained over the long term if the underlying condition cannot be eliminated.

4.5 EXPOSURE KERATOPATHY

SYMPTOMS

Ocular irritation, burning, foreign body sensation, and redness of one or both eyes. Usually worse in the morning.

SIGNS

Critical. Inadequate blinking or closure of the eyelids, leading to corneal drying. Punctate epithelial defects are found on the lower one third of the cornea or as a horizontal band in the region of the palpebral fissure.

Other. Conjunctival injection and chemosis, corneal erosion, infiltrate or ulcer, eyelid deformity, or abnormal eyelid closure.

ETIOLOGY

• Seventh nerve palsy [Orbicularis oculi weakness (e.g., Bell palsy). See 10.8, Isolated Seventh-Nerve Palsy.].

• Sedation or altered mental status (as in the intensive care unit).

• Eyelid deformity (e.g., ectropion or eyelid scarring from trauma, chemical burn, or herpes zoster ophthalmicus).

• Nocturnal lagophthalmos (Failure to close the eyes during sleep.).

• Proptosis (e.g., due to an orbital process, such as thyroid eye disease; see 7.1, Orbital Disease).

• After ptosis repair or blepharoplasty procedures.

• Floppy eyelid syndrome (see 6.5, Floppy Eyelid Syndrome).

WORKUP

1. History: Previous Bell palsy or eyelid surgery? Thyroid disease?

2. Evaluate eyelid closure and corneal exposure. Ask the patient to close his or her eyes gently (as if sleeping). Assess Bell phenomenon (the patient is asked to close the eyelids forcefully against resistance; abnormal when the eyes do not rotate upward). Check for eyelid laxity.

3. Check corneal sensation before instillation of anesthetic drops. When decreased corneal sensation present, higher risk for corneal complications.

4. Slit-lamp examination: Evaluate the tear film and corneal integrity with fluorescein dye. Look for signs of secondary infection (corneal infiltrate, anterior chamber reaction, severe conjunctival injection).

5. Investigate any underlying disorder (e.g., etiology of seventh nerve palsy).

TREATMENT

Prevention is critical. All patients who are sedated or obtunded are at risk for exposure keratopathy and should receive lubrication as recommended in the following.

In the presence of secondary corneal infection, see 4.11, Bacterial Keratitis.

1. Correct any underlying disorder.

2. Artificial tears (e.g., Refresh Plus, Thera-Tears, or Celluvisc) q1–6h.

3. Lubricating ointment (e.g., Refresh PM) q.h.s. or q.i.d.

4. Consider eyelid taping or patching q.h.s. to maintain the eyelids in the closed position. If severe, consider taping the lateral one third of the eyelids closed (leaving the visual axis open) during the day. (Taping is rarely a definitive therapy, but may be tried when the underlying disorder is thought to be temporary.)

5. When maximal medical therapy fails to prevent progressive corneal deterioration, one of the following surgical procedures may be beneficial:

—Eyelid reconstruction (e.g., for ectropion).

—Tarsorrhaphy or eyelid gold weight implant (e.g., for seventh nerve palsy).

—Orbital decompression (e.g., for proptosis).

—Conjunctival flap or amniotic membrane graft (for severe corneal decompensation if the preceding fail).

FOLLOW-UP

Reevaluate every 1 to 2 days in the presence of corneal ulceration. Less frequent examinations (e.g., in weeks to months) are required for less severe corneal disease.

4.6   NEUROTROPHIC KERATOPATHY

SYMPTOMS

Red eye, foreign body sensation, swollen eyelid.

SIGNS

Critical. Loss of corneal sensation, epithelial defects with fluorescein staining.

Other

• Early: Perilimbal injection progressing to corneal punctate epithelial defects.

• Late: Corneal ulcer with associated iritis. The ulcer often has a gray, heaped-up border, tends to be in the lower one half of the cornea, and is horizontally oval.

DIFFERENTIAL DIAGNOSIS

See 4.1, Superficial Punctate Keratitis.

ETIOLOGY

• Postinfection with varicella-zoster or herpes simplex virus (HSV).

• Stroke.

• Complication of trigeminal nerve surgery.

• Complication of irradiation to the eye or an adnexal structure.

• Tumor (especially an acoustic neuroma).

WORKUP

1. History: Previous episodes of a red and painful eye (herpes)? Previous surgery, irradiation, stroke, or hearing problem?

2. Test corneal sensation bilaterally with a sterile cotton wisp (before instillation of topical anesthesia).

3. Slit-lamp examination with fluorescein staining.

4. Check the skin for herpetic lesions or scars from a previous herpes zoster infection.

5. Look for signs of a corneal exposure problem (e.g., inability to close an eyelid, seventh nerve palsy, absent Bell phenomenon).

6. If suspicious of a central nervous system lesion, obtain a computed tomography scan (axial and coronal views) or magnetic resonance image of the brain.

TREATMENT

1. Mild to moderate punctate epithelial staining: Artificial tears (e.g., Refresh Plus, TheraTears, or Celluvisc) q2–4h and artificial-tear ointment (e.g., Refresh PM) q.h.s.

2. Small corneal epithelial defect: Antibiotic ointment (erythromycin or bacitracin) q.i.d. for 3 to 5 days or until resolved. Usually requires prolonged artificial tear treatment, as described previously.

3. Corneal ulcer: See 4.11, Bacterial Keratitis for the workup and treatment of an infected ulcer. If the ulcer is sterile, apply antibiotic ointment, cycloplegic drop, pressure patch, and reevaluate in 24 hours. Repeat procedure daily until healed. (Alternatively, antibiotic ointment q2h without patching may be used.) A tarsorrhaphy, bandage soft contact lens, conjunctival flap or amniotic membrane graft may be required.

Note: Patients with neurotrophic keratopathy and corneal exposure often do not respond to treatment unless a tarsorrhaphy is performed (eyelids partly sewn together). A temporary adhesive tape tarsorrhaphy (the lateral one third of the eyelid is taped closed) may be beneficial, pending more definitive treatment.

FOLLOW-UP

1. Mild to moderate epithelial staining: In 3 to 7 days.

2. Corneal epithelial defect: Every 1 to 2 days until improvement demonstrated, and then every 3 to 5 days until resolved.

3. Corneal ulcer: Daily until significant improvement is demonstrated. Hospitalization may be required for severe ulcers (see 4.11, Bacterial Keratitis).

4.7 THERMAL/ULTRAVIOLET KERATOPATHY

SYMPTOMS

Moderate to severe ocular pain, foreign body sensation, red eye, tearing, photophobia, blurred vision; often a history of welding or using a sunlamp without protective eyewear. The symptoms are typically worse 6 to 12 hours after the exposure, and are usually bilateral.

SIGNS

Critical. Confluent punctate epithelial defects in an interpalpebral distribution, seen with fluorescein staining.

Other. Conjunctival injection, mild to moderate eyelid edema, mild to no corneal edema, and relatively miotic pupils that react sluggishly.

DIFFERENTIAL DIAGNOSIS

- Toxic epithelial keratopathy from exposure to a chemical (e.g., solvents, alcohol) or drug (e.g., neomycin, gentamicin, antiviral agents).

- Exposure keratopathy (Poor eyelid closure. See 4.5, Exposure Keratopathy.).

- Nocturnal lagophthalmos (Eyelids remain partially open while asleep.).

- Floppy eyelid syndrome (Loose upper eyelids that evert easily during sleep. See 6.5, Floppy Eyelid Syndrome.).

WORKUP

1. History: Welding? Sunlamp use? Topical medications? Chemical exposure? Prior episodes?

2. Slit-lamp examination: Use fluorescein stain. Evert the eyelids to search for a foreign body.

3. If chemical exposure suspected, check pH of tear lake in lower conjunctival fornix. If not neutral (6.8 to 7.5), treat as chemical burn (see 3.1, Chemical Burn).

TREATMENT

1. Cycloplegic drop (e.g., cyclopentolate 1% to 2%, or scopolamine 0.25%).

2. Antibiotic ointment (e.g., erythromycin or bacitracin) three to four times per day.

3. Optional pressure patch for 24 hours on the more severely affected eye.

4. Oral analgesics (e.g., acetaminophen with or without codeine) as needed.

FOLLOW-UP

1. Reliable patients are asked to assess their own symptoms after 24 hours (if a patch was placed, it is removed at this time).

2. If much improved, the patient continues with topical antibiotics (e.g., erythromycin or bacitracin ointment q.i.d.).

3. If still significantly symptomatic, the patient should return for reevaluation. If significant punctate staining is still present, the patient is retreated with a cycloplegic, antibiotic, and possible pressure patch, as discussed previously.

4. Unreliable patients or those with an unclear etiology should be reexamined in 24 to 48 hours.

4.8 THYGESON SUPERFICIAL PUNCTATE KERATOPATHY

SYMPTOMS

Mild to moderate foreign body sensation, photophobia, tearing; no history of red eye. The disease is usually bilateral and has a chronic course with exacerbations and remissions.

SIGNS

Critical. Coarse punctate to stellate gray–white corneal epithelial opacities, often central and slightly elevated with minimal or no staining with fluorescein.

Other. No conjunctival injection, corneal edema, anterior chamber reaction, or eyelid abnormalities.

DIFFERENTIAL DIAGNOSIS

See 4.1, Superficial Punctate Keratitis.

TREATMENT

Mild

1. Artificial tears (e.g., Refresh Tears, Refresh Plus, GenTeal, or TheraTears) four to eight times per day.

---

2. Artificial tear ointment (e.g., Refresh PM) q.h.s.

Moderate-to-Severe

1. Mild topical steroid [e.g., fluorometholone 0.1%, q.i.d., or loteprednol 0.2% to 0.5% (e.g., Alrex or Lotemax), q.i.d.] for 1 to 4 weeks. Then taper very slowly. May need prolonged low-dose topical steroid therapy.

2. If no improvement with topical steroids, a therapeutic soft contact lens can be tried.

3. Cyclosporine 0.05% (e.g., Restasis q.d. to q.i.d.) may be an alternative treatment, especially in patients with side effects from steroids.

FOLLOW-UP

Every week during an exacerbation, then every 3 to 6 months. Patients receiving topical steroids require intraocular pressure (IOP) checks every 4 to 12 weeks.

4.9 PTERYGIUM/PINGUECULA

SYMPTOMS

Irritation, redness, decreased vision; may be asymptomatic.

SIGNS

Critical. One of the following, almost always located at the 3- or 9-o'clock position at the limbus.

• Pterygium: Wing-shaped fold of fibrovascular tissue arising from the interpalpebral conjunctiva and extending onto the cornea. Usually nasal in location.

• Pinguecula: Yellow–white, flat or slightly raised conjunctival lesion, usually in the interpalpebral fissure adjacent to the limbus, but not involving the cornea.

Other. Either lesion may be highly vascularized and injected or may be associated with superficial punctate keratitis or dellen (thinning of the cornea secondary to drying). An iron line (Stocker line) may be seen in the cornea just beyond the leading edge of a pterygium.

DIFFERENTIAL DIAGNOSIS

• Conjunctival intraepithelial neoplasia [Unilateral jelly-like, velvety, or leukoplakic (white) mass, often elevated, vascularized, not in a wing-shaped configuration, not in the typical 3- or 9-o'clock location of a pterygium or pinguecula. See 5.12, Conjunctival Tumors.].

• Limbal dermoid (Congenital rounded white lesion, usually at the inferotemporal limbus. May be a manifestation of Goldenhar syndrome if accompanied by preauricular skin tags or vertebral skeletal defects. See 5.12, Conjunctival Tumors.).

• Other conjunctival tumors (e.g., papilloma, nevus, melanoma; see 5.12, Conjunctival Tumors).

• Pannus (Blood vessels growing into the cornea, often secondary to contact lens wear, blepharitis, ocular rosacea, herpes keratitis, phlyctenular keratitis, atopic disease, trachoma, trauma, and others. Usually at the level of Bowman membrane with minimal to no elevation.).

ETIOLOGY

Elastotic degeneration of deep conjunctival layers, related to sunlight exposure and chronic irritation. More common in individuals from equatorial regions.

WORKUP

Slit-lamp examination to identify the lesion and evaluate the adjacent corneal integrity and thickness.

TREATMENT

1. Protect the eyes from sun, dust, and wind (e.g., sunglasses or goggles if appropriate).

2. Lubrication with artificial tears (e.g., Refresh Plus or TheraTears four to eight times per day) to reduce ocular irritation.

3. For an inflamed pinguecula:

   —Mild: Artificial tears q.i.d.

   —Moderate to severe: A mild topical steroid [e.g., fluorometholone 0.1% q.i.d., or loteprednol 0.2% to 0.5% (e.g., Alrex or Lotemax) q.i.d.]. A topical nonsteroidal anti-inflammatory medication [ketorolac (e.g., Acular) q.i.d.] can be added for a short time only.

3. If a delle is present, then apply artificial tear ointment (e.g., Refresh PM) q.h.s.

4. Surgical removal is indicated when:

   —The pterygium progresses toward the visual axis.

   —The patient is experiencing excessive irritation not relieved by the previously mentioned treatment.

   —The lesion is interfering with contact lens wear.

   *Note: Pterygia can recur after surgical excision. Bare sclera dissection with a conjunctival autograft reduces the recurrence rate.

FOLLOW-UP

1. Asymptomatic patients may be checked every 1 to 2 years.

2. Pterygia should be measured periodically (every 3 to 6 months, initially) to determine the rate at which they are growing toward the visual axis.

3. If treating with a topical steroid, check after a few weeks to monitor inflammation and IOP. Taper and discontinue the steroid drop over several weeks once the inflammation has abated. The nonsteroidal drop may be used periodically for short times for recurrent inflammation.

4.10 BAND KERATOPATHY

SYMPTOMS

Decreased vision, foreign body sensation, white spot on the cornea; may be asymptomatic.

SIGNS

Critical. Anterior corneal plaque of calcium at the level of Bowman membrane, within the interpalpebral fissure, and separated from the limbus by clear cornea. Holes are often present in the plaque, giving it a Swiss-cheese appearance. The plaque usually begins at the 3- and 9-o'clock positions, adjacent to the limbus, and can extend across the cornea.

Other. May have other signs of chronic eye disease.

ETIOLOGY

More common. Chronic uveitis (e.g., juvenile rheumatoid arthritis), interstitial keratitis (IK), corneal edema, phthisis bulbi, long-standing glaucoma, ocular surgery (especially retinal detachment repair with silicone oil).

Less common. Hypercalcemia (may result from hyperparathyroidism, sarcoidosis, Paget disease, vitamin D intoxication, and others), gout, corneal dystrophy, long-term exposure to irritants (e.g., mercury fumes), renal failure, and others.

WORKUP

1. History: Chronic eye disease? Previous ocular surgery? Chronic exposure to environmental irritants? Systemic disease?

2. Slit-lamp examination.

3. If no signs of chronic anterior segment disease or long-standing glaucoma are present and the band keratopathy cannot be accounted for, then consider the following workup:

—Serum calcium, albumin, magnesium, and phosphate levels, blood urea nitrogen, and creatinine.

—Uric acid level if gout is suspected.

TREATMENT

Mild (i.e., Foreign Body Sensation)

Artificial tears (e.g., Refresh Plus, TheraTears, GenTeal gel, or Celluvisc) four to six times per day and artificial tear ointment (e.g., Refresh PM) q.h.s. or q.i.d. as needed.

Severe (e.g., Obstruction of Vision, Irritation Not Relieved by Lubricants, Cosmetic Problem)

Removal of the calcium may be performed at the slit lamp or under the operating microscope by chelation using disodium ethylenediamine tetraacetic acid (EDTA):

1. Dilute a solution of 15% EDTA (e.g., Endrate) to create a 3% mixture by mixing in a 1.0-mL tuberculin syringe 0.2 mL of 15% EDTA with 0.8 mL of 0.9% normal saline.

2. Anesthetize the eye with a topical anesthetic (e.g., proparacaine) and place an eyelid speculum.

3. Debride the corneal epithelium with a sterile scalpel or a sterile cotton-tipped applicator dipped in topical anesthetic or EDTA solution.

4. Wipe a cellulose sponge or cotton swab saturated with the 3% disodium EDTA solution over the band keratopathy until the calcium clears (which may take 10 to 30 minutes).

5. Irrigate with normal saline, place an antibiotic ointment (e.g., erythromycin), a cycloplegic drop (e.g., cyclopentolate, 1% to 2%), and a pressure patch on the eye for 24 hours.

6. Consider giving the patient an analgesic (e.g., acetaminophen with codeine).

FOLLOW-UP

1. If surgical removal has been performed, the patient should be examined every 1 to 2 days with repatching (optional), frequent antibiotic ointment, and a cycloplegic until the epithelial defect heals.

2. Residual anterior stromal scarring may be amenable to excimer laser PTK.

3. The patient should be checked every 3 to 12 months, depending on the severity of symptoms. Surgical removal can be repeated if the band keratopathy recurs.

4.11 BACTERIAL KERATITIS

SYMPTOMS

Red eye, mild to severe ocular pain, photophobia, decreased vision, discharge, new contact lens intolerance.

SIGNS

Critical. Focal white opacity (infiltrate) in the corneal stroma. An ulcer exists if there is also stromal loss with an overlying epithelial defect that stains with fluorescein.

Note: An examiner using a slit beam cannot see through an infiltrate/ulcer to the iris, whereas stromal edema and inflammation are more transparent.

Other. Epithelial defect, mucopurulent discharge, stromal edema, anterior chamber reaction with or without hypopyon formation (which, in the absence of globe perforation, usually represents sterile inflammation), conjunctival injection, corneal thinning, folds in

Descemet membrane, upper eyelid edema. Posterior synechiae, hyphema, and glaucoma may occur in severe cases.

DIFFERENTIAL DIAGNOSIS

• Fungal [Must be considered after any traumatic corneal injury, particularly from vegetable matter (e.g., a tree branch), which may lead to filamentous fungal keratitis. Infiltrates commonly have feathery borders and may be surrounded by satellite lesions. *Candida* infections occur in eyes with preexisting ocular surface disease. See 4.12, Fungal Keratitis.].

• Acanthamoeba [This protozoan causes an extremely painful stromal infiltrate. It usually occurs in a soft contact lens wearer who practices poor lens hygiene or has a history of swimming while wearing contact lenses. In the late stages (3 to 8 weeks), the infiltrate becomes ring-shaped. See 4.13, *Acanthamoeba*.].

• HSV (May have eyelid vesicles or corneal epithelial dendrites. A history of recurrent eye disease or known ocular herpes is common. Bacterial superinfections may develop in patients with chronic herpes simplex keratitis. See 4.14, Herpes Simplex Virus.).

• Atypical mycobacteria [Usually follows ocular injuries or surgery, such as cataract extraction, corneal grafts, and refractive surgery (especially LASIK). Culture plates must be kept for 8 weeks.].

• Sterile corneal thinning and ulcers (Usually less painful, minimal or no discharge, iritis or corneal edema, and negative cultures. See 4.21, Peripheral Corneal Thinning/Ulceration.).

• Staphylococcal hypersensitivity (Peripheral corneal infiltrates, sometimes with an overlying epithelial defect, usually multiple, often bilateral, with a clear space between the infiltrate and the limbus. There is minimal to no anterior chamber reaction. Often with coexisting blepharitis. See 4.17, Staphylococcal Hypersensitivity.).

• Sterile corneal infiltrates (From an immune reaction to contact lenses, solutions, or hypoxia. Usually, multiple, small subepithelial infiltrates with an intact overlying epithelium and minimal or no anterior chamber reaction. Usually a diagnosis of exclusion after ruling out an infectious process. Similar lesions can occur after adenoviral conjunctivitis. See 5.1, Acute Conjunctivitis.).

• Residual corneal foreign body or rust ring (May be accompanied by corneal stromal inflammation, edema, and, sometimes, a sterile infiltrate. There may be a mild anterior chamber reaction. The infiltrate and inflammation usually clear after the foreign body and rust ring are removed.).

• Topical anesthetic abuse (Failure of the presenting condition to respond to appropriate therapy. In the late stages of anesthetic abuse, the corneal appearance may mimic an infectious process despite negative cultures. A large ring opacity, edema, and anterior chamber reaction are characteristic. Healing, with or without scarring, typically occurs when the exposure to anesthetic is stopped.).

ETIOLOGY

Bacterial organisms are the most common cause of infectious keratitis. In general, corneal infections are assumed to be bacterial until proven otherwise by laboratory studies or until a therapeutic trial is unsuccessful. At Wills Eye Hospital, the most common causes of bacterial keratitis are *Staphylococcus*, *Streptococcus*, *Pseudomonas*, and *Moraxella* species. Clinical findings vary widely depending on the severity of disease and, to a lesser extent, on the organism involved. The following clinical characteristics may be helpful in determining the etiology of a bacterial ulcer. However, clinical impression should never take the place of appropriate laboratory evaluation, as detailed later.

• Staphylococcal ulcers typically have a well defined, gray–white stromal infiltrate that may enlarge to form a dense stromal abscess.

• Streptococcal infiltrates may be either very purulent or crystalline. Severe anterior chamber reaction and hypopyon formation are common in the former.

• Pseudomonal keratitis typically presents as a rapidly progressive, suppurative, necrotic infiltrate associated with a hypopyon and mucopurulent discharge in the setting of contact lens use.

• *Moraxella* may cause infectious keratitis in patients with preexisting ocular surface disease and in patients who are immunocompromised. Infiltrates are typically indolent, located in the inferior portion of the cornea, and accompanied by a mild anterior uveitis.

WORKUP

1. History: Contact lens wear and lens care regimen? Overnight lens wear (overnight wear greatly increases the risk of bacterial keratitis and should be strongly discouraged). Swim with lenses? Trauma or corneal foreign body? Eye care before visit (e.g., antibiotics or topical steroids)? Previous corneal disease? Systemic illness?

2. Slit-lamp examination: Stain with fluorescein to determine if there is epithelial loss overlying the infiltrate; document the size, depth, and location of the corneal infiltrate; assess the anterior chamber reaction; and measure the IOP.

3. Corneal scrapings for smears and cultures are performed as described later.

4. In contact lens wearers suspected of having an infectious ulcer, the contact lenses and case are cultured if at all possible. Explain to the patient that the cultured contact lenses are to be discarded.

CULTURE PROCEDURE

Indications

Small, nonstaining infiltrates may be treated empirically with commercially available broad-spectrum antibiotics without prior scraping. We routinely culture infiltrates larger than 1 to 2 mm, in the visual axis, unresponsive to initial treatment, or if we suspect an unusual organism based on history or examination.

Equipment

Slit lamp; sterile Kimura spatula, knife blade, or moistened calcium alginate swab (i.e., with sterile saline, or thioglycolate or trypticase soy broth); culture media; microscopy slides; alcohol lamp.

Procedure

1. Anesthetize the cornea with topical drops (proparacaine is best because it appears to be less bactericidal than others).

2. At the slit lamp, scrape the ulcer base (unless significant corneal thinning has occurred) and the leading edge of the infiltrate firmly with the spatula, blade, or swab. Place the specimen on the slides first, then the culture media. Sterilize the spatula over the flame of the alcohol lamp between each separate culture or slide. Be certain that the spatula tip temperature has returned to normal before touching the cornea again.

Media

Routine:

1. Blood agar (most bacteria).

2. Sabouraud dextrose agar without cycloheximide; place at room temperature (fungi).

3. Thioglycolate broth (aerobic and anaerobic bacteria).

4. Chocolate agar; place into a CO_2 jar (*Haemophilus* species, *Neisseria gonorrhoeae*).

Optional:

1. Löwenstein–Jensen medium (mycobacteria, *Nocardia* species) should be included in patients with a history of LASIK.

2. Nonnutrient agar with *Escherichia coli* overlay (*Acanthamoeba*).

Slides

Routine:

1. Gram stain (bacteria, fungi).

2. Calcofluor white; a fluorescent microscope is needed (*Acanthamoeba*, fungi).

Optional:

1. Giemsa stain (bacteria, fungi, *Acanthamoeba*).

2. Acid-fast stain (mycobacteria, *Nocardia* species).

3. Gomori methenamine silver stain, periodic acid-Schiff (PAS) stain (*Acanthamoeba*, fungi).

Note: When a fungal infection is suspected, deep scrapings into the base of the ulcer are essential. Sometimes a corneal biopsy is necessary to obtain diagnostic information for fungal, atypical mycobacterial, and Acanthamoeba infections.

TREATMENT

Ulcers and infiltrates are usually treated as bacterial initially unless there is a high index of suspicion of another form of infection.

1. Cycloplegic drops for comfort and to prevent synechiae formation (e.g., scopolamine 0.25%, t.i.d.), or when a hypopyon is present (atropine 1%, t.i.d.).

2. Topical antibiotics according to the following algorithm:

Low risk of visual loss

Small, nonstaining peripheral infiltrate with at most minimal anterior chamber reaction and minimal discharge:

—Non–contact lens wearer: Broad-spectrum topical antibiotics [e.g., fluoroquinolone (moxifloxacin, gatifloxacin, ciprofloxacin) drops q2–4h].

—Contact lens wearer: Fluoroquinolone (ciprofloxacin, moxifloxacin, or gatifloxacin) drops q2–4h; can add tobramycin or ciprofloxacin ointment q.h.s.

Borderline risk

Medium size (1- to 1.5-mm diameter) peripheral infiltrate, or any smaller infiltrate with an associated epithelial defect, mild anterior chamber reaction, or moderate discharge:

Fluoroquinolone (e.g., ciprofloxacin, moxifloxacin, or gatifloxacin) q1h around the clock.

Vision threatening

Current practice at Wills is to start fortified antibiotics for most ulcers meeting the indications listed previously for diagnostic scrapings and cultures. (See Appendix 9 for directions on making fortified antibiotics.)

Fortified tobramycin or gentamicin (15 mg/mL) every 30 to 60 minutes, alternating with fortified cefazolin (50 mg/mL) or vancomycin (25 mg/mL) q1h. This means that the patient will be placing a drop in the eye every one-half hour around the clock. Vancomycin drops should be reserved for resistant organisms and for patients who are allergic to penicillin or cephalosporins.

An alternative choice for smaller (less than 1.5 mm), peripheral ulcers, or for when a formulating pharmacy is not available to compound fortified antibiotics, is intensive topical fluoroquinolone therapy (e.g., moxifloxacin, gatifloxacin, or ciprofloxacin drops).

Note: All patients with borderline risk of visual loss or severe vision-threatening ulcers are initially treated with loading doses of antibiotics using the following regimen: 1 drop every 5 minutes for five doses, then every 15 minutes for three doses, then every 30 to 60 minutes around the clock.

3. Topical corticosteroids are used in some cases only after the organism is identified, the infection is under control, and severe inflammation persists. Infectious keratitis may worsen significantly with topical corticosteroids, especially when caused by fungus or atypical mycobacteria.

4. Eyes with corneal thinning should be protected by a shield without a patch (a patch is *never* placed over an eye thought to have an infection).

5. No contact lens wear.

6. Oral pain medication as needed (e.g., acetaminophen with or without codeine).

7. Oral fluoroquinolones [e.g., ciprofloxacin 500 mg p.o., b.i.d.; moxifloxacin 400 mg p.o., q.d.; gatifloxacin 400 mg p.o., q.d.; or levo-

floxacin 500 mg p.o., q.d.] penetrate the cornea well. These may have added benefit for patients with scleral extension of infection or for those with frank or impending perforation. Systemic antibiotics are also necessary for *Neisseria* and *Haemophilus* infections [e.g., ceftriaxone 1 g, intravenously (i.v.) or intramuscularly (i.m.), q12–24h].

8. Admission to the hospital may be necessary if:

—There is a sight-threatening infection.

—The patient is unable to give himself or herself the antibiotics at the prescribed frequency without difficulty.

—There is a likelihood of noncompliance.

—The patient is unable or unwilling to return daily.

—Intravenous antibiotics are needed (e.g., corneal perforation, scleral extension of the infection, gonococcal conjunctivitis with corneal involvement).

—The patient is suspected of abusing topical anesthetic drops.

9. For atypical mycobacteria, consider prolonged treatment (q1h for 1 week, then gradually tapering) with one of the following topical agents: fluoroquinolones (e.g., moxifloxacin or gatifloxacin), amikacin (15 mg/mL), clarithromycin (1% to 4%), or tobramycin (15 mg/mL). Consider oral treatment with clarithromycin 500 mg b.i.d.

FOLLOW-UP

1. Daily evaluation at first, including repeated measurements of the size of the infiltrate and epithelial defect. The most important criteria in evaluating the response to treatment include the amount of pain, the size of the epithelial defect over the infiltrate, the size and depth of the infiltrate, and the anterior chamber reaction. Less pain, a smaller epithelial defect and infiltrate, and a less-inflamed eye are all favorable responses. The IOP must be checked and glaucoma treated, if present (see 9.4, Inflammatory Open-Angle Glaucoma).

2. If the ulcer is improving, the antibiotic regimen is gradually tapered. Otherwise, the antibiotic regimen is adjusted according to the culture and sensitivity results.

3. If the infiltrate or ulcer was not cultured originally and subsequently worsens, then cultures, stains, and treatment with fortified antibiotics are needed. Hospitalization is considered.

4. Reculture the ulcer (with the addition of optional media and stains) if it does not seem to be responding to the current antibiotic regimen and the original cultures are negative.

5. A corneal biopsy may be required if the condition is worsening and infection is still suspected despite negative cultures.

6. For an impending or a complete corneal perforation, a corneal transplant or patch graft is considered. Cyanoacrylate tissue glue may also work in a treated corneal ulcer that has perforated despite infection control. Glue should not be applied over an area of active infectious keratitis.

Note: Outpatients are told to return immediately if the pain increases or the vision decreases.

4.12 FUNGAL KERATITIS

Fungal keratitis may be seen after ocular trauma (typically filamentous fungi) or in eyes with preexisting chronic corneal surface disease (typically nonfilamentous fungi).

SYMPTOMS

Pain, photophobia, red eye, tearing, discharge, foreign body sensation; a history of trauma, particularly with vegetable matter (e.g., a tree branch), chronic eye disease, often a history of poor response to conventional antibacterial therapy. Fungal keratitis usually follows a more indolent course than bacterial keratitis.

SIGNS

Critical

• Filamentous fungi: Corneal stromal gray–white opacity (infiltrate) with a feathery border. The epithelium over the infiltrate may be elevated above the remainder of the corneal surface, or there may be an epithelial defect with stromal thinning (ulcer).

• Nonfilamentous fungi: A gray–white stromal infiltrate similar to a bacterial ulcer.

Other. Satellite lesions surrounding the primary infiltrate, conjunctival injection, mucopurulent discharge, anterior chamber reaction, hypopyon.

DIFFERENTIAL DIAGNOSIS

See 4.11, Bacterial Keratitis.

ETIOLOGY

• Filamentous fungi (e.g., *Fusarium* or *Aspergillus* species) (Usually from trauma with vegetable matter in previously healthy eyes.)

• Nonfilamentous fungi (e.g., *Candida* species) (Usually in previously diseased eyes, e.g., dry eyes, herpes keratitis, exposure keratopathy, chronic use of corticosteroid drops.)

WORKUP

See 4.11, Bacterial Keratitis for complete workup and culture procedure.

*Notes

1. *Be certain to obtain a Giemsa stain when a fungus is suspected (PAS, Gomori methenamine silver, and calcofluor white stains also can be used), and to scrape deep into the base of the ulcer for material.*

2. *If all cultures are negative, yet an infectious etiology is still suspected, consider a corneal biopsy to obtain further diagnostic information.*

TREATMENT

In general, corneal infiltrates and ulcers of unknown etiology are treated as bacterial until proven otherwise by laboratory studies (see 4.11, Bacterial Keratitis). If the stains or cultures indicate a fungal keratitis, institute the following measures:

1. Admission to the hospital may be necessary, unless the patient is very reliable. It may take weeks to achieve complete healing.

2. Natamycin 5% drops (especially for filamentous fungi) or amphotericin B 0.15% drops (especially for *Candida*), initially q1–2h around the clock, then taper over 4 to 6 weeks.

   Note: Natamycin is the only commercially available topical antifungal agent; all others must be made from i.v. solutions with proper approval and sterile techniques. Other medications such as fluconazole, ketoconazole, and itraconazole have been used systemically in fungal infections.

3. Cycloplegic (e.g., scopolamine 0.25%, t.i.d.).

4. No topical steroids. If the patient is currently taking steroids, they should be tapered rapidly.

5. Consider adding oral antifungal agents (e.g., itraconazole or fluconazole, 200 to 400 mg loading dose, then 100 to 200 mg p.o., q.d.).

6. Consider epithelial debridement to facilitate penetration of antifungal medications. (Topical antifungal medications do not penetrate into the cornea well, especially through an intact epithelium.)

7. Treat glaucoma if present (see 9.4, Inflammatory Open-Angle Glaucoma).

8. An eye shield, without a patch, may be advisable when the cornea is thinned.

FOLLOW-UP

As with all infectious corneal ulcers, patients must be reexamined daily. However, the clinical response to treatment of fungal keratitis is very different from that of bacterial keratitis. The initial response to treatment in fungal keratitis is slower than that in bacterial keratitis. Failure of the infection to worsen after initiation of treatment is often a favorable sign. Unlike for bacterial ulcers, epithelial healing in fungal keratitis is not always a sign of positive response to treatment. Fungal infections in deep corneal stroma are frequently recalcitrant to therapy. Fungal ulcers may require weeks to months of treatment, and corneal transplantation may be necessary for infection that progresses despite maximal medical therapy. A corneal transplant or patch graft may also be required in an impending or complete corneal perforation.

4.13 *ACANTHAMOEBA*

Corneal infection with *Acanthamoeba* should be considered in any patient with a history of soft contact lens wear; poor contact lens hygiene (e.g., using tap water to clean lenses, infrequent disinfection); or swimming, fishing, or hot-tub use while wearing contact lenses. Heat disinfection and hydrogen peroxide systems with at least 8 hours' contact time are effective in killing *Acanthamoeba* cysts and trophozoites, whereas thimerosal, sorbic acid, EDTA, and quaternary ammonium compounds are mostly ineffective against *Acanthamoeba*. The best approach to prevention is to use daily disposable (single-use) lenses.

SYMPTOMS

Severe ocular pain (often out of proportion to the early clinical findings), redness, and photophobia over a period of several weeks.

SIGNS

Critical

• Early: Less corneal and anterior segment inflammation than would be expected for the degree of pain the patient is experiencing, subepithelial infiltrates (sometimes along corneal nerves, producing a radial keratoneuritis), pseudodendrites on the epithelium.

• Late (3 to 8 weeks): A corneal stromal infiltrate in the shape of a ring.

Note: Cultures for bacteria are negative. The condition usually does not improve with antibiotic or antiviral medications and commonly follows a chronic, progressive, downhill course.

Other. Eyelid swelling, conjunctival injection (especially circumcorneal), cells and flare in the anterior chamber. Usually little discharge or corneal vascularization. Corneal ulceration may occur later in the course.

DIFFERENTIAL DIAGNOSIS

See 4.11, Bacterial Keratitis.

WORKUP

See 4.11, Bacterial Keratitis for a general workup. One or more of the following are obtained when *Acanthamoeba* is suspected:

1. Corneal scrapings for Giemsa, PAS, and Gram stains (Giemsa and PAS stains may show typical cysts).

2. Calcofluor white stain if available (requires a fluorescent microscope).

3. Culture on nonnutrient agar with *E. coli* overlay.

4. Consider a corneal biopsy if the stains and cultures are negative and the condition is not improving on the current regimen.

5. Consider cultures and smears of contact lens and case.

TREATMENT

One or more of the following are usually used in combination, sometimes in the hospital initially:

1. Polyhexamethyl biguanide 0.02% (PHMB, e.g., Baquacil) drops, q1h. The treatment of *Acanthamoeba* is more successful since the advent of PHMB. Chlorhexidine 0.02% can be used as an alternative to PHMB.

2. Propamidine isethionate 0.1% (e.g., Brolene) drops, every 30 minutes to 2 hours. Dibromopropamidine isethionate 0.15% (e.g., Brolene) ointment is also available.

3. Polymyxin B/neomycin/gramicidin (e.g., Neosporin) drops, every 30 minutes to 2 hours.

4. Itraconazole, 400 mg p.o. for one loading dose, then 100 to 200 mg p.o., q.d., or ketoconazole 200 mg p.o., q.d.

   Additional therapy includes clotrimazole 1% drops, miconazole 1% drops, or paromomycin drops, q2h. Low-dose corticosteroid drops may be helpful in reducing inflammation after the infection is controlled, but this is controversial.

All patients:

5. Discontinue contact lens wear.

6. Cycloplegic (e.g., atropine 1%, t.i.d.).

7. Oral nonsteroidal antiinflammatory agent (e.g., naproxen 250 to 500 mg p.o., b.i.d.) for pain and for scleritis, if present. Additional oral analgesics (e.g., acetaminophen with codeine) if needed.

Corneal transplantation may be indicated for medical failures, but this procedure can be complicated by recurrent infection.

FOLLOW-UP

Every 1 to 2 days until the condition is consistently improving. Medication may then be tapered judiciously. Treatment is usually continued for 3 months after resolution of inflammation, which may take up to 12 months in some cases.

Notes

1. *Brolene is available in the United Kingdom and may be obtained in the United States with U.S. Food and Drug Administration approval.*

2. *PHMB is available in the United Kingdom as Cosmocil; it can be prepared by a compounding pharmacy in the United States from Baquacil, a swimming pool disinfectant.*

4.14 HERPES SIMPLEX VIRUS

SYMPTOMS

Red eye, pain, photophobia, tearing, decreased vision, skin (e.g., eyelid) rash; history of previous episodes; usually unilateral.

SIGNS

Primary HSV infection is usually not apparent clinically. However, neonatal primary herpes infection is a rare, potentially devastating disease associated with localized skin, eye, or oral infection, and severe central nervous system and multiorgan system infection (see 8.9, Ophthalmia Neonatorum). In older children or adolescents, primary HSV infection may be suggested by a history of recent contact with HSV and by the presence of fever or flulike symptoms. Triggers for recurrent infections are commonly thought to include fever, stress, trauma, and ultraviolet light exposure [although this clinical suspicion was not confirmed by the Herpetic Eye Disease Study (HEDS)]. Infection may be characterized by any or all of the following:

Eyelid/Skin Involvement

Clear vesicles on an erythematous base that progress to crusting.

Conjunctivitis

Conjunctival injection with acute unilateral follicular conjunctivitis.

Corneal Epithelial Disease

May be seen as SPK, dendritic keratitis (a thin, linear, branching lesion with club-shaped terminal bulbs at the end of each branch), or a geographic ulcer (a large, amoeba-shaped corneal ulcer with a dendritic edge). The edges of herpetic lesions are heaped up with swollen epithelial cells that stain well with rose bengal or lissamine green; the central ulceration stains well with fluorescein. Corneal sensitivity may be decreased. Scars (ghost dendrites) may develop underneath the epithelial lesions.

Neurotrophic Ulcer

A sterile ulcer with smooth epithelial margins over an area of interpalpebral stromal disease that persists or worsens despite antiviral therapy. May be associated with stromal melting and perforation.

Corneal Stromal Disease

• Disciform keratitis (nonnecrotizing keratitis): Disc-shaped stromal edema with an intact epithelium. A mild iritis with localized granulomatous keratic precipitates is typical, and in-creased IOP may be present. No necrosis or corneal neovascularization is present.

• Necrotizing IK (uncommon): Appearance of multiple or diffuse, whitish corneal stromal infiltrates with or without an epithelial defect, often accompanied by stromal inflammation, thinning, and neovascularization. Concomitant iritis, hypopyon, or glaucoma may be present. Bacterial superinfection must be ruled out.

Uveitis

An anterior chamber reaction may develop as a result of severe corneal stromal involvement. Less commonly, anterior chamber reaction can develop without active corneal disease and may be associated with very high IOP.

Retinitis

Rare. In neonates, it is usually associated with a severe systemic HSV infection and is often bilateral.

DIFFERENTIAL DIAGNOSIS

(Conditions that produce dendritic-appearing corneal lesions)

• Herpes zoster virus (HZV): (Frequently painful skin vesicles are found along a dermatomal distribution of the face, not crossing the midline. Pain may be present before vesicles appear. The pseudodendrites in this condition are raised mucous plaques. They do not have true terminal bulbs and do not stain well with fluorescein. See 4.15, Herpes Zoster Virus.).

• Recurrent corneal erosion (A healing erosion often has a dendriform appearance. Patients often provide a history of a corneal abrasion in the involved eye or have underlying anterior basement membrane dystrophy. Pain frequently develops on awakening from sleep. See 4.2, Recurrent Corneal Erosion.).

• *Acanthamoeba* keratitis pseudodendrites (History of soft contact lens wear, pain out of proportion to inflammation, chronic course. See 4.13, *Acanthamoeba*.).

• Vaccinia keratitis (Recent history of smallpox vaccination or contact with recent vaccinee. May have skin vesicles, papillary conjunctivitis, epithelial or stromal keratitis. See 4.29, Ocular Vaccinia.).

WORKUP

1. History: Previous episodes? History of corneal abrasion; contact lens wear; or previous nasal, oral, or genital sores? Recent topical or systemic steroids? Immune deficiency state?

2. External examination: Note the distribution of skin vesicles if present. The lesions are more suggestive of HSV than HZV if concentrated around the eye without extension onto forehead and scalp.

3. Slit-lamp examination with IOP measurement.

4. Check corneal sensation (before instillation of topical anesthetic), which may be decreased in HSV and HZV.

5. Most cases of herpes simplex are diagnosed clinically and require no confirmatory laboratory tests. However, if the diagnosis is in doubt, any of the following tests may be supportive of the diagnosis:

—Scrapings of a corneal or skin lesion (scrape the edge of a corneal ulcer or the base of a skin lesion) for Giemsa stain, which shows multinucleated giant cells. Enzyme-linked immunosorbent assay testing also is available.

—Viral culture: A sterile, cotton-tipped applicator is used to swab the cornea, conjunctiva, or skin (after unroofing vesicles with a sterile needle) and is then placed into the viral transport medium.

Note: Smears and cultures for bacteria should be taken if a corneal ulceration suddenly worsens (see 4.11, Bacterial Keratitis).

TREATMENT

The treatment of HSV eye disease has been refined by the findings of the HEDS. Treatment modalities supported by evidence from HEDS are indicated by an asterisk (*).

Eyelid/Skin Involvement

1. Antibiotic ointment (e.g., erythromycin or bacitracin ophthalmic ointment) b.i.d. to the skin lesions. Topical acyclovir ointment, five times per day, is an option, although it has not been proven effective. (Topical acyclovir ointment is a skin preparation and should not be placed in the eye.)

2. Warm or cool soaks to skin lesions t.i.d.

3. If the eyelid margin is involved, add trifluridine 1% drops (e.g., Viroptic), five times per day, to the eye. [Vidarabine 3% ointment (e.g., Vira-A) five times per day is useful for small children but is currently available only in Canada and Europe.]

These medications are continued for 7 to 14 days until resolution of the symptoms.

Note: Oral acyclovir, 200 to 400 mg p.o., five times per day, for 7 to 14 days, is given by some physicians to adults suspected of having primary herpetic disease.

Conjunctivitis

Trifluridine 1% drops [e.g., Viroptic; or vidarabine 3% ointment (e.g., Vira-A) when available], five times per day. Discontinue the antiviral agent when the conjunctivitis has resolved after 7 to 14 days.

Corneal Epithelial Disease

1. Trifluridine 1% drops (e.g., Viroptic), nine times per day [or vidarabine 3% ointment (e.g., Vira-A), five times per day]. Oral antiviral agents (e.g., acyclovir 400 mg p.o., five times per day, for 7 to 10 days) may be used to avoid the toxicity of topical antiviral drops.

2. Cycloplegic agent (e.g., scopolamine 0.25%, t.i.d.) if an anterior chamber reaction is present.

3. Patients taking topical steroids should have them tapered rapidly.

4. Consider gentle debridement of the infected epithelium as an adjunct to the antiviral agents.

—Technique: After topical anesthesia, a sterile, moistened (with anesthetic drops or sterile saline), cotton-tipped applicator or semisharp instrument is used carefully to peel off the lesions at the slit lamp. After debridement, antiviral treatment should be instituted as described earlier.

5. For epithelial defects that do not resolve after 1 to 2 weeks, topical antiviral toxicity or a neurotrophic ulcer should be suspected. At that point, the topical antiviral agent should be discontinued, and a nonpreserved artificial tear ointment (e.g., Refresh PM) or an antibiotic ointment (e.g., erythromycin) should be used four to eight times per day for several days with careful follow-up.

Note: Oral acyclovir does not prevent stromal keratitis or uveitis in patients with HSV epithelial keratitis. However, a short course of systemic acyclovir may be used when frequent topical antivirals cannot be given.

Neurotrophic Ulcer

See 4.6, Neurotrophic Keratopathy.

Corneal Stromal Disease

1. Disciform keratitis

   Mild. Cycloplegic (e.g., scopolamine 0.25%, t.i.d.) alone.

   Severe or central (i.e., vision is reduced)

   —Cycloplegic as previously.

   —Topical steroid (e.g., prednisolone acetate 1%, q.i.d.).*

   —Antiviral drops for prophylaxis [e.g., trifluridine 1% (e.g., Viroptic), t.i.d. to q.i.d.).* Oral acyclovir alone is not effective treatment of stromal keratitis.* However, oral antivirals may be used instead of topical antivirals as prophylaxis when topical steroids are used for HSV keratouveitis (e.g., acyclovir 400 mg, b.i.d.).

   —Adjunctive medications sometimes required include antibiotic prophylaxis (e.g., erythromycin ointment q.h.s.) in the presence of epithelial defects, and aqueous suppressants for increased IOP.

2. Necrotizing IK: Treated as severe disciform keratitis. The first priority is to treat any associated overlying epithelial defect and bacterial superinfection with antibiotic drops or ointment (see 4.11, Bacterial Keratitis). Corneal transplantation may be required if the cornea perforates.

   Notes

   1. *Topical steroids are contraindicated in those with infectious epithelial disease.*

   2. *Rarely, a systemic steroid (e.g., prednisone, 40 to 60 mg p.o., q.d., tapered rapidly) is given to patients with severe stromal disease accompanied by an epithelial defect.*

   3. *Oral antivirals (e.g., acyclovir, famciclovir, and valacyclovir) have not been shown to be beneficial in the treatment of stromal disease but may be beneficial in the treatment of herpetic uveitis* (see 12.1, Anterior Uveitis).*

   4. *The persistence of an ulcer in the presence of stromal inflammation commonly is due to the underlying inflammation (requiring cautious steroid therapy); however, it may be due to antiviral toxicity or active HSV epithelial infection. When an ulcer deepens, a new infiltrate develops, or the anterior chamber reaction increases, smears and cultures should be taken for bacteria and fungi (see 4.11, Bacterial Keratitis).*

FOLLOW-UP

1. Patients are reexamined in 2 to 7 days to evaluate the response to treatment and then every 7 to 14 days, depending on the clinical findings. The following clinical parameters are evaluated: the size of the epithelial defect and ulcer, the corneal thickness and the depth to which the cornea is involved, the anterior chamber reaction, and the IOP (see 9.4, Inflammatory Open-Angle Glaucoma, for glaucoma management).

2. Antiviral medications for corneal dendrites and geographic ulcers should be continued five to eight times per day for 7 to 14 days and then tapered over 1 week.

3. Topical steroids used for corneal stromal disease are tapered slowly (often over months to years). The initial concentration of the steroid (e.g., prednisolone acetate 1%) is eventually reduced (e.g., prednisolone acetate 0.125%). Prophylactic topical (e.g., trifluridine 1%, t.i.d.) or systemic (e.g., acyclovir 400 mg, b.i.d.) antiviral agents are used. Antiviral coverage is probably not needed when the steroid is given once a day or less.

4. Corneal transplantation may eventually be necessary in stromal disease if inactive postherpetic scars significantly affect vision.

5. Consider long-term oral antiviral prophylaxis (e.g., acyclovir 400 mg, b.i.d.) if a patient has had multiple episodes of herpetic epithelial or stromal disease.*

*Note: Topical antivirals can cause a local toxic or allergic reaction (usually a papillary or follicular conjunctivitis) typically after at least 3 weeks of therapy. If such a reaction should occur, the antiviral agent should be replaced with an oral antiviral agent.

BIBLIOGRAPHY

Barron BA, Gee L, Hauck WW, et al. Herpetic Eye Disease Study. A controlled trial of oral acyclovir for herpes simplex stromal keratitis. *Ophthalomology* 1994;101:1871–1882.

Herpetic Eye Disease Study Group. A controlled trial of oral acyclovir for the prevention of stromal keratitis or iritis in patients with herpes simplex virus epithelial keratitis. The Epithelial Keratitis Trial. *Arch Ophthalmol* 1997;115:703–712.

Herpetic Eye Disease Study Group. Acyclovir for the prevention of recurrent herpes simplex virus eye disease. *N Engl J Med* 1998;339:300–306.

Herpetic Eye Disease Study Group. Oral acyclovir for herpes simplex virus eye disease: effect on prevention of epithelial keratitis and stromal keratitis. *Arch Ophthalmol* 2000;118:1030–1036.

Wilhelmus KR, Gee L, Hauck WW, et al. Herpetic Eye Disease Study. A controlled trial of topical corticosteroids for herpes simplex stromal keratitis. *Ophthalmology* 1994;101:1883–1895.

4.15 HERPES ZOSTER VIRUS

SYMPTOMS

Skin rash, skin discomfort, and paresthesias. May be preceded by headache, fever, malaise, blurred vision, eye pain, and red eye.

SIGNS

Critical. Acute vesicular skin rash that follows a dermatome of the fifth cranial nerve and can progress to scarring. Characteristically, the rash appears on one side of the forehead and scalp, does not cross the midline, and involves the upper eyelid only. Hutchinson sign (rash involving the tip of the nose in the distribution of nasociliary branch of ophthalmic division) may predict higher risk of ocular involvement.

Other. Less commonly, the rash involves the lower eyelid and cheek on one side, and, rarely, one side of the jaw. Conjunctivitis, corneal involvement [e.g., multiple small epithelial dendrites early, followed by larger pseudodendrites (raised mucous plaques), SPK, immune stromal keratitis, neurotrophic keratitis], uveitis, sectorial iris atrophy, scleritis, retinitis, choroiditis, optic neuritis, cranial nerve palsy, and elevated IOP can occur. Late postherpetic neuralgia also may occur.

Note: Corneal disease may follow the acute skin rash by many months to years. Occasionally, it can precede the skin rash.

DIFFERENTIAL DIAGNOSIS

HSV (The rash neither follows a dermatome nor obeys the midline. Patients are often young. Corneal dendrites of HSV have true terminal bulbs and stain well with fluorescein; pseudodendrites of HZV usually appear stuck on the epithelium, do not have true terminal bulbs, and stain poorly with fluorescein. See 4.14, Herpes Simplex Virus.).

WORKUP

1. History: Duration of rash and pain? Immunocompromised or risk factors for acquired immunodeficiency syndrome?

2. Complete ocular examination, including a slit-lamp evaluation with fluorescein staining, IOP check, and dilated optic nerve and retinal examination.

3. Systemic evaluation:

   —Patients younger than 40 years: Medical evaluation to determine whether the patient may be immunocompromised.

   —Patients aged 40 to 60 years: None (unless immunodeficiency is suspected from the history).

   —Patients older than 60 years: If systemic steroid therapy is to be instituted, obtain a steroid workup as required (see Drug Glossary for systemic steroid workup).

   Note: Immunocompromised patients should not receive systemic steroids.

TREATMENT

See 13.4, Acquired Immunodeficiency Syndrome for the treatment of HZV in immunocompromised patients.

Skin Involvement

1. Adults with an acute moderate to severe skin rash for less than 72 hours in which active skin lesions are present.

   —Oral antiviral agent[1] (e.g., acyclovir 800 mg p.o., five times per day; famciclovir 500 mg p.o., t.i.d.; or valacyclovir 1,000 mg p.o., t.i.d.) for 7 to 10 days; if the condition is severe or the patient is systemically ill, hospitalize and prescribe acyclovir 5 to 10 mg/kg i.v., q8h, for 5 to 10 days.

   —Bacitracin or erythromycin ointment to the skin lesions b.i.d.

   —Warm compresses to periocular skin t.i.d. (to keep it clean).

2. Adults with a skin rash of more than 3 days' duration or without active skin lesions.

   —Warm compresses to periocular skin t.i.d.

   —Bacitracin or erythromycin ointment to skin lesions b.i.d.

3. Children: Treat as in (2) unless there is evidence of systemic spread. For systemic spread, hospitalize and prescribe acyclovir 500 mg/m^2/day in three divided doses for 7 days. The hospital pharmacy should have a conversion chart for height, weight, and surface area in square meters. The patient is usually transferred to the pediatric service.

Ocular Involvement

1. Conjunctival involvement: Cool compresses and erythromycin ointment to the eye b.i.d.

2. Corneal pseudodendrites or SPK: Lubrication with preservative-free artificial tears (e.g., Refresh Plus or TheraTears) q1–2h and ointment (e.g., Refresh PM) q.h.s. Topical steroids (e.g., prednisolone acetate 1%, q.i.d.) are occasionally helpful.

[1]See Drug Glossary for systemic antiviral drug precautions.

3. Immune stromal keratitis: Topical steroid (e.g., prednisolone acetate 1%, q1–6h), tapering over months to years.

4. Uveitis (with or without immune stromal keratitis): Topical steroid (e.g., prednisolone acetate 1%) q1–6h, cycloplegic (e.g., cyclopentolate, 1% to 2%, t.i.d.), and erythromycin ointment q.h.s. (see 12.1, Anterior Uveitis).

5. Neurotrophic keratitis: Treat mild epithelial defects with erythromycin or preservative-free artificial tear ointment q.i.d. If corneal ulceration occurs, obtain appropriate smears and cultures to rule out infection (see 4.11, Bacterial Keratitis). If the ulcer is sterile, and there is no response to ointment and patching, consider a tarsorrhaphy or conjunctival flap (see 4.6, Neurotrophic Keratopathy).

6. Scleritis: Treat as any other scleritis (see 5.7, Scleritis).

7. Retinitis, choroiditis, optic neuritis, or cranial nerve palsy: Acyclovir, 5 to 10 mg/kg i.v., q8h for 1 week, and prednisone 60 mg p.o., for 3 days, then tapering over 1 week.[2] Consider neurologic consultation to rule out central nervous system involvement.

8. Increased IOP: May be caused by the uveitis or steroids. If uveitis is present, increase the frequency of the steroid administration for a few days. If IOP remains increased, substitute fluorometholone 0.1% (e.g., FML), rimexolone 1% (e.g., Vexol), or loteprednol 0.5% (e.g., Lotemax) drops for prednisolone acetate, and attempt to taper the dose. Topical aqueous suppressants (e.g., timolol 0.5%, b.i.d.; brimonidine 0.2%, t.i.d.; or dorzolamide 2%, t.i.d.) also help reduce IOP (see 9.4, Inflammatory Open-Angle Glaucoma and 9.5, Steroid-Response Glaucoma).

Note: Pain may be severe during the first 2 weeks, and analgesics (e.g., acetaminophen with or without codeine) may be required. An antidepressant (e.g., amitriptyline 25 mg p.o., t.i.d.) may be beneficial because depression frequently develops during the acute phase of HZV infection. Antidepressants also may help postherpetic neuralgia. Capsaicin 0.025% (e.g., Zostrix) or doxepin (e.g., Zonalon) ointment t.i.d. to q.i.d. may be applied to the skin (not around the eyes) for postherpetic neuralgia after the initial skin lesions heal. Management of postherpetic neuralgia should involve the patient's primary medical doctor.

FOLLOW-UP

If ocular involvement is present, examine the patient every 1 to 7 days, depending on the severity. Patients without ocular involvement can be followed every 1 to 4 weeks. After the acute episode resolves, check the patient every 3 to 6 months because relapses may occur months to years later, particularly as steroids are tapered. Systemic steroid administration requires collaboration with the patient's medical doctor.

Note: HZV is contagious for children and adults who have not had chickenpox or the chickenpox vaccine: It can be spread by inhalation. Pregnant women who have not had chickenpox must be especially careful to avoid contact with an HZV-infected patient.

[2]See Drug Glossary for systemic antiviral drug precautions.

4.16 INTERSTITIAL KERATITIS

Acute symptomatic IK most commonly occurs within the first or second decade of life. Signs of old IK often persist throughout life.

SYMPTOMS (ACUTE PHASE)

Pain, tearing, photophobia, red eye.

SIGNS

Acute Phase

Critical. Corneal stromal blood vessels and edema.

Other. Anterior chamber cells and flare, fine keratic precipitates on the corneal endothelium, conjunctival injection.

Nonacute Phase

Deep corneal haze or scarring, often corneal stromal blood vessels containing minimal or no blood (ghost vessels), corneal stromal thinning.

ETIOLOGY

• *More common.* Congenital syphilis (usually bilateral, often occurs in first or second decade of life, affects both eyes within one year of each other).

• *Less common.* Acquired syphilis (unilateral, often sectorial); tuberculosis (TB) (unilateral, often sectorial); Cogan syndrome [bilateral involvement, vertigo, tinnitus, hearing loss, negative syphilis serologies, often associated with systemic vasculitis (typically polyarteritis nodosa), can occur at any age]; leprosy; HSV; and Lyme disease.

WORKUP

For active IK and old, previously untreated IK:

1. History: Venereal disease in the mother during pregnancy or in the patient? Difficulty hearing or tinnitus?

2. External examination: Look for saddle-nose deformity, Hutchinson teeth, frontal bossing, or other signs of congenital syphilis. Look for hypopigmented or anesthetic skin lesions and thickened skin folds, loss of the temporal eyebrow, and loss of eyelashes, as in leprosy.

3. Slit-lamp examination: Note whether the corneal nerves are segmentally thickened, like beads on a string, and whether iris nodules are present (leprosy). Look for patchy hyperemia of the iris with fleshy, pink nodules (syphilis). Check IOP.

4. Dilated fundus examination: Look for the classic salt-and-pepper chorioretinitis or optic atrophy of syphilis.

5. Venereal Disease Research Laboratory test (VDRL) or rapid plasma reagin (RPR); fluorescent treponemal antibody absorption (FTA-ABS) or microhemagglutination–*Treponema pallidum* (MHA-TP).

6. Purified protein derivative (PPD) with anergy panel.

7. Chest radiograph if negative FTA-ABS (or MHA-TP) or positive PPD.

8. Consider erythrocyte sedimentation rate, antinuclear antibody, rheumatoid factor, Lyme titer.

TREATMENT

1. Acute disease

—Topical cycloplegic.

—Topical steroid (e.g., prednisolone acetate 1%, q1–6h, depending on the degree of inflammation).

—Treat any underlying disease.

2. Old inactive disease: Corneal transplantation surgery may improve vision when it has been impaired by central corneal scarring and minimal amblyopia is present.

3. Acute, or old inactive disease

—If FTA-ABS is positive and the patient has not been treated for syphilis in the past (or is unsure about treatment), there are signs of active syphilitic disease (e.g., active chorioretinitis or papillitis), or the VDRL or RPR titer is positive and has not declined the expected amount after treatment, then treatment for syphilis is indicated (see 8.8, Congenital Syphilis, or 13.5, Acquired Syphilis).

—If PPD is positive and the patient is younger than 35 years and has not been treated for TB in the past, or there is evidence of active systemic TB (e.g., positive finding on chest radiograph), then refer the patient to a medical internist for treatment of TB.

—If Cogan syndrome is present, then refer the patient to an ear, nose, and throat specialist and consider rheumatologic follow-up.

FOLLOW-UP

1. Acute disease: Every 3 to 7 days initially, and then every 2 to 4 weeks. The frequency of steroid administration is slowly reduced as the inflammation subsides over the course of months (may take up to 2 years). IOP is monitored closely and reduced with medication when it is thought to be high enough to cause optic nerve damage (e.g., more than 30 mm Hg in a patient with a healthy optic nerve; see 9.4, Inflammatory Open-Angle Glaucoma).

2. Old inactive disease: Routine follow-up every year unless treatment is required for underlying etiology.

4.17 STAPHYLOCOCCAL HYPERSENSITIVITY

SYMPTOMS

Acute photophobia, mild pain, red eye, chronic eyelid crusting and itching; history of recurrent acute episodes.

SIGNS

Critical. Usually multiple, often bilateral, peripheral corneal stromal infiltrates with a clear space between the infiltrates and the limbus, and minimal to no staining with fluorescein. The anterior chamber is usually quiet, and only a sector of the conjunctiva is typically injected.

Other. Blepharitis, inferior SPK, phlyctenule (a wedge-shaped, raised, sterile infiltrate near the limbus), peripheral scarring and corneal neovascularization in the contralateral eye.

DIFFERENTIAL DIAGNOSIS

• Infectious corneal infiltrates (A dense, white–gray stromal infiltrate, often central, painful, and associated with a marked anterior chamber reaction. Not usually multiple and recurrent. See 4.11, Bacterial Keratitis.).

• Other causes of marginal thinning/infiltrates (See 4.21, Peripheral Corneal Thinning/Ulceration.).

ETIOLOGY

Likely related to staphylococcal blepharitis. (Infiltrates are believed to be a noninfectious reaction of the host's antibodies to the staphylococcal antigens.)

Note: Patients with ocular rosacea (e.g., telangiectases of the eyelids, nose, cheeks, and forehead that may progress to rhinophyma) are especially susceptible to this condition.

WORKUP

1. History: Recurrent episodes? Contact lens wearer (a risk of infection)?

2. Slit-lamp examination with fluorescein staining and IOP check.

3. If an infectious infiltrate is suspected, then corneal scrapings for cultures and smears should be obtained. See 4.11, Bacterial Keratitis.

TREATMENT

Mild

Warm compresses, eyelid hygiene, and erythromycin or bacitracin ointment q.h.s. (see 5.8, Blepharitis/Meibomianitis).

Moderate to Severe

Treat as described earlier, but add a topical steroid (e.g., prednisolone acetate 0.125%, or loteprednol 0.2% to 0.5%, q.i.d.) or a combination antibiotic/steroid (e.g., dexamethasone/tobramycin, q.i.d.). Maintain until the symptoms improve, and then slowly taper. If recurrent episodes are not prevented by eyelid hygiene, consider systemic tetracycline (250 mg p.o., q.i.d., for 2 weeks, then b.i.d. for 1 month, and then q.d.) or doxycycline (100 mg p.o., b.i.d., for 2 weeks, and then q.d. for 1 month, and then 50 to 100 mg q.d., titrated as necessary) until the ocular disease is controlled for several months. These medications have an antiinflammatory effect on the sebaceous glands in addition to their antimicrobial action. Low-dose antibiotics may have to be maintained indefinitely.

Note: Tetracycline and doxycycline are contraindicated in children younger than 8 years, pregnant women, and breast-feeding mothers. Erythromycin in the same dose as tetracycline can be substituted, but may not be as effective.

FOLLOW-UP

In 2 to 7 days, depending on the clinical picture. IOP is monitored while patients are taking topical steroids.

4.18 PHLYCTENULOSIS

SYMPTOMS

Tearing, irritation, pain, mild to severe photophobia; history of similar episodes. Corneal phlyctenules cause more severe symptoms than conjunctival phlyctenules.

SIGNS

Critical

• Conjunctival phlyctenule: A small, white nodule on the bulbar conjunctiva in the center of a hyperemic area. Often occurs at the limbus.

• Corneal phlyctenule: A small, white nodule, initially at the limbus, with dilated conjunctival blood vessels bordering it. The phlyctenule may be associated with epithelial ulceration and may migrate toward the center of the cornea, producing wedge-shaped corneal neovascularization and scarring behind the leading edge of the lesion. Can be bilateral.

Other. Conjunctival injection, blepharitis, corneal scarring.

DIFFERENTIAL DIAGNOSIS

• Inflamed pinguecula (Located in the palpebral fissure. Connective tissue is often seen to extend from the lesion to the limbus. Usually bilateral. See 4.9, Pterygium/Pinguecula.).

• Infectious corneal ulcer [Corneal phlyctenules that migrate from the limbus toward the center of the cornea may produce a sterile ulcer surrounded by a white infiltrate. When an infectious ulcer is suspected (e.g., increased pain, anterior chamber reaction), appropriate antibiotic treatment and diagnostic smears and cultures are necessary. See 4.11, Bacterial Keratitis.].

- Ocular rosacea (Corneal neovascularization with thinning and subepithelial infiltration may develop in an eye with rosacea. Telangiectases, erythema, or pustules are found on the cheeks, nose, forehead, and eyelid margins. See 5.9, Ocular Rosacea.).

- Herpes simplex keratitis (May produce corneal neovascularization associated with a stromal infiltrate. A history of recurrent herpes is often elicited. Usually unilateral. See 4.14, Herpes Simplex Virus.).

ETIOLOGY

Delayed hypersensitivity reaction usually as a result of one of the following:

- *Staphylococcus* (Often related to blepharitis. See 4.17, Staphylococcal Hypersensitivity.).

- Tuberculosis.

- Rarely, another infectious agent (e.g., coccidioidomycosis, candidiasis, lymphogranuloma venereum).

WORKUP

1. History: TB or recent infection?

2. Slit-lamp examination: Inspect the eyelid margin for signs of blepharitis and rosacea.

3. PPD (tuberculin skin test) in patients without blepharitis who have not had a positive PPD in the past.

4. Chest radiograph if the PPD is positive or TB is suspected.

TREATMENT

Indicated for symptomatic patients.

1. Topical steroid [e.g., loteprednol 0.5% (e.g., Lotemax) or prednisolone acetate 1%, four times per day, depending on severity of symptoms].

2. Topical antibiotic in presence of corneal ulcer (see 4.11, Bacterial Keratitis).

3. Eyelid hygiene b.i.d. to t.i.d. for blepharitis (see 5.8, Blepharitis/Meibomianitis).

4. Artificial tears (e.g., Refresh Plus or TheraTears) four to six times per day.

5. Antibiotic ointment q.h.s. (e.g., bacitracin or erythromycin ointment).

6. In severe cases of blepharitis, use doxycycline 100 mg p.o., b.i.d., or erythromycin 250 mg p.o., b.i.d. (see 5.8, Blepharitis/Meibomianitis).

7. If the PPD or chest radiograph is positive for TB, refer the patient to a medical internist or infectious disease specialist for appropriate treatment.

FOLLOW-UP

Recheck in several days. Healing occurs usually over a 10- to 14-day period, with residual stromal scar. When the symptoms have significantly improved, start tapering the steroid. Maintain the antibiotic ointment q.h.s., continue eyelid hygiene indefinitely, and continue oral antibiotics for 6 months.

4.19 CONTACT LENS–RELATED PROBLEMS

SYMPTOMS

Pain, photophobia, foreign body sensation, decreased vision, red eye, itching, discharge, burning.

Note: Any contact lens wearer with pain or redness should remove the lens immediately and have a thorough ophthalmic examination as soon as possible, if symptoms persist or worsen.

SIGNS

See the distinguishing characteristics of each etiology.

ETIOLOGY

- Infectious corneal infiltrate/ulcer (bacterial, fungal, *Acanthamoeba*). (White corneal lesion that may stain with fluorescein. Must always be ruled out in contact lens patients with eye pain. See 4.11, Bacterial Keratitis, 4.13, *Acanthamoeba*, and 4.12, Fungal Keratitis.).

- Giant papillary conjunctivitis (Itching, mucus discharge, and lens intolerance in a patient with large superior tarsal conjunctival papillae. See 4.20, Contact Lens–Induced Giant Papillary Conjunctivitis.).

- Hypersensitivity/toxicity reactions to preservatives in solutions [Conjunctival injection and ocular irritation typically develop shortly after lens cleaning and insertion, but can be present chronically. A recent change from one type or brand of solution to another often is elicited in the history. Commonly occurs in patients using older preserved solutions (e.g., thimerosal or chlorhexidine as a component), also occasionally with newer "all-purpose" solutions. May be due to inadequate rinsing of lenses after enzyme use. Signs include SPK, conjunctival injection, bulbar conjunctival follicles, subepithelial or stromal corneal infiltrates, epithelial irregularity, and superficial scarring.].

- Contact lens deposits (Multiple small deposits on the contact lens, leading to corneal and conjunctival irritation. The contact lens is often old and may not have been cleaned or enzyme-treated properly in the past.).

- Tight lens syndrome [Symptoms may be severe and often develop within 1 or 2 days of being fit with the responsible contact lens (usually a soft lens), especially if patient sleeps overnight with daily wear lenses. The lens does not move with blinking and appears "sucked-on" to the cornea (this can occur after rewearing a soft lens that has dried out and then been rehydrated). An imprint in the conjunctiva is often observed after the lens is removed. Corneal edema (usually anterior "brawny" edema), SPK, anterior chamber reaction, and sometimes a sterile hypopyon may develop.].

- Corneal warpage (Seen predominantly in long-term polymethylmethacrylate hard contact lens wearers. Initially, the vision becomes blurred with glasses but remains good with contact lenses. Gradually, blurred vision and sometimes discomfort develop with contact lenses. There may or may not be SPK. Keratometry reveals distorted mires and computed corneal topography may show irregular astigmatism that resolves after lens discontinuation.).

- Corneal neovascularization [Patients are often asymptomatic until the visual axis is involved. Superficial corneal neovascularization for 1 to 2 mm is common and usually not concerning in aphakic contact lens wearers (with the exception of corneal transplant recipients, who are at a greater risk for graft rejection). With any sign of chronic hypoxia, the goal is to increase oxygen permeability, increase movement, and discontinue extended wear lens.].

- Inadequate/incomplete blinking (Can lead to chronic inflammation and staining at the 3- and 9-o'clock positions.).

- Contact lens keratopathy (pseudo-superior limbic keratoconjunctivitis). [Hyperemia and fluorescein staining of the superior bulbar conjunctiva, particularly at the limbus. SPK, subepithelial infiltrates, haze, and irregularity may be found on the superior cornea. This may represent a hypersensitivity or toxicity reaction to a solution or contact lens–related product (classically thimerosal, but newer preservatives as well). Unlike superior limbic keratoconjunctivitis unassociated with contact lenses, there are no corneal filaments, papillary reaction, or association with thyroid disease.].

- Displaced contact lens (Most commonly the lens has actually fallen out of the eye and been lost, but if still present in the eye is usually found in the superior fornix. May require double-eversion of the upper eyelid to remove. Fluorescein will stain a soft lens to aid in finding it.)

- Others [Contact lens inside out, corneal abrasion (see 3.2, Corneal Abrasion), poor lens fit, damaged contact lens, change in refractive error.].

WORKUP

1. History: What is the main complaint [severe pain (scale 1 to 10), mild discomfort, itching]? What kind of contact lens does the patient wear (soft, hard, gas-permeable, daily-wear, extended-wear, or frequent replacement/disposable)? How old are the lenses? For how many continuous hours/days/weeks are the lenses worn? Does the patient sleep in lenses? How are the lenses cleaned and disinfected? Are enzyme tablets used? Are the products preservative free? Any recent changes in contact lens habits or solutions? When is the pain in relation to wearing time? Is the pain relieved by removal of the lens?

2. In noninfectious conditions, while the contact lens is still in the eye, evaluate its fit and examine its surface for deposits and defects at the slit lamp.

3. Remove lens and examine the eye with fluorescein. Evert the upper eyelids of both eyes and inspect the superior tarsal conjunctiva for papillae.

4. Smears and cultures are taken when an infectious corneal ulcer is suspected with infiltrate greater than 1 mm or when an unusual organism is suspected (i.e., *Acanthamoeba*). (See 4.11, Bacterial Keratitis, 4.13, *Acanthamoeba*, and 4.12, Fungal Keratitis.)

5. The contact lenses and lens case are cultured occasionally, when an infectious corneal process is suspected.

TREATMENT

When the diagnosis of infection is suspected:

1. Discontinue contact lens wear (if patient has not already done so).

2. Antibiotic treatment regimen varies with diagnosis as follows:

   —Possible corneal ulcer (corneal infiltrate, epithelial defect, anterior chamber reaction, pain):

   a. Obtain appropriate smears and cultures.

   b. Start intensive topical antibiotics, either fortified or a fluoroquinolone (given every 30 minutes initially), and a cycloplegic (see 4.11, Bacterial Keratitis).

   —Small subepithelial infiltrates, corneal abrasion, or diffuse SPK.

   a. Topical antibiotic (e.g., a fluoroquinolone) drops six to eight times per day and a cycloplegic.

   b. Can also add tobramycin or ciprofloxacin ointment q.h.s. Beware of toxicity with long-term use (especially tobramycin).

3. Never pressure patch a contact lens wearer: Doing so risks rapid development of *Pseudomonas* infection.

When a specific contact lens problem is suspected, it may be treated as follows:

1. Giant papillary conjunctivitis (see 4.20, Contact Lens–Induced Giant Papillary Conjunctivitis).

2. Hypersensitivity/toxicity reaction

   —Discontinue contact lens wear.

   —Preservative-free artificial tears (e.g., Refresh Plus or TheraTears drops four to six times per day).

   —On resolution of the condition, the patient may return to new contact lenses. Preferably, the patient is switched to daily disposable contact lenses. If the patient wishes to stay with frequent-replacement or conventional lenses, preservative-free solutions or hydrogen peroxide–based systems are recommended, and appropriate lens hygiene is reviewed.[3]

[3]The following regimen for contact lens care is one we recommend.
1. Daily cleaning and disinfection with removal of lenses while sleeping for all lens types, including those approved for "extended wear."
2. Daily cleaning regimen:
   —Preservative-free daily cleaner (e.g., MiraFlow).
   —Preservative-free saline (e.g., Unisol).
   —Disinfectant—preferably hydrogen peroxide type.
3. Weekly treatment with enzyme tablets (not necessary in disposable lenses replaced every 2 weeks or less).

3. Contact lens deposits

—Discontinue contact lens wear.

—Replace with a new contact lens once the symptoms resolve. Consider changing the brand of contact lens, or change to daily disposable or frequent replacement lens.

—Teach proper contact lens care, stressing weekly enzyme treatments for lenses replaced less frequently than every 2 weeks.

4. Tight lens syndrome

—Discontinue contact lens wear.

—Consider a topical cycloplegic (e.g., scopolamine 0.25%, t.i.d., or atropine 1%, t.i.d.) in the presence of an anterior chamber reaction.

—Patients should be refit with a flatter and more oxygen-permeable contact lens after the symptoms and signs resolve. Extended-wear contact lenses should be discontinued.

—If a soft lens has dried out, discard and refit.

Note: Patients do not need to be cultured for hypopyon when tight lens syndrome is highly suspected (i.e., if surface intact, with edema but no infiltrate).

5. Corneal warpage

—Discontinue contact lens wear. It is explained to patients that vision may be poor for the following 2 to 4 weeks, and that they may require a change in spectacle prescription.

—A gas-permeable hard contact lens should be refit when the refraction and keratometric readings have returned to normal (obtain the original keratometric readings and old spectacle prescription).

6. Corneal neovascularization

—Discontinue contact lens wear.

—Consider a topical steroid (e.g., prednisolone acetate 1%, q.i.d. or loteprednol 0.5%, q.i.d.) for extensive deep neovascularization (rarely necessary).

—Refit carefully with a highly oxygen-transmissible daily-wear contact lens that moves adequately over the cornea.

7. Corneal epithelial changes

—Discontinue contact lens wear.

—Use preservative-free artificial tears.

—Consider a new contact lens when the epithelial changes resolve, which may take weeks or months.

—Consider daily disposable lenses or preservative-free solutions.

8. Inadequate/incomplete blinking: Frequently apply preservative-free artificial tears (e.g., Refresh Plus or TheraTears). Consider punctal plugs if the patient has dry eyes (based on Schirmer testing).

9. Pseudo-superior limbic keratoconjunctivitis: Treated as described for hypersensitivity/toxicity reactions. When a large subepithelial opacity extends toward the visual axis, topical steroids may be added cautiously (e.g., loteprednol 0.5%, q6h), but they are often ineffective.

10. Displaced lens: Inspect lens carefully for damage. If undamaged, clean and disinfect lens, then recheck fit when symptoms have resolved. If damaged, discard and refit.

FOLLOW-UP

1. When a corneal infection cannot be ruled out, patients are reevaluated the following day. Treatment is maintained until the condition clears.

2. In noninfectious conditions, patients are reevaluated in 1 to 4 weeks, depending on the clinical situation. Contact lens wear is resumed when the condition resolves. Patients using topical steroids should be followed up more closely and their IOP monitored.

4.20 CONTACT LENS–INDUCED GIANT PAPILLARY CONJUNCTIVITIS

SYMPTOMS

Itching, mucus discharge, decreased lens-wearing time, increased lens awareness, excessive lens movement.

SIGNS

Critical. Giant papillae on the superior tarsal conjunctiva.

*Note: The upper eyelid must be everted to make the diagnosis. Upper eyelid eversion should be part of the routine eye examination in any patient who wears contact lenses.

Other. Contact lens coatings, high-riding lens, mild conjunctival injection, ptosis (usually a late sign).

WORKUP

1. History: Details of contact lens use, including age of lenses and cleaning and enzyme treatment regimen.
2. Slit-lamp examination: Evert the upper eyelids and examine for large papillae.

TREATMENT

1. Start a topical mast cell stabilizer, either lodoxamide (e.g., Alomide) q.i.d., olopatadine (e.g., Patanol) b.i.d., ketotifen fumarate (e.g., Zaditor) b.i.d., cromolyn sodium (e.g., Crolom or Opticrom) q.i.d., nedocromil 2% (e.g., Alocril) b.i.d., azelastine 0.05% (e.g., Optivar) b.i.d., or pemirolast 0.1% (e.g., Alamast) q.i.d.
2. Modify contact lens regimen as follows:

   a. Mild to moderate giant papillary conjunctivitis

   —Replace the contact lens. Refit with a new brand of soft contact lens (consider planned-replacement or daily disposable lenses).

   —Reduce contact lens wearing time (switch from extended-wear contact lens to daily wear).

   —Have the patient clean the lenses more thoroughly, preferably by using preservative-free solutions (e.g., MiraFlow daily cleaner), preservative-free saline (e.g., Unisol), or hydrogen peroxide–based disinfection systems.

   —Increase enzyme use (use at least every week).

   b. Severe giant papillary conjunctivitis

   —Suspend contact lens wear.

   —Restart with a new contact lens when the symptoms clear (usually 1 to 4 months), preferably with daily disposable soft or rigid gas-permeable lenses.

   —Careful lens hygiene as described earlier.

FOLLOW-UP

In 2 to 4 weeks. Mast cell stabilizers are continued until signs are resolved, then used as needed.

*Note: Giant papillary conjunctivitis also can result from an exposed suture or ocular prosthesis. Exposed sutures are removed. Prostheses should be cleaned and polished. A coating (e.g., Biocoat) can be placed on the prosthesis to reduce giant papillary conjunctivitis. Otherwise, these entities are treated as described earlier.

4.21 PERIPHERAL CORNEAL THINNING/ULCERATION

SYMPTOMS

Pain, photophobia, red eye; may be asymptomatic.

SIGNS

Corneal thinning (best seen with a narrow beam from the slit lamp), may have a sterile infiltrate or ulcer.

DIFFERENTIAL DIAGNOSIS

Infectious infiltrate or ulcer. (A dense, gray–white stromal infiltrate or ulcer that stains with fluorescein. The conjunctiva is injected and an anterior chamber reaction is usually present. Often lesions are treated as infectious until cultures are noted to be negative. See 4.11, Bacterial Keratitis.).

ETIOLOGY

• Connective tissue disease (e.g., rheumatoid arthritis, Wegener granulomatosis, relapsing polychondritis, polyarteritis nodosa, systemic lupus erythematosus, others). (Peripheral, unilateral or bilateral, corneal thinning/ulcers, possibly with inflammatory infiltrates. May progress circumferentially to involve the entire peripheral cornea. Perforation may occur. This may be the first manifestation of systemic disease.).

• Terrien marginal degeneration [Often asymptomatic, usually bilateral, slowly progressive thinning of the peripheral cornea, sparing the limbus, typically superiorly, more often in men. The anterior chamber is quiet, and the eye is typically not injected. A yellow line (lipid) may appear, with a fine pannus over the thinned areas of involvement. The ulceration may slowly spread circumferentially. Irregular and against-the-rule astigmatism is often present. The epithelium usually remains intact, but perforation may occur with minor trauma.].

• Mooren ulcer (Unilateral or bilateral, idiopathic, painful corneal thinning and ulceration with inflammation, initially involving a focal area of peripheral cornea nasally or temporally without an adjacent perilimbal lucid zone, but later extending circumferentially or centrally. An epithelial defect, stromal thinning, and a leading undermined edge are present. Limbal blood vessels may grow into the ulcer, and perforation can occur. This diagnosis can be made only after other etiologies are ruled out. Mooren-like ulcer has been associated with systemic hepatitis C virus infection.).

• Pellucid marginal degeneration [Painless, bilateral corneal thinning of the inferior peripheral cornea (usually from the 4- to 8-o'clock portions). There is no anterior chamber reaction, conjunctival injection, lipid deposition, or vascularization. The epithelium is intact. Corneal protrusion may be seen above the area of thinning. The thinning may slowly progress.].

• Furrow degeneration (Painless corneal thinning just peripheral to an arcus senilis, typically in the elderly. There is neither vascular infiltration nor ocular inflammation, and perforation is rare. Usually nonprogressive and does not require treatment.).

• Dellen (Painless oval corneal thinning resulting from corneal drying and stromal dehydration adjacent to an abnormal conjunctival or corneal elevation. The epithelium is usually intact. See 4.22, Dellen.).

• Staphylococcal hypersensitivity/marginal keratitis (Mildly painful, peripheral, white corneal infiltrate separated from the limbus by a zone of clear cornea. Often multiple, bilateral infiltrates that may stain with fluorescein, may be mildly thinned, and are typically associated with blepharitis. See 4.17, Staphylococcal Hypersensitivity.).

• Dry-eye syndrome (Peripheral corneal ulcers may result from severe cases of dry eye. Patients may demonstrate a poor tear lake, decreased tear breakup time, SPK inferiorly or centrally, and corneal filaments. May be associated with a connective tissue disease. See 4.3, Dry-Eye Syndrome.).

• Exposure/neurotrophic keratopathy (Typically, a sterile oval ulcer develops inferiorly on the cornea without signs of significant inflammation. An eyelid abnormality, a fifth or seventh cranial nerve defect, or proptosis is common. The ulcer may become superinfected. See 4.5, Exposure Keratopathy and 4.6, Neurotrophic Keratopathy.).

• Sclerokeratitis (Corneal ulceration is associated with severe ocular pain radiating to the temple or jaw because of accompanying scleritis. The sclera develops a blue hue, scleral vessels are engorged, and scleral edema with or without nodules is present. An underlying connective tissue disease, especially Wegener granulomatosis, must be ruled out. See 5.7, Scleritis.).

• Vernal keratoconjunctivitis (Superior, shallow, shield-shaped, sterile corneal ulcer, accompanied by giant papillae on the superior tarsal conjunctiva or limbal papillae. The conjunctivitis is usually bilateral, often occurs in children, and recurs during the summer months, but it can occur anytime in warm climates. See 5.1, Acute Conjunctivitis.).

• Ocular rosacea (Typically affects the inferior cornea in middle-aged patients. Erythema and telangiectases of the eyelid margins, nose, forehead, and cheeks are characteristic, and can progress to rhinophyma. See 5.9, Ocular Rosacea.).

• Others (Cataract surgery, inflammatory bowel disease, and leukemia can rarely cause peripheral corneal thinning/ulceration.).

WORKUP

1. History: Contact lens wearer or previous HSV or HSZ keratitis (infectious)? Known connective tissue disease or inflammatory bowel disease? Other systemic symptoms? Seasonal conjunctivitis with itching (vernal)?

2. External examination: Old facial scars of HSZ? Eyelid-closure problem causing exposure? Blue tinge to the sclera? Rosacea facies?

3. Slit-lamp examination: Look for infiltrate, corneal ulcer, hypopyon, uveitis, scleritis, old herpetic scarring, poor tear lake, SPK, blepharitis. Look for giant papillae on the superior tarsal conjunctiva or limbal papillae. Measure IOP.

4. Schirmer test (see 4.3, Dry-Eye Syndrome).

5. Dilated fundus examination: Look for cotton-wool spots consistent with connective tissue disease or evidence of posterior scleritis (e.g., vitreitis, subretinal fluid, chorioretinal folds, exudative retinal detachment).

6. Corneal scrapings and cultures when infection is suspected (see 4.11, Bacterial Keratitis).

7. Serum antinuclear antibody, rheumatoid factor, erythrocyte sedimentation rate, and complete blood count with differential to rule out connective tissue disease and leukemia, if suspected. Serum anti-neutrophilic cytoplasmic antibody levels can be obtained if Wegener granulomatosis is suspected.

8. Scleritis workup, when present (see 5.7, Scleritis).

9. Refer to an internist (or rheumatologist) when connective tissue disease or leukemia is suspected.

TREATMENT

The treatment of dellen, staphylococcal hypersensitivity, dry-eye syndrome, exposure and neurotrophic keratopathies, scleritis, vernal conjunctivitis, and ocular rosacea are discussed elsewhere in this book. See appropriate sections.

1. **Corneal thinning due to connective tissue disease:** Management is usually coordinated with a rheumatologist or internist.

    —Antibiotic ointment (e.g., erythromycin ointment) and a pressure patch q.h.s.

    —Ocular lubricants while awake (e.g., Refresh Plus or TheraTears q1h or Refresh PM ointment q2h).

—Cycloplegic drops (e.g., scopolamine 0.25% or atropine 1%) when an anterior chamber reaction or pain is present.

—Systemic steroids (e.g., prednisone, 60 to 100 mg p.o., q.d.; the dosage is adjusted according to the response) and a histamine type 2 receptor (H_2) blocker (e.g., ranitidine 150 mg p.o., b.i.d.) are used for significant and progressive corneal thinning, but not for perforation.

—An immunosuppressive agent such as cyclophosphamide is often required, especially for Wegener granulomatosis. This should be done in coordination with the patient's internist or rheumatologist.

—Excision of adjacent inflamed conjunctiva is occasionally helpful when the condition progresses despite treatment.

—Punctal occlusion if dry-eye syndrome also is present. Typical cyclosporine 0.05% (e.g., Restasis) b.i.d. also may be helpful.

—Consider cyanoacrylate tissue adhesive or corneal transplantation surgery for an impending or actual corneal perforation. A conjunctival flap or amniotic membrane graft can also be used for an impending corneal perforation.

—Patients with significant corneal thinning should wear their glasses [or protective glasses (e.g., polycarbonate lens)] during the day and an eye shield at night.

Note: Topical steroids are usually not used when significant corneal thinning is present because of the risk of perforation due to inhibition of a proper healing response. Topical steroids should be gradually tapered if the patient is already taking them. Corneal thinning due to relapsing polychondritis, however, seems to improve with topical steroids (e.g., prednisolone acetate 1%, q1–2h).

2. **Terrien marginal degeneration:** Correct astigmatism with glasses or contact lenses if possible. Protective eyewear (e.g., polycarbonate lens) during the day and an eye shield at night should be worn to prevent traumatic perforation if significant thinning

is present. Lamellar grafts can be used if thinning is extreme.

3. **Mooren ulcer:** Underlying systemic diseases must be ruled out before this diagnosis can be made. A stepwise approach to treatment is taken, using any or all of the following therapeutic modalities. If the epithelial defect over the ulcer is not healing within a few days of initiating treatment, more aggressive therapy is pursued. Some cases are resistant to all forms of treatment.

—Topical antibiotic drops [e.g., trimethoprim/polymyxin B (e.g., Polytrim) or a fluoroquinolone q.i.d.] to prevent secondary bacterial infection.

—Cycloplegic (e.g., atropine 1%, t.i.d.).

—Glasses during the day and an eye shield at night because of the risk of perforation with minor trauma.

—Topical steroid (e.g., prednisolone acetate 1%, q1–6h).

—Systemic steroid (e.g., prednisone, 60 to 100 mg p.o., q.d.) and an H_2 blocker (e.g., ranitidine 150 mg p.o., b.i.d.) if unresponsive to topical steroid alone.

—Consider conjunctival excision, conjunctival flap, amniotic membrane graft, or cryotherapy, if the ulceration progresses.

—Immunosuppressive agents (e.g., cyclophosphamide, methotrexate) for severe disease, in conjunction with an internist or other specialist to assist in monitoring for systemic toxicity. Topical cyclosporine also may be beneficial.

—Systemic interferon treatment has been shown to be effective in hepatitis C–related Mooren ulcer.

—Cyanoacrylate tissue adhesive or corneal surgery for actual or imminent corneal perforation.

4. **Pellucid marginal degeneration:** See 4.23, Keratoconus.

5. **Furrow degeneration:** No treatment is required.

Note: If systemic steroid therapy is to be instituted, obtain a steroid workup (see *Drug Glossary*) as indicated, and involve the patient's primary medical doctor.

FOLLOW-UP

Patients with severe disease are examined daily in the hospital or as outpatients if compliant; those with milder conditions are checked less frequently. Watch carefully for signs of superinfection (e.g., increased pain, stromal infiltration, anterior chamber cells and flare, conjunctival injection), increased IOP, and progressive corneal thinning. Treatment is maintained until the epithelial defect over the ulcer heals and is then gradually tapered. As long as an epithelial defect is present, there is risk of progressive thinning and perforation.

4.22 DELLEN

SYMPTOMS

Usually asymptomatic; irritation, foreign body sensation.

SIGNS

Critical. Corneal thinning, usually at the limbus, often in the shape of an ellipse, accompanied by an adjacent focal conjunctival or corneal elevation.

Other. Fluorescein pooling in the area, but minimal staining. No infiltrate, no anterior chamber reaction, often no hyperemia.

DIFFERENTIAL DIAGNOSIS

See 4.21, Peripheral Corneal Thinning/Ulceration.

ETIOLOGY

Poor spread of the tear film over a focal area of cornea (with resultant stromal dehydration) due to an adjacent surface elevation (e.g., chemosis, conjunctival hemorrhage, filtering bleb from glaucoma surgery, pterygium, tumor, after muscle surgery).

WORKUP

1. History: Previous eye surgery?

2. Slit-lamp examination with fluorescein staining: Look for an adjacent area of elevation.

TREATMENT

1. Lubricating or antibiotic ointment (e.g., Refresh PM, erythromycin ointment) and a pressure patch for 24 hours.

2. Lubricating ointment q.h.s. after removal of the pressure patch. Maintain the ointment until the adjacent elevation is eliminated.

3. If the cause cannot be removed (e.g., filtering bleb), lubricating ointment should be applied nightly, and artificial tear drops (e.g., Refresh Plus or TheraTears) used four to eight times per day, over the long term. (Most conjunctival elevations regress with patching.)

FOLLOW-UP

Unless there is severe thinning, reexamination can be performed in 1 to 7 days, at which time the cornea can be expected to be of normal thickness. If it is not, full-time patching and lubrication should again be instituted.

4.23 KERATOCONUS

SYMPTOMS

Progressive decreased vision, usually beginning in adolescence and continuing into middle age. Acute corneal hydrops can cause a sudden decrease in vision, pain, red eye, photophobia, and profuse tearing.

SIGNS

Critical. Slowly progressive irregular astigmatism resulting from paracentral thinning and bulging of the cornea (maximal thinning near the apex of the protrusion), vertical tension lines in the posterior cornea (Vogt striae), an irregular corneal retinoscopic reflex, and egg-shaped mires on keratometry. Inferior steepening is seen on corneal topographic evaluation. Usually bilateral but often asymmetric.

Other. Fleischer ring (epithelial iron deposits at the base of the cone), bulging of the lower eyelid when looking downward (Munson sign), superficial corneal scarring. Corneal hydrops (sudden development of corneal edema) results from a rupture in Descemet membrane.

ASSOCIATIONS

Keratoconus is associated with Down syndrome, atopic disease, and mitral valve prolapse. It may be related to chronic eye rubbing.

DIFFERENTIAL DIAGNOSIS

• Pellucid marginal degeneration (Corneal thinning in the inferior periphery. The cornea protrudes superior to the band of thinning.).

• Keratoglobus (Rare. Uniform circularly thinned cornea with maximal thinning in the mid-periphery of the cornea. The cornea protrudes central to the area of maximal thinning.).

   Treatment for these two conditions is the same as for keratoconus, except corneal transplantations are technically more difficult and have a higher failure rate.

WORKUP

1. History: Duration and rate of decreased vision? Frequent change in eyeglass prescriptions? History of eye rubbing? Medical problems? Allergies?

2. Slit-lamp examination

   Note: Fleischer ring is sometimes best seen with the cobalt blue light of the slit lamp.

3. Retinoscopy and refraction. Look for irregular astigmatism and a waterdrop or scissors red reflex.

4. Computed corneal topography (can show central and inferior steepening) and keratometry (irregular mires and steepening).

TREATMENT

1. Patients are instructed not to rub their eyes.

2. Correct refractive errors with glasses (for mild cases) or rigid gas-permeable contact lenses (successful in most cases).

3. Corneal transplantation surgery is usually indicated when contact lenses cannot be tolerated or no longer produce satisfactory vision.

4. Thermokeratoplasty, epikeratophakia, lamellar keratoplasty, and intracorneal ring segments are rarely used.

5. For eyes with corneal hydrops

   —Cycloplegic agent (e.g., scopolamine 0.25%), sodium chloride 5% ointment, and occasionally a pressure patch.

   —Patients are instructed to remove the pressure patch in 24 to 48 hours and start sodium chloride 5% ointment, b.i.d., until resolved (usually several weeks to months).

   —Glasses or a shield should be worn by patients at risk for trauma or by those who cannot be relied on to avoid vigorous eye rubbing.

Note: Acute hydrops is not an indication for emergency corneal transplantation, except in the extremely rare case of corneal perforation (reported cases are associated with minor trauma or topical steroid use).

Every 3 to 12 months, depending on the progression of symptoms. After an episode of hydrops, examine the patient every 1 to 4 weeks until resolved (which can take several months).

4.24   CORNEAL DYSTROPHIES

Bilateral, inherited, progressive corneal disorders showing no signs of inflammation or corneal vascularization and without associated systemic disease.

ANTERIOR CORNEAL DYSTROPHIES

• Anterior basement membrane dystrophy (map–dot–fingerprint dystrophy): Diffuse gray patches (maps), large or tiny creamy white cysts (dots), or fine refractile lines (fingerprints) in the corneal epithelium, best seen with retroillumination or a broad slit-lamp beam angled from the side. Spontaneous corneal epithelial defects (erosions) and associated pain and photophobia may develop, particularly on opening the eyes after sleep. May also cause decreased vision. See 4.2, Recurrent Corneal Erosion for treatment.

• Meesmann dystrophy: Rare, autosomal dominant epithelial dystrophy that is seen in the first years of life, but is usually asymptomatic until middle age. Retroillumination shows discrete, tiny epithelial vesicles diffusely involving the cornea but concentrated in the palpebral fissure. Although treatment is usually not required, bandage soft contact lenses, superficial keratectomy, or lamellar corneal transplantation may be beneficial if significant photophobia is present or if visual acuity is severely affected.

• Reis–Bücklers dystrophy: Autosomal dominant, progressive dystrophy that appears early in life. Subepithelial, gray reticular opacities are seen primarily in the central cornea. Painful

episodes from recurrent erosions are relatively common and require treatment. Corneal transplantation surgery may be necessary to improve vision, but the dystrophy often recurs in the graft. Superficial lamellar keratectomy or excimer laser PTK may be adequate treatment in some cases.

CORNEAL STROMAL DYSTROPHIES

Patients with reduced vision from these conditions usually benefit from a corneal transplant or PTK.

• Lattice dystrophy: Refractile branching lines, white subepithelial dots, and scarring of the corneal stroma centrally, best seen with retroillumination. Recurrent erosions are common (see 4.2, Recurrent Corneal Erosion). The corneal periphery is clear. Autosomal dominant. Tends to recur more rapidly than granular or macular dystrophy after PTK or corneal transplantation.

• Granular dystrophy: White anterior stromal deposits in the central cornea, separated by discrete clear intervening spaces. The corneal periphery is spared. Appears in the first decade of life but rarely becomes symptomatic before middle age. Erosions uncommon. Autosomal dominant. Also may recur after PTK or corneal transplantation within 3 to 5 years.

• Macular dystrophy: Gray–white stromal opacities with ill-defined edges extending from limbus to limbus with cloudy intervening spaces. Can involve the full thickness of the stroma, more superficial centrally and deeper peripherally. Causes decreased vision more commonly than recurrent erosions. Autosomal recessive. May recur very slowly, many years after corneal transplantation.

• Central crystalline dystrophy of Schnyder: Fine, yellow–white anterior stromal crystals located in the central cornea. Later develop full-thickness central haze and a dense arcus senilis. Can be associated with hyperlipidemia and hypercholesterolemia. Autosomal dominant. Workup includes fasting serum cholesterol and triglyceride levels. Rarely compromises vision enough to require transplantation.

CORNEAL ENDOTHELIAL DYSTROPHIES

• Fuchs dystrophy: See 4.25, Fuchs Endothelial Dystrophy.

• Posterior polymorphous dystrophy: Changes at the level of Descemet membrane, including vesicles arranged in a linear or grouped pattern, gray haze, or broad bands with irregular, scalloped edges. Iris abnormalities, including iridocorneal adhesions and a decentered pupil, may be present and are occasionally associated with corneal edema. Glaucoma may occur. Autosomal dominant with marked variability. See 8.12, Developmental Anterior Segment and Lens Anomalies for differential diagnosis.

• Congenital hereditary endothelial dystrophy: Bilateral corneal edema with normal corneal diameter, normal IOP, and no cornea guttata. See 8.11, Congenital Glaucoma for differential diagnosis. Some patients may benefit from a corneal transplant. Two distinct types distinguished by clinical presentation and genetics:

—Autosomal recessive: Present at birth, nonprogressive, nystagmus present. Pain or photophobia uncommon.

—Autosomal dominant: Is first seen during childhood, slowly progressive, no nystagmus. Pain, tearing, and photophobia are common.

4.25 FUCHS ENDOTHELIAL DYSTROPHY

SYMPTOMS

Glare and blurred vision, especially on awakening, that may progress to severe pain. Symptoms rarely develop before 50 years of age. May be autosomal dominant.

SIGNS

Critical. Cornea guttata and corneal stromal edema. Bilateral, but may be asymmetric.

*Note: Central cornea guttata without stromal edema is called endothelial dystrophy. This condition may progress to Fuchs dystrophy.

Other. Fine pigment dusting on the endothelium, central epithelial edema and bullae, folds in Descemet membrane, subepithelial scar tissue.

DIFFERENTIAL DIAGNOSIS

• Aphakic or pseudophakic bullous keratopathy: (History of cataract surgery, unilateral. See 4.26, Aphakic Bullous Keratopathy/Pseudophakic Bullous Keratopathy.).

• Congenital hereditary endothelial dystrophy (Bilateral corneal edema at birth. See 4.24, Corneal Dystrophies.).

• Posterior polymorphous dystrophy (Autosomal dominant, seen early in life. Corneal endothelium shows either grouped vesicles, geographic gray lesions, or broad bands. Occasionally associated with corneal edema. Iridocorneal adhesions and pupillary abnormalities may be present. See 4.24, Corneal Dystrophies.).

• Iridocorneal endothelial syndrome ("Beaten metal" corneal endothelial appearance, with corneal edema, increased IOP, possible iris thinning, and pupil distortion. Typically unilateral, in young to middle-aged adults. See 9.15, Iridocorneal Endothelial Syndrome.).

WORKUP

1. History: Previous cataract surgery?

2. Slit-lamp examination: Cornea guttata are often best seen with retroillumination. Fluorescein staining may demonstrate ruptured bullae.

3. Measure IOP.

4. Consider corneal pachymetry to determine the central corneal thickness.

TREATMENT

1. Topical sodium chloride 5% drops, q.i.d. and ointment q.h.s.

2. May gently blow warm air from a hair dryer at arm's length toward the eyes for 5 to 10 minutes every morning to dehydrate the cornea.

3. Reduce the IOP with antiglaucoma medications if greater than 20 to 22 mm Hg (e.g., timolol or levobunolol, 0.25% to 0.5%, b.i.d.), if no systemic contraindications.

4. Ruptured corneal bullae are painful and should be treated as a corneal abrasion (see 3.2, Corneal Abrasion).

5. Corneal transplantation surgery is usually indicated when visual acuity decreases or the disease becomes advanced and painful.

FOLLOW-UP

Every 3 to 12 months to check IOP and assess corneal edema. The condition progresses very slowly, and visual acuity typically remains good until epithelial edema develops.

4.26 APHAKIC BULLOUS KERATOPATHY/PSEUDOPHAKIC BULLOUS KERATOPATHY

SYMPTOMS

Decreased vision, pain, tearing, photophobia, red eye; history of cataract surgery in the involved eye.

SIGNS

Critical. Corneal edema in an eye in which the natural lens has been removed.

Other. Corneal bullae, corneal neovascularization, preexisting corneal endothelial guttata. Cystoid macular edema (CME) may be present.

ETIOLOGY

Often results from a combination of the following factors: corneal endothelial damage, intraocular inflammation, vitreous or subluxed intraocular lens touching (or intermittently touching) the cornea.

WORKUP

1. Slit-lamp examination: Stain the cornea with fluorescein to check for denuded epithelium, check the position of the intraocular lens if present, determine whether vitreous is touching the corneal endothelium, and evaluate the eye for inflammation. Evaluate the contralateral eye for corneal endothelial dystrophy.

2. Check IOP.

3. Dilated fundus examination: Look for CME or vitreous inflammation.

4. Consider a fluorescein angiogram to help detect CME.

TREATMENT

1. Topical sodium chloride 5% drops, q.i.d. and ointment q.h.s., if epithelial edema is present.

2. Reduce IOP with antiglaucoma medications if increased (e.g., more than 20 mm Hg). Avoid epinephrine derivatives and prostaglandin analogs, if possible, because of the risk of CME (see 9.1, Primary Open-Angle Glaucoma).

3. Ruptured epithelial bullae (producing corneal epithelial defects) may be treated with an antibiotic ointment (e.g., erythromycin), a cycloplegic (e.g., scopolamine 0.25%), and pressure patching for 24 to 48 hours. Alternatively, the antibiotic ointment can be used frequently (e.g., q2h) without patching. A bandage soft contact lens, anterior stromal puncture, or PTK can be used for recurrent ruptured epithelial bullae (see 4.2, Recurrent Corneal Erosion).

4. Corneal transplantation surgery (possibly including intraocular lens repositioning, replacement, or removal or vitrectomy) is indicated when vision fails or when the disease becomes advanced and painful. Conjunctival flap or amniotic membrane graft surgery may be indicated for a painful eye with poor visual potential.

5. See 11.18, Cystoid Macular Edema, for treatment of CME.

Note: Although both CME and corneal disease may contribute to decreased vision, the precise role of each is often difficult to determine.

FOLLOW-UP

In 24 to 48 hours, until the epithelial defect heals. Otherwise, every 1 to 6 months, depending on the symptoms.

4.27 CORNEAL GRAFT REJECTION

SYMPTOMS

Decreased vision, mild pain, redness, and photophobia in an eye that has undergone a prior corneal transplantation, usually several weeks to years previously. Some patients may be asymptomatic.

SIGNS

Critical. Any of the following suggest corneal graft rejection: new keratic precipitates or a fine line of white blood cells on the corneal endothelium (endothelial rejection line), stromal edema or cellular infiltration, subepithelial infiltrates, epithelial edema, an irregularly elevated epithelial line (epithelial rejection line).

Other. Conjunctival injection (particularly circumcorneal injection), anterior chamber cells and flare, neovascularization growing up to or extending onto the graft (typically the rejection starts near a blood vessel adjacent to the graft wound). Tearing may occur, but discharge is not present.

DIFFERENTIAL DIAGNOSIS

• Suture abscess or corneal infection [May have a corneal infiltrate, hypopyon, or a purulent discharge. Remove the suture (by pulling the contaminated portion through the shortest track possible) and obtain smears and cultures, including a culture of the suture. Steroid frequency is usually reduced slowly rather than increased. Patients are treated with intensive topical fluoroquinolone or fortified antibiotics and monitored closely, sometimes in the hospital. See 4.11, Bacterial Keratitis.].

• Uveitis (May produce anterior chamber cells and flare with keratic precipitates. Often, a previous history of uveitis is obtained. It is best to treat uveitis as if it were a graft rejection.).

- Increased IOP (A markedly increased IOP may produce epithelial corneal edema, but few to no other signs of graft rejection are present, and the edema often clears after the IOP is reduced.).

- Other causes of graft failure [Corneal endothelial decompensation in the graft, recurrent disease in the graft (e.g., herpes keratitis, corneal dystrophy)].

WORKUP

1. History: Time since corneal transplantation? Current eye medications? Recent change in topical steroid regimen? Previous ocular disease leading to the corneal transplantation (e.g., HSV)?

2. Slit-lamp examination, looking for the critical signs listed previously: Look carefully for endothelial rejection line, keratic precipitates, and subepithelial infiltrates.

TREATMENT

1. Topical steroids (e.g., prednisolone acetate 1%, q1h while awake and dexamethasone 0.1% ointment, q.h.s.) if significant endothelial rejection is present. If only subepithelial infiltrates, keratic precipitates, or an epithelial rejection is present, use twice the current level of topical steroids or use prednisolone acetate 1%, q.i.d. (whichever is more).

2. Cycloplegic agent (e.g., scopolamine 0.25%, b.i.d. to t.i.d.).

3. Consider systemic steroids (e.g., prednisone 40 to 80 mg p.o., q.d.) or, rarely, subconjunctival steroids (e.g., betamethasone, 3 mg in 0.5 mL) to be used additionally when the graft rejection does not respond to topical steroids alone, or for recurrent rejection.

4. Control IOP if increased (see 9.4, Inflammatory Open-Angle Glaucoma).

5. For multiple rejection episodes or severe rejection, consider hospitalization and a single-pulse dose of methylprednisolone 500 mg i.v., along with prednisolone acetate 1%, q1h, topically.

FOLLOW-UP

Treatment must be instituted immediately to maximize the likelihood of graft survival. Examine the patient every 3 to 7 days. Once improvement is noted, the steroids are tapered very slowly and may need to be maintained at low doses for months to years. IOP must be checked regularly in patients taking topical steroids.

4.28 REFRACTIVE SURGERY COMPLICATIONS

The basic principle of corneal refractive surgery is to induce a change in curvature of the cornea to correct a preexisting refractive error.

COMPLICATIONS OF SURFACE ABLATION PROCEDURES (PHOTOREFRACTIVE KERATECTOMY AND LASER SUBEPITHELIAL KERATECTOMY)

In photorefractive keratectomy (PRK), the surgeon removes the corneal epithelium and partially ablates the corneal stroma by using an argon–fluoride excimer laser (193 nm, ultraviolet) to correct a refractive error. In laser subepithelial keratectomy (LASEK), the epithelium is separated from the Bowman layer, moved to the side before laser ablation of the stroma, and then repositioned centrally.

SYMPTOMS

Early (1 to 14 days). Decreasing visual acuity, increased pain.

Note: There is a normal element of pain caused by an induced epithelial defect at surgery, which usually takes a few days to heal.

Later (2 weeks to several months). Decreasing visual acuity, severe glare, monocular diplopia.

SIGNS

Corneal infiltrate, central corneal scar.

ETIOLOGY

Early

- Dislocated bandage soft contact lens (see 4.19, Contact Lens–Related Problems).

- Nonhealing epithelial defect (see 3.2, Corneal Abrasion).

- Corneal ulcer (see 4.11, Bacterial Keratitis).

- Medication allergy (see 5.1, Acute Conjunctivitis).

Later

- Corneal haze (scarring) noted in anterior corneal stroma.

- Irregular astigmatism (e.g., central island, decentered ablation).

- Regression or progression of refractive error.

- Steroid-induced glaucoma (see 9.5, Steroid-Response Glaucoma).

WORKUP

1. Complete ophthalmic examination, including IOP. IOP may be underestimated given decreased corneal thickness.

2. Refraction if change in refractive error suspected. Refraction with hard contact lens may correct irregular astigmatism.

3. Corneal topography if irregular astigmatism is suspected.

TREATMENT AND FOLLOW-UP

1. Epithelial defect (see 3.2, Corneal Abrasion).

2. Corneal infiltrate (see 4.11, Bacterial Keratitis).

3. Corneal haze. Increase steroid drop frequency. Follow-up 1 to 2 weeks. Cases of severe haze may respond to PTK with or without mitomycin C.

4. Refractive error or irregular astigmatism. Appropriate refraction. Consider PRK or LASEK enhancement. If irregular astigmatism, may need repeated PRK or LASEK or hard contact lens.

5. Steroid-induced glaucoma (see 9.5, Steroid-Response Glaucoma).

COMPLICATIONS OF LASER IN SITU KERATOMILEUSIS

In LASIK, the surgeon creates a hinged, partial-thickness corneal flap by using a microkeratome or femtosecond laser, and then ablates the underlying stroma with an excimer laser to correct refractive error. The corneal flap is repositioned over the corneal stroma without sutures.

SYMPTOMS

Early (1 to 14 days). Decreasing visual acuity, increased pain.

Later (2 weeks to several months). Decreasing visual acuity, severe glare, monocular diplopia, dry-eye symptoms.

SIGNS

Severe conjunctival injection, corneal infiltrate, large fluorescein-staining epithelial defect, dislocated corneal flap, central corneal scar, SPK.

ETIOLOGY

Early

- Flap dislocation or lost corneal flap.

- Large epithelial defect.

- Diffuse lamellar keratitis. Also known as "sands of the Sahara" because of its appearance (multiple fine inflammatory infiltrates in the flap interface). Usually occurs within 5 days of surgery.

- Corneal ulcer/infection in flap interface (see 4.11, Bacterial Keratitis).

- Medication allergy (see 5.1, Acute Conjunctivitis).

Later

- Epithelial ingrowth into flap interface.

- Corneal haze (scarring): Less common than in PRK.

- Irregular astigmatism (e.g., decentered ablation, central island, flap irregularity, ectasia).

- Regression or progression of refractive error.

- Dry-eye syndrome/neurotrophic keratopathy.

WORKUP

1. Complete slit-lamp examination, including IOP measurement and fluorescein staining.

2. Schirmer test, as needed.

3. Refraction if irregular astigmatism or change in refractive error is suspected. Refraction with hard contact lens.

4. Corneal topography if irregular astigmatism is suspected.

TREATMENT AND FOLLOW-UP

1. Flap dislocation: Requires urgent surgical repositioning.

2. Lost corneal flap: Treat as epithelial defect (see 3.2, Corneal Abrasion).

3. Epithelial defect (see 3.2, Corneal Abrasion).

4. *SPK* (see 4.1, Superficial Punctate Keratitis and 4.3, Dry-Eye Syndrome).

5. Diffuse lamellar keratitis: Aggressive treatment with frequent topical steroids (e.g., prednisolone acetate 1%, q1h). If severe, may also require lifting of flap and irrigation of interface.

6. Corneal infiltrate (see 4.11, Bacterial Keratitis).

7. Epithelial ingrowth: Observation if not affecting vision and very peripheral. Surgical debridement if dense, approaching visual axis, or affecting vision.

8. Corneal haze: Increase steroid drop frequency. Follow-up 1 to 2 weeks.

9. Refractive error or irregular astigmatism: Appropriate refraction. Consider repositioning flap or LASIK enhancement. If irregular astigmatism, may need LASIK enhancement or hard contact lens.

COMPLICATIONS OF RADIAL KERATOTOMY

In radial keratotomy (RK), the surgeon makes partial-thickness, spokelike cuts in the peripheral cornea using a diamond blade (often 90% to 95% depth), which results in a flattening of the central cornea and correction of myopia. Astigmatic keratotomy (AK) is a similar procedure in which arcuate or tangential incisions are made to correct astigmatism.

SYMPTOMS

Early (1 to 14 days). Decreasing visual acuity, increased pain.

Later (2 weeks to years). Decreasing visual acuity, severe glare, monocular diplopia.

Note: Because the corneal integrity is weakened with RK, patients are at higher risk for a ruptured globe with trauma.

SIGNS

Corneal infiltrate, large fluorescein-staining epithelial defect, rupture at RK incision site after trauma, anterior chamber reaction.

ETIOLOGY

Early

- Large epithelial defect (see 3.2, Corneal Abrasion).

- Corneal ulcer/infection in RK incision (see 4.11, Bacterial Keratitis).

- Medication allergy (see 5.1, Acute Conjunctivitis).

- Very rarely, endophthalmitis (see 12.10, Postoperative Endophthalmitis).

Later

- RK incisions approaching the visual axis causing glare and starbursts.

- Irregular astigmatism.

- Regression or progression of refractive error.

- Ruptured globe at RK incision site after trauma (see 3.14, Ruptured Globe and Penetrating Ocular Injury).

WORKUP

1. Complete slit-lamp examination, including IOP measurement and fluorescein staining.

2. Refraction if irregular astigmatism or change in refractive error is suspected. Refraction with hard contact lens.

3. Corneal topography if irregular astigmatism suspected.

TREATMENT AND FOLLOW-UP

1. Corneal infiltrate (see 4.11, Bacterial Keratitis).

2. Epithelial defect (see 3.2, Corneal Abrasion).

3. Endophthalmitis (see 12.10, Postoperative Endophthalmitis).

4. Refractive error or irregular astigmatism. Appropriate refraction. Consider enhancement of RK incisions or AK. If irregular astigmatism, may require a hard contact lens.

5. Ruptured globe at RK incision. Requires surgical repair (see 3.14, Ruptured Globe and Penetrating Ocular Injury).

4.29 OCULAR VACCINIA

SYMPTOMS

Red eye, pain, photophobia, tearing, itching, decreased vision, eyelid swelling, vesicular or pustular skin rash; malaise, fever, history of recent smallpox vaccination or exposure to someone recently vaccinated.

SIGNS

Eyelid/Skin Involvement

Acute blepharitis: Vesicles (which do not obey a dermatomal distribution) progress into pustules, which umbilicate and indurate. Severe eyelid edema and erythema may mimic orbital cellulitis. Lymphadenopathy may be present.

Conjunctivitis

Acute papillary conjunctivitis, often with muco-purulent discharge and inflammatory membrane. Ulcers of the conjunctiva are common. Symblepharon may follow.

Keratitis (Uncommon)

Similar to HSV: SPK, corneal dendrites, or a geographic epithelial ulcer. Focal or diffuse stromal edema; stromal infiltrate/ulceration, sometimes with necrosis and rarely perforation; late corneal scarring/clouding may develop; secondary uveitis and elevated IOP may occur.

DIFFERENTIAL DIAGNOSIS

- HSV (The rash neither follows a dermatome nor obeys the midline. Unlike vaccinia, the vesicles do not become pustules. Patients are often young. Corneal dendrites of HSV have true terminal bulbs and stain well with fluorescein. See 4.14, Herpes Simplex Virus.).

- HZV (Frequently painful skin vesicles are found along a dermatomal distribution of the face, not crossing the midline. Pain may be present before vesicles appear. The pseudodendrites in this condition are raised mucous plaques. They do not have true terminal bulbs and do not stain well with fluorescein. See 4.15, Herpes Zoster Virus.).

- Chicken pox (Varicella zoster) [Systemic illness, common during childhood. See 13.7, Chicken Pox (Varicella Zoster Virus).].

- Molluscum contagiosum (Skin lesions are umbilicated, but not vesicular/pustular. See 5.2, Chronic Conjunctivitis.).

ETIOLOGY

Vaccinia may be shed from the inoculation site for 3 weeks from the time of inoculation. The virus is spread by contact (e.g., by hands or clothes) and replicates at a new site. The most common sites for inadvertent vaccinia inoculation are the eye and ocular adnexae. Patients with past or current inflammatory diseases of the skin (e.g., atopic dermatitis, seborrheic dermatitis) are at higher risk. The incubation period before symptoms appear is 5 to 19 days. Approximately one per 40,000 vaccinations results in ocular vaccinia.

WORKUP

1. History: Recent smallpox vaccination? Exposure to someone recently vaccinated? History of previous nasal, oral, or genital sores? History of exposure to chicken pox? Recent topical or systemic steroids? Immune deficiency state? History of atopic dermatitis?

2. External examination: Note the distribution of skin vesicles, if present. Lesions following a dermatomal distribution, extending onto the forehead and scalp, are suggestive of HZV.

3. Slit-lamp examination with IOP measurement.

4. Check corneal sensation (before instillation of topical anesthetic), which may be decreased in HSV and HZV.

5. Most cases of ocular vaccinia are diagnosed clinically and require no confirmatory laboratory tests. However, if the diagnosis is in doubt, viral studies may be obtained (including culture, polymerase chain reaction, and restriction endonuclease analysis).

Note: Smears and cultures for bacteria should be taken to rule out superinfection if a corneal ulceration suddenly worsens. See 4.11, Bacterial Keratitis.

TREATMENT

Ocular vaccinia is usually self-limiting. The goal of treatment is to decrease the severity of the disease. To prevent spread of the disease, all patients are counseled on contact precautions.

Eyelid/Skin Involvement (Without Keratitis)

1. Trifluridine 1% drops (e.g., Viroptic) five times per day for 2 weeks [may substitute vidarabine 3% (e.g., Vira-A) ointment five times per day for children, if available.].

2. Topical antibiotic ointment (e.g., bacitracin) to skin lesions b.i.d.

3. If severe (e.g., with cellulitis and fever), add vaccinia immune globulin (VIG) 100 mg/kg i.m. Repeat in 48 hours if not improved.

Conjunctivitis (Without Keratitis)

1. Trifluridine 1% drops (e.g., Viroptic) eight times per day for 2 weeks [may substitute vidarabine 3% (e.g., Vira-A) ointment five times per day for children, if available.].

2. Topical antibiotic ointment (e.g., bacitracin) b.i.d.

3. VIG 100 mg/kg i.m.

4. If severe (e.g., with ulceration, membrane, fever) and no improvement in 48 hours, VIG 100 mg/kg i.m. may be repeated.

Keratitis

1. Trifluridine 1% drops (e.g., Viroptic) eight times per day for 2 weeks [may substitute vidarabine 3% (e.g., Vira-A) ointment five times per day for children, if available.].

2. Topical antibiotic ointment (e.g., bacitracin) q.d. or q.i.d. (if epithelial defect).

3. If severe (e.g., with infiltrate or ulcer), add

—Cycloplegic agent (e.g., scopolamine 0.25%, t.i.d.).

—After the epithelium heals, cautiously add topical steroid (dose depends on severity) and slowly taper (while using prophylactic topical antivirals).

4. VIG is relatively contraindicated for patients with isolated vaccinia keratitis. However, it should not be withheld from patients when keratitis accompanies a serious nonocular indication (e.g., progressive vaccinia, eczema vaccinatum).

Note: VIG is currently available only through the Centers for Disease Control and Prevention (CDC).

FOLLOW-UP

1. Vaccinia dermatitis and conjunctivitis usually resolve in 7 days. Patients are reexamined in 2 to 7 days to evaluate the response to treatment and then every 7 to 14 days, depending on the clinical findings.

2. The following clinical parameters are evaluated: the size of the epithelial defect and ulcer, the corneal thickness and the depth to which the cornea is involved, the anterior chamber reaction, and the IOP (see 9.4, Inflammatory Open-Angle Glaucoma, for glaucoma management).

3. Topical antiviral medications should be continued for 2 weeks.

4. Topical steroids used for corneal stromal disease are tapered slowly. Prophylactic topical antiviral agents are used while on steroids.

5. A corneal transplant may eventually be necessary in stromal disease if inactive scars significantly affect vision.

CHAPTER 5

CONJUNCTIVA/SCLERA/IRIS/ EXTERNAL DISEASE

5.1 ACUTE CONJUNCTIVITIS

SYMPTOMS

"Red eye" (conjunctival hyperemia), discharge, eyelids sticking (worse in morning), foreign body sensation, *less than 4-week* duration of symptoms (otherwise, see 5.2, Chronic Conjunctivitis). See Figure 5.1.

GONOCOCCAL CONJUNCTIVITIS

SIGNS

Critical. Severe purulent discharge, hyperacute onset (within 12 to 24 hours).

Other. Conjunctival papillae, marked chemosis, preauricular adenopathy, eyelid swelling.

*Note: A follicular response is not seen with neonatal conjunctivitis (see 8.9, Ophthalmia Neonatorum).

WORKUP

1. Examine the entire cornea for peripheral ulcers (especially superiorly) because of the risk for rapid perforation.

2. Conjunctival scrapings for *immediate* Gram stain and for routine culture and sensitivities [e.g., blood agar, chocolate agar (37°C, 10% CO_2)].

TREATMENT

Initiated if the Gram stain shows gram-negative intracellular diplococci or there is a clinically high suspicion of gonococcal conjunctivitis.

1. Ceftriaxone, 1 g intramuscularly (i.m.), in a single dose. If corneal involvement exists, or cannot be excluded because of chemosis and eyelid swelling, then hospitalize the patient and treat with ceftriaxone, 1 g intravenously, every 12 to 24 hours. The duration of treatment depends on the clinical response. In penicillin-allergic patients, may consider ciprofloxacin 500 mg orally (p.o.), single dose, or ofloxacin 400 mg p.o., single dose, and consider consulting infectious disease specialist (fluoroquinolones are contraindicated in pregnant women and children).

2. Topical bacitracin ointment q.i.d. or ciprofloxacin drops q2h. If the cornea is involved, use topical ciprofloxacin, levofloxacin, gentamicin, or tobramycin q1h.

3. Eye irrigation with saline q.i.d. until the discharge is eliminated.

4. Treat for possible coinfection with chlamydia (e.g., azithromycin 1 g p.o., single dose, or doxycycline 100 mg p.o., b.i.d. for 7 days.).

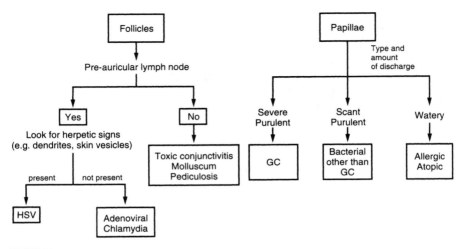

FIGURE 5.1

5. Treat sexual partners with oral antibiotics for both gonococcal conjunctivitis and chlamydia as described previously.

FOLLOW-UP

Daily, until consistent improvement is noted, and then examine every 2 to 3 days until the condition resolves. The patient and sexual partners should be evaluated by their medical doctors for other sexually transmitted diseases.

VIRAL CONJUNCTIVITIS (USUALLY ADENOVIRAL)

SYMPTOMS

Itching, burning, foreign body sensation; history of recent upper respiratory tract infection or sick contact. It usually starts in one eye and involves the fellow eye a few days later.

SIGNS

Critical. Inferior palpebral conjunctival follicles, palpable preauricular lymph node.

Other. Watery, mucous discharge, red and edematous eyelids, palpable preauricular node, pinpoint subconjunctival hemorrhages, membrane/

pseudomembrane. Subepithelial infiltrates (SEIs) may develop 1 to 2 weeks after the onset of the conjunctivitis.

WORKUP

No conjunctival cultures or swabbings are indicated unless discharge is excessive or the condition becomes chronic (see 5.2, Chronic Conjunctivitis).

TREATMENT·

1. Artificial tears (e.g., Refresh Tears) four to eight times per day for 1 to 3 weeks.

2. Cool compresses several times per day for 1 to 2 weeks.

3. Vasoconstrictor/antihistamine (e.g., naphazoline/pheniramine) q.i.d., if itching is severe.

4. If a membrane/pseudomembrane is present, it is gently peeled.

5. If a membrane/pseudomembrane is present or if SEIs reduce vision, use topical steroids (e.g., fluorometholone 0.1% to 0.25%, loteprednol 0.2% to 0.5%, or prednisolone acetate 0.125%, q.i.d.). Steroid treatment is maintained for 1 week and then slowly tapered. SEIs may recur during or after tapering.

6. Counsel the patient that viral conjunctivitis is a self-limited condition that typically gets worse for the first 4 to 7 days after onset and may not resolve for 2 to 3 weeks.

7. Viral conjunctivitis is very contagious, usually for 10 to 12 days from the day of onset. Patients should avoid touching their eyes, shaking hands with other people, sharing towels, and so forth. Restrict work and school for patients with significant exposure to others as long as the eyes are red and weeping.

8. Frequent handwashing.

   Note: Routine use of topical antibiotics or steroids for viral conjunctivitis is discouraged.

FOLLOW-UP

In 1 to 2 weeks, but sooner if the condition worsens significantly.

VARIANTS (TREATED THE SAME AS PRECEDING)

• Pharyngoconjunctival fever: As earlier, but associated with pharyngitis and fever; usually in children.

• Acute hemorrhagic conjunctivitis: As earlier, but associated with a large subconjunctival hemorrhage. Associated with enterovirus and lasts 1 to 2 weeks. Tends to occur in tropical regions.

Note: Many systemic viral syndromes (e.g., measles, mumps influenza) can cause a nonspecific conjunctivitis. The underlying condition should be managed appropriately; the eyes are treated with artificial tears four to eight times per day.

HERPES SIMPLEX VIRUS CONJUNCTIVITIS

Patients may have a known history of ocular herpes simplex or perioral cold sores. May be triggered by such environmental stressors as fever, ultraviolet light exposure, or psychological stress.

SYMPTOMS

Foreign body sensation, pain, burning (rarely itching).

SIGNS

Unilateral (sometimes recurrent) follicular conjunctival reaction; occasionally, concurrent herpetic skin vesicles along the eyelid margin or periocular skin; a palpable preauricular node.

TREATMENT

If the cornea or skin is involved, see 4.14, Herpes Simplex Virus.

1. Antiviral therapy [e.g., trifluridine 1% drops, five times per day; or vidarabine 3% ointment, five times per day (if available)].

2. Cool compresses several times per day.

FOLLOW-UP

Every 2 to 5 days initially, to monitor for corneal involvement and to taper topical medications, then every 1 to 2 weeks until resolved. Usually better in 1 week.

Note: After vaccination for smallpox, vaccinia virus can cause conjunctivitis with periocular dermatitis similar to that caused by herpes simplex virus (see 4.29, Ocular Vaccinia).

ALLERGIC CONJUNCTIVITIS (E.G., HAY FEVER)

SYMPTOMS

Itching, watery discharge, and a history of allergies are typical.

SIGNS

Chemosis, red and edematous eyelids, conjunctival papillae; a preauricular node is not palpable.

TREATMENT

1. Eliminate the inciting agent.

2. Cool compresses several times per day.

3. Topical drops, depending on the severity.

   —Mild: Artificial tears (e.g., Refresh Tears or TheraTears) four to eight times per day.

   —Moderate: Vasoconstrictor/antihistamine q.i.d. (e.g., naphazoline/pheniramine). Be aware of rebound vasodilation after prolonged use. Olopatadine 0.1%, lodoxamide 0.1%, nedocromil 2%, or ketotifen 0.025%, b.i.d. may help relieve itching. Ketorolac 0.5% q.i.d. may occasionally reduce symptoms.

   —Severe: Mild topical steroid (e.g., loteprednol 0.2% or fluorometholone 0.1%, q.i.d., for 1 to 2 weeks) in addition to the preceding medications.

4. Oral antihistamine (e.g., fexofenadine 60 mg p.o., b.i.d., loratadine 10 mg p.o., q.d., cetirizine 5 to 10 mg p.o., q.d., or diphenhydramine 25 mg p.o., t.i.d. to q.i.d.) in moderate to severe cases can be very helpful.

Note: Routine use of topical antibiotics or steroids for allergic conjunctivitis is discouraged.

FOLLOW-UP

In 2 weeks. If topical steroids are being used, patients should be monitored for steroid side effects. The steroids should be slowly tapered.

VERNAL/ATOPIC CONJUNCTIVITIS

SYMPTOMS

Itching, thick, ropy discharge, seasonal (spring/summer) recurrences, history of atopy. Usually seen in young patients, especially boys.

SIGNS

Critical. Large conjunctival papillae seen under the upper eyelid or along the limbus (limbal vernal).

Other. Superior corneal "shield" ulcer (a well-delineated, sterile, gray–white infiltrate), limbal or palpebral raised white dots (Horner–Trantas dots) of degenerated eosinophils, superficial punctate keratitis (SPK).

TREATMENT

1. Treat as for allergic except add either topical cromolyn sodium 4%, q.i.d.; lodoxamide 0.1%, q.i.d.; olopatadine 0.1%, nedocromil 2%, or ketotifen 0.025%, b.i.d.; for 2 to 3 weeks before the season starts.

2. If a shield ulcer is present, add:

   —Topical steroid (e.g., fluorometholone 0.1% to 0.25%, loteprednol 0.5%, prednisolone acetate 1%, or dexamethasone 0.1% ointment) four to six times per day.

   —Topical antibiotic (e.g., erythromycin ointment q.i.d.).

   —Cycloplegic agent (e.g., scopolamine 0.25%, t.i.d.).

   —Add antiallergy drops as for allergic conjunctivitis if not already using.

3. Cool compresses q.i.d.

4. Consider cyclosporin 0.05% (e.g., Restasis) b.i.d. if not responding to the preceding treatment.

5. If atopic conjunctivitis is associated with atopic dermatitis of eyelids, may use topical steroid ophthalmic ointment such as fluorometholone 0.1%, q.i.d. or topical FK506 (Tacrolimus) 0.03% to 0.1% b.i.d. to the affected skin.

FOLLOW-UP

Every 1 to 3 days in the presence of a shield ulcer; otherwise, every few weeks. Topical medications are tapered slowly as improvement is noted. Antiallergy drops are maintained for the duration of the season and are often reinitiated a few weeks before the next spring. Patients on topical steroids should be monitored regularly to check intraocular pressure (IOP). Cyclosporine may take several weeks to months to have a significant effect.

BACTERIAL CONJUNCTIVITIS (OTHER THAN GONOCOCCAL)

SYMPTOMS

Redness, foreign body sensation; itching is much less prominent.

SIGNS

Critical. Purulent discharge of mild to moderate degree.

Other. Conjunctival papillae, chemosis, typically without preauricular adenopathy.

ETIOLOGY

Common organisms are *Staphylococcus aureus* (often associated with blepharitis, phlyctenules, and marginal sterile infiltrates), *Staphylococcus epidermidis*, *Streptococcus pneumoniae*, and *Haemophilus influenzae* (especially in children).

*Note: If hyperacute onset suspect for gonococcal conjunctivitis, see Gonococcal Conjunctivitis (earlier in this section).

WORKUP

Conjunctival swab, if severe, for routine cultures and sensitivities (blood and chocolate agar) and Gram stain.

TREATMENT

1. Use topical antibiotic therapy [e.g., trimethoprim/polymyxin B (e.g., Polytrim) or fluoroquinolone drops q.i.d.; or bacitracin or ciprofloxacin ointment q.i.d.] for 5 to 7 days.

2. *H. influenzae* conjunctivitis should be treated with oral amoxicillin/clavulanate (20 to 40 mg/kg/day in three divided doses) because of occasional extraocular involvement (i.e., otitis media, pneumonia, and meningitis).

FOLLOW-UP

Every 2 days initially, then every 3 to 5 days until resolved. Antibiotic therapy is adjusted according to culture and sensitivity results if the condition does not respond.

PEDICULOSIS (LICE, CRABS)

Typically develops from contact with pubic lice (usually sexually transmitted). May be unilateral or bilateral.

SYMPTOMS

Itching, minimal injection.

SIGNS

Critical. Adult lice, nits, and blood-tinged debris on the eyelids and eyelashes.

Other. Conjunctival follicles.

TREATMENT

1. Mechanical removal of lice and eggs with jeweler's forceps.

2. Any bland ophthalmic ointment (e.g., erythromycin or bacitracin) to the eyelids t.i.d. for 10 days to smother the lice and nits. Physostigmine 0.25% (e.g., Eserine) ointment to the eyelids, two applications 1 week apart, may be used instead, but this therapy has ocular side effects.

3. Antilice (e.g., Kwell, Nix, Rid) lotion and shampoo as directed to *non*ocular areas for patient and close contacts.

4. Thoroughly wash and dry all clothes and linens.

For chlamydial, toxic, and molluscum contagiosum–related conjunctivitis, see 5.2, Chronic Conjunctivitis.

Also see related sections: 8.9, Ophthalmia Neonatorum; 13.10, Stevens–Johnson Syndrome; and 5.10, Ocular Cicatricial Pemphigoid.

5.2 CHRONIC CONJUNCTIVITIS

SYMPTOMS

Discharge, eyelids sticking (worse in morning), red eye (conjunctival hyperemia), foreign body sensation, duration *greater than 4 weeks* (otherwise see 5.1, Acute Conjunctivitis).

DIFFERENTIAL DIAGNOSIS

- Parinaud oculoglandular conjunctivitis (see 5.3, Parinaud oculoglandular conjunctivitis).

- Silent dacryocystitis (see 6.8, Dacryocystitis).

- Verruca vulgaris papilloma.

- Contact lens related (see 4.19, Contact Lens–Related Problems).

CHLAMYDIAL INCLUSION CONJUNCTIVITIS

Sexually transmitted, typically found in young adults. A history of vaginitis, cervicitis, or urethritis may or may not be present.

SIGNS

Inferior tarsal or bulbar conjunctival follicles, superior corneal pannus, palpable preauricular node, or tiny, gray–white peripheral SEIs. A stringy, mucous discharge is typical.

WORKUP

1. History: Determine duration of red eye, any prior treatment, concomitant vaginitis, cervicitis, or urethritis. Sexual contacts with chlamydia?

2. Slit-lamp examination.

3. In adults, direct chlamydial immunofluorescence test or chlamydial culture of conjunctiva. (Chlamydia polymerase chain reaction is available but not yet validated for ocular use.)

   Note: Topical fluorescein can interfere with immunofluorescence tests.

4. Consider conjunctival scraping for Giemsa stain: shows basophilic intracytoplasmic inclusion bodies in epithelial cells, polymorphonuclear leukocytes, and lymphocytes in newborns.

TREATMENT

1. Azithromycin 1 g p.o., single dose; doxycycline 100 mg p.o., b.i.d., or erythromycin 500 mg p.o., q.i.d., for 7 days is given to the patient and sexual partners.

2. Topical erythromycin, tetracycline, or sulfacetamide ointment b.i.d. to t.i.d. for 2 to 3 weeks.

FOLLOW-UP

In 1 to 3 weeks, depending on the severity. The patient and sexual partners should be evaluated by their medical doctors for other sexually transmitted diseases and should be treated to prevent reinfection (although they may be asymptomatic).

TRACHOMA

Principally occurs in developing countries in areas of poor sanitation and crowded conditions.

SIGNS

MacCallan Classification

- Stage 1: Superior tarsal immature follicles, mild superior SPK and pannus, often preceded by purulent discharge and tender preauricular node.

- Stage 2: Florid superior tarsal follicular reaction (2a) or papillary hypertrophy (2b) associated with superior corneal SEIs, pannus, and limbal follicles.

- Stage 3: Follicles and scarring of superior tarsal conjunctiva.

- Stage 4: No follicles, extensive conjunctival scarring.

- Late complications: Severe dry eyes, trichiasis, entropion, keratitis, corneal scarring, superficial fibrovascular pannus, Herbert pits (scarred limbal follicles), corneal bacterial superinfection, and ulceration.

World Health Organization (WHO) Classification

- TF (Trachomatous inflammation: follicular): More than five follicles on the upper tarsus.

- TI (Trachomatous inflammation: intense): Inflammation with thickening obscuring more than 50% of the tarsal vessels.

- TS (Trachomatous scarring): Cicatrization of tarsal conjunctiva with fibrous white bands.

- TT (Trachomatous trichiasis): Trichiasis of at least one eyelash.

- CO (Corneal opacity): Corneal opacity involving at least part of the pupillary margin.

WORKUP

1. History of exposure to areas in which it is endemic (i.e., North Africa, Middle East, India, Southeast Asia, rarely in United States).

2. Examination and diagnostic studies as noted for chlamydial inclusion conjunctivitis, described previously.

TREATMENT

1. Azithromycin 20 mg/kg p.o. single dose; doxycycline 100 mg p.o., b.i.d.; erythromycin 500 mg p.o., q.i.d.; or tetracycline 250 mg p.o., q.i.d. for 2 weeks.

2. Tetracycline, erythromycin, or sulfacetamide ointment b.i.d. to q.i.d. for 3 to 4 weeks.

   Note: The tetracyclines are contraindicated in children younger than 8 years, pregnant women, and nursing mothers.

FOLLOW-UP

Every 2 to 3 weeks initially, then as needed. Although the previously described treatment is usually curative, reinfection is common if hygienic conditions do not improve.

MOLLUSCUM CONTAGIOSUM

SIGNS

Critical. Dome-shaped, usually multiple, umbilicated shiny nodules on the eyelid or eyelid margin.

Other. Follicular conjunctival response from toxic viral products, corneal pannus. If many lesions are present, consider the possibility of human immunodeficiency virus.

TREATMENT

Removal of lesions by simple excision, incision and curettage, or cryosurgery.

FOLLOW-UP

Every 2 to 4 weeks until the conjunctivitis resolves.

TOXIC CONJUNCTIVITIS (EYE DROPS)

SIGNS

Inferior papillary reaction, especially with aminoglycosides, antivirals, and preserved drops. With long-term use, usually more than 1 month, a follicular response may be seen with atropine, brimonidine, miotics, epinephrine agents, antibiotics, and antivirals. Inferior SPK and scant discharge may be noted.

TREATMENT

Discontinuing the offending eye drop is usually sufficient. Artificial tears without preservatives (e.g., Refresh Plus or TheraTears) four to eight times per day may help as well.

FOLLOW-UP

In 1 to 2 weeks, as needed.

5.3 PARINAUD OCULOGLANDULAR CONJUNCTIVITIS

SYMPTOMS

Red eye, mucopurulent discharge, foreign body sensation.

SIGNS

Critical. Granulomatous nodule(s) on the palpebral conjunctiva, visibly swollen preauricular or submandibular lymph node on the same side.

Other. Fever, rash, follicular conjunctivitis.

ETIOLOGY

• Cat-scratch disease from *Bartonella henselae* (most common cause): (Often a history of being scratched or licked by a kitten within 2 weeks before the onset of symptoms.).

• Tularemia (History of contact with rabbits, other small wild animals, or ticks. Patients have severe headache, fever, and other systemic manifestations.).

• Tuberculosis and other mycobacteria.

• Rare causes: Syphilis, leukemia, lymphoma, mumps, mononucleosis, fungi, sarcoidosis, and others.

WORKUP

Initiated when etiology is not known (e.g., no recent cat scratch).

1. Conjunctival biopsy with scrapings for Gram, Giemsa, and acid-fast stains.

2. Conjunctival cultures on blood, Löwenstein–Jensen, Sabouraud, and thioglycolate media.

3. Complete blood count, rapid plasma reagin (RPR), fluorescent treponemal antibody, absorbed (FTA-ABS), and, if the patient is febrile, blood cultures.

4. Chest radiograph, purified protein derivative (PPD), and anergy panel.

5. If tularemia is suspected, serologic titers are necessary.

6. If diagnosis of cat-scratch disease is uncertain, cat-scratch serology and cat-scratch skin test (Hanger–Rose) may be performed.

TREATMENT

1. Warm compresses for tender lymph nodes.

2. Antipyretics as needed.

3. Specifically:

—Cat-scratch disease: The disease generally resolves spontaneously in 6 weeks. Consider tetracycline 250 mg p.o., q.i.d.; trimethoprim/sulfamethoxazole DS p.o., b.i.d.; or ciprofloxacin 250 mg p.o., b.i.d., for 4 weeks. Use a topical antibiotic (e.g., bacitracin/polymyxin B ointment or gentamicin drops, q.i.d.) for 4 weeks. The cat does not need to be removed.

—Tularemia: Streptomycin 1 g i.m., b.i.d., for 7 days. Gentamicin drops, q2h, for 1 week, and then five times per day until resolved. Refer to a medical internist for systemic management.

—Tuberculosis: Refer to an internist for antituberculosis medication.

—Syphilis: Systemic penicillin (dose depends on the stage of the syphilis) and topical tetracycline ointment (see 13.5, Acquired Syphilis).

FOLLOW-UP

Repeat the ocular examination in 1 to 2 weeks. Conjunctival granulomas and lymphadenopathy may take 4 to 6 weeks to resolve for cat-scratch disease.

5.4 SUPERIOR LIMBIC KERATOCONJUNCTIVITIS

SYMPTOMS

Red eye, burning, foreign body sensation, pain, tearing, mild photophobia, frequent blinking. The course may be chronic with exacerbations and remissions.

SIGNS

Critical. Thickening and inflammation of the superior bulbar conjunctiva, especially at the limbus.

Other. Fine papillae on the superior palpebral conjunctiva; fine punctate fluorescein staining on the superior cornea, limbus, and conjunctiva; superior corneal micropannus and filaments. Usually bilateral.

WORKUP

1. History: Recurrent episodes? History of dysthyroid disease (present in 50% of patients with superior limbic keratoconjunctivitis)?

2. Slit-lamp examination with fluorescein staining, particularly of the superior cornea and adjacent conjunctiva. The upper eyelid often must be lifted by the examiner to see the superior limbal area, and then should be everted to visualize the tarsus. Sometimes the localized hyperemia of the superior bulbar conjunctiva is best appreciated by direct inspection without a slit lamp by raising the eyelids of the patient while he or she looks down.

3. Thyroid function tests.

TREATMENT

Mild

1. Aggressive lubrication with artificial tears (e.g., Refresh Plus or TheraTears) four to eight times per day and artificial tear ointment (e.g., Refresh PM) q.h.s.

2. May consider punctal occlusion.

3. Treat any concurrent blepharitis.

4. Consider treatment with cyclosporine 0.05% (e.g., Restasis) b.i.d. if not responding to lubrication.

Moderate to Severe (in addition to preceding)

1. Silver nitrate 0.5 to 1.0% *solution* (from wax ampules) applied on a cotton-tipped applicator for 10 to 20 seconds to the superior tarsal and superior bulbar conjunctiva after topical anesthesia (e.g., proparacaine). Then irrigation and antibiotic ointment (e.g., erythromycin) q.h.s. for 1 week.

   Note: Do not *use silver nitrate cautery sticks, which cause severe ocular burns.*

2. If significant amounts of mucus or filaments are present, then acetylcysteine 10% drops (e.g., Mucomyst), three to five times per day are usually added.

3. If two to three separate silver nitrate solution applications are unsuccessful, consider cautery or surgical resection or recession of the superior bulbar conjunctiva.

FOLLOW-UP

Every 1 to 2 weeks during an exacerbation. If signs and symptoms persist, a reapplication of silver nitrate solution, as described previously, may be performed at the weekly follow-up visit.

5.5 SUBCONJUNCTIVAL HEMORRHAGE

SYMPTOMS

Red eye, may have mild irritation, usually asymptomatic.

SIGNS

Blood underneath the conjunctiva, often in a sector of the eye. The entire view of the sclera may be obstructed by blood.

DIFFERENTIAL DIAGNOSIS

• Kaposi sarcoma. [Red or purple lesion beneath the conjunctiva, usually elevated slightly. These patients should be evaluated for acquired immunodeficiency syndrome (AIDS).]

• Other conjunctival neoplasms (e.g., lymphoma) with secondary hemorrhage.

ETIOLOGY

• Valsalva (e.g., coughing or straining).

• Traumatic (May be isolated or associated with a retrobulbar hemorrhage or ruptured globe.).

• Hypertension.

• Bleeding disorder.

• Hemorrhage due to orbital mass (rare).

• Idiopathic.

WORKUP

1. History: Bleeding or clotting problems? Medications (e.g., aspirin, warfarin)? Eye rubbing, trauma, heavy lifting, or Valsalva? Recurrent subconjunctival hemorrhage? Acute or chronic cough?

2. Ocular examination: Rule out a conjunctival lesion and check IOP. Check extraocular motility and resistance to retropulsion. In traumatic cases, rule out a ruptured globe (abnormally deep anterior chamber, significant subconjunctival hemorrhage, hyphema, vitreous hemorrhage, or prolapse of uveal tissue), a retrobulbar hemorrhage (associated with proptosis, increased IOP, and occasionally, chemosis), or orbital fracture (limited extraocular motility, enophthalmos or proptosis, periorbital crepitus, hypesthesia, and stepoff of inferior orbital rim).

3. Check blood pressure.

4. If the patient has recurrent subconjunctival hemorrhages or a history of bleeding problems, a bleeding time, prothrombin time, partial thromboplastin time, complete blood count (to evaluate for leukemia) with platelets, and protein C and S should be obtained.

5. If orbital signs are present (proptosis, decreased extraocular motility, elevated IOP) in atraumatic cases, perform axial and coronal computed tomography scanning of the orbits with and without contrast to evaluate for an orbital mass (e.g., neuroblastoma in children or lymphangioma in adults). In traumatic cases, image as appropriate (see 3.8, Orbital Blow-out Fracture).

TREATMENT

None required. Artificial tear drops (e.g., Refresh Tears) q.i.d. can be given if mild ocular irritation is present. In addition, elective use of aspirin products and nonsteroidal antiinflammatory drugs (NSAIDs) should be discouraged if possible in the context of coexisting medical conditions.

FOLLOW-UP

This condition usually clears spontaneously within 1 to 2 weeks. Patients are told to return if the blood does not fully resolve or if they experience a recurrence. Referral to an internist or family physician should be made as indicated for hypertension or a bleeding diathesis. If workup reveals an orbital mass, refer to an oculoplastics specialist.

5.6 EPISCLERITIS

SYMPTOMS

Acute onset of redness and mild pain in one or both eyes, typically in young adults; a history of recurrent episodes is common. No discharge.

SIGNS

Critical. Sectorial (and, less commonly, diffuse) redness of one or both eyes, mostly due to engorgement of the episcleral vessels. These vessels are large and run in a radial direction beneath the conjunctiva.

Other. Mild to moderate tenderness over the area of episcleral injection or a nodule that can be moved slightly over the underlying sclera may be seen. Associated anterior uveitis and corneal involvement are rare. Vision is normal.

DIFFERENTIAL DIAGNOSIS

• Scleritis [Pain is deep, severe, and often radiates to the ipsilateral side of the head or face. The sclera may have a bluish hue when observed in natural light. Scleral (and deep episcleral) vessels, as well as conjunctival and superficial episcleral vessels, are injected. The scleral vessels do not blanch on application of topical phenylephrine 2.5%. Corneal involvement may be present. See 5.7, Scleritis.].

• Iritis (Cells and flare are present in the anterior chamber. May be present with scleritis.).

• Conjunctivitis (Characterized by a discharge, and inferior tarsal conjunctival follicles or papillae. See 5.1, Acute Conjunctivitis, and 5.2, Chronic Conjunctivitis.).

• Contact lens overwear or tight contact lens syndrome (Increasing contact lens intolerance, history of sleeping in contact lenses, prolonged contact lens wear with ill-fitting contact lens, possible protein buildup, and con-

junctival hyperemia on slit-lamp examination. See 4.19, Contact Lens–Related Problems.).

ETIOLOGY

• Idiopathic (Most common).

• Connective tissue disease (e.g., rheumatoid arthritis, polyarteritis nodosa, systemic lupus erythematosus, Wegener granulomatosis).

• Gout (Serum uric acid increased.).

• Infectious [e.g., herpes zoster virus (scars from an old facial rash may be present), herpes simplex virus, Lyme disease, syphilis (FTA-ABS positive), hepatitis B].

• Others (e.g., inflammatory bowel disease, rosacea, atopy, and thyroid disease).

WORKUP

1. History: Assess for a history of rash, arthritis, venereal disease, recent viral illness, other medical problems.

2. External examination in natural light: Look for the bluish hue of scleritis.

3. Slit-lamp examination: Anesthetize (e.g., topical proparacaine) and move the conjunctiva with a cotton-tipped applicator to determine the depth of the injected blood vessels. Evaluate for any corneal or anterior chamber involvement. Check IOP.

4. Place a drop of phenylephrine 2.5% in the affected eye and reexamine the vascular pattern 10 to 15 minutes later. Episcleral vessels should blanch.

5. If the history suggests an underlying etiology, the appropriate laboratory tests should be obtained [e.g., antinuclear antibody (ANA), rheumatoid factor, erythrocyte sedimentation rate (ESR), serum uric acid level, RPR, FTA-ABS, anti-neutrophil cytoplasmic antibody (ANCA)].

TREATMENT

- If mild, treat with artificial tears (e.g., Refresh Tears) q.i.d.

- If moderate to severe, a mild topical steroid (e.g., fluorometholone 0.1% to 0.25% or loteprednol 0.2% to 0.5%) q.i.d. often relieves the discomfort. Rarely, more potent or frequent topical steroid application is necessary.

- Oral NSAIDs often help (e.g., ibuprofen 200 to 600 mg p.o., t.i.d. to q.i.d., or naproxen 250 to 500 mg p.o., b.i.d., with food or antacids).

Some physicians prefer oral NSAIDs to topical steroids as initial therapy.

FOLLOW-UP

Patients treated with artificial tears need not be seen for several weeks for their episcleritis unless it worsens or discomfort continues. Patients taking topical steroids are checked every 1 to 4 weeks (including an IOP check) until their symptoms have resolved. The frequency of steroid administration is then tapered. Patients are informed that episcleritis may recur in the same or contralateral eye.

5.7 SCLERITIS

SYMPTOMS

Severe and boring eye pain (most prominent feature), which may radiate to the forehead, brow, or jaw, and may awaken the patient at night. Usually, gradual onset with red eye and insidious decrease in vision. Recurrent episodes are common. Scleromalacia perforans may have minimal symptoms.

SIGNS

Critical. Inflammation of scleral, episcleral, and conjunctival vessels (scleral vessels are large, deep vessels that cannot be moved with a cotton swab and do not blanch with topical phenylephrine) can be sectorial or diffuse. The sclera has a characteristic bluish hue (best seen in natural light by gross inspection) and may be thin or edematous.

Other. Scleral nodules, corneal changes (peripheral keratitis, limbal guttering, or keratolysis), glaucoma, subretinal granuloma, uveitis, exudative retinal detachment, cataract, proptosis (posterior scleritis), or rapid-onset hyperopia (posterior scleritis).

*Note: The patient should be examined in all directions of gaze in daylight or with adequate room illumination without a slit lamp.

DIFFERENTIAL DIAGNOSIS

- Episcleritis: (Sclera not involved. Blood vessels blanch with topical phenylephrine. More acute onset than scleritis. Patients tend to be younger and have very mild symptoms, if any. See 5.6, Episcleritis.)

ETIOLOGY

Fifty percent of patients with scleritis have an associated systemic disease.

- *More common.* Connective tissue disease (e.g., rheumatoid arthritis, Wegener granulomatosis, relapsing polychondritis, systemic lupus erythematosus, Reiter syndrome, polyarteritis nodosa, ankylosing spondylitis), herpes zoster ophthalmicus, syphilis, status postocular surgery, gout.

- *Less common.* Tuberculosis, other bacteria (*Pseudomonas* species), Lyme disease, sarcoidosis, hypertension, foreign body, parasite.

CLASSIFICATION

1. Diffuse anterior scleritis: Widespread inflammation of the anterior segment.

2. Nodular anterior scleritis: Immovable inflamed nodule(s).

3. Necrotizing anterior scleritis with inflammation:

—Extreme pain.

—The sclera becomes transparent (choroidal pigment visible) because of necrosis.

—High level of association with systemic inflammatory diseases.

4. Necrotizing anterior scleritis without inflammation (scleromalacia perforans):

—Almost complete lack of symptoms.

—Mainly seen in patients with long-standing rheumatoid arthritis.

5. Posterior scleritis:

—May start posteriorly or may be an extension of anterior scleritis.

—May simulate an amelanotic choroidal mass.

—Exudative retinal detachment, disc swelling, retinal hemorrhage, choroidal folds, choroidal detachment.

—Restricted extraocular movements.

—Proptosis, pain, tenderness.

—Usually unrelated to systemic disease.

WORKUP

1. History: Previous episodes? Medical problems?

2. Examine the sclera in all directions of gaze by gross inspection in natural light or adequate room light.

3. Slit-lamp examination with a red-free filter (green light) to determine whether avascular areas of the sclera exist. Check for corneal or anterior chamber involvement.

4. Dilated fundus examination to rule out posterior involvement.

5. Complete physical examination (especially joints, skin, cardiovascular and respiratory systems, often performed by an internist or rheumatologist).

6. Complete blood count, ESR, uric acid, RPR, FTA-ABS, rheumatoid factor, ANA, fasting blood sugar, angiotensin-converting enzyme, CH 50, C3, C4, and serum ANCA.

7. Other tests if clinical suspicion warrants additional workup: PPD with anergy panel, chest radiograph, radiograph of sacroiliac joints, B-scan ultrasonography to detect posterior scleritis, and magnetic resonance imaging or computed tomography scan if indicated.

TREATMENT

1. **Diffuse and nodular scleritis:** One or more of the following may be required. Concurrent antacid or histamine type 2 receptor blocker (e.g., ranitidine 150 mg p.o., b.i.d.) is advisable.

—NSAIDs (e.g., ibuprofen, 400 to 600 mg p.o., q.i.d.; indomethacin, 25 mg p.o., t.i.d.; naproxen, 250 to 500 mg, p.o. b.i.d., or others): Three separate NSAIDs may be tried before nonsteroidal therapy is considered a failure. If still no improvement, consider systemic steroids.

—Systemic steroids: Prednisone, 60 to 100 mg p.o., q.d. for 1 week, followed by a taper to 20 mg, q.d. over the next 2 to 3 weeks, followed by a slower taper. The addition of an NSAID often facilitates the tapering of the steroid. If steroids are unsuccessful, consider immunosuppressive therapy. See Drug Glossary before prescribing systemic steroids.

—Immunosuppressive therapy (e.g., cyclophosphamide, methotrexate, cyclosporine, azathioprine): If one drug is ineffective or not tolerated, another should be tried, up to two to three different drugs. Systemic steroids may be used in conjunction. Immunosuppressive therapy is given in conjunction with an internist or a rheumatologist. The role of topical cyclosporine drops is unclear.

2. **Necrotizing scleritis:**

—Systemic steroid and immunosuppressive therapies are used as in (1).

—For scleromalacia perforans, abundant lubrication is also important.

—Scleral patch grafting may be necessary, if there is significant risk of perforation.

3. **Posterior scleritis:** Therapy is controversial and may include systemic aspirin, NSAIDs, steroids, or immunosuppressive therapy as described previously.

4. **Infectious etiologies:** Treat with appropriate topical and systemic antimicrobials. If a foreign body is present, surgical removal is indicated.

5. Glasses or eye shield should be worn at all times if there is significant thinning and risk of perforation.

Notes

1. *Topical steroids are not effective in scleritis.*

2. *Subconjunctival steroids are usually contraindicated, especially in necrotizing scleritis, and may lead to scleral thinning and perforation.*

FOLLOW-UP

Depends on the severity of the symptoms and the degree of scleral thinning. Decreased pain is a sign of response to treatment, even if inflammation appears unchanged.

5.8 BLEPHARITIS/MEIBOMIANITIS

SYMPTOMS

Itching, burning, mild pain, foreign body sensation, tearing, crusting around the eyes on awakening.

SIGNS

Critical. Crusty, red, thickened eyelid margins with prominent blood vessels (blepharitis) or inspissated oil glands at the eyelid margins (meibomianitis).

Other. Conjunctival injection, swollen eyelids, mild mucous discharge, SPK; acne rosacea may be present. Corneal infiltrates and phlyctenules may be present.

TREATMENT

See 5.9, Ocular Rosacea for treatment options in the presence of acne rosacea.

1. Scrub the eyelid margins twice a day with mild shampoo (e.g., Johnson's baby shampoo) on a cotton-tipped applicator or a wash cloth.

2. Warm compresses for 10 to 15 minutes, t.i.d. to q.i.d.

3. If associated with dry eyes, use artificial tears (e.g., Refresh Plus or TheraTears) four to eight times per day.

4. If moderately severe, add erythromycin or bacitracin ointment to the eyelids q.h.s.

5. Recurrent meibomianitis can be treated with tetracycline 250 mg p.o., q.i.d., or doxycycline 100 mg p.o., b.i.d., for 1 to 2 weeks, then taper slowly.

Note: Tetracycline and doxycycline should not be used in pregnant women, nursing mothers, or children younger than 8 years. Erythromycin 250 mg p.o., q.i.d., can be used instead.

FOLLOW-UP

In 3 to 4 weeks as needed. Eyelid scrubs and warm compresses may be reduced to q.d. as the condition improves. They often need to be maintained indefinitely.

Note: Rarely, intractable, unilateral, or asymmetric blepharitis is the only manifestation of sebaceous gland carcinoma of the eyelid.

5.9 OCULAR ROSACEA

SYMPTOMS

Bilateral chronic ocular irritation, redness, burning, photophobia, and foreign body sensation. Patients are typically middle-aged adults, but it can be found in children. More common in women.

SIGNS

Critical. Telangiectases, pustules, papules, or erythema of the cheeks, forehead, and nose. The findings may be subtle and are often best seen in natural light. Superficial or deep corneal vascularization, particularly in the inferior cornea, is sometimes seen, and it may extend into a stromal infiltrate.

Other. Rhinophyma of the nose occurs in the late stages of the disease, especially in men. Blepharitis (telangiectases of the eyelid margin with inflammation) and chalazia are common. Conjunctival injection, SPK, phlyctenules, perilimbal infiltrates of staphylococcal hypersensitivity, iritis, or even corneal perforation may occur.

DIFFERENTIAL DIAGNOSIS

• Herpes simplex keratitis: (Usually unilateral. Stromal keratitis with neovascularization may appear similar. The typical facial lesions of rosacea are absent. See 4.14, Herpes Simplex Virus.).

• See 4.1, Superficial Punctate Keratitis for additional differential diagnoses.

ETIOLOGY

Unknown, but signs and symptoms are often induced by certain environmental/local factors, including coffee, tea, alcohol, and the like.

WORKUP

1. External examination: Look at the face for the characteristic skin findings and inspect the eyelids for chalazia.

2. Slit-lamp examination: Look for telangiectases of the eyelid margins, conjunctival injection, and corneal scarring and vascularization, especially inferiorly.

TREATMENT

1. Warm compresses and eyelid hygiene for blepharitis or meibomianitis (see 5.8, Blepharitis/Meibomianitis). Treat dry eyes if present (see 4.3, Dry-Eye Syndrome).

2. Avoidance of exacerbating foods, beverages, and environmental factors.

3. Tetracycline 250 mg p.o., q.i.d., or doxycycline 100 mg p.o., b.i.d., for 2 to 6 weeks; taper the dose slowly once relief of symptoms is obtained. Some patients are maintained on low-dose tetracycline (e.g., 250 mg p.o., q.d.) or doxycycline (e.g., 40 to 50 mg p.o., q.d.) indefinitely, if active disease recurs when the patient is off medication. Erythromycin, in the same dose as tetracycline, may be substituted if tetracycline or doxycycline cannot be used (e.g., in a pregnant woman, nursing mother, or child younger than 8 years).

Note: Patients diagnosed with ocular rosacea who are asymptomatic and who do not demonstrate progressively worsening eye disease need not be treated with oral antibiotics.

4. Facial lesions can be treated with metronidazole gel (0.75%) application b.i.d.

5. Treat chalazia as needed (see 6.1, Chalazion/Hordeolum).

6. Corneal perforations may be treated with cyanoacrylate tissue adhesive if small, whereas larger perforations may require surgical correction. (Tetracycline is usually administered in the preoperative and postoperative periods.)

7. If infiltrates stain with fluorescein, infectious corneal ulcer may be present. Smears,

cultures, and antibiotic treatment may be necessary (see 4.11, Bacterial Keratitis).

FOLLOW-UP

Variable; depends on the severity of disease. Patients without corneal involvement are seen weeks to months later. Those with corneal disease are examined more often. Patients with moderate to severe facial disease should also seek dermatologic consultation.

Note: Tetracycline and doxycycline should not be given to pregnant women, nursing women, or children younger than 8 years. Patients should be told to take the tetracycline on an empty stomach and should be warned of susceptibility to sunburn while taking tetracycline and doxycycline.

5.10 OCULAR CICATRICIAL PEMPHIGOID

SYMPTOMS

Insidious onset of redness, foreign body sensation, tearing, and photophobia. Bilateral involvement. The course is characterized by remissions and exacerbations. Usually occurs in patients older than 55 years.

SIGNS

Critical. Inferior symblepharon (linear folds of conjunctiva connecting the palpebral conjunctiva of the lower eyelid to the inferior bulbar conjunctiva), foreshortening and tightness of the lower fornix.

Other. Secondary bacterial conjunctivitis, SPK, corneal ulcer. Later, poor tear film, resulting in severe dry-eye syndrome; entropion; trichiasis; corneal opacification with pannus and keratinization; obliteration of the fornices, with eventual limitation of ocular motility; and ankyloblepharon may occur.

Systemic. Mucous membrane (nose, oral cavity, pharynx, larynx, esophagus, anus, vagina, urethra) vesicles, scarring or strictures; ruptured or formed bullae; denuded epithelium. In the mouth, a desquamative gingivitis is common. Vesicles and bullae also may be noted on the skin, sometimes with erythematous plaques or scars near affected mucous membranes.

DIFFERENTIAL DIAGNOSIS

• Stevens–Johnson syndrome (erythema multiforme major) [Acute onset, usually with fever and malaise. Similar ocular involvement as ocular pemphigoid. The lips are typically swollen and crusted, and target lesions of the skin (red centers surrounded by a pale zone) are often found. Often precipitated by drugs (e.g., sulfa, penicillin, other antibiotics, Dilantin) or infections (e.g., herpes and mycoplasma). See 13.10, Stevens–Johnson Syndrome.].

• Membranous conjunctivitis with scarring (Usually adenovirus or beta hemolytic streptococcus. Symblepharon can follow any severe membranous/pseudomembranous conjunctivitis.).

• Severe chemical burn (see 3.1, Chemical Burn).

• Chronic topical medicine [e.g., glaucoma medications (especially epinephrine and pilocarpine), antiviral agents].

• Others (e.g., atopic keratoconjunctivitis, radiation treatment, squamous cell carcinoma).

WORKUP

1. History: Long-term topical medications? Acute onset of severe systemic illness in the past? Recent systemic medications?

2. Skin and mucous membrane (especially the mouth) examination.

3. Slit-lamp examination: Especially examine for inferior symblepharon. (Pull down the lower eyelid and have the patient look up.) Check IOP.

4. Gram stain and culture of the cornea or conjunctiva if secondary bacterial infection is suspected.

5. Consider a conjunctival biopsy for immunofluorescence studies.

6. Dermatology; ear, nose, and throat; gastrointestinal; and pulmonary consults if needed.

TREATMENT

(Often needs to be coordinated with an internist, rheumatologist, or a dermatologist. Early diagnosis of the ocular involvement is critical for optimal management.)

1. Artificial tears (e.g., Refresh Plus, Thera-Tears) 4 to 10 times per day. Can add an artificial tear ointment (e.g., Refresh PM) b.i.d. to q.i.d. and q.h.s.

2. Treat blepharitis vigorously with eyelid hygiene, warm compresses, and antibiotic ointment (e.g., bacitracin, t.i.d.). Oral tetracycline/doxycycline can be used if eyelid disease is severe (see 5.8, Blepharitis/Meibomianitis).

3. Goggles or glasses with sides to provide a moist environment for the eyes.

4. Punctal occlusion if puncta are not already closed by scarring.

5. Topical steroids (e.g., prednisolone acetate 1%, q.i.d.) may rarely help in suppressing acute exacerbations, but be cautious of corneal melting.

6. Systemic steroids (e.g., prednisone 60 mg p.o., q.d.) may also help in suppressing acute exacerbations but are largely ineffective when used without other immune modulators.

7. Dapsone is often used for progressive disease. Starting dose is 25 mg p.o., for 3 to 7 days; increase by 25 mg every 4 to 7 days until the desired result is achieved (usually 100 to 150 mg p.o., q.d.). Dapsone is maintained for several months and tapered slowly.

   Note: Dapsone can cause a dose-related hemolysis; therefore, complete blood count and glucose-6-phosphate dehydrogenase (G-6-PD) must be checked before administration. Dapsone should be avoided in patients with G-6-PD deficiency. A complete blood count with reticulocyte count is obtained weekly as the dose is increased, every 3 to 4 weeks until blood counts are stable, and then every few months.

8. Immunosuppressive agents (e.g., cyclophosphamide, methotrexate, or azathioprine) are typically used for progressive disease.

9. Consider surgical correction of entropion and cryotherapy or electrolysis of trichiasis. (This is best done in the absence of any active inflammation, but it carries a risk of further scarring.)

10. Mucous membrane grafts (e.g., buccal) can be used to reconstruct the fornices if needed.

11. Consider a keratoprosthesis in an end-stage eye with apparently good macular and optic nerve function.

FOLLOW-UP

Every 1 to 2 weeks during acute exacerbations, and every 1 to 3 months during remissions.

5.11 CONTACT DERMATITIS

SYMPTOMS

Sudden onset of a periorbital rash or eyelid swelling, mild watery discharge.

SIGNS

Critical. Periorbital edema, erythema, vesicles, lichenification of the skin. Conjunctival chemosis out of proportion to injection and papillary response.

Other. Watery discharge; crusting of the skin may develop when secondary infection arises.

ETIOLOGY

Most commonly, eye drops and cosmetics, including nail polish.

TREATMENT

1. Avoid the offending agent(s).

2. Cool compresses four to six times per day.

3. Preservative-free artificial tears (e.g., Refresh Plus or TheraTears) four to eight times per day and topical antihistamines (e.g., levocabastine, q.i.d.).

4. Consider a mild steroid cream (e.g., dexamethasone cream, 0.05%) applied to the periocular area b.i.d. to t.i.d. for 4 to 5 days for skin involvement.

5. Consider an oral antihistamine [e.g., diphenhydramine (e.g., Benadryl) 25 to 50 mg p.o., t.i.d. to q.i.d. for several days.

FOLLOW-UP

Reexamine within 1 week.

5.12 CONJUNCTIVAL TUMORS

The following are the most common and important conjunctival tumors. Phlyctenulosis and pterygium/pinguecula are discussed in 4.9 and 4.10, respectively.

AMELANOTIC LESIONS

LIMBAL DERMOID

Congenital benign tumor, usually located in the inferotemporal quadrant of the limbus; it may involve the cornea. Lesions are white, solid, fairly well circumscribed, elevated, and may have hair arising from their surface. They may enlarge, particularly at puberty. They may be associated with eyelid colobomas, preauricular skin tags, and vertebral abnormalities (Goldenhar syndrome). Surgical removal may be performed for cosmetic purposes or if they are affecting the visual axis, although a white corneal scar may persist after surgery.

Note: The cornea or sclera underlying a dermoid may be very thin or even absent, and penetration of the eye can occur with surgical resection.

DERMOLIPOMA

Congenital benign tumor, usually occurring under the bulbar conjunctiva temporally. It appears as a yellow–white, solid tumor and may have hair arising from its surface. Surgical removal is avoided, if possible, because of the frequent extension of this tumor into the orbit, involving orbital structures. If necessary, partial resection of the anterior portion can usually be done without difficulty.

PYOGENIC GRANULOMA

Benign, deep-red, pedunculated mass. It typically develops at a site of prior surgery, trauma, or chalazion. It may respond to topical steroids. A topical steroid–antibiotic combination (e.g., prednisolone acetate/tobramycin, q.i.d., for 1 to 2 weeks) may be helpful because infection may be present. The tumor often must be excised if it persists.

LYMPHANGIOMA

Probably congenital, but often not detected until years after birth. The lesion is benign yet slowly progressive and appears as a diffuse, multiloculated, cystic mass. This lesion is seen most commonly between birth and young adulthood, often before 6 years of age. Hemorrhage into the cystic spaces may produce a "chocolate cyst." Lymphangiomas may enlarge, sometimes due to an upper respiratory tract infection. Concomitant eyelid, orbital, facial, nasal, or oropharyngeal lymphangiomas may be present. Surgical excision may be performed for cosmetic or functional purposes, but it often must be repeated because it is difficult to remove the entire tumor with one surgical procedure. Lesions often stabilize in early adulthood. These lesions do not regress like the capillary hemangiomas.

GRANULOMA

May occur at any age, predominantly on the tarsal conjunctiva. No distinct clinical appearance, but patients may have an associated embedded foreign body, sarcoidosis, tuberculosis, or another granulomatous disease. Management often includes a course of topical corticosteroids or excisional biopsy.

PAPILLOMA

1. Viral [Frequently multiple pedunculated or sessile lesions in children and young adults. These lesions can occur on palpebral or bulbar conjunctiva. They are benign and are usually left untreated because of their high recurrence rate (which is often multiple) and their tendency for spontaneous resolution. They may also be treated with oral cimetidine 30 mg/kg/day in children, 150 mg p.o., b.i.d. in adults because of the drug's immune-stimulating properties.].

2. Nonviral (Typically, a single sessile or pedunculated lesion found in older patients. These are located more commonly near the limbus and may represent precancerous lesions with malignant potential. Complete excisional biopsy flush with the surface is the preferred treatment. Supplemental cryotherapy may be applied.).

Note: In dark-skinned individuals, papillomas may appear pigmented and may be mistaken for malignant melanoma (MM).

KAPOSI SARCOMA

Malignant, subconjunctival nodule, usually red or purple. Patients should be evaluated for AIDS (see 13.4, Acquired Immunodeficiency Syndrome).

CONJUNCTIVAL INTRAEPITHELIAL NEOPLASIA (DYSPLASIA AND CARCINOMA IN SITU)

Typically occurs in middle-aged to elderly people. The lesion is a leukoplakic or gray–white, gelatinous lesion that usually begins at the limbus. Occasionally, a papillomatous, fernlike appearance develops. The lesions are usually unilateral and unifocal. They may evolve into invasive squamous cell carcinoma if not treated early and successfully. They can spread over the cornea or, less commonly, invade the eye or metastasize. A complete excisional biopsy followed by supplemental cryotherapy to the remaining adjacent conjunctiva is the preferred treatment. Excision may require lamellar dissection into the corneal stroma and sclera in recurrent or long-standing lesions. Topical mitomycin C drops also have been used. Periodic follow-up examinations are required to detect recurrences.

LYMPHOID TUMORS (RANGE FROM BENIGN REACTIVE LYMPHOID HYPERPLASIA TO LYMPHOMA)

Occurs in young to middle-aged adults. Usually appears as a light pink, salmon-colored lesion. It may appear in the bulbar conjunctiva, where it is typically oval, or in the fornix, where it is usually horizontal, conforming to the contour of the fornix. Excisional or incisional biopsy is performed for immunohistochemical studies (may require nonfixed tissue). Symptomatic benign reactive lymphoid hyperplasia may be treated by excisional biopsy, low-dose radiation, cryotherapy, or topical steroid drops. Lymphomas should be completely excised, without damage to the extraocular muscle or excessive sacrifice of conjunctiva. Otherwise, an incisional biopsy is justified. Patients are referred to an internist or oncologist for systemic evaluation. Systemic lymphoma may or may not develop, if it is not already present.

EPIBULBAR OSSEOUS CHORISTOMA

Congenital, benign, hard, bony mass, usually on the superotemporal bulbar conjunctiva. Surgical removal may be performed for cosmetic purposes.

AMYLOID

Smooth, waxy, yellow masses seen especially in the lower fornix when the conjunctiva is involved. Often there are associated small hemorrhages. Definitive diagnosis is made with biopsy. Consider workup for systemic amyloidosis.

AMELANOTIC MELANOMA

Pigmentation of conjunctival melanoma is variable. Look for bulbar or limbal lesions with significant vascularity to help make this difficult diagnosis.

SEBACEOUS GLAND CARCINOMA

Although usually involving the palpebral conjunctiva, this tumor can involve the bulbar conjunctiva (when there is pagetoid invasion of the conjunctiva). This diagnosis should always be considered in older patients with refractory unilateral blepharoconjunctivitis.

MELANOTIC LESIONS

OCULAR OR OCULODERMAL MELANOCYTOSIS

Congenital episcleral (not conjunctival) lesion, as demonstrated (after topical anesthesia) by moving the conjunctiva back and forth over the area of pigmentation with a sterile, cotton-tipped swab. (Conjunctival pigmentation will move with the conjunctiva.) Typically, the lesion is unilateral, blue–gray, and often accompanied by a darker ipsilateral iris and choroid. In oculodermal disease, also called nevus of Ota, the periocular skin is also pigmented. These lesions may become pigmented at puberty. Both conditions predispose to MM of the uveal tract, orbit, and brain (most commonly in whites).

PRIMARY ACQUIRED MELANOSIS

Appears in middle-aged adults as flat, brown patches of pigmentation without small cysts in the conjunctiva. These tumors usually arise during or after middle age and almost always occur in whites. (Overall, approximately one fifth of these lesions develop into MM of the conjunctiva.) Malignant transformation should be suspected when an elevation or increase in vascularity in one of these areas develops. Management options include careful observation with photographic comparison for any change and incisional or excisional biopsy followed by cryotherapy for suggestive lesions.

NEVUS

Commonly develops during puberty, most often within the palpebral fissure on the bulbar conjunctiva. It is usually well demarcated and may or may not be pigmented. The degree of pigmentation may also change with time. A key sign in the diagnosis is the presence of small cysts in the lesion. Benign nevi may enlarge; however, MM may occasionally develop from a nevus, and enlargement may be an early sign of malignant transformation. Nevi of the palpebral conjunctiva are rare; primary acquired melanosis and MM must be considered in such lesions. A baseline photograph of the nevus should be taken, and the patient should be observed every 6 to 12 months. Surgical excision is elective.

MALIGNANT MELANOMA

Typically occurs in middle-aged to elderly patients. The lesion is a nodular brown mass. The tumor is well vascularized, and a large conjunctival vessel can often be seen feeding the tumor. It may develop from a nevus or primary acquired melanosis, but it may also develop *de novo*. Check for an underlying ciliary body melanoma (dilated fundus examination, transillumination, and B-scan ultrasonography). Intraocular and orbital extension may occur. Excisional biopsy (often with supplemental cryotherapy) is performed unless intraocular

or orbital involvement is present. In advanced cases, exenteration is necessary.

OTHER, LESS COMMON CAUSES OF INCREASED PIGMENTATION

1. **Ochronosis with alkaptonuria** (Autosomal recessive enzyme deficiency. Occurs in young adults with arthritis and dark urine. Pigment is at the level of the sclera.).

2. **Argyrosis** (Silver deposition causes black discoloration. Patients have a history of long-term use of silver nitrate drops.).

3. **Hemochromatosis** (Bronze diabetes. This condition can cause increased conjunctival pigmentation.).

4. **Ciliary staphyloma** (Scleral thinning with uveal show.).

5. **Adrenochrôme deposits** [Long-term epinephrine or dipivefrin (e.g., Propine) use.].

6. **Mascara deposits** (Usually occurs in the inferior fornix and becomes entrapped in epithelium or cysts.).

5.13 MALIGNANT MELANOMA OF THE IRIS

Malignant melanoma of the iris may occur as a localized or diffuse pigmented (melanotic) or nonpigmented (amelanotic) lesion.

SIGNS

Critical. Unilateral brown or translucent iris mass lesion exhibiting slow growth. It is more common in the inferior half of the iris and in light-skinned individuals. Rare in blacks.

Other. A localized MM is usually greater than 3 mm in diameter at the base and greater than 1 mm in depth and sometimes has a prominent feeder vessel. It may produce secondary glaucoma. It may cause a sector cortical cataract, ectropion iridis, spontaneous hyphema, seeding

of tumor cells into the anterior chamber, or direct invasion of tumor into the trabecular meshwork. A diffuse MM causes progressive darkening of the involved iris, loss of iris crypts, and increased IOP. Focal iris nodules may be present.

DIFFERENTIAL DIAGNOSIS

Melanotic Masses

• Nevi [Typically become clinically apparent at puberty, usually flat or minimally elevated (i.e., less than 1 mm) and uncommonly exceed 3 mm in diameter. Can cause ectropion iridis, sector cortical cataract, or secondary glaucoma. Usually not vascular. More common in the inferior half of the iris. Nevi do not usually grow.].

- Tumors of the iris pigment epithelium (Usually black, in contrast to melanomas, which are often brown or amelanotic.).

Amelanotic Masses

- Metastasis (Grows rapidly. More likely to be multiple or bilateral than is MM. Frequently liberates cells and produces a pseudohypopyon. Involves the superior and inferior halves of the iris equally.).

- Leiomyoma (Transparent and vascular. May be difficult to distinguish from an amelanotic melanoma.).

- Iris cyst (Unlike MM, most transmit light with transillumination.).

- Inflammatory granuloma (e.g., sarcoidosis, tuberculosis, or juvenile xanthogranuloma). (Often have other signs of inflammation such as keratic precipitates, synechiae, and posterior subcapsular cataracts. A history of iritis or a systemic inflammatory disease may be elicited.).

Diffuse Lesions

- Congenital iris heterochromia (The darker iris is present at birth or in early childhood. It is nonprogressive and usually is not associated with glaucoma. The iris has a smooth appearance.).

- Fuchs heterochromic iridocyclitis (Asymmetry of iris color, mild iritis in the eye with the lighter-colored iris, usually unilateral. Often associated with a cataract or glaucoma.).

- Iris nevus syndrome (Corneal edema, peripheral anterior synechiae, iris atrophy, or an irregular pupil may be present along with multiple iris nodules and glaucoma.).

- Pigment dispersion [Usually bilateral. The iris is rarely heavily pigmented (although the trabecular meshwork may be), and iris transillumination defects are often present.].

- Hemosiderosis (A dark iris may result after iron breakdown products from old blood deposit on the iris surface. Patients have a history of a traumatic hyphema or vitreous hemorrhage.).

WORKUP

1. History: Previous cancer, ocular surgery or trauma? Weight loss? Anorexia?

2. Slit-lamp examination: Carefully evaluate the irides. Check IOP.

3. Gonioscopy of the anterior chamber angle.

4. Dilated fundus examination using indirect ophthalmoscopy.

5. Transillumination (used to differentiate between epithelial cysts that transmit light and pigmented lesions that do not).

6. Photograph the lesion and accurately draw it in the chart, including dimensions. Ultrasonographic biomicroscopy may be helpful.

TREATMENT/FOLLOW-UP

1. Observe the patient with periodic examinations and photographs every 3 to 12 months, depending on suspicion of malignancy.

2. Surgical resection is indicated if growth is documented, the tumor interferes with vision, or it produces intractable glaucoma.

3. Diffuse iris MM with secondary glaucoma may require enucleation.

4. Avoid filtering surgery for glaucoma associated with possible MM because of the risk of tumor dissemination.

CHAPTER 6

EYELID

6.1 CHALAZION/HORDEOLUM

SYMPTOMS

Acute or chronic eyelid lump, swelling, pain, tenderness, erythema.

SIGNS

Critical. Visible, or palpable, well-defined subcutaneous nodule in the eyelid. In some cases, a nodule cannot be identified.

Other. Blocked meibomian orifice, eyelid swelling and erythema, localized eyelid tenderness, associated blepharitis or acne rosacea. May also note "pointing" of mucopurulent material on the anterior eyelid.

DIFFERENTIAL DIAGNOSIS

• Preseptal cellulitis (Eyelid erythema, edema, and warmth. Often there is a periorbital skin abrasion, laceration, or site of infection. Patients may be febrile. See 6.10, Preseptal Cellulitis.).

• Sebaceous gland carcinoma (Should be suspected in recurrent chalazion, thickening of both the upper and lower eyelids, chronic unilateral blepharitis, or a chalazion associated with loss of the eyelashes. It usually develops in older patients. See 6.11, Malignant Tumors of the Eyelid.).

• Pyogenic granuloma (Benign, deep red, pedunculated lesion often associated with chalazia, hordeola, trauma, or surgery. May be excised or treated with a topical antibiotic–steroid combination such as sulfacetamide/prednisolone acetate q.i.d. for 1 to 2 weeks. Intraocular pressure must be monitored if topical steroids are used.).

WORKUP

1. History: Previous ocular surgery or trauma? Previous chalazia or eyelid lesions?

2. External examination: Palpate the involved eyelid for a nodule.

3. Slit-lamp examination: Evaluate the meibomian glands for inspissation and evert the eyelid to rule out other etiologies.

TREATMENT

1. Warm compresses for 10 minutes q.i.d. with light massage over the lesion.

2. Consider a topical antibiotic (e.g., bacitracin or erythromycin ointment b.i.d.).

3. If the chalazion fails to resolve after 3 to 4 weeks of appropriate medical therapy and the patient wishes to have it removed, inci-

sion and curettage are performed. Occasionally an injection of steroid (e.g., 0.2 to 1.0 mL of triamcinolone, 40 mg/mL, usually mixed 1:1 with 2% lidocaine with epinephrine) into the lesion is performed instead of minor surgery, especially if the chalazion is near the lacrimal apparatus. The total dosage depends on the size of the lesion. All recurrent or unusual chalazia must be sampled for biopsy.

Note: A steroid injection can lead to permanent depigmentation or atrophy of the skin at the injection site.

FOLLOW-UP

Patients are not seen after instituting medical therapy unless the lesion persists beyond 3 to 4 weeks. Patients who have incision and curettage are usually reexamined in 1 week or as needed.

6.2 ECTROPION

SYMPTOMS

Tearing, eye or eyelid irritation. May be asymptomatic.

SIGNS

Critical. Outward turning of the eyelid margin.

Other. Superficial punctate keratitis (SPK) from corneal exposure; conjunctival injection, thickening, and eventual keratinization from chronic conjunctival dryness. Scarring of skin may be seen in cicatricial cases. Facial hemiparesis and lagophthalmus may be seen in paralytic cases.

ETIOLOGY

• Involutional (Aging).

• Paralytic (Seventh nerve palsy).

• Cicatricial (Due to chemical burn, surgery, eyelid laceration scar, skin diseases, and others).

• Mechanical (Due to herniated orbital fat, eyelid tumor, and others).

• Allergic (Contact dermatitis).

• Congenital (Facial dysmorphic syndromes or isolated abnormality).

WORKUP

1. History: Previous surgery, trauma, chemical burn, or seventh nerve palsy?

2. External examination: Check orbicularis oculi function, look for an eyelid tumor, eyelid scarring, herniated orbital fat, and other causes.

3. Slit-lamp examination: Check for SPK due to exposure and evaluate conjunctival integrity.

TREATMENT

1. Treat exposure keratopathy with lubricating agents (see 4.5, Exposure Keratopathy).

2. Treat an inflamed, exposed eyelid margin with warm compresses and antibiotic ointment (e.g., bacitracin or erythromycin t.i.d.). A short course of combination antibiotic–steroid ointment (e.g., sulfacetamide/prednisolone acetate) may be helpful if close follow-up is ensured.

3. Taping the eyelids into position with adhesive tape may be a temporizing measure.

4. Definitive treatment usually requires surgery. Surgery is delayed for 3 to 6 months in patients with a seventh nerve palsy because the ectropion may resolve spontaneously (see 10.8, Isolated Seventh Nerve Palsy).

FOLLOW-UP

Patients with signs of corneal or conjunctival drying are examined in 1 to 2 weeks to evaluate the efficacy of therapy. Otherwise, follow-up is not urgent.

6.3 ENTROPION

SYMPTOMS

Ocular irritation, foreign body sensation, tearing, redness.

SIGNS

Critical. Inward turning of the eyelid margin that pushes otherwise normal lashes onto the globe.

Other. SPK from eyelashes contacting the cornea, conjunctival injection. In severe cases, corneal thinning and ulceration are possible.

ETIOLOGY

- Involutional (Aging).

- Cicatricial (Due to conjunctival scarring in ocular cicatricial pemphigoid, Stevens–Johnson syndrome, chemical burns, trauma, trachoma, and others).

- Spastic (Due to surgical trauma, ocular irritation, or blepharospasm).

- Congenital

WORKUP

1. History: Previous surgery, trauma, chemical burn, severe eye disease?

2. Slit-lamp examination: Check for corneal involvement as well as conjunctival and eyelid scarring.

TREATMENT

If blepharospasm is present, see 6.6, Blepharospasm.

1. Antibiotic ointment (e.g., erythromycin or bacitracin t.i.d.) for SPK.

2. Everting the eyelid margin away from the globe and taping it in place with adhesive tape may be a temporizing measure.

3. For spastic ectropion, a Quickert suture may be placed at bedside or office immediately to resolve the eyelid malposition.

4. Surgery is often required for permanent correction.

FOLLOW-UP

If the cornea is relatively healthy, the condition does not require urgent attention. If the cornea is significantly damaged, aggressive treatment is indicated (see 4.1, Superficial Punctate Keratitis).

6.4 TRICHIASIS

SYMPTOMS

Ocular irritation, foreign-body sensation, tearing, redness.

SIGNS

Critical. Misdirected eyelashes rubbing against the globe.

Other. SPK, conjunctival injection.

DIFFERENTIAL DIAGNOSIS

- Entropion (Inward turning of the entire eyelid margin that pushes otherwise normal lashes onto the globe. See 6.3, Entropion.).

- Epiblepharon (Congenital or familial condition in which an extra lower eyelid skin fold redirects lashes into a vertical position, where they may contact the globe. Most common in Asian children.).

- Distichiasis (Aberrant second row of lashes that emanates from meibomian gland openings. Most commonly acquired in the setting of chronic inflammation. Rarely congenital.).

ETIOLOGY

- Idiopathic

- Chronic blepharitis (Thickened, crusted, erythematous, or inflamed eyelid margin with mild discharge and telangiectatic blood vessels. See 5.8, Blepharitis/Meibomianitis.).

- Cicatricial (Due to eyelid scarring from trauma, surgery, ocular cicatricial pemphigoid, trachoma, and others.).

WORKUP

1. History: Recurrent episodes? Severe systemic illness in the past? Previous trauma?

2. Slit-lamp examination: Evert the eyelids and inspect the palpebral conjunctiva. Check the cornea for abrasions and SPK.

TREATMENT

1. Epilation: Remove the misdirected lashes.

   —A few misdirected lashes: Remove them at the slit lamp with fine forceps. Recurrence is common, and cooperative patients may be instructed to epilate themselves carefully at home.

   —Diffuse, severe, or recurrent trichiasis: Can attempt to epilate as described; however, definitive therapy usually requires electrolysis, cryotherapy, or surgery.

2. Treat SPK with antibiotic ointment (e.g., erythromycin or bacitracin t.i.d.) for several days.

3. Treat any underlying blepharitis (see 5.8, Blepharitis/Meibomianitis).

FOLLOW-UP

As needed based on symptoms if the cornea is healthy. Closer follow-up is needed if evidence of SPK or corneal abrasion.

6.5 FLOPPY EYELID SYNDROME

SYMPTOMS

Chronically red, irritated eye with mild mucous discharge, often worst on awakening from sleep. Often unilateral but may be bilateral. Patients are typically obese with short, thick necks and sleep apnea syndrome.

SIGNS

Critical. Upper eyelids are easily everted without an accessory finger or cotton-tipped applicator exerting counterpressure.

Other. Soft and rubbery superior tarsal plate, superior tarsal papillary conjunctivitis, SPK, ptosis. May have associated keratoconus.

DIFFERENTIAL DIAGNOSIS

All of the following may produce superior tarsal papillary conjunctivitis, but none has eyelids that evert as easily as described above.

- Vernal conjunctivitis (Seasonal, itching, ropy discharge, giant papillary reaction. See 5.2, Chronic Conjunctivitis.).

- Giant papillary conjunctivitis (Often related to contact lens wear or an exposed suture. See 4.20, Contact Lens–Induced Giant Papillary Conjunctivitis.).

- Superior limbic keratoconjunctivitis (Hyperemia and thickening of the superior bulbar conjunctiva, often with filaments and corneal pannus. See 5.4, Superior Limbic Keratoconjunctivitis.).

• Toxic keratoconjunctivitis (Papillae or follicles are usually more abundant on the inferior tarsal conjunctiva in a patient using eye drops. See 5.2, Chronic Conjunctivitis.).

ETIOLOGY

The symptoms are thought to result from spontaneous eversion of the upper eyelid during sleep, allowing the superior palpebral conjunctiva to rub against a pillow or sheets. Unilateral symptoms are often on the side on which the patient predominantly sleeps.

WORKUP

1. Pull the skin of the upper eyelid toward the patient's forehead, and watch to see if the eyelid spontaneously everts or is abnormally lax.

2. Conduct slit-lamp examination of the cornea and conjunctiva with fluorescein staining, looking for upper palpebral conjunctival papillae and SPK.

3. Ask family members whether patient snores severely.

TREATMENT

1. Topical antibiotics or lubricants for any mild corneal or conjunctival abnormality (e.g., erythromycin ointment b.i.d. to t.i.d.). May change to artificial tear ointment (e.g., Refresh PM q.h.s.) when corneal lesion resolves.

2. The eyelids may be taped closed during sleep, or an eye shield may be worn to protect the eyelid from rubbing against the pillow or bed. Patients are asked to refrain from sleeping face down. Asking patients to sleep on their contralateral side may be therapeutic as well as diagnostic.

3. An eyelid-tightening surgical procedure is often required.

FOLLOW-UP

1. Every 2 to 7 days initially, and then every few weeks to months as the condition stabilizes.

2. Refer to an internist, otolaryngologist, or pulmonologist for evaluation and management of possible sleep apnea syndrome. This evaluation is an important step in anesthesia risk assessment before eyelid surgery.

6.6 BLEPHAROSPASM

SYMPTOMS

Uncontrolled blinking, twitching, or closure of the eyelids. Always bilateral, but may briefly be unilateral at first onset.

SIGNS

Critical. Bilateral, episodic, involuntary contractions of the orbicularis oculi muscles.

Other. Disappears during sleep. May have uncontrollable orofacial, head, and neck movements (Meige syndrome).

DIFFERENTIAL DIAGNOSIS

• Hemifacial spasm [Unilateral contractures of the entire side of the face that do not disappear during sleep. Usually idiopathic, but may be related to prior cranial nerve VII palsy or injury at the level of the brainstem. Magnetic resonance imaging (MRI) of the cerebellopontine angle should be obtained in all patients because tumor is the underlying etiology in approximately 1% of cases. Treatment options include observation, botulinum toxin injections, or neurosurgical decompression of cranial nerve VII by the Jannetta procedure.].

- Tourette syndrome (Multiple compulsive muscle spasms associated with utterances of bizarre sounds or obscenities.).

- Tic douloureux (trigeminal neuralgia) (Acute episodes of pain in the distribution of the fifth cranial nerve, often causing a wince or tic.).

- Tardive dyskinesia (Orofacial dyskinesia, often with restlessness and dystonic movements of the trunk and limbs, typically from long-term use of antipsychotic medications.).

- Eyelid myokymia (Eyelid twitches, often brought on by stress and caffeine. Usually unilateral lower eyelid involvement. Typically self-limited. Can also be secondary to aberrant regeneration of cranial nerve VII after a facial palsy. In such cases, the twitching is sometimes associated with speaking or chewing.).

ETIOLOGY

- Idiopathic

- Ocular irritation (e.g., corneal or conjunctival foreign body, trichiasis, blepharitis, dry eye).

WORKUP

1. History: Unilateral or bilateral? Are the eyelids alone involved, or are the facial and limb muscles also involved? Medications?

2. Slit-lamp examination: Search for a local ocular disorder such as dry eyes, blepharitis, or a foreign body.

3. Neuroophthalmic examination to rule out other accompanying abnormalities.

4. MRI of the brain with attention to the posterior fossa in atypical cases.

TREATMENT

1. Treat any underlying eye disorder causing ocular irritation (See 4.3, Dry-Eye Syndrome and 5.8, Blepharitis/Meibomianitis.).

2. Consider botulinum toxin injections into the orbicularis muscles around the eyelids if the blepharospasm is severe.

3. If the spasm is not relieved with botulinum toxin injections, consider surgical excision of the orbicularis muscle from the upper eyelids and brow.

FOLLOW-UP

Not an urgent condition, but with severe blepharospasm, patients can be functionally blind.

6.7 CANALICULITIS

SYMPTOMS

Tearing or discharge, red eye, mild tenderness over the nasal aspect of the lower or upper eyelid.

SIGNS

Critical. Erythematous pouting of the punctum, erythema of the skin surrounding the punctum. Mucopurulent discharge or concretions may be expressed from the punctum when pressure is applied over the lacrimal sac in the nasal corner of the lower eyelid. Focal injection of the nasal conjunctiva is sometimes present.

Other. Recurrent conjunctivitis confined to the nasal aspect of the eye, gritty sensation on probing of the canaliculus.

DIFFERENTIAL DIAGNOSIS

- Dacryocystitis (Much more lacrimal sac swelling, tenderness, and pain than canaliculitis. Swelling of the skin is more prominent than pouting of the punctum. See 6.8, Dacryocystitis.).

- Nasolacrimal duct obstruction (Tearing, minimal to no erythema or tenderness around the punctum. Probing and irrigation of the lacrimal system are diagnostic. See 8.10, Congenital Nasolacrimal Duct Obstruction.).

- Conjunctivitis (Conjunctival follicles and/or papillae, discharge. No punctal pouting or discharge. See 5.1, Acute Conjunctivitis, and 5.2, Chronic Conjunctivitis.).

ETIOLOGY

- *Actinomyces israelii* (streptothrix) (Most common. Gram-positive rod with fine, branching filaments seen on Gram stain.).

- Other bacteria (e.g., *Fusobacterium* and *Nocardia* species).

- Fungal (e.g., *Candida*, *Fusarium*, and *Aspergillus* species).

- Viral (e.g., herpes simplex and varicella zoster).

WORKUP

1. Apply gentle pressure over the lacrimal sac with a cotton-tipped swab and roll it toward the punctum while observing for punctal discharge.

2. Smears and cultures of the material expressed from the punctum, including slides for Gram stain and Giemsa stain. Consider thioglycolate and Sabouraud cultures.

TREATMENT

1. Remove obstructing concretions. Can try expressing the concretions through the punctum at the slit lamp, but a surgical canaliculotomy (with marsupialization of the canaliculus) is usually required to remove them all.

2. After removing the concretions, irrigate the canaliculus with penicillin G solution 100,000 units/mL, or iodine 1% solution. The patient is irrigated while in the upright position so the solution drains out of the nose and not into the nasopharynx.

3. If a fungus is found on smears and cultures, nystatin 1:20,000 drops, t.i.d., and nystatin 1:20,000 solution, irrigation several times per week, may be effective. If evidence of herpes virus is found on smears, treat with trifluridine 1% drops (e.g., Viroptic) five times per day. Silicone intubation along with appropriate antiviral therapy is sometimes required in viral canaliculitis.

4. Apply warm compresses to the punctal area q.i.d.

5. More extensive surgical treatment is occasionally required.

FOLLOW-UP

This is usually not an urgent condition.

6.8 DACRYOCYSTITIS

(INFLAMMATION OF THE LACRIMAL SAC)

SYMPTOMS

Pain, redness, and swelling over the lacrimal sac in the innermost aspect of the lower eyelid. Also tearing, discharge, or fever. Symptoms may be recurrent.

SIGNS

Critical. Erythematous, tender, tense swelling centered over the nasal aspect of the lower eyelid and extending around the periorbital area nasally. A mucoid or purulent discharge can be expressed from the punctum when pressure is applied over the lacrimal sac.

Note: Swelling in dacryocystitis is below the medial canthal tendon. Suspect lacrimal sac tumor (rare) if mass is above the medial canthal tendon.

Other. Fistula formation from the skin beneath the medial canthal tendon. A lacrimal sac cyst or mucocele can occur in chronic cases. Can progress to a lacrimal sac abscess, and rarely orbital or facial cellulitis may develop.

DIFFERENTIAL DIAGNOSIS

• Facial cellulitis involving the medial canthus (Discharge cannot be expressed from the punctum by placing pressure over the lacrimal sac. The lacrimal drainage system is patent on irrigation and special lacrimal drainage system radiographic studies. See 6.10, Preseptal Cellulitis.).

• Dacryocystocele (Mild enlargement of a noninflamed lacrimal sac in an infant. Present at birth but may not be detected until later. Caused by nasolacrimal duct obstruction or entrapment of mucus or amniotic fluid in the lacrimal sac. Usually unilateral, but, if bilateral, breathing must be assessed to rule out nasal obstruction. Conservative therapy with antibiotic ointment and warm compresses is usually sufficient for nonobstructive cases.).

• Acute ethmoid sinusitis (Pain, tenderness, and erythema over the nasal bone, just medial to the inner canthus. Frontal headache and nasal obstruction are common. Patients are often febrile.).

• Acute frontal sinusitis (Inflammation predominantly involves the upper eyelid. The forehead is tender on palpation.).

ETIOLOGY

• Almost always related to nasolacrimal duct obstruction.

• Less commonly due to diverticula of the lacrimal sac, dacryoliths, nasal or sinus surgery, trauma, or, rarely, a lacrimal sac tumor.

• The most common organisms found are staphylococci, streptococci, and diphtheroids.

WORKUP

1. History: Previous episodes? Concomitant ear, nose, or throat infection?

2. External examination: Apply gentle pressure to the lacrimal sac in the nasal corner of the lower eyelid with a cotton-tipped swab in an attempt to express discharge from the punctum. This should be performed bilaterally to uncover a subtle contralateral dacryocystitis.

3. Ocular examination: Assess extraocular motility and possible proptosis for evidence of orbital cellulitis.

4. Obtain a Gram stain and blood agar culture (and chocolate agar culture in children) of any discharge expressed from the punctum.

5. Consider a computed tomography (CT) scan (axial and coronal views) of the orbit and paranasal sinuses in atypical cases, severe cases, and cases that do not respond to appropriate antibiotics.

Note: Do not attempt to probe or irrigate the lacrimal system during the acute stage of the infection.

TREATMENT

1. Systemic antibiotics in the following regimen

Children:

—Afebrile, systemically well, mild case, and reliable parent: Amoxicillin/clavulanate (e.g., Augmentin) 20 to 40 mg/kg/day orally (p.o.), in three divided doses.

—Alternative treatment: Cefaclor (e.g., Ceclor) 20 to 40 mg/kg/day p.o., in three divided doses.

—Febrile, acutely ill, moderate to severe case, or unreliable parent: Hospitalize and treat with cefuroxime, 50 to 100 mg/kg/day intravenously (i.v.), in three divided doses.

Adults:

—Afebrile, systemically well, mild case, and reliable patient: Cephalexin (e.g., Keflex) 500 mg p.o., q6h.

—Alternative treatment: Amoxicillin/clavulanate (e.g., Augmentin) 500 mg p.o., q8h.

—Febrile, acutely ill: Hospitalize and treat with cefazolin (e.g., Ancef), 1 g i.v. q8h.

—Alternative treatment: See 7.4, Orbital Cellulitis.

The antibiotic regimen is adjusted according to the clinical response and the culture and sensitivity results. The i.v. antibiotics can be changed to comparable p.o. antibiotics depending on the rate of improvement, but systemic antibiotic therapy should be continued for a full 10- to 14-day course.

2. Topical antibiotic drops [e.g., trimethoprim/polymyxin B (e.g., Polytrim), q.i.d.] may be used in addition to systemic therapy. Topical therapy alone is not adequate.

3. Apply warm compresses and gentle massage to the inner canthal region q.i.d..

4. Administer pain medication (e.g., acetaminophen with or without codeine) p.r.n.

5. Consider incision and drainage of a pointing abscess.

6. Consider surgical correction (e.g., dacryocystorhinostomy with silicone intubation) once the acute episode has resolved, particularly with chronic dacryocystitis.

FOLLOW-UP

Daily until improvement confirmed. If the condition of an outpatient worsens, hospitalization and i.v. antibiotics are recommended.

6.9 ACUTE INFECTIOUS DACRYOADENITIS
(INFECTION OF THE LACRIMAL GLAND)

SYMPTOMS

Unilateral pain, redness, and swelling over the outer one third of the upper eyelid, often with tearing or discharge. Typically occurs in children and young adults.

SIGNS

Critical. Erythema, swelling, and tenderness over the outer one third of the upper eyelid. May be associated with hyperemia of the palpebral lobe of the lacrimal gland.

Other. Ipsilateral preauricular lymphadenopathy, ipsilateral conjunctival chemosis temporally, fever, elevated white blood cell count (WBC).

DIFFERENTIAL DIAGNOSIS

• Chalazion (A palpable subcutaneous nodule or a blocked meibomian orifice may be present, afebrile, normal WBC. See 6.1, Chalazion/Hordeolum.).

• Adenoviral conjunctivitis (May produce eyelid swelling and erythema with preauricular lymphadenopathy and discharge. Typically produces inferior tarsal conjunctival follicles, often bilateral. See 5.1, Acute Conjunctivitis.).

• Preseptal cellulitis (Erythema, edema, and warmth of the eyelids and surrounding soft tissue. May have a periorbital skin laceration or site of infection. See 6.10, Preseptal Cellulitis.).

- Orbital cellulitis (Proptosis and limitation of ocular motility often accompany eyelid erythema and swelling. See 7.4, Orbital Cellulitis.).

- Orbital pseudotumor involving more than just the lacrimal gland (No preauricular lymphadenopathy. May have concomitant proptosis, downward displacement of the globe, or limitation of ocular motility. Typically afebrile with a normal WBC. Does not respond to antibiotics but improves dramatically with systemic steroids. See 7.3, Orbital Inflammatory Pseudotumor.).

- Rhabdomyosarcoma (Most common pediatric orbital malignancy. Presentation similar to orbital pseudotumor. See 7.5, Orbital Tumors in Children.).

- Malignant lacrimal gland tumor (Commonly produces displacement of the globe or proptosis. Often palpable, evident on CT scan. See 7.7, Lacrimal Gland Mass/Chronic Dacryoadenitis.).

ETIOLOGY

- Inflammatory (By far the most common. More indolent course in lymphoid proliferation and sarcoidosis. More acute presentation in orbital pseudotumor.).

- Bacterial (Rare. Usually due to *Staphylococcus aureus*, *Neisseria gonorrhoeae*, or streptococci.).

- Viral (Seen in mumps, infectious mononucleosis, influenza, and herpes zoster.).

WORKUP

The following is performed when an acute infectious etiology is suspected. When the disease does not respond to medical therapy or another etiology is being considered, see 7.7, Lacrimal Gland Mass/Chronic Dacryoadenitis.

1. History: Acute or chronic? Fever? Discharge? Systemic infection or viral syndrome?

2. Palpate the eyelid and along the orbital rim for a mass.

3. Evaluate the resistance of each globe to retropulsion.

4. Look for proptosis by Hertel exophthalmometry.

5. Complete ocular examination, particularly extraocular motility assessment.

6. Obtain smears and bacterial cultures of any discharge.

7. Examine the parotid glands (Often, but not always, enlarged in mumps, sarcoidosis, tuberculosis, lymphoma, and syphilis.).

8. If the patient is febrile, a complete blood count with differential, and sometimes blood cultures are obtained.

9. Perform CT scan of the orbit and brain (axial and coronal views) with contrast when proptosis or a motility restriction is present or a mass is suspected.

TREATMENT

1. Bacterial or infectious (but unidentified) etiology

   If mild-to-moderate:

   Amoxicillin/clavulanate (e.g., Augmentin)

   Children: 20 to 40 mg/kg/day p.o., in three divided doses.

   Adults: 250 to 500 mg p.o., q8h.

   or

   Cephalexin (e.g., Keflex)

   Children: 25 to 50 mg/kg/day p.o., in four divided doses.

   Adults: 250 to 500 mg p.o., q6h.

   If moderate-to-severe, hospitalize and treat with:

   Ticarcillin/clavulanate (e.g., Timentin)

   Children: 200 mg/kg/day i.v., in four divided doses.

   Adults: 3.1 g i.v., q4–6h.

   or

   Cefazolin (e.g., Ancef)

   Children: 50 to 100 mg/kg/day i.v., in three to four divided doses.

Adults: One g i.v., q8h.

The antibiotic regimen should be adjusted according to the clinical response and culture and sensitivity test results. Intravenous antibiotics can be changed to comparable oral antibiotics depending on the rate of improvement, but systemic antibiotics should be continued for a full 7- to 14-day course. If an abscess develops, incision and drainage are necessary.

2. Viral (e.g., mumps, infectious mononucleosis)

—Cool compresses to the area of swelling and tenderness.

—Analgesic as needed (e.g., acetaminophen 650 mg p.o., q4h p.r.n.).

3. Inflammatory

—See treatment for 7.3, Orbital Inflammatory Pseudotumor.

—Analgesic as needed.

Note: Do not give aspirin to children with a viral syndrome because of the risk of Reye syndrome.

FOLLOW-UP

Daily until improvement confirmed. Watch for signs of orbital involvement, such as decreased motility or proptosis. Outpatients are admitted to the hospital for i.v. antibiotic therapy and an orbital CT scan if the condition worsens. Patients who fail to respond to medical therapy are managed similarly to those with chronic dacryoadenitis (See 7.7, Lacrimal Gland Mass/Chronic Dacryoadenitis.).

6.10 PRESEPTAL CELLULITIS

SYMPTOMS

Tenderness, redness, and swelling of the eyelid and periorbital area. Often history of sinusitis or local skin abrasions and insect bites. May be a mild fever.

SIGNS

Critical. Eyelid erythema, tense edema, warmth, tenderness. No proptosis, no optic neuropathy, no restriction of extraocular motility, and no pain with eye movement (unlike orbital cellulitis). The patient may not be able to open the eye because of the eyelid edema.

Other. Tightness of the eyelid skin or fluctuant lymphedema of the eyelids. The eye itself may be slightly injected but is relatively uninvolved.

DIFFERENTIAL DIAGNOSIS

• Orbital cellulitis (Proptosis, pain with eye movement, restricted motility, decreased sensa-

tion along the first division of the trigeminal nerve, decreased vision, fever, or chemosis. See 7.4, Orbital Cellulitis.).

• Other orbital disorders (Proptosis, globe displacement, or restricted ocular motility. See 7.1, Orbital Disease.).

• Necrotizing fasciitis (Due to group A β-hemolytic *Streptococcus*. Rapidly progressive with eschar formation and sepsis. Typically grayish–purplish discoloration of the eyelids with local hypesthesia or anesthesia. Emergency debridement may be necessary.).

• Chalazion (Focal eyelid inflammation, palpable mass, inspissated meibomian gland. See 6.1, Chalazion/Hordeolum.).

• Allergic eyelid swelling (Sudden onset, bright-red eyelid discoloration, prominent itching, absence of tenderness, positive history of contact allergies or new eye or skin medication. More often bilateral with boggy edema. See 5.11, Contact Dermatitis.).

• Viral conjunctivitis with eyelid swelling (Conjunctival follicles, palpable preauricular lymph node, itching, tearing, eyelid sticking, or watery discharge. See 5.1, Acute Conjunctivitis.).

• Cavernous sinus thrombosis (Proptosis; paresis of the third, fourth, and sixth cranial nerves out of proportion with the eyelid swelling; decreased sensation of the first and second division of the trigeminal nerve; chemosis; conjunctival hyperemia; typically bilateral. See 10.9, Cavernous Sinus and Associated Syndromes.).

• Erysipelas (Rapidly advancing streptococcal cellulitis, often with a clear demarcation line, high fever, and chills.).

• Ocular vaccinia (From recent smallpox vaccination or from contact with recent vaccinees. Results in unilateral or bilateral erythema and edema of the eyelids. Often accompanied by blepharoconjunctivitis, skin vesicles, or keratitis. See 4.29, Ocular Vaccinia.).

• Others (Insect bite, angioedema, trauma, maxillary osteomyelitis, and others.).

ETIOLOGY

• Adjacent infection (e.g., extension from sinusitis or dacryocystitis).

• Trauma (e.g., after puncture wound, laceration, insect bite).

ORGANISMS

S. aureus and streptococci are most common, but *Haemophilus influenzae* should be considered in nonimmunized children. Suspect anaerobes if a foul-smelling discharge or necrosis is present or there is a history of an animal or human bite. Consider a viral cause if preseptal cellulitis is associated with a skin rash (e.g., herpes simplex or herpes zoster).

WORKUP

1. History: Pain with eye movements? Prior trauma or cancer? Sinus congestion or purulent nasal discharge? Recent smallpox vaccine?

2. Complete ocular examination: Look carefully for restriction of ocular motility or proptosis. An eyelid speculum or Desmarres eyelid retractor may facilitate the ocular examination if the eyelids are excessively swollen.

3. Check facial sensation in the distribution of first and second divisions of the trigeminal nerve.

4. Palpate the periorbital area and the head and neck lymph nodes for a mass.

5. Check vital signs.

6. Obtain Gram stain and culture of any open wound or drainage.

7. Perform CT scan of the brain and orbits (axial and coronal views) with contrast if there is a history of significant trauma or a concern about the possibility of an orbital or intraocular foreign body, orbital cellulitis, a subperiosteal abscess, paranasal sinusitis, cavernous sinus thrombosis, or cancer.

8. Consider obtaining a complete blood count with differential and blood cultures in severe cases or when a fever is present.

TREATMENT

1. Antibiotic therapy

   a. Mild preseptal cellulitis, older than 5 years, afebrile, reliable patient/parent:

   Amoxicillin/clavulanate (e.g., Augmentin)

   Children: 20 to 40 mg/kg/day p.o., in three divided doses.

   Adults: 500 mg p.o., q8h.

   or

   Cefaclor (e.g., Ceclor)

   Children: 20 to 40 mg/kg/day p.o., in three divided doses; maximum dose, 1 g/day.

   Adults: 250 to 500 mg, p.o. q8h.

   If the patient is allergic to penicillin, then

Trimethoprim/sulfamethoxazole (e.g., Bactrim)

Children: 8 to 12 mg/kg/day trimethoprim with 40 to 60 mg/kg/day sulfamethoxazole, p.o., in two divided doses.

Adults: 160 to 320 mg trimethoprim with 800 to 1,600 mg sulfamethoxazole (1 to 2 double strength tablets), p.o. b.i.d.

Note: Oral antibiotics are maintained for 10 days.

b. Moderate to severe preseptal cellulitis, or any one of the following:

- Patient appears toxic.

- Patient may be noncompliant with outpatient treatment and follow-up.

- Child 5 years of age or younger.

- No noticeable improvement, or worsening after a few days of oral antibiotics.

Admit to the hospital for i.v. antibiotics as follows

Ampicillin/sulbactam (e.g., Unasyn)

Children: 100 to 200 mg/kg/day i.v., in four divided doses.

Adults: 1.5 to 3.0 g i.v., q6h.

or

Ceftriaxone (e.g., Rocephin)

Children: 100 mg/kg/day i.v., in two divided doses.

Adults: 1 to 2 g i.v., q12h.

or if methicillin-resistant S. aureus is suspected as the underlying etiology

Vancomycin

Neonates: 15 mg/kg load, then 10 mg/kg q12h.

Children: 40 mg/kg/day i.v., in three to four divided doses.

Adults: 0.5 to 1 g i.v., q12h.

Note: Intravenous antibiotics can be changed to comparable oral antibiotics after significant improvement is observed. Systemic antibiotics are maintained for a complete 10- to 14-day course. See 7.4, Orbital Cellulitis, for alternative treatment.

2. Warm compresses to the inflamed area t.i.d., p.r.n.

3. Polymyxin B/bacitracin ointment (e.g., Polysporin) to the eye q.i.d., if secondary conjunctivitis is present.

4. Tetanus toxoid if needed (see Appendix 10).

5. Nasal decongestants if sinusitis is present.

6. Exploration and debridement of the lesion if a fluctuant mass or abscess is present. Incise over the mass or reopen a healing laceration with a scalpel, fully explore the wound, and Gram stain and culture any drainage. Avoid the orbital septum if possible. A drain may need to be placed.

FOLLOW-UP

Daily until clear and consistent improvement is demonstrated, then every 2 to 7 days until the condition has totally resolved. If a preseptal cellulitis progresses despite antibiotic therapy, the patient is admitted to the hospital and a repeated (or initial) orbital CT scan is obtained. For patients taking p.o. antibiotics, i.v. antibiotic treatment is started (see 7.4, Orbital Cellulitis). Consultation with an infectious disease specialist may be helpful.

6.11 MALIGNANT TUMORS OF THE EYELID

SYMPTOMS

Asymptomatic or mildly irritating eyelid lump.

SIGNS

Skin ulceration and inflammation with distortion of the normal eyelid anatomy are common findings in malignant lesions. Abnormal color, texture, or persistent bleeding suggests malignancy. Loss of eyelashes (madarosis) or whitening of eyelashes (poliosis) over the lesion may occur. Feeder vessels may be seen.

DIFFERENTIAL DIAGNOSIS

(Benign eyelid masses)

• Seborrheic keratosis (Middle-aged or elderly patients. Brown–black, well-circumscribed, crustlike lesion, usually elevated slightly and uninflamed. May be removed by shave biopsy if desired.).

• Hordeolum (Acute, erythematous, tender, well-circumscribed lesion, often associated with blepharitis. See 6.1, Chalazion/Hordeolum.).

• Chalazion (A chronically obstructed meibomian gland. See 6.1, Chalazion/Hordeolum.).

• Keratoacanthoma (1 to 2 cm, elevated with a large central ulcer. Can resemble basal and squamous cell carcinomas. Rapid growth with slow regression and even spontaneous resolution is distinctive. Lesions that involve the eyelid or eyelash margin can be destructive and are excised.).

• Cysts (Well-circumscribed white or yellow lesions on the eyelid margin or underneath the skin. Ultrasound may help differentiate a cyst from a solid lesion. Epidermal inclusion cysts, sebaceous cysts, and eccrine and apocrine hydrocystomas may be excised.).

• Molluscum contagiosum (Frequently multiple small papules with umbilicated centers. Viral in origin. Found mostly in younger patients, but can be severe in human immunodeficiency virus–positive patients. May produce a chronic follicular conjunctivitis. If treatment is desired, these lesions are usually surgically excised, but cryotherapy or other methods may also be used. See 5.2, Chronic Conjunctivitis.).

• Nevus (Light to dark brown, sometimes amelanotic, well-circumscribed lesion, sometimes with hair arising from the surface. It does not grow in size.).

• Xanthelasma (Multiple, often bilateral, soft yellow plaques of lipid in the upper and sometimes the lower eyelids. Patients younger than 40 years of age should have a serum cholesterol and lipid profile evaluation to rule out hypercholesterolemia. Diabetes also may be present. Surgical excision can be performed as desired for cosmesis.).

• Squamous papilloma (Soft, elevated, or flat, benign skin-colored lesion. May enlarge slowly over time. Often spontaneously regresses. Some squamous carcinomas can appear papillomatous. Excisional biopsy should be performed for suggestive lesions.).

• Actinic keratosis (Round, premalignant lesion with scaly surface. Found in sun-exposed areas of skin. Treated with excisional biopsy.).

• Others (Verrucae from human papillomavirus, benign tumors of hair follicles or sweat glands, inverted follicular keratosis, neurofibroma, neurilemoma, capillary hemangioma, cavernous hemangioma, and pseudoepitheliomatous hyperplasia. Necrobiotic xanthogranuloma nodules of multiple myeloma appear as yellow plaques or nodules often mistaken for xanthelasma.).

ETIOLOGY

• Basal cell carcinoma (Most common malignant eyelid tumor, usually occurs on the lower eyelid of middle-aged or elderly patients. Rarely metastasizes, but may be locally invasive, particularly when it is present in the medial canthal region.) There are two forms:

Nodular. Indurated, firm mass, commonly with telangiectases over the tumor margins. Sometimes the center of the lesion is ulcerated.

Morpheaform. Firm, flat, subcutaneous lesion with indistinct borders.

—Squamous cell carcinoma (Variable presentation, often appearing similar to a basal cell carcinoma. Metastasis may occur but is uncommon. A premalignant lesion, actinic keratosis, may appear as a scaly, erythematous flat lesion or as a cutaneous horn.).

—Sebaceous gland carcinoma (Usually occurs in middle-aged or elderly patients. Most common on the upper eyelid, but may be multifocal, involving both the upper and lower eyelids. Often confused with recurrent chalazia or intractable blepharitis. Loss of eyelashes and destruction of the meibomian gland orifices in the region of the tumor may occur. Metastasis or orbital extension is possible.).

—Others (Malignant melanoma; lymphoma; sweat gland carcinoma; metastasis, usually breast or lung; and others.).

WORKUP

1. History: How long has the lesion been present? Rapid or slow growth? Previous malignant skin lesion?

2. External examination: Check the skin for additional lesions, palpate the preauricular and submaxillary nodes for metastasis.

3. Slit-lamp examination: Look for telangiectases on nodular tumors, evaluate for loss of eyelashes in the region of the tumor, and inspect the meibomian orifices to determine whether they have been destroyed. Eyelid eversion is important in all patients with eyelid complaints.

4. Photograph or draw the lesion and its location for documentation.

5. Perform a biopsy of the lesion: An incisional biopsy is most commonly performed when a malignancy is suspected, although an exci-

sional biopsy with wide margins on all sides is preferable to detect malignant melanoma. Margins of potential malignant melanoma are sent for permanent section. Histopathologic confirmation must precede any extensive procedures.

6. When a sebaceous gland carcinoma is suspected, the pathologist should be alerted, and frozen or nonfixed tissue must be obtained for lipid stains (e.g., oil red-O). Patients confirmed to have this tumor are referred to a medical internist for a metastatic workup with attention to the lymph nodes, lungs, brain, liver, and bone.

TREATMENT

1. **Basal cell carcinoma:** Surgical excision with histologic evaluation of the tumor margins either by frozen sections or Mohs techniques. Cryotherapy and radiation are used rarely. Patients are informed about the etiologic role of the sun and are advised to avoid sunlight when possible and to use protective sunscreens.

2. **Squamous cell carcinoma:** Same as for basal cell carcinoma. Radiation therapy is the second-best treatment after surgical excision. Patients are informed about the etiologic role of the sun. Referral to oncologist or internist for systemic workup and surveillance is important.

3. **Sebaceous gland carcinoma:** Surgical excision, taking wide margins of normal tissue on all sides. Not responsive to radiation. Frozen-section evaluation of the margins is recommended. Referral to oncologist or internist for systemic workup and surveillance is important.

FOLLOW-UP

Initial follow-up is every 1 to 4 weeks to ensure proper healing of the surgical site. Patients are then reevaluated every 6 to 12 months. Patients who have had one skin malignancy are at greater risk for additional malignancies.

CHAPTER 7

ORBIT

7.1 ORBITAL DISEASE

This introductory section provides an overview to aid in distinguishing a variety of orbital diseases. Specific details on individual disease entities are covered in the remainder of the chapter.

SYMPTOMS

Eyelid swelling, bulging eye(s), and double vision are common. Pain and decreased vision can occur.

SIGNS

Critical. Proptosis and restriction of ocular motility, which can be confirmed by forced duction testing (see Appendix 5). There is often resistance on attempted retropulsion of the globe.

Other. See the individual entities.

DIFFERENTIAL DIAGNOSIS

• Arteriovenous fistula (e.g., carotid–cavernous fistula) [May mimic orbital disease. It follows trauma or can occur spontaneously. A bruit is sometimes heard by the patient and may be detected if ocular auscultation is performed. Arterialized conjunctival vessels and chemosis may be present. Computed tomography (CT) scan: Enlarged superior ophthalmic vein, sometimes accompanied by enlarged extraocular muscles. Orbital color Doppler ultrasonography: reversed, arterialized flow in superior ophthalmic vein.].

• Cavernous sinus thrombosis (Orbital cellulitis signs, plus decreased sensation of the fifth cranial nerve, dilated and sluggish pupil, paresis of the third, fourth, and sixth cranial nerves out of proportion to the degree of orbital edema, decreasing level of consciousness, nausea, and vomiting. Usually bilateral with rapid progression.).

• Cranial nerve palsy (May produce mild proptosis with limitation of eye movement in specific directions. No resistance to retropulsion, negative forced-duction testing result. Orbital CT scan is negative.).

• Enlarged globe (e.g., myopia) (May produce pseudoproptosis. Large, myopic eyes frequently have tilted discs and peripapillary crescents, and ultrasonography reveals a long axial length.).

• Enophthalmos of the fellow eye (e.g., after an orbital floor fracture). (May produce pseudoproptosis.).

ETIOLOGY

One or more of the critical signs is usually present, but it is the specific characteristics listed that help to distinguish the individual entities.

- Thyroid eye disease (Eyelid retraction and eyelid lag. Painless unless exposure keratopathy develops. Often bilateral. CT scan: Thickening of the extraocular muscles without involvement of the associated tendons.).

- Orbital inflammatory pseudotumor [Often painful. The patient is usually afebrile with a normal white blood cell count (WBC). CT scan: Extraocular muscles are commonly thickened, with involvement of the associated tendons. The sclera, orbital fat, or lacrimal gland may be involved. Acute disease usually responds dramatically to systemic steroids.].

- Orbital cellulitis (Patients are usually febrile and often have an elevated WBC. CT scan: Sinusitis, especially ethmoid sinusitis, is usually present.).

- Orbital tumors [A palpable mass may be present. The globe may be displaced away from the location of the tumor. CT or magnetic resonance imaging (MRI) scan: A mass lesion is evident.].

- Lacrimal gland tumors (Tumor is located in the outer one third of the upper eyelid. The globe usually is displaced inferiorly and medially with ptosis of the involved eyelid. CT or MRI scan: A mass lesion is present in the lacrimal gland.).

- Trauma (e.g., intraorbital foreign body, retrobulbar hemorrhage) (An intraorbital foreign body may not produce orbital signs for a long period. Retrobulbar hemorrhage can result in optic nerve compression. CT scan with or without orbital ultrasonography can be diagnostic. If wood foreign body is suspected, then MRI is preferred.).

- Orbital vasculitis (e.g., Wegener granulomatosis, polyarteritis nodosa) [Systemic signs and symptoms of vasculitis (especially sinus, renal, pulmonary, and skin disease), fever, markedly increased erythrocyte sedimentation rate (ESR).].

- Mucormycosis (Orbital, nasal, and sinus disease in a diabetic, immunocompromised, or debilitated patient. Rapidly progressive and potentially life-threatening. See 10.9, Cavernous Sinus and Associated Syndromes.).

- Varix [A large, dilated vein in the orbit that produces proptosis when it fills and dilates (e.g., during a Valsalva maneuver or with the head in a dependent position). When the vein is not engorged, the proptosis disappears, and enophthalmos may even be present. CT scan: Demonstrates the dilated vein if an enhanced scan is performed during a Valsalva maneuver. MRI with gadolinium may be done if CT scan is negative.].

WORKUP

1. History: Rapid or slow onset? Pain? Ocular bruit? Fever, chills, systemic symptoms? History of cancer, diabetes, pulmonary disease, or renal disease? Skin rash? Trauma?

2. External examination:

   —Look from over the patient's forehead to examine for proptosis. Measure the amount with a Hertel exophthalmometer. Normal upper limits for proptosis are approximately 22 mm in whites and 24 mm in blacks. There should be no more than a 2-mm difference between the two eyes.

   —Look for displacement of the globe. Measure from the bridge of the nose with a ruler.

   —Test for resistance to retropulsion. Have the patient close his or her eyes while gently pushing each globe back into the orbit with your thumb. Assess the resistance of each eye in the orbit.

   —Feel along the orbital rim for a mass.

   —Measure any ocular misalignment with prisms (see Appendix 2).

3. Ocular examination: Specifically check the pupils, visual fields, color vision (by using color plates), intraocular pressure (IOP), optic nerve, and peripheral retina.

4. Imaging studies: Orbital CT scan (axial and coronal views) or MRI with surface coil, depending on suspected etiology. When ordering CT scans, specify that axial *and* coronal cuts should be performed through the orbits. When ordering MRI, specify performance with surface coil and T1-weighted fat suppression. Occasionally, orbital ultrasonogra-

phy with or without color Doppler imaging is useful if the diagnosis is uncertain or when a cystic or vascular lesion is identified. (See Chapter 14 for more information on ophthalmic imaging.)

5. Vital signs, particularly temperature.

6. Laboratory tests when appropriate: triiodothyronine (T₃), thyroxine (T₄), thyroid-stimulating hormone (TSH), complete blood count (CBC), ESR, antinuclear antibody (ANA), blood urea nitrogen (BUN), creati-

nine, fasting blood sugar, blood cultures, others.

7. Consider a forced-duction test (see Appendix 5 for technique).

8. Consider an excisional, incisional, or fine-needle biopsy, as dictated by the working diagnosis.

Additional workup, treatment, and follow-up vary according to the suspected diagnosis. See individual sections.

7.2 THYROID-RELATED ORBITOPATHY

(GRAVES DISEASE)

OCULAR SYMPTOMS

Prominent eyes, chemosis, eyelid swelling, double vision, foreign body sensation, pain, photophobia, and decreased vision in one or both eyes.

SIGNS

Critical. Retraction of the eyelids, eyelid lag on downward gaze, and, often, unilateral or bilateral proptosis. When extraocular muscles are involved, elevation and abduction are commonly restricted. There is resistance on forced-duction testing. Orbital CT scan shows thickening of the involved extraocular muscles with sparing of the tendon.

Note: Optic nerve compression caused by thickened extraocular muscles at the orbital apex can produce an afferent pupillary defect, reduced color vision, visual field and visual acuity loss. The optic disc may be swollen. Optic nerve compression can develop in the presence of minimal exophthalmos. Involvement of more than one muscle with restriction of both elevation and horizontal eye movements is an indication that the patient is at risk for this complication.

Other. Reduced frequency of blinking (stare), injection of the blood vessels over the insertion sites of involved extraocular muscles, resistance

to retropulsion, superficial punctate keratopathy, or ulceration from exposure keratopathy.

Systemic signs. Hyperthyroidism common [rapid pulse, hot and dry skin, diffusely enlarged thyroid gland (goiter), weight loss, muscle wasting with proximal muscle weakness, hand tremor, pretibial dermopathy or myxedema, and, sometimes, cardiac arrhythmias]. Some patients are euthyroid, and some are hypothyroid taking replacement therapy. Concomitant myasthenia gravis with fluctuating double vision and ptosis is rarely present.

DIFFERENTIAL DIAGNOSIS

See 7.1, Orbital Disease, for conditions that produce proptosis.

• Previous eyelid surgery may produce eyelid retraction or eyelid lag. Rarely, the same eyelid signs may be seen in the following two conditions.

• Third cranial nerve palsy with aberrant regeneration (The upper eyelid may elevate with downward gaze, simulating eyelid lag. Ocular motility may be limited, but results of forced-duction testing and orbital CT scan are normal.).

• Parinaud syndrome (Eyelid retraction and limitation of upward gaze may accompany mildly dilated pupils that react poorly to light, but react normally to convergence.).

WORKUP

See 7.1, Orbital Disease, for a general workup of proptosis of unknown etiology.

1. History: Duration of symptoms? Pain? Known thyroid disease or cancer?

2. Complete ocular examination to establish the diagnosis and to determine whether the patient is developing exposure keratopathy (slit-lamp examination with fluorescein staining) or optic nerve compression (pupillary assessment and evaluation of color vision by using color plates). Diplopia is measured with prisms (see Appendix 2) and proptosis is measured with a Hertel exophthalmometer. Check IOP in both primary and upgaze; thyroid eye disease is associated with increased IOP in upgaze.

3. CT scan of the orbit (axial and coronal views) is performed when the diagnosis is uncertain (e.g., proptosis is present without other signs of thyroid disease) or surgery is planned. Intravenous (i.v.) contrast is *not* needed to establish the diagnosis.

4. Forced-duction testing as needed to establish the diagnosis (see Appendix 5).

5. Formal visual field examination when signs or symptoms of optic nerve compression are present (e.g., Humphrey, Octopus, or Goldmann).

6. Thyroid function tests (T_3, T_4, TSH, selective TSH).

7. Edrophonium chloride (e.g., Tensilon) test for suspected myasthenia gravis (see 10.10, Myasthenia Gravis).

TREATMENT

1. Refer the patient to a medical internist or endocrinologist for management of systemic thyroid disease, if present.

2. Treat exposure keratopathy with artificial tears and lubricating ointment (e.g., Refresh Plus drops q1h to q6h or Refresh PM ointment each evening to t.i.d.) or by taping eye-lids closed at night (see 4.5, Exposure Keratopathy).

3. Elevate the head of the bed at night if eyelid edema is developing.

4. Orbital disease may need to be treated more aggressively when exposure keratopathy is worsening despite treatment (or is already severe), bothersome diplopia is present (particularly when looking straight ahead or reading), or optic nerve compression is developing.

The following recommendations are somewhat controversial:

1. Proptosis and corneal ulceration: Prednisone, 100 mg orally (p.o.), q.d., up to 2 weeks followed by orbital decompression surgery.

2. Acute disturbing double vision with an inflamed eye: Prednisone, 60 to 100 mg p.o., q.d., which may be tapered slowly as the condition improves. If no improvement occurs within 10 days, then quickly taper and discontinue the steroids. Orbital irradiation also may be considered as an alternative to steroid treatment. When thyroid disease is no longer active and orbital disease is stable, extraocular muscle surgery may be performed as needed.

3. Visual loss from optic neuropathy: Treat immediately. Options include prednisone, 100 mg p.o., q.d., radiation therapy, and posterior orbital decompression surgery. Often prednisone is started immediately in preparation for radiation or surgical therapy. If the vision does not improve or continues to deteriorate after 2 to 7 days of systemic steroids, posterior orbital decompression surgery is recommended if it can be performed by a surgeon very familiar with the technique.

4. Orbital irradiation as a steroid-sparing modality has gained increasing acceptance, and its use continues to evolve. It is best performed according to strict protocols with carefully controlled dosage and shielding, under the supervision of a radiation oncologist familiar with the technique. Typically, a total dose of 2,000 cGy is administered in ten fractions over 2 weeks. Improvement in orbitopathy is often seen within 2 weeks af-

ter completion of treatment, but it may take several months to attain maximum benefit. It is unusual for radiation to succeed if steroids have failed.

Irradiation improves swelling, motility, and optic nerve compression but does not improve proptosis. It does not seem to prevent progression.

5. A stepwise approach is used for surgical treatment, starting with orbital decompression (if needed), followed by strabismus surgery (for diplopia, if present), followed by eyelid surgery. Alteration of this sequence leads to unpredictable results.

FOLLOW-UP

1. Optic nerve compression is the most urgent ocular complication of thyroid eye disease; it requires immediate attention.

2. Patients with advanced exposure keratopathy and severe proptosis also require prompt attention.

3. Patients with minimal to no exposure problems and mild to moderate proptosis are reevaluated every 1 to 2 months.

4. Patients in whom fluctuating diplopia or ptosis develops should be evaluated for myasthenia gravis.

7.3 ORBITAL INFLAMMATORY PSEUDOTUMOR

(NONSPECIFIC ORBITAL INFLAMMATORY DISEASE)

SYMPTOMS

May be acute, recurrent, or chronic. Pain, prominent red eye, double vision, or decreased vision are common in acute disease. Children may have concomitant constitutional symptoms (including fever), which are not typical in adults. Asymptomatic proptosis may develop in chronic disease.

SIGNS

Critical. Proptosis or restriction of ocular motility, usually unilateral. Orbital CT scan shows a thickened posterior sclera (or a ring of scleral thickening 360 degrees around the globe), orbital fat or lacrimal gland involvement, or thickening of extraocular muscles (including the tendons). Bone destruction is very rare.

Other. Eyelid erythema and edema, lacrimal gland enlargement or a palpable orbital mass, decreased vision, uveitis, increased IOP, hyperopic shift, optic nerve swelling or atrophy, decreased sensitivity of the first division of the trigeminal nerve, conjunctival chemosis, and injection.

*Note: Bilateral pseudotumor in adults can occur, but should prompt a careful evaluation to rule out a systemic cause (e.g., sarcoidosis, Wegener granulomatosis, polyarteritis nodosa, and lymphoma). Bilateral pseudotumor is more common in children than in adults.

ETIOLOGY

Idiopathic.

DIFFERENTIAL DIAGNOSIS

See 7.1, Orbital Disease.

WORKUP

See 7.1, Orbital Disease, for general orbital workup.

1. History: Previous episodes? Any other systemic symptoms or diseases? History of cancer?

2. Complete ocular examination, including ocular motility, exophthalmometry, IOP, and optic nerve evaluation.

3. Vital signs, particularly temperature.

4. Orbital CT scan (axial and coronal views) with contrast.

5. Blood tests as needed (e.g., bilateral or atypical cases): ESR, CBC with differential, ANA, BUN, creatinine (to rule out vasculitis), and fasting blood sugar (before instituting systemic steroids). Consider checking angiotensin-converting enzyme (ACE) levels or a gallium scan if sarcoidosis is suspected and checking anti-neutrophilic cytoplasmic antibody if Wegener granulomatosis is suspected.

6. Orbital biopsy (fine-needle aspiration or incisional biopsy) when the diagnosis is uncertain, the case is atypical, the patient has a history of cancer, or a patient with an acute case does not respond to systemic steroids within a few days.

TREATMENT

Prednisone, 80 to 100 mg p.o., q.d., with an antiulcer medication (e.g., ranitidine, 150 mg p.o., b.i.d.). Low-dose radiation therapy may be used when the patient does not respond to systemic steroids, when disease recurs as steroids are tapered, or when steroids pose a significant risk to the patient, after the diagnosis is confirmed by biopsy.

FOLLOW-UP

Reevaluate in 3 to 5 days. Patients who respond to the systemic steroids are maintained at the initial dose for several weeks and then tapered off of them slowly, usually over several months. Patients who do not respond to the steroids usually undergo biopsy, and low-dose radiation may be considered. The IOP must be followed closely in patients being treated with steroids.

7.4 ORBITAL CELLULITIS

SYMPTOMS

Red eye, pain, blurred vision, headache, double vision.

SIGNS

Critical. Eyelid edema, erythema, warmth, tenderness. Conjunctival chemosis and injection, proptosis, and restricted ocular motility with pain on attempted eye movement are usually present.

Other. Decreased vision, retinal venous congestion, optic disc edema, purulent discharge, decreased periorbital sensation, fever. CT scan usually shows a sinusitis (typically an ethmoid sinusitis).

DIFFERENTIAL DIAGNOSIS

See 7.1, Orbital Disease.

ETIOLOGY

• Direct extension from a sinus infection (especially ethmoiditis), focal orbital infection (e.g., dacryoadenitis, dacryocystitis, panophthalmitis), orbital fracture, or dental infection.

• Complication of orbital trauma (e.g., blowout fracture or penetrating trauma).

• Complication of eye surgery (especially orbital surgery) or paranasal sinus surgery.

• Vascular extension (e.g., seeding from a systemic bacteremia, or locally from facial cellulitis via venous anastomoses).

Note: When a foreign body is retained, the cellulitis may develop months after injury.

ORGANISMS

Staphylococcus species, *Streptococcus* species, *Haemophilus influenzae* (rarely in vaccinated children), bacteroides, gram-negative rods (especially after trauma).

WORKUP

See 7.1, Orbital Disease for a nonspecific orbital workup.

1. History: Trauma? Ear, nose, throat, or systemic infection? Stiff neck or mental status changes? Diabetes or an immunosuppressive illness?

2. Complete ophthalmic examination: Look for an afferent pupillary defect, limitation of or pain with eye movements, proptosis, decreased skin sensation, or an optic nerve or fundus abnormality.

3. Check vital signs, mental status, and neck flexibility.

4. CT scan of the orbits and sinuses (axial and coronal views, with and without contrast, if possible) to confirm the diagnosis and to rule out a foreign body, orbital or subperiosteal abscess, and sinus disease.

5. CBC with differential.

6. Blood cultures.

7. Explore and debride wound, if present, and obtain a Gram stain and culture of any drainage (e.g., blood and chocolate agars, Sabouraud dextrose agar, thioglycolate broth).

8. Obtain a lumbar puncture for suspected meningitis. Consider a neurology and infectious disease consult.

Note: Mucormycosis, a life-threatening disease, must be considered in all diabetic or immunocompromised patients with orbital cellulitis. Immediate action may need to be taken. See 10.9, Cavernous Sinus and Associated Syndromes.

TREATMENT

1. Admit the patient to the hospital.

2. Broad-spectrum i.v. antibiotics to cover gram-positive, gram-negative, and anaerobic organisms are required for at least 72 hours, followed by p.o. medication for 1 week. The specific recommendations frequently change. We currently prefer the following (or equivalent) drugs:

Children (Age 1 Month to 13 Years)

Ampicillin/sulbactam (e.g., Unasyn), 100 to 200 mg/kg/day in four divided doses (not to exceed 4 g/day)

or

Ceftriaxone, 100 mg/kg/day i.v., in two divided doses (maximum, 4 g/day) *plus* vancomycin, 40 mg/kg/day i.v., in two to three divided doses.

Note: Consult infectious disease and pediatrics specialists to confirm the most current antibiotics and dosages.

Adults

Ampicillin/sulbactam (e.g., Unasyn), 1.5 to 3 g i.v. q6h

or

Ceftriaxone, 1 to 2 g i.v., q12h *plus* vancomycin, 1 g i.v., q12h

In addition to the above, consider adding metronidazole, 15 mg/kg i.v. load over 1 hour, and then 7.5 mg/kg i.v. q6h for adults with chronic orbital cellulitis or when an anaerobic infection is suspected (not to exceed 4 g/day).

For Adults Who Are Allergic to Penicillin/Cephalosporin

Vancomycin, 1 g i.v., q12h *plus* gentamicin, 5.0 mg/kg i.v., q.d. (in adults)

or

Clindamycin, 300 mg i.v. q6h *plus* gentamicin, 5.0 mg/kg i.v., q.d. (in adults)

Note: Antibiotic dosages may need to be reduced in the presence of renal insufficiency or failure. Peak and trough levels of vancomycin and gentamicin are usually monitored, and dosages are adjusted as needed. BUN and creatinine levels are monitored closely.

3. Otolaryngology consult for surgical drainage of the sinuses as needed, usually after the initial episode is treated.

4. Nasal decongestant spray (e.g., Afrin, b.i.d.) as needed.

5. Erythromycin ointment, q.i.d., for corneal exposure if there is severe proptosis.

FOLLOW-UP

Reevaluate every day in the hospital; may take 24 to 36 hours to show improvement.

1. Progress may be monitored by

—Temperature and WBC.

—Visual acuity.

—Ocular motility.

—Degree of proptosis and any displacement of the globe (significant displacement may indicate an abscess).

If any of these are worsening, then a CT scan of the orbit and brain with contrast should be repeated to look for an abscess. If an abscess is found, surgical drainage may be required. Other conditions that must be considered when the patient is not improving are cavernous sinus thrombosis and meningitis.

2. Evaluate the cornea for signs of exposure.

3. Check IOP.

4. Examine the retina and optic nerve for signs of posterior compression (e.g., choroidal folds), inflammation, or exudative retinal detachment.

5. When orbital cellulitis is clearly and consistently improving, then the regimen can be changed to oral antibiotics (depending on the culture and sensitivity results) to complete a total 14-day course. We often use:

Amoxicillin/clavulanate (i.e., Augmentin)

—20 to 40 mg/kg/day in three divided doses in children older than 1 month;

—250 to 500 mg, t.i.d., in adults

or

Cefaclor (i.e., Ceclor)

—20 to 40 mg/kg/day in three divided doses in children older than 1 month;

—250 to 500 mg, t.i.d., in adults

The patient is examined every few days as an outpatient until the condition resolves.

7.5 ORBITAL TUMORS IN CHILDREN

SIGNS

Critical. Proptosis or globe displacement.

Other. See the specific etiologies for additional presenting signs and imaging characteristics (Table 7.1).

ETIOLOGY

• Dermoid and epidermoid cysts [Present from birth to young adulthood and progresses slowly, unless the cyst ruptures. May develop in the orbit (especially superotemporally) or

TABLE 7.1 CHILDHOOD ORBITAL LESIONS SEEN ON COMPUTED TOMOGRAPHY OR MAGNETIC RESONANCE IMAGING

Well circumscribed	Dermoid cyst, rhabdomyosarcoma, optic nerve glioma, plexiform neurofibroma, capillary hemangioma
Diffuse/infiltrating	Lymphangioma, leukemia, pseudotumor, capillary hemangioma, neuroblastoma, teratoma

outside of the orbit in the temporal upper eyelid or brow. When external to the orbit, the cyst is usually a smooth, round, nontender mass. CT scan: Well-defined lesion that may mold the bone of the orbital walls. MRI with contrast: Well-defined mass; T1-weighted image (T1W): hypointense to orbital fat, contrast enhances capsule only; T2-weighted image (T2W): isointense/hypointense to fat, can sometimes see fat/fluid level in lesion. Ultrasonography (B-scan): Cystic lesion with good transmission of echoes.].

• Capillary hemangioma [Seen first from birth to early infancy, slow progression, usually in the superonasal orbit. May be observed through the eyelid as a bluish mass or be accompanied by a red hemangioma of the skin (strawberry nevus), which blanches with pressure. Proptosis may be exacerbated by crying. It can enlarge over the first year but spontaneously regresses over the following several years. CT scan: Irregular, contrast-enhancing, usually extraconal lesion. MRI with fat suppression: Fairly well-defined mass; T1W, hypointense to fat, hyperintense to muscle; T2W, hyperintense to fat and muscle.].

• Rhabdomyosarcoma (Average age of presentation is 7 years, but may occur from infancy to adulthood. Malignant and may metastasize. Rapid onset and progression. May have edema of the eyelids, a palpable superonasal eyelid or subconjunctival mass, or a history of nosebleeds. *Must be managed by urgent biopsy.* CT scan: Bone destruction is typical. The mass may be well circumscribed and is commonly in the superior orbit, especially nasally. MRI with contrast and fat suppression: Well-circumscribed mass; T1W, hypointense to fat, hyperintense to muscle, enhances with contrast; T2W, hyperintense to fat and muscle.).

• Lymphangioma [Usually seen in the first decade of life with a slowly progressive course, but may abruptly worsen if the tumor bleeds. Proptosis may be intermittent and exacerbated by upper respiratory infections. This mass may present as atraumatic eyelid or orbital ecchymosis. Concomitant conjunctival, eyelid, or oropharyngeal lymphangiomas may be noted (a

conjunctival lesion appears as a multicystic mass). CT scan: Nonencapsulated, irregular mass. MRI with contrast and fat suppression: Cystic, possibly multiloculated, nonhomogeneous mass; T1W, hypointense to fat, hyperintense to muscle, diffuse contrast enhancement; T2W, markedly hyperintense to fat and muscle. MRI is often diagnostic. Ultrasonography (B-scan): Cystic spaces are often seen.].

• Optic nerve glioma (Juvenile pilocytic astrocytoma) [Usually first seen at age 2 to 6 years and is slowly progressive. Decreased visual acuity and a relative afferent pupillary defect usually develop. Optic atrophy or optic nerve swelling may be present. May be associated with neurofibromatosis (in which case, it may be bilateral). CT scan: Fusiform enlargement of the optic nerve. The optic canal or chiasm may be involved. MRI with contrast: tubular or fusiform mass; T1W, hypointense to gray matter, variable contrast enhancement; T2W, homogeneous hyperintensity.].

• Leukemia (Granulocytic sarcoma) (Seen first in the first decade of life with rapidly evolving unilateral or bilateral proptosis and occasionally, swelling of the temporal fossa area due to a mass. Typically, these lesions precede blood or bone marrow signs of leukemia, usually acute myelogenous leukemia, by several months. CT scan: Irregular mass, sometimes with bony erosion. There may also be extension of the mass into the temporal fossa.).

Note: Acute lymphoblastic leukemia also can produce unilateral or bilateral proptosis.

• Metastatic neuroblastoma (Seen first in the first few years of life. Abrupt presentation with unilateral or bilateral proptosis, eyelid ecchymosis, and globe displacement. The child is usually systemically ill. The vast majority of patients have already been diagnosed with abdominal cancer. CT scan: Poorly defined mass with bony destruction, especially of the lateral orbital wall.).

• Plexiform neurofibroma (First seen in the first decade of life and is pathognomonic of neurofibromatosis. Ptosis, eyelid hypertrophy, S-shaped deformity of the upper eyelid, or pulsating proptosis may be present. Facial asymmetry and a palpable anterior orbital mass may also be evident. CT scan: Diffuse, irregular, soft tissue mass. A defect in the orbital roof may be seen. MRI: Well-circumscribed oval or fusiform mass; T1W, isointense or slightly hyperintense to muscle; T2W, hyperintense to fat and muscle. See 13.17, Neurofibromatosis.).

• Teratoma (Seen at birth with severe unilateral proptosis that may progress. Vision is often lost from increased IOP, optic nerve atrophy, and corneal exposure. The mass transilluminates. CT scan: Multiloculated soft tissue mass and enlarged orbit; intracranial extension is possible.).

• See 7.1, Orbital Disease.

WORKUP

1. History: Determine the age of onset and the rate of progression. Does the proptosis vary in degree (e.g., with crying)? Nosebleeds? Systemic illness?

2. External examination: Look for an anterior orbital mass, a skin hemangioma, or a temporal fossa lesion. Measure any proptosis (Hertel exophthalmometer) or globe displacement (measure from the bridge of the nose with a ruler). Conduct abdominal examination to rule out mass or organomegaly.

3. Complete ocular examination, including visual acuity, pupillary assessment, color vision, IOP, refraction, and optic nerve evaluation.

4. CT scan (axial and coronal views) of the orbit and brain or orbital MRI (with gadolinium-DTPA contrast and fat suppression if indicated).

5. Orbital ultrasonography with or without color Doppler imaging, if needed to define the lesion further.

6. In cases of acute onset and rapid progression, an emergency incisional biopsy for frozen, permanent, and electron microscopic evaluation is indicated to rule out an aggressive malignancy (e.g., rhabdomyosarcoma).

7. Other tests as determined by the working diagnosis (usually performed in conjunction with a pediatric oncologist):

—Rhabdomyosarcoma: Physical examination (look especially for enlarged lymph nodes), chest and bone radiographs, bone marrow aspiration, lumbar puncture, liver function studies.

—Leukemia: CBC with differential, bone marrow studies, others.

—Neuroblastoma: Abdominal CT scan, urine for vanillylmandelic acid.

Note: If clinical suspicion for rhabdomyosarcoma is high, emergency biopsy and initiation of therapy is indicated.

TREATMENT

1. **Dermoid and epidermoid cysts:** Complete surgical excision with the capsule intact. If the cyst ruptures, the contents can incite an acute inflammatory response.

2. **Capillary hemangioma:** Observe if mild. A local steroid injection (e.g., betamethasone, 6 mg, and triamcinolone, 40 mg) may be given to shrink the lesion if necessary. Treatment is often indicated if strabismus, anisometropia, or amblyopia develop (see 8.6, Amblyopia). The natural history is involution after the first year of life.

3. **Rhabdomyosarcoma** (managed by urgent referral to a pediatric oncologist in most cases): Local radiation therapy and systemic chemotherapy are given once the diagnosis is confirmed by biopsy.

4. **Lymphangioma:** Most are managed by observation. Surgical excision is performed for a significant cosmetic deformity, ocular dysfunction (e.g., strabismus and amblyopia), or compressive optic neuropathy from acute orbital hemorrhage. Incidence of hemorrhage into lesion is increased after surgery. May recur after excision.

5. **Optic nerve glioma:** Controversial. Observation, surgery, and radiation are used variably on a case-by-case basis.

6. **Leukemia (managed by a pediatric oncologist in most cases):** Systemic chemotherapy for the leukemia. Some physicians administer orbital radiation therapy alone when systemic leukemia cannot be confirmed on bone marrow studies.

7. **Metastatic neuroblastoma (managed by a pediatric oncologist in most cases):** Local radiation and systemic chemotherapy.

8. **Plexiform neurofibroma:** Surgical excision is reserved for patients with significant symptoms or disfigurement.

9. Teratoma: Surgical excision (sometimes with the help of a neurosurgeon). Aspiration of the cyst may facilitate complete removal of large lesions. Preservation of ocular function may be possible.

FOLLOW-UP

1. Tumors with rapid onset and progression require urgent attention to rule out malignancy.

2. Tumors that progress more slowly may be managed less urgently.

7.6 ORBITAL TUMORS IN ADULTS

SYMPTOMS

Prominent eye, double vision, pain, decreased vision; may be asymptomatic.

SIGNS

Critical. Proptosis, displacement of the globe away from the location of the tumor, orbital mass on palpation, mass found with neuroimaging.

Other. A palpable mass, limitation of ocular motility, optic disc edema, or choroidal folds may be present. See the individual etiologies for more specific findings and imaging characteristics (Table 7.2).

ETIOLOGY

• Metastatic [Most common orbital mass in adults. Usually occurs in middle-aged to elderly people with a rapid onset of orbital signs. Common primary sources include the breast (most common), lung, genitourinary tract (especially prostate), and gastrointestinal tract. Enophthalmos (not proptosis) may be seen with scirrhous breast carcinoma. CT scan: Poorly defined, diffuse tumor that may conform to the shape of the adjacent orbital structures; bone destruction may be seen. MRI with contrast: Diffuse, infiltrating, nonencapsulated mass; T1W, hypointense to fat, isointense to muscle, moderate to marked contrast enhancement; T2W, hyperintense to fat and muscle.].

• Cavernous hemangioma [Most common benign orbital mass in adults. Typically occurs in young adulthood to middle age, with a slow onset of orbital signs. CT scan: Well-defined mass, usually within the muscle cone. MRI with contrast: Well-circumscribed homogeneous mass; T1W, isointense/hyperintense to muscle, diffuse

TABLE 7.2 ADULT ORBITAL LESIONS ON COMPUTED TOMOGRAPHY OR MAGNETIC RESONANCE IMAGING

Well circumscribed	Cavernous hemangioma, neurolemoma, fibrous histiocytoma, solitary neurofibroma, hemangiopericytoma, mucocele, optic nerve sheath meningioma
Diffuse/infiltrating	Pseudotumor, lymphoid tumors, lymphangioma, metastasis

contrast enhancement; T2W, hyperintense to muscle and fat. Ultrasonography (A-scan): High-amplitude internal echoes.].

• Mucocele (Often a frontal headache and a history of chronic sinusitis or sinus trauma. Usually nasally or superonasally located. CT scan: A frontal or ethmoid sinus cyst usually seen extending through eroded bone into the orbit; affected sinuses may be opacified.).

• Lymphoid tumors (Usually occurs in middle-aged to elderly adults. Slow onset and progression. Typically develops superiorly in the anterior aspect of the orbit. May be accompanied by a subconjunctival, salmon-colored lesion. Less responsive to systemic steroids than orbital pseudotumor. Can occur without evidence of systemic lymphoma. CT scan: Irregular mass conforming to the shape of the orbital bones or globe, no bony erosion. MRI with contrast: Nonspecific, irregular mass; T1W, hypointense to fat, isointense/hyperintense to muscle, moderate to marked contrast enhancement; T2W, hyperintense to muscle.).

• Optic nerve sheath meningioma [Typically occurs in middle-aged women with painless, slowly progressive visual loss, often with mild proptosis. An afferent pupillary defect develops with visual loss. Ophthalmoscopy can reveal optic nerve swelling, optic atrophy, or abnormal collateral vessels around the disc (optociliary shunt vessels). Meningiomas arising intracranially can produce a temporal fossa mass. CT scan with contrast: Tubular enlargement of the optic nerve, sometimes with a "railroad-track" appearance (a linear shadow is seen in the lesion). MRI with contrast and fat suppression: Variable-intensity lesion surrounding optic nerve; T1W, marked contrast enhancement, difficult to differentiate from orbital fat unless fat suppression is used.].

• Localized neurofibroma [Occurs in young to middle-aged adults with slow development of orbital signs. Some have neurofibromatosis, but most do not. CT scan: Well-defined mass in the superior orbit (rarely inferiorly). MRI: Well-circumscribed, possibly heterogeneous mass; T1W, isointense/hyperintense to muscle; T2W, hyperintense to fat and muscle.].

• Neurilemoma (benign schwannoma). (Progressive painless proptosis. Rarely associated with neurofibromatosis. CT scan: Well-circumscribed fusiform or ovoid mass, usually located in the superior orbit. MRI with contrast: Well-circumscribed mass; T1W, isointense/hyperintense to muscle, variable contrast enhancement; T2W, variable intensity.).

• Fibrous histiocytoma [Occurs at any age. Cannot be distinguished from a hemangiopericytoma before biopsy (see the following entry). CT scan: Well-circumscribed mass anywhere in the orbit. MRI with contrast: Heterogeneous mass; T1W, hypointense to fat, isointense/hyperintense to muscle, irregular contrast enhancement; T2W, hypointense areas similar to T1W.].

• Hemangiopericytoma [Occurs at any age. Relatively slow development of signs. Usually superiorly located. CT scan: May appear well defined and indistinguishable from a cavernous hemangioma or fibrous histiocytoma. Sometimes extends through the orbital bones into the temporal fossa and cranial cavity. MRI: Well-circumscribed mass; T1W, hypointense to fat, isointense/hyperintense to muscle, moderate diffuse contrast enhancement; T2W, variable. Ultrasound (A-scan): Low to medium internal reflectivity.].

• Others (Dermoid cyst, osteoma, hematocele, lymphangioma, extension of an ocular or periocular tumor, others).

• See 7.1, Orbital Disease, and 7.7, Lacrimal Gland Mass.

WORKUP

1. History: Determine the age of onset and rate of progression. Headache or chronic sinusitis? History of cancer? Trauma (e.g., hematocele, orbital foreign body, ruptured dermoid)?

2. Complete ocular examination, particularly visual acuity, pupillary response, ocular motility, color vision and visual field of each eye, measurement of globe displacement (from the bridge of the nose with a ruler) and proptosis (Hertel exophthalmometer), IOP, and optic nerve evaluation.

3. CT scan (axial and coronal views) of the orbit and brain or orbital MRI with surface coil/fat suppression, depending on suspected etiology.

4. Orbital ultrasonography with or without color Doppler imaging as needed to define the lesion further.

5. When a metastasis is suspected and primary tumor is unknown, the following should be performed:

—Fine-needle aspiration biopsy or incisional biopsy to confirm the diagnosis, with estrogen receptor assay if breast carcinoma is suspected.

—Breast examination and palpation of axillary lymph nodes.

—Medical workup as directed by the biopsy result (e.g., chest radiograph, mammogram).

6. When a lymphoma is suspected, a medical consult is obtained and a systemic workup is instituted (e.g., CBC with differential, serum protein electrophoresis, bone marrow biopsy, CT scan of the abdomen and brain). If the workup is negative, an incisional biopsy is performed (often need nonfixed tissue for special studies, e.g., flow cytometry). If the workup is positive, the systemic lymphoma is treated and the orbital lesion is observed for its response to treatment. Occasionally a fine-needle biopsy is performed to confirm the orbital diagnosis.

TREATMENT

1. **Metastatic disease:** Systemic chemotherapy as required for the primary malignancy. Radiation therapy is often used palliatively for the orbital mass. Carcinoid tumors are occasionally resected.

2. **Cavernous hemangioma:** Complete surgical excision is performed when there is compromised visual function or for cosmetic purposes. If the patient is asymptom-

atic, he or she can be followed every 6 to 12 months.

3. **Mucocele:** Systemic antibiotics (e.g., ampicillin/sulbactam 3g i.v., q6h) followed by surgical drainage of the mucocele and exenteration of the involved sinus.

4. **Lymphoid tumors:** Lymphoid hyperplasia and orbital lymphoma without systemic involvement are treated with local radiation therapy. Systemic lymphoma is treated with chemotherapy.

5. **Optic nerve sheath meningioma:** Surgery or stereotactic radiation therapy is usually indicated when the tumor is growing and producing visual loss. Otherwise, the patient may be followed every 3 to 6 months with serial clinical examinations and imaging studies (CT scan or MRI) as needed.

6. **Localized neurofibroma:** Surgical removal is performed for enlarging tumors that are producing symptoms.

7. **Neurilemoma:** Same as for cavernous hemangioma (see earlier).

8. **Fibrous histiocytoma:** Complete surgical removal. Recurrences are usually more aggressive and more malignant, sometimes necessitating orbital exenteration.

9. **Hemangiopericytoma:** Complete surgical excision (because there is a potential for malignant transformation and metastasis).

FOLLOW-UP

1. Variable: Referral for treatment is not an emergency, except when optic nerve compromise is present.

2. Metastatic disease requires workup without much delay.

Note: See also 7.7, Lacrimal Gland Mass, especially if the mass is in the outer one third of the upper eyelid, and 7.5, Orbital Tumors in Children.

7.7 LACRIMAL GLAND MASS/CHRONIC DACRYOADENITIS

SYMPTOMS

Persistent or progressive swelling of the outer one third of the upper eyelid. Pain or double vision may or may not be present.

SIGNS

Critical. Chronic eyelid swelling and erythema, predominantly in the outer one third of the upper eyelid, with or without proptosis and displacement of the globe inferiorly and medially.

Other. A palpable mass may be present in the outer one third of the upper eyelid. Extraocular motility may be restricted.

ETIOLOGY

- Sarcoidosis (May be bilateral. May have concomitant lung, skin, or ocular disease. Lymphadenopathy, parotid gland enlargement, or seventh-nerve palsy may be present. More common in blacks. Serum ACE level may be increased.).

- Orbital inflammatory pseudotumor (Commonly, pain and swelling develop acutely, with or without limitation of ocular motility, displacement of the globe, or proptosis. CT scan may show stranding of orbital fat if not confined to lacrimal gland. A rapid response to systemic steroids is typical in acute cases.).

- Benign mixed epithelial tumor (pleomorphic adenoma) (Slowly progressive, painless proptosis or displacement of the globe in middle-aged adults. CT scan may show a well-circumscribed mass with pressure-induced remodeling and enlargement of the lacrimal gland fossa. No bony erosion occurs.).

- Dermoid (Typically a painless, subcutaneous cystic mass that enlarges slowly and is found in a child. May rarely rupture, causing acute swelling and inflammation. Well-defined, extraconal mass noted on CT scan.).

- Lymphoid tumor (Slowly progressive proptosis and globe displacement in a middle-aged patient. May have a pink–white "salmon-patch" area of subconjunctival extension. CT scan shows an irregularly shaped lesion that conforms to the globe and lacrimal fossa. Bony erosion is not usually found.).

- Adenoid cystic carcinoma (Acute onset of pain and proptosis, which progress rapidly. Globe displacement, ptosis, and a motility disturbance are common. This highly malignant lesion often exhibits perineural invasion. CT scan shows an irregular mass, often with bony erosion.).

- Malignant mixed epithelial tumor (pleomorphic adenocarcinoma) (Occurs primarily in elderly patients, acutely producing pain and progressing rapidly. Usually develops within a long-standing benign mixed epithelial tumor, or secondarily, as a recurrence of a previously resected benign mixed tumor. CT scan findings are similar to those for adenoid cystic carcinoma.).

- Lacrimal gland cyst (dacryops) (Usually an asymptomatic mass that may fluctuate in size. Typically occurs in a young adult or middle-aged patient.).

- Others (Tuberculosis, syphilis, leukemia, mumps, mucoepidermoid carcinoma, plasmacytoma, others).

Note: *Primary neoplasms (except lymphoma) are almost always unilateral; inflammatory disease may be bilateral. Lymphoma is more commonly unilateral, but may be bilateral.*

WORKUP

1. History: Determine the duration of the abnormality and rate of progression. Associated pain, tenderness, double vision? Weak-

ness, weight loss, fever, or other signs of systemic malignancy? Breathing difficulty, skin rash, or history of uveitis (sarcoidosis)? Any known medical problems? Prior lacrimal gland biopsy or surgery?

2. Complete ocular examination: Specifically look for keratic precipitates, iris nodules, posterior synechiae, and old retinal periphlebitis from sarcoidosis.

3. Orbital CT scan (axial and coronal views): MRI is rarely required.

4. Consider a chest radiograph or chest CT (may diagnose sarcoidosis and, rarely, tuberculosis).

5. Consider CBC with differential, ACE, rapid plasma reagin, fluorescent treponemal antibody, absorbed, and purified protein derivative with anergy panel if clinical history suggests a specific etiology.

6. Systemic workup by an internist or hematologist/oncologist when a lymphoma is suspected (e.g., abdominal and head CT scan, bone marrow biopsy).

7. Lacrimal gland biopsy is indicated when a malignant tumor is suspected, or if the diagnosis is uncertain and a malignancy or inflammatory etiology is probable. (Biopsy may be unnecessary when a lymphoma is suspected clinically and is confirmed on systemic workup.)

Note: Do not perform a biopsy on lesions thought to be benign mixed tumors or dermoids. Incomplete excision of a benign mixed tumor may lead to a recurrence with or without malignant transformation. Rupture of a dermoid cyst may lead to a severe inflammatory reaction. These two lesions must be completely excised without rupturing the capsule or pseudocapsule.

TREATMENT

1. **Sarcoidosis:** Systemic steroids (see 12.6, Sarcoidosis).

2. **Orbital inflammatory pseudotumor:** Systemic steroids (see 7.3, Orbital Inflammatory Pseudotumor).

3. **Benign mixed epithelial tumor:** Complete surgical removal.

4. **Dermoid cyst:** Complete surgical removal.

5. **Lymphoid tumor:**

   —Confined to the orbit: Orbital irradiation.

   —Systemic involvement: Chemotherapy (orbital irradiation is usually withheld until the response of the orbital lesion to chemotherapy can be evaluated).

6. **Adenoid cystic carcinoma:** Consider orbital exenteration with irradiation. (Rarely, chemotherapy is used.)

7. **Malignant mixed epithelial tumor:** Same as for adenoid cystic carcinoma.

8. **Lacrimal gland cyst:** Excise if symptomatic.

FOLLOW-UP

Depends on the specific cause.

CHAPTER 8

PEDIATRICS

8.1 LEUKOCORIA

DEFINITION

A white pupillary reflex.

ETIOLOGY

• Retinoblastoma [A malignant tumor of the retina that appears as a white, nodular mass extending into the vitreous (endophytic), as a mass lesion underlying a retinal detachment (exophytic), or as a diffusely spreading lesion simulating uveitis (diffuse infiltrating). Iris neovascularization is common. Pseudohypopyon and vitreous seeding may occur. Cataract is uncommon, and the eye is normal in size. May be bilateral, unilateral, or multifocal. Diagnosis is usually made between 12 and 24 months of age. A family history may be elicited.].

• Toxocariasis [A nematode infection that may appear as a localized, white, elevated granuloma in the retina or as a diffuse endophthalmitis. Localized inflammation of ocular structures also may be seen. Vitreous traction bands associated with macular dragging may occur, traction retinal detachment may occur, and cataract may develop secondary to the inflammation. It is rarely bilateral and is usually diagnosed between 6 months and 10 years of age. Paracentesis of the anterior chamber may reveal eosinophils, and a serum enzyme-linked immunosorbent assay (ELISA) test for *Toxocara* organisms is positive. The patient may have a history of contact with puppies or eating dirt.].

• Coats disease (A retinal vascular abnormality resulting in small multifocal outpouchings of the retinal vessels, associated with yellow intraretinal and subretinal exudate. An exudative retinal detachment may account for the leukocoria. It usually develops in boys during the first two decades of life; more severe cases occur in the first decade of life. Coats disease is rarely bilateral, and there is no family history.).

• Persistent hyperplastic primary vitreous (PHPV) (A developmental ocular abnormality consisting of a varied degree of fibroglial and vascular proliferation in the vitreous cavity. It is usually associated with a slightly small eye. Other findings can include cataract, a fibrovascular membrane behind the lens that places traction on the ciliary processes, glaucoma, and retinal detachment. The condition is present at birth but may not be detected until later in childhood. It is rarely bilateral and there is no family history.).

• Congenital cataract (Opacity of the lens present at birth; may be unilateral or bilateral. There may be a family history or an associated systemic disorder. See 8.7, Congenital Cataract.).

- Retinal astrocytoma (A sessile to slightly elevated, yellow–white retinal mass that may be calcified and is often associated with tuberous sclerosis, and rarely neurofibromatosis. May be associated with giant drusen of the optic nerve in patients with tuberous sclerosis.).

- Retinopathy of prematurity (ROP) (Predominantly occurs in premature children, who may have received supplemental oxygen therapy. Leukocoria is usually the result of a retinal detachment. See 8.2, Retinopathy of Prematurity.).

- Others [e.g., retinochoroidal coloboma, retinal detachment, familial exudative vitreoretinopathy (FEVR), myelinated nerve fibers, uveitis, incontinentia pigmenti].

WORKUP

1. History: Age at onset? Family history of one of the conditions mentioned? Prematurity? Contact with puppies or habit of eating dirt?

2. Complete ocular examination, including a measurement of corneal diameters (look for a small eye), an examination of the iris (look for neovascularization), and an inspection of the lens (look for a cataract). A dilated fundus examination and anterior vitreous examination are essential.

3. Any or all of the following may be helpful in diagnosis and planning treatment:

   —B-scan ultrasonography (retinoblastoma, PHPV, cataract).

   —Intravenous fluorescein angiogram (Coats disease, ROP, retinoblastoma).

   —Computed tomography (CT) scan or magnetic resonance imaging (MRI) of the orbit and brain (retinoblastoma), particularly for bilateral cases or those with a family history.

   —Serum ELISA test for *Toxocara* (positive at 1:8 in the vast majority of infected patients).

   —Systemic examination (retinal astrocytoma, retinoblastoma).

   —Anterior chamber paracentesis (toxocariasis). Note that paracentesis in a patient with

a retinoblastoma can possibly lead to tumor cell dissemination.

4. Consider examination under anesthesia (EUA) in young or uncooperative children, particularly when retinoblastoma, toxocariasis, Coats disease, or ROP is being considered as a diagnosis.

See 8.7, Congenital Cataract, for a more specific cataract workup.

TREATMENT

1. **Retinoblastoma:** Enucleation, irradiation, photocoagulation, cryotherapy, chemoreduction, chemothermotherapy, or occasionally other therapeutic modalities. Systemic chemotherapy is used in metastatic disease.

2. **Toxocariasis:**

   —Steroids (Topical, periocular depot injection, or systemic routes may be used, depending on the severity of the inflammation.)

   —Consider a surgical vitrectomy when vitreoretinal traction bands form or when the condition does not improve or worsens with medical therapy.

   —Consider laser photocoagulation of the nematode if it is visible.

3. **Coats disease:** Laser photocoagulation or cryotherapy to leaking vessels; surgery may be required for a retinal detachment.

4. **PHPV**

   —Cataract extraction.

   —Possible vitreal membrane excision.

   —Treat any amblyopia.

5. **Congenital cataract:** See 8.7, Congenital Cataract.

6. **Retinal astrocytoma:** Observation.

7. **ROP:** See 8.2, Retinopathy of Prematurity.

FOLLOW-UP

Variable, depending on the diagnosis.

8.2 RETINOPATHY OF PREMATURITY

RISK FACTORS

· Prematurity (especially less than 32 weeks of gestation).

· Birthweight less than 1,500 g (3 lb, 5 oz), especially less than 1,250 g (2 lb, 12 oz).

· Supplemental oxygen therapy, hypoxemia, hypercarbia, and concurrent illness.

SIGNS

Critical. An avascular peripheral retina.

Other. Extraretinal fibrovascular proliferation, plus disease (see classification later), vitreous hemorrhage, retinal detachment, or leukocoria, usually bilateral. Poor pupillary dilation despite mydriatic drops with engorgement of iris vessels. In older children and adults, decreased visual acuity, myopia, strabismus, retinal dragging, lattice-like vitreoretinal degeneration, or retinal detachment may occur.

DIFFERENTIAL DIAGNOSIS

· FEVR (Appears similar to ROP, except FEVR is autosomal dominant, although family members may be asymptomatic; asymptomatic family members often show peripheral retinal vascular abnormalities. There usually is no history of prematurity or oxygen therapy.).

· Incontinentia pigmenti in girls.

· See 8.1, Leukocoria, for additional differential diagnoses.

CLASSIFICATION

Location

Zone 1: *Posterior pole:* Two times the disc–fovea distance, centered around the disc. (Poorest prognosis.)

Zone 2: From zone 1 to the nasal periphery, temporally equidistant from the disc.

Zone 3: The remaining temporal periphery.

Extent

Number of clock hours (30-degree sectors) involved.

Severity

Stage 1: Flat demarcation line separating the vascular posterior retina from the avascular peripheral retina.

Stage 2: Ridged demarcation line.

Stage 3: Ridged demarcation line with extraretinal fibrovascular proliferation.

Stage 4A: Extrafoveal retinal detachment.

Stage 4B: Subtotal retinal detachment involving the macula.

Stage 5: Total retinal detachment.

"Plus" Disease

Engorged veins and tortuous arteries in the posterior pole. If plus disease is present, a + is placed after the stage (e.g., stage 3+). Zone 1 ROP with plus disease indicates high risk for rapid progression ("rush" disease).

WORKUP

1. Dilated retinal examination with scleral depression at gestational age 31 to 32 weeks (number of weeks after date of last menstrual period), or as soon as feasible before discharge from the hospital.

2. Can dilate with phenylephrine, 1.0%, tropicamide, 0.2%.

TREATMENT (BASED ON SEVERITY)

1. **Stages 1 and 2:** No treatment necessary.

2. **Stage 3:** Laser photocoagulation or cryotherapy if threshold disease present, defined as at least five contiguous or eight accumulated clock hours of stage 3+ disease in zone 1 or 2. Treatment of the avascular zone should be instituted within 72 hours.

3. **Stages 4 and 5:** Surgical repair of retinal detachment by scleral buckling, vitrectomy surgery, or both.

FOLLOW-UP

1. The initial eye examination should be conducted by 31 weeks postmenstrual age or 4 weeks chronologic age, whichever is later. If prethreshold disease is detected [(a) any stage less than threshold in zone 1, or (b) stage 2+ or 3 ROP in zone 2], then perform repeated examinations at least weekly, depending on the tempo of the disease. If regression of ROP is noted, follow-up should be every 1 to 2 months at first and every 6 to 12 months later.

2. Children who have had ROP have a higher incidence of myopia, strabismus, amblyopia, macular dragging, cataracts, glaucoma, and retinal detachment. An untreated fully vascularized fundus needs examinations only at age 6 months to rule out these complications.

3. Acute-phase ROP screening can be discontinued when any of the three signs listed in the following is present, indicating that the risk of visual loss form ROP is minimal or passed:

—Zone III retinal vascularization attained without previous zone I or II ROP assuming no examiner error. If there is doubt about the zone or if the postmenstrual age is unexpectedly young, confirmatory examinations may be warranted.

—Full retinal vascularization.

—Postmenstrual age of 45 weeks and no prethreshold ROP or worse present.

BIBLIOGRAPHY

Cryotherapy for Retinopathy of Prematurity Cooperative Group. Multicenter trial of cryotherapy for retinopathy of prematurity: one year outcome: structure and function. *Arch Ophthalmol* 1990;108:1408.

Laser ROP Study Group. Laser therapy for retinopathy of prematurity. *Arch Ophthalmol* 1994;112:154.

8.3 ESODEVIATIONS IN CHILDREN

SIGNS

Critical. Either eye is turned inward (i.e., "cross-eyed"). The nonfixating eye turns outward to refixate straight ahead when the fixating eye is covered during the cover–uncover test (see Appendix 2).

Other. Amblyopia, overreaction of the inferior oblique muscles.

DIFFERENTIAL DIAGNOSIS

• Pseudoesotropia (The eyes appear esotropic; however, there is no ocular misalignment detected during cover–uncover testing. Usually, the child has a wide nasal bridge, prominent epicanthal folds, or a small interpupillary distance.).

• See 8.5, Strabismus Syndromes.

TYPES

Concomitant Esotropic Deviations

A manifest convergent misalignment of the eye (or eyes) in which the measured angle of esodeviation is nearly constant in all fields of gaze at distance fixation.

1. Congenital (infantile) esotropia [Manifests by age 6 months, the angle of esodeviation is usually large (more than 40 to 50 prism diopters) and equal at distance and near

fixation. Refractive error is usually normal for age (slightly hyperopic). Amblyopia is often present in those who do not cross-fixate. The patient may have a family history of the condition, and often develops latent nystagmus and dissociated vertical deviation.].

2. Accommodative esotropia (Convergent misalignment of the eyes associated with activation of the accommodative reflex. Average age of onset is 2.5 years.).

Subtypes:

—Refractive accommodative esotropia [These children are hyperopic (farsighted) in the range of +3.00 to +10.00 diopters (average, +4.75). The measured angle of esodeviation is usually moderate (20 to 30 prism diopters) and is equal at distance and near fixation. Full hyperopic correction eliminates the esodeviation. The accommodative convergence/accommodation ratio (AC/A) is normal. Amblyopia is common.].

—Nonrefractive accommodative esotropia [The measured angle of esodeviation is greater at near fixation than at distance fixation. The refractive error is similar to that of normal children of similar age (slightly hyperopic). The AC/A ratio is high. Amblyopia is common.].

—Partial or decompensated accommodative esotropia (Refractive and nonrefractive accommodative esotropias that demonstrate a significant reduction in the esodeviation when given full hyperopic correction, but still have a residual esodeviation. The residual esodeviation is the nonaccommodative component. This condition often occurs when there is a delay between the onset of the accommodative esotropia and the use of full hyperopic correction.).

3. Sensory-deprivation esotropia [An esodeviation that occurs in a patient with a monocular or binocular lesion or a condition that prevents good vision (e.g., corneal opacity, cataract, retinal scars, inflammations, tumors, optic neuropathy, anisometropia).].

4. Divergence insufficiency (A convergent ocular misalignment that is greater at distance fixation than at near fixation. This is a diagnosis of exclusion and must be differentiated from divergence paralysis, which can be associated with pontine tumors, neurologic trauma, and other conditions.).

Incomitant Esodeviations

The measured angle of esodeviation varies with the direction of gaze at distance fixation.

1. Serious neurologic disorder (Acute onset and new onset of nystagmus may suggest tumor, hydrocephalus, or other causes of increased intracranial pressure.).

2. Medial rectus restriction (e.g., thyroid disease, medial orbital wall fracture).

3. Lateral rectus weakness (e.g., isolated sixth cranial nerve palsy, slipped or detached lateral rectus from trauma or previous surgery).

WORKUP

1. History: Ascertain age of onset of crossing, frequency of crossing, history of glasses, and any history of patching or trauma.

2. Visual acuity of each eye separately, with correction and pinhole, to evaluate for amblyopia. Note any nystagmus.

3. Ocular motility examination; observe for restricted movements or oblique overactions.

4. Measure the distance deviation in all fields of gaze and the near deviation in the primary position (straight ahead) using prisms (see Appendix 2).

5. Manifest and cycloplegic refractions.

6. Pupillary, slit-lamp, and fundus examinations; look for causes of sensory deprivation.

7. If divergence insufficiency or paralysis or if acute-onset incomitant esotropia is present, a head CT scan (axial and coronal views) or an MRI scan and a neurologic evaluation are necessary to rule out an intracranial mass lesion.

8. With incomitant esodeviation, consider thyroid function tests or a workup for myasthenia gravis, or look for characteristics of strabismus syndromes (see 8.5, Strabismus Syndromes).

TREATMENT

In all cases, correct refractive errors of +2.00 diopters or more, and treat any amblyopia by patching the better-seeing eye (see 8.6, Amblyopia).

1. **Congenital esotropia:** When equal vision is obtained in the two eyes, corrective muscle surgery is usually performed.

2. **Accommodative esotropia:** Glasses must be worn full time.

   a. If the patient is younger than 5 to 6 years, correct the hyperopia with the full cycloplegic refraction.

   b. If the patient is older than 5 to 6 years, push plus lenses during the manifest (noncycloplegic) refraction until distance vision blurs, and give the most plus lenses without blurring distance vision.

   c. If the patient's eyes are straight at distance with full correction, but still esotropic at near distance (high AC/A ratio), treatment options include:

      —Bifocals (executive type) +2.50 or +3.00 diopter add, with top of the bifocal crossing the lower pupillary border.

      —Extraocular muscle surgery: There is no consensus on this treatment.

   d. Nonaccommodative esotropia or decompensated accommodative esotropia: Muscle surgery is usually performed to correct any significant esotropia that remains when glasses are worn.

   e. Sensory-deprivation esotropia:

—Attempt to correct the cause of poor vision.

—Give the full cycloplegic correction.

—Muscle surgery to correct the manifest esotropia.

—All patients with very poor vision in one eye need to wear protective polycarbonate lens glasses at all times.

FOLLOW-UP

At each visit, evaluate for amblyopia and measure the degree of deviation with prisms (with glasses worn).

1. If amblyopia is present, see 8.6, Amblyopia, for management.

2. If amblyopia is not present, the child is reevaluated in 3 to 6 weeks after a new prescription is given or in 1 to 6 months if no changes are made and the eyes are straight.

3. When a residual esotropia is present while the patient wears glasses, an attempt is made to add more plus power to the current prescription. Children younger than 6 years should receive a new cycloplegic refraction; plus lenses are pushed without cycloplegia in older children. The maximal additional plus lens that does not blur distance vision is prescribed. If the eyes cannot be straightened with more plus power, then a decompensated accommodative esotropia has developed (see preceding).

4. Hyperopia (farsightedness) often decreases slowly after age 5 to 7 years, and the strength of the glasses may need to be reduced so as not to blur distance vision. If the strength of the glasses must be reduced to improve visual acuity and the esotropia returns, then this is a decompensated accommodative esotropia (see earlier).

8.4 EXODEVIATIONS IN CHILDREN

SIGNS

Critical. Either eye is constantly or intermittently turned outward (i.e., "wall-eyed"). On the cover–uncover test, when the fixating eye is covered, the uncovered eye turns inward to fixate (see Appendix 2).

Other. Amblyopia, overaction of the superior or inferior oblique muscles (producing an "A" or a "V" pattern), vertical deviation.

DIFFERENTIAL DIAGNOSIS

Pseudoexotropia (The patient appears to have an exodeviation, but no movement is noted on cover–uncover testing despite good vision in each eye. A wide interpupillary distance or temporal dragging of the macula from ROP, toxocariasis, or other retinal disorders may be responsible.).

TYPES

1. Intermittent exotropia (The most common type of exodeviation in children. Onset is usually from infancy to age 4 years, and it often increases in frequency over time. Amblyopia is rare.) There are three phases:

   —Phase 1: One eye turns out at distance fixation, spontaneously or when it is covered. Primarily occurs when the patient is fatigued, sick, or not concentrating. The eyes become straight within one to two blinks of the cover being removed. The eyes are straight at near fixation. Patient often has diplopia and closes one eye to relieve symptoms.

   —Phase 2: Increasing frequency of exotropia at distance fixation. Exotropia begins to occur at near fixation.

   —Phase 3: There is a constant exotropia at distance and near fixations.

2. Sensory-deprivation exotropia (An eye that does not see well, for any reason, may turn outward.).

3. Duane syndrome, type 2 (Limitation of adduction of one eye, with globe retraction and narrowing of the palpebral fissure on attempted adduction. Rarely bilateral. See 8.5, Strabismus Syndromes.).

4. Third nerve palsy (Limitation of eye movement superiorly, medially, and inferiorly, usually with ptosis. See 10.5, Isolated Third Nerve Palsy.).

5. Orbital disease (e.g., tumor, orbital pseudotumor). (Proptosis and restriction of ocular motility are usually evident. See 7.1, Orbital Disease.).

6. Myasthenia gravis (Ptosis and limitation of eye movement can vary throughout the day. See 10.10, Myasthenia Gravis.).

7. Convergence insufficiency (Usually occurs in patients older than 10 years. Blurred near vision, headaches when reading. An exodeviation at near fixation, but straight at distance fixation. Must be differentiated from convergence paralysis. See 13.8, Convergence Insufficiency.).

WORKUP

1. Evaluate visual acuity of each eye, with correction and pinhole, to evaluate for amblyopia.

2. Perform motility examination; observing for restricted eye movements or signs of Duane's syndrome.

3. Measure the exodeviation in all fields of gaze at distance and in primary position (straight ahead) at near, using prisms (see Appendix 2).

4. Check for proptosis with Hertel exophthalmometry when appropriate.

5. Perform pupillary, slit-lamp, and fundus examinations; check for causes of sensory deprivation.

6. Manifest and cycloplegic refractions.

7. Consider workup for myasthenia gravis when suspected.

8. Consider a CT scan (axial and coronal views) or an MRI of the orbit and brain, as needed.

TREATMENT

In all cases, correct significant refractive errors and treat amblyopia (see 8.6, Amblyopia).

1. **Intermittent exotropia:**

—Phase 1: Follow patient closely.

—Phase 2: Muscle surgery may be indicated to maintain normal binocular vision.

—Phase 3: Muscle surgery is often considered at this point. Bifixation and peripheral fusion can occasionally be attained.

2. **Sensory-deprivation exotropia:**

—Correct the underlying cause, if possible.

—Treat any amblyopia.

—Muscle surgery may be performed for manifest exotropia.

—When one eye has very poor vision, protective glasses (polycarbonate lens glasses) should be worn at all times to protect the good eye.

3. **Duane syndrome:** See 8.5, Strabismus Syndromes.

4. **Third nerve palsy:** See 10.5, Isolated Third Nerve Palsy.

5. **Convergence insufficiency:** See 13.8, Convergence Insufficiency.

FOLLOW-UP

1. If amblyopia is being treated, see 8.6, Amblyopia.

2. If no amblyopia is present, then reexamine every 4 to 6 months. The parents and patient are told to return sooner if the deviation increases or becomes more frequent.

8.5 STRABISMUS SYNDROMES

Motility disorders that demonstrate typical features of a particular syndrome. Specific entities include the following:

SYNDROMES

• Duane syndrome (A congenital motility disorder, usually unilateral, characterized by limited abduction, limited adduction, or both. The globe may retract and the eyelid fissure narrow on adduction. There is often a face-turn to allow the patient to use both eyes together.) Duane syndrome may be classified into three types:

—Type 1: Limited abduction (most common).

—Type 2: Limited adduction.

—Type 3: Limited abduction and adduction.

• Brown syndrome (A motility disorder characterized by limitation of elevation in adduction. Elevation in abduction is normal. Typically, eyes are straight in primary gaze. Usually congenital, but may be acquired secondary to trauma, surgery, or inflammation in the area of the trochlea. Bilateral in 10% of patients.).

• Double-elevator palsy (Congenital unilateral limitation of elevation in all fields of gaze. There may be hypotropia of the involved eye when the other eye fixes in primary gaze. Ptosis or pseudoptosis may be present in primary gaze. The child may assume a chin-up position to maintain fusion in downgaze.).

• Möbius syndrome (Congenital unilateral or bilateral limitation of horizontal eye movements with a unilateral or bilateral, partial or complete facial nerve palsy. Other cranial nerve palsies as well as deformities of the hands or feet may also occur.).

• Congenital fibrosis syndrome [Congenital stationary bilateral ptosis and external ophthalmoplegia with limited horizontal gaze. The eyes cannot be elevated to primary gaze (straight ahead), so the patient maintains a chin-up position.].

WORKUP

1. History: Age of onset? History of trauma? Family history? History of other ocular or systemic diseases?

2. Complete ophthalmic examination, including alignment in all fields of gaze. Note if a compensatory head posture is present. Look for retraction of globe and narrowing of interpalpebral fissure in adduction.

3. Pertinent physical examination, including cranial nerve evaluation.

4. Radiologic studies (e.g., MRI or CT scan) may be indicated for acquired, atypical, or progressive motility disturbances.

TREATMENT

1. Treatment is usually indicated for significant abnormal head position, or if a cosmetically noticeable horizontal or vertical deviation exists in primary gaze.

2. Surgery, when indicated, depends on the particular motility disorder, extraocular muscle function, and the degree of abnormal head position.

FOLLOW-UP

Follow-up depends on the condition or conditions being treated.

8.6 AMBLYOPIA

SYMPTOMS

Usually asymptomatic or decreased vision in one eye. A history of patching, strabismus, or muscle surgery as a child may be elicited.

Note: Amblyopia occasionally occurs bilaterally as a result of bilateral visual deprivation (e.g., congenital cataracts, high refractive errors).

SIGNS

Critical. Poorer vision in one eye that is not improved with refraction and not entirely explained by an organic lesion. The decrease in vision develops during the first decade of life and does not deteriorate thereafter. Amblyopia occasionally occurs bilaterally as a result of bilateral visual deprivation such as in congenital cataracts.

Other. Crowding phenomenon occurs when individual letters can be read better than a whole line. A neutral-density filter significantly reduces vision in organic disease, but usually does not in pure amblyopia.

Note: Amblyopia, when severe, may cause a mild relative afferent pupillary defect.

ETIOLOGY

• Anisometropia (A large difference in refractive error between the two eyes.).

• Strabismus (The eyes are not straight. Vision is worse in the nonfixating eye. Strabismus can lead to, or be the result of, amblyopia.).

• Occlusion [Such as from ptosis; congenital or secondary (e.g., eyelid hemangioma) or iatrogenic (e.g., patching).].

• Organic [Such as a media opacity (e.g., cataract, corneal scar, PHPV, retinal or macular lesion).].

WORKUP

1. History: Eye problem in childhood, particularly misaligned eyes? Patching or muscle surgery as a child?

2. Ocular examination to rule out an organic cause for the reduced vision. Carefully check the pupils, optic disc, and macula.

3. Cover–uncover test to evaluate eye alignment (see Appendix 2).

4. Refraction; cycloplegic in children too young to cooperate.

TREATMENT

1. Patients younger than 9 to 11 years:

   —Appropriate spectacle correction.

   —Full-time patching over the eye with better vision for 1 week per year of age (e.g., 3 weeks for a 3-year-old), followed by a repeated eye examination. Pirate patches and patches worn over glasses are less effective than patches placed directly over the eye and adhering to the skin. If a patch causes local irritation, use tincture of benzoin on the skin before applying the patch and use warm water compresses on the patch before removal.

   —Continue patching until the vision is equalized or shows no improvement after three compliant cycles of patching. If a recurrence of amblyopia is likely, then use part-time patching to maintain improved vision.

   —If occlusion amblyopia (i.e., a decrease in vision in the patched eye) develops, patch the opposite eye for a short period (e.g., 1 day per year of age), and repeat the examination.

   —In strabismic amblyopia, delay strabismus surgery until the vision in the two eyes is equal, or maximal vision has been obtained in the amblyopic eye.

2. Patients older than 11 years of age: A trial of patching may be considered if patching has never been done. Otherwise no treatment is available. Protective glasses (e.g., polycarbonate lenses) should be worn at all times if there is only one good eye.

8.7 CONGENITAL CATARACT

SIGNS

Critical. Opacity of the lens.

Other. A white fundus reflex (leukocoria), absent red pupillary reflex, or abnormal eye movements (nystagmus) in one or both eyes. Infants with bilateral cataracts may be noted to be visually inattentive. Eye misalignment (strabismus), nystagmus, or a blunted red reflex may be present. In patients with a monocular cataract, the involved eye is often smaller. A cataract alone does not cause a relative afferent pupillary defect.

DIFFERENTIAL DIAGNOSIS

See 8.1, Leukocoria.

ETIOLOGY

• Idiopathic (most common).

• Familial, autosomal dominant.

• Galactosemia (Cataract may be the sole manifestation when galactokinase deficiency is responsible. A deficiency of galactose-1-phosphate uridyl transferase may produce mental retardation and symptomatic cirrhosis along with cataracts. The typical oil-droplet opacity may or may not be seen.).

• PHPV (Unilateral. The involved eye is usually slightly smaller than the normal fellow eye. Examination after pupil dilatation may reveal a plaque of fibrovascular tissue behind the lens with elongated ciliary processes extending to it.

Progression of the lens opacity often leads to angle-closure glaucoma.).

• Rubella (Nuclear cataract, "salt-and-pepper" chorioretinitis, a smaller involved eye than the normal contralateral eye. Associated hearing defects and heart abnormalities are common.).

• Lowe syndrome (oculocerebrorenal syndrome) (Opaque lens, congenital glaucoma, renal disease, and mental retardation. X-linked recessive. Patients' mothers may have small cataracts.).

• Others (Chromosomal disorders, systemic syndromes, other intrauterine infections, trauma, drugs, other metabolic abnormalities.).

TYPES

1. Polar: Opacity of the lens capsule and adjacent cortex on the anterior or posterior pole of the lens.

2. *Zonular* (lamellar): White opacities that surround the nucleus with alternating clear and white cortical lamella like an onion skin.

3. Nuclear: Opacity within the embryonic/fetal nucleus.

4. Posterior lenticonus: A posterior protrusion, usually opacified, in the posterior capsule (most common cause of nontraumatic congenital cataract).

WORKUP

1. History: Maternal illness or drug ingestion during pregnancy? Systemic or ocular disease in the infant or child? Radiation exposure or trauma? Family history of congenital cataracts?

2. Visual assessment of each eye alone, by using illiterate E's, pictures, or by following small toys or a light.

3. Ocular examination: Attempt to determine the visual significance of the cataract. Evaluate the size and location of the cataract and whether the retina can be seen with a direct ophthalmoscope when looking through an undilated pupil. Cataracts 3 mm or more in diameter usually affect vision, although cataracts less than 3 mm may cause ambly-

opia secondary to anisometropia. A portable slit lamp is helpful when available, as is a retinoscope (a blunted retinoscopic reflex suggests the cataract is visually significant). Check for signs of associated glaucoma (e.g., large corneal diameter, corneal edema, breaks in Descemet membrane) and examine the optic nerve and retina for abnormalities, if possible.

4. Cycloplegic refraction.

5. B-scan ultrasonography may be helpful when the fundus view is obscured.

6. Medical examination by a pediatrician looking for associated abnormalities.

7. Red blood cell (RBC) galactokinase activity (galactokinase levels) with or without RBC galactose-1-phosphate uridyl transferase activity to rule out galactosemia. This test is performed routinely on all infants in the United States.

8. Other tests as suggested by the systemic or ocular examination. (The chance that one of these conditions is present in a healthy child is remote.)

—Blood: Calcium and phosphorus levels (hypocalcemia, hypoparathyroidism), glucose levels (hypoglycemia, diabetes mellitus).

—Urine: Amino acid quantitation (Alport syndrome), amino acid content (Lowe syndrome).

—Antibody titers for rubella.

TREATMENT

1. Referral to a pediatrician to treat any underlying disorder.

2. Treat associated ocular diseases (e.g., glaucoma; see 8.11, Congenital Glaucoma).

3. Cataract extraction, usually within days to weeks of discovery to prevent irreversible amblyopia, is performed in the following circumstances:

—Vision is obstructed, and the eye's visual development is at risk.

—The lens is responsible for intraocular disease (e.g., lens-related glaucoma, uveitis).

—Cataract progression threatens the health of the eye (e.g., in PHPV).

4. After cataract extraction, treat amblyopia in children younger than 9 to 11 years.

5. A dilating agent (e.g., phenylephrine, 2.5%, t.i.d., homatropine, 2%, t.i.d., or scopolamine, 0.25%, q.d.) may be used as a temporizing measure, allowing peripheral light rays to pass around the lens opacity and reach the retina. This rarely is successful.

6. Unilateral cataracts that are not large enough to obscure the visual axis and thus require removal may still result in amblyopia. Treat amblyopia in children younger than 9 to 11 years (see 8.6, Amblyopia).

FOLLOW-UP

1. Young children who do not undergo surgery are monitored closely for cataract progression and amblyopia.

2. Amblyopia is less likely to develop in older children even if the cataract progresses; they are followed on a 6- to 12-month basis.

Note: Children with rubella must be isolated from pregnant women.

8.8 CONGENITAL SYPHILIS

SIGNS

Critical

• Interstitial keratitis: Usually presents acutely in the first or second decade of life with cellular infiltration and superficial and deep vascularization of the cornea (corneal "salmon patch"). Both eyes eventually become affected. As the inflammation resolves, the cornea may thin, opacify, or exhibit blood vessels containing no blood in their lumens (ghost vessels).

• Anterior uveitis: Cells and flare in the anterior chamber.

• Secondary cataracts.

• Chorioretinitis: Typically appears as a salt-and-pepper fundus (pigmented areas interspersed among atrophic white areas). Pseudoretinitis pigmentosa.

• Optic atrophy: A pale optic nerve.

Systemic. Widely spaced, peg-shaped teeth (Hutchinson teeth), frontal bossing, depressed nasal bridge (saddle nose), nerve deafness, recurrent arthropathy, linear scars at the angles of the mouth, mental retardation, others.

DIFFERENTIAL DIAGNOSIS

Other congenital infections [Toxoplasmosis, rubella, cytomegalovirus, herpes simplex or herpes zoster virus, rubeola (measles). Specific serologic titers usually are positive; rapid plasma reagin (RPR) and fluorescent treponemal antibody, absorbed (FTA-ABS) usually are negative.].

WORKUP

1. History: Maternal syphilis? Medical problems since birth (persistent runny nose, rash, deafness, scars on the skin, others)? Previous treatment for syphilis?

2. Complete ocular examination, including a pupillary assessment, a slit-lamp examination if possible, and a dilated fundus examination (in interstitial keratitis, the fundus may not be well visualized).

3. B-scan ultrasonography should be considered when no fundus view is obtained to rule out a retinal detachment and mass lesion.

4. Blood tests (may also test on placenta and umbilical cord): RPR [or Venereal Disease Re-

search Laboratory (VDRL)] and FTA-ABS [or microhemagglutination–*Treponema pallidum* (MHA-TP)]; consider viral and *Toxoplasma* titers when the diagnosis is uncertain.

Note: Passively transferred maternal treponemal antibodies can be present in an infant until age 15 months, so both the RPR/ VDRL and FTA-ABS can be positive in a syphilis-free infant born to a mother with the disease.

5. Consider dark-field examination of scrapings from skin lesions, if available.

6. Lumbar puncture for routine studies, including a VDRL, is indicated in all cases of active disease or in cases of inactive disease not previously treated.

7. Long bone radiographic studies may assist in systemic diagnosis.

TREATMENT

See 13.5, Acquired Syphilis, for serology determinations.

1. In general, treatment is indicated for a positive blood VDRL and one of the following:

—Clinical evidence of syphilis (see Signs, Systemic).

—Long bone radiographic changes.

—Positive cerebrospinal fluid (CSF) VDRL.

—Unexplained increased CSF protein or white blood cells (WBCs).

—Blood VDRL four times mother's serology.

—Positive FTA-ABS immunoglobulin M.

2. Systemic antibiotics (one of the following):

Younger than 1 month of age (according to Centers for Disease Control and Prevention):

—Aqueous crystalline penicillin G, 50,000 U/kg/dose intravenously (i.v.) q12h during the first 7 days of life and q8h thereafter for a total of 10 days.

—Procaine penicillin G, 50,000 U/kg/dose intramuscularly (i.m.) q.d. for 10 days.

—Penicillin-allergic patients should be desensitized and then treated with penicillin because data are insufficient regarding the use of other antimicrobial agents.

Older than 1 month of age:

—Aqueous crystalline penicillin G, 50,000 U/kg/dose q4–6h for 10 days.

Note: If more than 1 day of therapy is missed, the entire course should be restarted.

3. In the presence of acute interstitial keratitis or anterior chamber inflammation, a topical steroid (prednisolone acetate, 1%, four to eight times per day) and a cycloplegic (e.g., scopolamine, 0.25%, t.i.d.) should be used.

4. Intraocular pressure (IOP) control [e.g., if greater than 30 mm Hg, consider levobunolol or timolol, 0.25% to 0.5%, b.i.d., or acetazolamide, 5 mg/kg orally (p.o.), q6h, or both].

FOLLOW-UP

1. Patients are seen daily until their systemic therapy is completed, and then in 1 to 2 weeks.

2. All seroreactive infants should receive careful follow-up examinations and serologic testing every 2 to 3 months until the test becomes nonreactive or the titer has decreased fourfold. Nontreponemal antibody titers decline by age 3 months and should be nonreactive by 6 months in disease-free infants or in infants infected but adequately treated. The serologic response after therapy may be slower for infants treated after the neonatal period.

3. When the results of lumbar puncture are abnormal (e.g., positive CSF VDRL, WBC count more than 5 WBCs/mm^3 or protein greater than 45 mg/dL), follow-up is as described for neurosyphilis (see 13.5, Acquired Syphilis).

8.9 OPHTHALMIA NEONATORUM
(NEWBORN CONJUNCTIVITIS)

SIGNS

Critical. Purulent, mucopurulent, or mucoid discharge from one or both eyes in the first month of life, with diffuse conjunctival injection.

Other. Eyelid edema, chemosis.

DIFFERENTIAL DIAGNOSIS

• Dacryocystitis (Swelling and erythema of the inner canthus. Purulent discharge may be expressed from the punctum by rolling a finger from the lacrimal sac to the punctum. Nasal conjunctival injection may be present, but diffuse injection is typically not present. See 6.8, Dacryocystitis.).

• Nasolacrimal duct obstruction (Tearing, may have a mild mucopurulent discharge from the punctum, minimal to no conjunctival injection or eyelid swelling. See 8.10, Congenital Nasolacrimal Duct Obstruction.).

• Congenital glaucoma (Corneal enlargement greater than 12 mm horizontally, photophobia, Haab stria, corneal edema, buphthalmos, tearing but not discharge. See 8.11, Congenital Glaucoma.).

ETIOLOGY

• Chemical [Seen within a few hours of instilling a prophylactic agent (e.g., silver nitrate), lasts no more than 24 to 36 hours. Rarely seen now that erythromycin is used routinely.].

• *N. gonorrhoeae* (May see gram-negative intracellular diplococci on Gram stain. Typically seen within the first few days of life.).

• *Chlamydia trachomatis* (May see basophilic intracytoplasmic inclusion bodies in conjunctival epithelial cells, polymorphonuclear leukocytes, or lymphocytes on Giemsa stain. Presentation in the second week of life is common.).

• Bacteria (Staphylococci, streptococci, and gram-negative species may be seen on Gram stain.).

• Herpes simplex virus (May have typical herpetic vesicles on the eyelid margins, can see multinucleated giant cells on Giemsa stain.).

WORKUP

1. History: Previous or concurrent venereal disease in the mother? Were cervical cultures performed during pregnancy? If so, obtain the results.

2. Ocular examination with a penlight and then a blue light after fluorescein instillation; look for corneal involvement.

3. Conjunctival scrapings for two slides: Gram and Giemsa stain.

   —Technique: Irrigate the discharge out of the fornices, place a drop of topical anesthetic (e.g., proparacaine) in the eye, and scrape the palpebral conjunctiva of the lower eyelid with a flame-sterilized spatula after it cools off, or use a calcium alginate swab. Place the scrapings on the slides.

4. Conjunctival cultures for blood and chocolate agars: Chocolate agar should be placed in an atmosphere of 2% to 10% carbon dioxide immediately after being plated.

   —Technique: Reanesthetize the eye if necessary. Moisten a calcium alginate swab (a cotton-tipped applicator is a less desirable alternative) with liquid broth media, and vigorously rub it along the inferior palpebral conjunctiva. Plate it directly on the culture dish. Repeat the procedure for additional cultures.

5. Scrape the conjunctiva for the chlamydial immunofluorescent antibody test or polymerase chain reaction if available.

6. Viral culture: Moisten another cotton-tipped applicator and roll it along the palpebral conjunctiva. Break off the end of the applicator and place it into the viral transport medium.

TREATMENT

Initial therapy is based on the results of the Gram and Giemsa stains, if they can be examined immediately. Therapy is then modified according to the culture results and the clinical response.

1. No information from stains, no particular organism suspected: Erythromycin ointment q.i.d. plus erythromycin elixir, 50 mg/kg/day, for 2 to 3 weeks.

   Note: Erythromycin elixir is divided into four doses daily and added to the infant's formula.

2. Suspect chemical (e.g., silver nitrate) toxicity: No treatment or preservative-free artificial tears q.i.d. Reevaluate in 24 hours.

3. Suspect chlamydial infection: Erythromycin elixir, 50 mg/kg/day, for 2 to 3 weeks, plus erythromycin ointment q.i.d. If confirmed by culture or immunofluorescent stain, treat the mother and her sexual partner or partners with one of the following:

   —Tetracycline, 250 to 500 mg p.o., q.i.d., or doxycycline, 100 mg p.o., b.i.d., for 7 days (for men and mothers who are neither breast-feeding nor pregnant) or azithromycin 1 g as a single dose; or

   —Erythromycin, 250 to 500 mg p.o., q.i.d., for 7 days (for breast-feeding or pregnant women).

   Note: Inadequately treated chlamydial conjunctivitis in a neonate can lead to chlamydial otitis or pneumonia.

4. Suspect N. gonorrhoeae: Treatment is not well established. We favor the following:

   —Hospitalize and evaluate for disseminated gonococcal infection with careful physical examination (especially of joints). Blood and CSF cultures are obtained if a culture-proven infection is present.

   —Ceftriaxone 25 to 50 mg/kg i.v. or i.m. (not to exceed 125 mg), as a single dose or cefotaxime 100 mg/kg i.v. or i.m. as a single dose. In penicillin- or cephalosporin-allergic patients, an infectious disease consult is obtained.

   —Bacitracin ointment, every 2 to 4 hours.

   —Topical saline lavage to remove any discharge, q.i.d.

   —All neonates with gonorrhea should also be treated for chlamydial infection with erythromycin elixir, 50 mg/kg/day for 14 days.

   Note: If GC is confirmed by culture, the mother and her sexual partner or partners should be treated for 7 days in accordance with the sensitivity results. If sensitivities are not initially available, ceftriaxone is the first choice. In addition, chlamydial infection should be treated as outlined earlier.

5. Gram-positive bacteria on Gram stain, with no suspicion of gonorrhea and no corneal involvement: Bacitracin ointment, q.i.d., for 2 weeks.

6. Gram-negative bacteria on Gram stain, but no suspicion of gonorrhea, and no corneal involvement: Gentamicin, tobramycin, or ciprofloxacin (Ciloxan) ointment, q.i.d., for 2 weeks.

7. Bacteria on Gram stain and corneal involvement: Hospitalize, workup, and treat as 4.11, Bacterial Keratitis.

8. Suspect herpes simplex virus: The neonate, regardless of the presenting ocular findings, should be treated with acyclovir i.v. as well as vidarabine 3% ointment (e.g., Vira-A), if available, or trifluridine (e.g., Viroptic) drops. Vidarabine should be administered five times per day and trifluridine nine times a day, after which the dosage should be cut in half for 1 week. In full-term infants, the dosage for acyclovir is 45 to 60 mg/kg/day divided in three doses, given i.v. for 14 days if limited to the skin, eye, and mouth and for 21 days if the disease is disseminated or involves the central nervous system. For children

with recurrent ocular lesions, oral suppressive therapy with acyclovir (20 mg/kg q6h) may be of benefit.

FOLLOW-UP

1. Initially, examine daily as an inpatient or outpatient.

2. If the condition worsens (e.g., corneal involvement develops), reculture and hospitalize. As mentioned, therapy is tailored according to the clinical response and the culture results. The frequency of follow-up visits may be reduced once improvement is clearly demonstrated.

8.10 CONGENITAL NASOLACRIMAL DUCT OBSTRUCTION

SIGNS

Critical. Wet-looking eye or tears flowing over the eyelid; moist or dried mucopurulent material on the eyelashes (predominantly medially), and reflux of mucoid or mucopurulent material from the punctum when pressure is applied over the lacrimal sac, where the lower eyelid abuts the nose.

Other. Erythema (irritation) of the surrounding skin; redness and swelling of the medial canthus. Preseptal cellulitis or dacryocystitis may rarely develop.

Note: Nasolacrimal duct obstruction may be associated with an otitis or pharyngitis.

DIFFERENTIAL DIAGNOSIS

• Conjunctivitis (Red eye, discharge. Usually acute. Follicles or papillae may or may not be present on the inferior tarsal conjunctiva. Tearing is not chronic.).

• Congenital anomalies of the upper lacrimal drainage system (Atresia of the lacrimal puncta or canaliculus.).

• Mucocele of the lacrimal sac (Bluish, cystic, nontender mass located just below the medial canthal angle. Caused by both a distal and a proximal obstruction of the nasolacrimal apparatus.).

• Other causes of tearing (e.g., entropion/trichiasis, corneal defects, foreign body under the upper eyelid, congenital glaucoma). (See 8.11, Congenital Glaucoma.)

ETIOLOGY

Usually the result of an imperforate membrane at the distal end of the nasolacrimal duct.

WORKUP

1. Exclude other causes of tearing with slit-lamp or penlight examination. Make sure the corneal diameter is not large, and ruptures in Descemet membrane are not present (congenital glaucoma).

2. Palpate over the lacrimal sac; reflux of mucoid or mucopurulent discharge from the punctum confirms the diagnosis.

TREATMENT

1. Digital pressure to canalicular system b.i.d. to q.i.d. The parent is taught to place his or her index finger over the child's common canaliculus (inner corner of the eye) and to apply pressure several times a day.

2. Erythromycin ointment b.i.d., as needed, to control mucopurulent discharge if present.

3. In the presence of acute dacryocystitis, a systemic antibiotic is needed (see 6.8, Dacryocystitis).

Most cases open spontaneously with this regimen by 1 year of age. If this is not the case:

4. Nasolacrimal duct probing is usually performed after age 13 months, earlier if recurrent or persistent infections of the lacrimal system develop, or at the request of the parents. Most obstructions are corrected after the initial probing; others may require repeated probings. If patency is not established after two probings, place silicone tubing in the nasolacrimal duct and leave it in place for weeks to months.

FOLLOW-UP

Follow up by phone calls. The child returns if the situation becomes worse or acute dacryocystitis is present, or if the parents are unsure.

8.11 CONGENITAL GLAUCOMA

SIGNS

Critical. Enlarged globe and corneal diameter (horizontal corneal diameter greater than 12 mm before age 1 year is suggestive), corneal edema, increased IOP, increased cup/disc ratio, commonly bilateral.

Other. Linear tears in Descemet membrane of the cornea (Haab striae), usually running horizontally or concentric to the limbus; corneal stromal scarring; conjunctival injection; myopic shift in refractive error.

DIFFERENTIAL DIAGNOSIS

• Congenital megalocornea (Bilateral horizontal corneal diameter greater than 13 mm, with normal corneal thickness and endothelium. IOP and cup/disc ratio are normal.).

• Trauma from forceps during delivery (May produce tears in Descemet membrane and localized corneal edema; however, the tears are typically vertical or oblique, and the corneal diameter is normal. Birth trauma is usually unilateral and may often be obtained from the history.).

• Congenital hereditary endothelial dystrophy (Bilateral corneal edema at birth with a normal corneal diameter and normal IOP.).

• Mucopolysaccharidoses and cystinosis (Some inborn errors of metabolism produce cloudy corneas in infancy or early childhood, but usually not at birth; the corneal diameter and IOP are normal.).

• Nasolacrimal duct obstruction (Tearing, sometimes with a mild mucopurulent discharge from the punctum. The cornea is clear and not enlarged. The IOP is normal. See 8.10, Congenital Nasolacrimal Duct Obstruction.).

ETIOLOGY

Common:

• Primary congenital glaucoma (Not associated with other ocular or systemic disorders.).

Less Common:

• Sturge–Weber syndrome (Usually unilateral; may have a port wine stain, cerebral calcifications, and seizures; not familial.).

Rare:

• Developmental anterior segment abnormality (e.g., Axenfeld syndrome, Rieger anomaly/syndrome, Peters anomaly, others). (Bilateral. Abnormalities of the cornea, iris, and anterior chamber angle.).

• Lowe syndrome (oculocerebrorenal syndrome) (Cataract, glaucoma, and renal disease; X-linked recessive.).

• Rubella (Glaucoma, cataracts, "salt-and-pepper" chorioretinopathy, hearing and cardiac defects.).

- Aniridia (Iris hypoplasia, often with only a rudimentary iris stub visible on gonioscopy, cataracts, glaucoma, foveal hypoplasia, nystagmus.).

- Others (e.g., neurofibromatosis, homocystinuria, PHPV, secondary glaucoma from anteriorly displaced lens–iris diaphragm).

WORKUP

1. History: Other systemic abnormalities? Rubella infection during pregnancy? Birth trauma?

2. Ocular examination, including a visual acuity assessment of each eye separately (can the child fixate and follow?), a penlight examination to detect corneal enlargement and haziness, and retinoscopy to estimate refractive error. IOP measurement by Tono-Pen or Schiötz tonometry is attempted. A dilated fundus examination is performed to evaluate the optic disc and retina. Examination with a retinoscope or hand-held portable slit lamp is sometimes used in uncertain cases to look for tears in Descemet membrane and corneal edema.

3. EUA is performed in suggestive cases and in those for whom surgical treatment is planned. The horizontal corneal diameter and IOP are measured; retinoscopy, gonioscopy, and ophthalmoscopy are performed. Ultrasonography is often used to measure axial length. At 40 gestational weeks, the mean axial length is 17 mm. This increases to 20 mm on average by age 1 year. Axial length progression also may be monitored by successive cycloplegic refractions.

Note: IOP may be reduced substantially by general anesthesia, particularly halothane; an IOP of 20 mm Hg or more under halothane anesthesia is suggestive of glaucoma. An exception is ketamine hydrochloride, which may increase IOP. In general, IOP is measured as soon as possible after general anesthesia is induced to achieve as accurate a measurement as possible.

TREATMENT

Definitive treatment is usually surgical. Medical therapy is temporary and is started initially, pending surgery.

1. Medical: (Any or all of the following may be used.)

   —Topical beta-blocker (e.g., levobunolol or timolol, 0.25% to 0.5%, b.i.d.).

   —Carbonic anhydrase inhibitor (e.g., acetazolamide, 5 to 10 mg/kg p.o., q6h).

   Note: Miotics are rarely effective in controlling and may increase IOP, but they sometimes are used to constrict the pupil in preparation for a surgical goniotomy.

2. Surgical: First choice, goniotomy (incising the trabecular meshwork with a blade under gonioscopic visualization) or trabeculotomy (opening Schlemm canal into the anterior chamber). These procedures are often repeated if they are unsuccessful at first attempt.

3. Other: Trabeculectomy.

   Note: Amblyopia may be superimposed on glaucoma and should be treated by patching (see 8.6, Amblyopia).

FOLLOW-UP

1. Repeated examinations, under anesthesia when needed, are necessary to monitor corneal diameter, IOP, cup/disc ratio, and axial length.

2. These patients must be followed throughout life to monitor for progression.

8.12 DEVELOPMENTAL ANTERIOR SEGMENT AND LENS ANOMALIES

SPECIFIC ENTITIES

Unilateral or bilateral congenital abnormalities of the cornea, iris, anterior chamber angle, and lens. Specific entities include the following:

• Megalocornea (A nonprogressive corneal enlargement): The horizontal corneal diameter is greater than 13 mm in the newborn. There are two types:

—Simple megalocornea: Bilateral, clear corneas of normal thickness; sporadic or autosomal dominant.

—Anterior megalophthalmos: Bilateral; associated with abnormalities of the iris, angle, and lens; may be associated with glaucoma; X-linked recessive.

• Microcornea [Horizontal corneal diameter less than 11 mm. May be isolated or associated with nanophthalmos (a small globe that is otherwise anatomically normal) and microphthalmos (a small globe with multiple anomalies).].

• Posterior embryotoxon (A prominent, anteriorly displaced Schwalbe ring. A normal variant.).

• Axenfeld anomaly (Posterior embryotoxon associated with iris strands that span the angle to insert into the prominent Schwalbe ring. Glaucoma develops in 50% to 60% of patients. Autosomal dominant or sporadic.).

• Rieger anomaly (Axenfeld anomaly plus iris thinning and abnormally shaped and displaced pupils. Glaucoma develops in 50% to 60% of patients. Autosomal dominant or sporadic.).

• Rieger syndrome (Rieger anomaly associated with dental, craniofacial, and skeletal abnormalities. May be associated with short stature caused by growth hormone deficiency, cardiac defects, deafness, and mental retardation. Autosomal dominant or sporadic.).

• Peters anomaly [Central corneal opacity, usually with iris strands that extend from the iris collarette to the margin of the corneal defect. The lens may be clear and normally positioned, cataractous and displaced anteriorly (making the anterior chamber shallow), or adherent to the corneal defect.].

• Microspherophakia (The lens is small and spherical in configuration. The lens can subluxate into the anterior chamber, causing a secondary glaucoma.).

• Anterior and posterior lenticonus (An anterior or posterior ectasia of the lens surface, posterior occurring more commonly than anterior. Often associated with cataract. Usually unilateral.).

• Ectopia lentis (May be associated with Marfan syndrome, homocystinuria, Weill–Marchesani syndrome, aniridia, and trauma. Simple ectopia lentis is either a sporadic or autosomal dominantly inherited condition with bilateral, usually superior, lens displacement. Glaucoma may occur because of displacement of the lens–iris diaphragm.).

• Ectopia lentis et pupillae (Lens displacement associated with pupillary displacement in the opposite direction. Glaucoma may occur. Autosomal recessive.).

• Aniridia (Bilateral, near-total absence of the iris. The pupil appears to occupy the entire area of the cornea. Glaucoma, foveal hypoplasia with poor vision, nystagmus, and corneal pannus can occur. At least two inheritance patterns are known to exist:

—Autosomal dominant in two thirds of patients: This type is not associated with Wilms tumor.

—Sporadic in one third of patients: Wilms tumor develops in 25% of children with sporadic aniridia.).

WORKUP

1. History: Family history of ocular disease? Associated systemic abnormalities?

2. Complete ophthalmic examination, including gonioscopy of the anterior chamber angle and IOP determination (may require EUA).

3. Complete physical examination by a primary care physician with blood pressure determination (may be elevated with renal abnormalities).

4. Chromosomal karyotype in patients with sporadic cases of aniridia. (There is an increased incidence of Wilms tumor in patients with a deletion of the short arm of chromosome 11.).

5. Renal ultrasonography and possibly i.v. pyelography in patients with sporadic aniridia to monitor for Wilms tumor. The frequency and duration of monitoring should be determined by a pediatrician or pediatric oncologist. One suggested schedule is to evaluate every 3 months up to age 5 years, and then every 6 months up to age 10, and then once per year up to age 16.

TREATMENT

1. Correct refractive errors and treat amblyopia if present (see 8.6, Amblyopia). Children with unilateral structural abnormalities often have improved visual acuity after amblyopia therapy.

2. Treat glaucoma if present. Beta-blockers and carbonic anhydrase inhibitors may be used. Pilocarpine and epinephrine compounds are not as effective and are not used in primary therapy (see 9.1, Primary Open-Angle Glaucoma). Surgery is often used initially (see 8.11, Congenital Glaucoma).

3. Consider cataract extraction if a significant cataract exists and a corneal transplant if a dense corneal opacity exists.

4. Provide genetic counseling.

5. Systemic abnormalities (e.g., Wilms tumor) are managed by pediatric specialists.

FOLLOW-UP

1. Ophthalmic examination every 6 to 12 months throughout life, checking for increased IOP and other signs of glaucoma.

2. If amblyopia exists, follow-up may need to be more frequent (see 8.6, Amblyopia).

8.13 CONGENITAL PTOSIS

SIGNS

Critical. Droopy eyelid(s).

Other. Amblyopia, strabismus, telecanthus.

DIFFERENTIAL DIAGNOSIS

• Simple congenital ptosis (Usually unilateral. Present at birth and stable throughout life. Indistinct or absent upper eyelid crease. Ptosis improves with downgaze. May have compensatory brow elevation or chin-up head position. Coexisting motility abnormality.).

• Blepharophimosis (Bilateral and severe. Autosomal dominant with high penetrance.) There are three types:

—Type I: All four eyelids phimotic with upper eyelid ptosis.

—Type II: Telecanthus, ptosis, and absent epicanthal folds.

—Type III: Telecanthus, ptosis, and present epicanthal folds. May also have flattened nasal bridge and low-set ears.

• Marcus Gunn jaw winking [Usually unilateral. Upper eyelid movement with contraction of muscles of mastication, resulting in "winking" while chewing. Upper eyelid crease intact with decreased or variable levator function. May have associated strabismus (hypotropia secondary to superior rectus paralysis).].

- Acquired ptosis (see Differential Diagnosis of Ptosis in Chapter 2).

- Pseudoptosis [Dermatochalasis, contralateral proptosis, enophthalmos, hypotropia (see Differential Diagnosis of Pseudoptosis in Chapter 2).].

ETIOLOGY

Defective function of either the levator or Muller neuromuscular complexes.

WORKUP

1. History: Age of onset? Duration and variability? Family history? History of trauma or prior surgery? Any crossing of eyes? Asymmetry in tearing? Facial flushing?

2. Visual acuity for each eye separately, with correction, to evaluate for amblyopia.

3. Manifest and cycloplegic refraction checking for anisometropia.

4. Pupillary examination

5. Ocular motility examination

6. Measure interpalpebral fissure distance, distance between corneal light reflex and upper eyelid margin, levator function (while manually fixing eyebrow), position and depth of upper eyelid crease. Check for Bell phenomenon.

7. Slit-lamp examination; look for signs corneal exposure.

8. Dilated fundus examination

TREATMENT

1. Observation if degree of ptosis mild, no evidence of amblyopia, and abnormal head positioning is not interfering with child's development. Surgery is optimally deferred until 3 to 5 years of age to allow for maturation of the eyelid and more accurate preoperative measurements.

2. Simple congenital ptosis: If levator function is poor, consider a frontalis suspension. If levator function is normal, consider a levator resection.

3. Blepharophimosis: Staged procedure initially repairing epicanthal folds and telecanthus followed by frontalis suspension.

4. Marcus Gunn jaw winking: No treatment if mild. If ptosis is moderate, levator resection may be performed. If ptosis is severe, consider ablation of levator followed by frontalis suspension.

FOLLOW-UP

1. If observing, patients should be reexamined every 3 to 12 months, depending on severity and age, to monitor for occlusion or anisometropic amblyopia.

2. After surgery, patients should be monitored for undercorrection or overcorrection and recurrence.

8.14 THE BLIND INFANT

SIGNS

An infant whose visual skills are far below those expected (e.g., an inability to fixate on and follow objects after several months of age). Obvious causes include bilateral central corneal opacities, congenital cataracts, or infectious retinal problems with macular scarring. The following are conditions that may not be obvious on clinical examination.

Conditions that usually produce a searching nystagmus

- Pupils react poorly to light.

—Any severe ocular disease or malformation (e.g., ROP, cataracts, aniridia, optic nerve atrophy, optic nerve hypoplasia) diagnosed by examination.

—Leber congenital amaurosis. [May have a normal-appearing fundus initially, but by age

1 to 3 years, may show narrowing of retinal blood vessels, optic disc pallor, and pigmentary retinal changes. The electroretinogram (ERG) is markedly abnormal or flat. Autosomal recessive.].

—Optic nerve hypoplasia [A small optic disc that can be difficult to detect when bilateral (compare disc with vessels). If unilateral, may be seen with strabismus, a relative afferent pupillary defect, and unilateral poor fixation instead of searching nystagmus. When present, a "double ring" sign (a pigmented ring at the inner and outer edge of peripapillary atrophy) is diagnostic. Usually idiopathic, but can be a result of maternal diabetes or quinine, phenytoin, alcohol, or lysergic acid diethylamide (LSD) use.].

Note: Optic nerve hypoplasia is rarely associated with septooptic dysplasia (de Morsier syndrome), which includes midline abnormalities of the brain and growth, thyroid, and other trophic hormone deficiencies. Growth retardation, seizures as a result of hypoglycemia, and diabetes insipidus may develop.

—Congenital optic atrophy (Rare. Pale, normal-sized optic disc, often associated with mental retardation or cerebral palsy. Normal ERG. Autosomal recessive or sporadic.).

—Congenital stationary night blindness (Visual acuity may even be normal, nystagmus less common, associated with myopia. ERG is abnormal. Autosomal dominant, recessive, and X-linked forms exist.).

• Pupils react briskly to light.

—Infantile nystagmus (Some patients with this condition have a severe visual deficit. The iris is normal. It may be accompanied by face turn, head nodding, or both.).

—Albinism with delayed maturation (Iris transillumination defects and foveal hypoplasia are seen.).

No nystagmus present and pupils react normally to light

• Diffuse cerebral dysfunction (Infants do not respond to sound or touch and are neurologically abnormal. Vision may slowly improve with time.).

• Delayed maturation of the visual system (Normal response to sound and touch, and neurologically normal. The ERG is normal, and vision usually develops between age 4 and 12 months.).

• Extreme refractive error (Diagnosed on cycloplegic refraction.).

• Achromatopsia (rod monochromatism) (Pupils react normally to light but have paradoxical pupil response. Normal fundus, but photopic ERG is markedly attenuated or nonrecordable. Scotopic ERG is normal.).

WORKUP

1. History: Premature? Normal development and growth? Maternal infection, diabetes, or drug use during pregnancy? Family history of eye disease?

2. Evaluate the infant's ability to fixate on an object and follow it with each eye individually (cover one eye and then the other).

3. Pupillary examination, noting both equality and briskness.

4. Look carefully for nystagmus.

5. Penlight examination of the anterior segment; check especially for iris transillumination defects with a slit lamp.

6. Dilated retinal and optic nerve evaluation.

7. Cycloplegic refraction.

8. ERG, especially if Leber congenital amaurosis is suspected.

9. Consider a CT scan or MRI of the brain in cases with other focal neurologic signs, seizures, failure to thrive, developmental delay, optic nerve hypoplasia, optic atrophy, or neurologically localizing nystagmus (e.g., see-saw, vertical, gaze paretic, vestibular). Consider including orbital cuts if optic atrophy is unilateral. Imaging is performed in these cases to rule out brain

tumors, hydrocephalus, infarctions, evidence of trauma, and brain malformations such as septooptic dysplasia.

10. Consider a sweep visual evoked potential for vision measurement.

11. Consider eye movement recordings to evaluate the nystagmus wave form, if available.

TREATMENT

1. Correct refractive errors and treat known or suspected amblyopia.

2. Parental counseling is necessary in all of these conditions with respect to the infant's visual potential, the likelihood of visual problems in siblings, and so forth.

3. Referral to educational services for the visually handicapped or blind may be helpful.

4. Provide genetic counseling.

5. If neurologic or endocrine abnormalities are found or suspected, the child should be referred to a pediatrician for appropriate workup or management.

CHAPTER 9

GLAUCOMA

9.1 PRIMARY OPEN-ANGLE GLAUCOMA

SYMPTOMS

Usually asymptomatic until the later stages both because of the slowly progressive nature of the disease and because the individual visual fields of each eye overlap quite significantly when both eyes are open. For symptoms to occur, the individual field defects must overlap. Patients with early symptoms may complain that parts of a page are missing. The classic symptom of tunnel vision does not occur until both visual fields are markedly damaged. Typically, central fixation is preserved until late in the disease. In the end stages of glaucoma, the remaining visual field is usually a temporal island.

SIGNS

Critical. Sixty to 70% of patients have an intraocular pressure (IOP) greater than average (more than 22 mm Hg); 30% to 40% have an IOP of less than 21 mm Hg. Open anterior chamber angle on gonioscopic evaluation. No peripheral anterior synechiae (PAS). Characteristic optic nerve appearance includes documented thinning of the neurosensory rim over time, acquired pit of the optic nerve, notching in the rim, nerve fiber layer hemorrhage that crosses the disc margin (i.e., Drance hemorrhage), nerve fiber layer defect, cup/disc (C/D) asymmetry greater than 0.2 in the absence of a

cause such as anisometropia, thinner rim superiorly or inferiorly than temporally, or thinner rim nasally than temporally, bayoneting (quick angulation in the course of the blood vessels as they exit the nerve), enlarged C/D ratio (greater than 0.6; less specific). Characteristic visual field loss: Nasal step (respects the horizontal midline), paracentral scotoma, or an arcuate scotoma extending from the blind spot nasally (defects usually respect the horizontal midline, or are greater in one hemifield than the other). Late finding may show only a temporal island of vision remaining.

Other. Large fluctuations in IOP, absence of microcystic corneal edema, an uninflamed eye.

DIFFERENTIAL DIAGNOSIS

• Ocular hypertension (Elevated IOP, with normal optic nerve and visual field. See 9.2, Ocular Hypertension.).

• Physiologic optic nerve cupping (Enlarged C/D ratio, but no change over time, no neurosensory rim notching, no visual field loss, and usually a normal IOP.).

• Secondary open-angle glaucoma [Lens-induced, inflammatory, exfoliative, pigmentary, steroid-induced, developmental anterior segment abnormalities, angle recession, traumatic (as a result of direct injury, blood, or debris), glaucoma related to increased episcleral venous pressure (e.g., Sturge–Weber syndrome, carotid–cavernous fistula), glaucoma related to intraocular tumors.].

• Secondary angle-closure glaucoma [e.g., iridocorneal endothelial (ICE) syndrome].

• Chronic angle-closure glaucoma (CACG) [Findings of primary open-angle glaucoma (POAG) except PAS are present on gonioscopy. CACG has an insidious onset, and may be associated with secondary causes of PAS such as uveitis, central retinal vein occlusion, and previous attack of angle closure leaving PAS.].

• Previous glaucomatous damage (e.g., from steroids, uveitis, glaucomatocyclitic crisis, trauma) in which the inciting agent has been removed.

• Optic atrophy [Chiasmal tumors, syphilis, ischemic optic neuropathy, drugs, retinal vascular or degenerative disease, others. IOP is usually not increased in these conditions unless a secondary or unrelated glaucoma also is present. These conditions are differentiated by optic nerve pallor in greater proportion than optic nerve cupping. Visual field defects are usually larger than expected, given the degree of optic nerve cupping. Glaucomatous-appearing visual fields are possible. Altitudinal defects are less typical of glaucoma and are more characteristic of anterior ischemic optic neuropathies. Altitudinal defects that respect the vertical midline are more typical of intracranial lesions (e.g., tumor, hemorrhage, ischemia) in the visual pathways.].

• Congenital optic nerve defects (Myopic discs, colobomas, optic nerve pits. IOP is usually not increased in these conditions, unless a secondary or unrelated glaucoma also is present. Visual field defects may be present, but do not progress.).

• Optic nerve drusen [Visual field defects may remain stable or progress unrelated to IOP. Optic nerves are usually not cupped, and drusen are often visible on examination. Characteristic calcified lesions seen on B-scan ultrasonography and on computed tomography (CT).].

WORKUP

1. History: Presence of risk factors (e.g., family history of blindness or visual loss from glaucoma, hypertension, age, black race, myopia). Previous history of increased IOP or chronic steroid use? Medical problems such as asthma, congestive heart failure, heart block, renal stones, allergies?

2. Complete ocular examination including slit lamp, gonioscopy, and dilated fundus examination with special attention to the optic nerve.

3. Baseline documentation of the optic nerves (e.g., stereoscopic disc photos, red-free photographs, image analysis, or meticulous drawings), corneal pachymetry, and formal visual field testing (preferably automated, e.g., Humphrey or Octopus). Goldmann visual field tests may be helpful in patients unable to take the automated tests adequately. Color vision testing indicated in those suspected of a neurologic disorder.

4. Central corneal pachymetry (CCT), identified in the Ocular Hypertension Treatment Study (OHTS) to be a strong predictor for development of POAG, may be measured to aid in risk factor stratification for a patient. The IOP should be adjusted based on corneal thickness algorithms.

5. Atypical cases may warrant a further evaluation for other causes of optic nerve damage. Aspects that may warrant further evaluation include the following.

—Optic nerve pallor out of proportion to the degree of cupping.

—Visual field defects greater than expected based on amount of cupping.

—Visual field patterns not typical of glaucoma (e.g., defects respecting the vertical midline, hemianopic defects, enlarged blind spot, central scotoma).

—IOP within the average range (less than 21 mm Hg).

—Unilateral progression despite equal IOP in both eyes.

—Decreased visual acuity out of proportion to the amount of cupping or field loss.

—Color vision loss, especially in the red–green axis.

If any of these are present, further evaluation may include:

—History: Acute episodes of eye pain or redness? Steroid use? Acute visual loss? Ocular trauma? Surgery, systemic trauma, heart attack, or other event that may lead to hypotension?

—Diurnal IOP curve consisting of multiple IOP checks during the course of the day.

—Complete blood count, erythrocyte sedimentation rate, rapid plasma reagin, fluorescent treponemal antibody, absorbed, possibly antinuclear antibody.

—If visual field defect patterns are more indicative of neurologic disease or if other neurologic signs/symptoms are present, may consider CT (axial and coronal, preferably with contrast if no contraindications are present) or magnetic resonance imaging of orbit and brain with gadolinium and fat suppression (if no contraindications are present).

—Consider referral to the primary care physician for a complete cardiovascular evaluation.

TREATMENT

General Considerations

1. Who to treat?

The clinician must evaluate the appropriateness of treatment for each individual case, because not all three elements of pressure, optic nerve damage, and visual field loss may be present in every case. Treatment must be based on the patient's overall physical and social health. Some general guidelines are suggested.

—Consideration should be given to the amount of damage already present, the rate of damage progression, and the estimated duration of time further damage may accumulate (i.e., an estimation of the patient's life expectancy).

—Treatment decisions regarding patients with an IOP greater than 24 mm Hg, without optic nerve or visual field changes, are difficult. Some clinicians may elect to monitor these patients with close observation because some patients may never get worse. Some clinicians may elect to treat these patients, given the statistical possibility that visual field loss will develop in approximately 50% in 5 to 10 years. Factors to consider when deciding whether to proceed with treatment include degree of IOP increase (e.g., the higher the IOP, the more likely visual loss is to develop), presence of risk factors (particularly family history of visual loss and black race), estimation of the duration of time damage may develop (i.e., the patient's life expectancy), and risks of the various treatment options.

2. What is the treatment goal?

The goal of treatment is to enhance or at least maintain the patient's health. This is accomplished by halting optic nerve damage and not causing problems through the treatments. The only proven method of stopping or slowing optic nerve damage is reducing IOP. It appears necessary to reduce the IOP by approximately 30% to have the best chance of preventing optic nerve damage. When optic nerve damage is marked, pressure reduction may need to be even greater for the destruction to be halted; some have suggested setting 15 mm Hg as the maximal tolerable IOP in such cases. Another method of calculating the IOP goal is the use of formula: [IOP d − (IOP d × IOP d)]/100 = goal, where IOP d represents the level of pressure known to be associated with damage. Some have suggested that if IOP can be lowered below 40%, visual field restoration can occur.

3. How to treat?

The main treatment options for glaucoma include medications, argon laser trabeculoplasty (ALT), selective laser trabeculoplasty

(SLT), and guarded filtration surgery (trabeculectomy). For many patients, medications are the first-line therapy. ALT or SLT is often an appropriate initial therapy, especially in elderly, ill, or demented patients with 2+, 3+, or 4+ posterior trabecular meshwork pigmentation. Surgery as first-line therapy is being investigated. Results of a prospective, randomized, multicenter trial (Collaborative Initial Glaucoma Treatment Study) at 5-year follow-up have shown the same visual field outcome for surgical and medical therapy; however, further follow-up is needed to form conclusions as to whether current treatment approaches to POAG should be revised.

The type and aggressiveness of treatment are determined by the amount of damage already present, the rate of destruction, and the anticipated duration of the disease. When the rate of destruction is rapid and damage is advanced, surgery is usually needed.

Additional treatment modalities, such as tube-shunt procedures (with either Molteno, Baerveldt, Krupin, Ahmed, or Schocket implants), laser cyclophotocoagulation of the ciliary body [with yttrium aluminum garnet (YAG) laser, diode laser, or endolaser], cyclocryotherapy, and cyclodialysis are typically reserved for IOP uncontrolled by other methods such as medications, laser, and traditional filtering procedures.

Medications

Unless there are extreme circumstances, such as an IOP greater than 40 mm Hg or an impending risk to central fixation, treatment is started by using one type of drop in only one eye (one-eyed therapeutic trial). This is done by initiating therapy with the new medication in only one eye with reexamination in 3 to 6 weeks to check for effectiveness. Effectiveness is determined by comparing the difference in IOP in the two eyes before therapy with the differences in IOP after initiating therapy.

For example, if IOP is 30 mm Hg OD and 33 mm Hg OS before treatment, and, after treatment of the right eye, the IOP is 20 mm Hg OD and 23 mm Hg OS, the drug is not having any effect. If the IOP after starting treatment is 25 mm Hg OD and 34 mm Hg OS, then the drug is having an effect.

1. Beta-blockers (e.g., levobunolol or timolol 0.25% to 0.5% q.i.d. or b.i.d. metipranolol, 0.3%; or carteolol, 1% b.i.d.) often effectively reduce IOP, but should be used with caution in patients with asthma/chronic obstructive pulmonary disease (COPD), heart block, congestive heart failure, depression, or myasthenia gravis. Betaxolol, 0.25% to 0.5% b.i.d., is less likely to cause pulmonary complications. The pulse is usually checked before and after initiating therapy. Diabetic patients should be warned of the possibility of decreased sensitivity to the symptoms of hypoglycemia.

2. Selective α_2-receptor agonists (brimonidine, 0.15% or 0.2% t.i.d. or b.i.d.) are also often effective at reducing IOP. These agents should not be given to patients currently taking monoamine oxidase inhibitors because of the possibility of hypertensive crisis. Commonly encountered side effects include allergy, dry mouth, dry eye, lethargy, mydriasis, and hypotension. Apraclonidine, 0.5% t.i.d., also may be used for short-term therapy (3 months), but tends to lose its effectiveness and has a relatively high allergy rate.

3. Topical carbonic anhydrase inhibitors (e.g., dorzolamide, 2%, or brinzolamide, 1% t.i.d., or b.i.d. if used in conjunction with a beta-blocker) can be used to reduce IOP. These drops have the same potential side effects as systemic carbonic anhydrase inhibitors, except that metabolic acidosis, hypokalemia, gastrointestinal symptoms, weight loss, and paresthesias are usually not seen. More commonly seen side effects include burning, bitter taste, and topical allergy.

4. Prostaglandin agonists (e.g., latanoprost, 0.005% q.h.s.; bimatoprost, 0.03% q.h.s.; travoprost, 0.004% q.h.s.; unoprostone isopropyl, 0.15%) also can be added to reduce IOP further. This type of agent is contraindicated in patients with active uveitis or cystoid macular edema (CME), and in pregnant women. Potential side effects include increased melanin pigmentation in the iris and

periorbital skin, conjunctival injection, stinging sensation, increase in eyelash length, viral upper respiratory tract infection symptoms, and CME.

5. Miotics (e.g., pilocarpine q.i.d.) are usually used in low strengths initially (e.g., 0.5% to 1.0%) and then built up to higher strengths (e.g., 4%). Commonly not tolerated in patients older than 40 years because of accommodative spasm. Miotics are usually contraindicated in patients with retinal holes and should be used cautiously in patients at risk for retinal detachment (e.g., high myopes and aphakes). Pilocarpine is also available as a 4% gel used nightly or as an ocular insert replaced each week; the latter may be most useful in young patients. Long-acting agents, such as echothiophate iodide, are often the preferred medication in aphakic or pseudophakic glaucoma patients.

6. Sympathomimetics (dipivefrin, 0.1%, b.i.d., or epinephrine, 0.5% to 2.0%, b.i.d.) rarely reduce IOP to the degree of the other drugs, but have few systemic side effects other than red eyes. They may cause CME in aphakic patients and cardiac arrhythmias.

7. Systemic carbonic anhydrase inhibitors [e.g., methazolamide, 25 to 50 mg orally (p.o.), b.i.d. to t.i.d., acetazolamide, 125 to 250 mg p.o., b.i.d. to q.i.d., or acetazolamide, 500 mg sequel p.o., b.i.d.] should usually not be given to patients with a sulfa allergy and should be avoided in patients with a history of renal stones. Potassium levels must be monitored if the patient is taking other diuretic agents or digitalis. Side effects, such as fatigue, nausea, confusion, and paresthesias, are common. Rare, but severe, hematologic side effects (e.g., aplastic anemia) have occurred.

Note: Digital punctal occlusion or passive eyelid closure should be used in every patient to decrease systemic absorption. All patients should be given specific instruction in this regard.

Argon Laser Trabeculoplasty

In some patients, as defined earlier, ALT may be used as first-line therapy. In addition, ALT may be considered first-line therapy in patients with demonstrated or suspected noncompliance. Approximately 10% of patients have some increase of pressure each year, so the average effective duration is approximately 5 years.

Selective Laser Trabeculoplasty

As a primary laser therapy, studies show that the IOP-lowering effect of SLT is equivalent to ALT. SLT, however, is repeatable and may be more effective than ALT after previous ALT therapy.

Guarded Filtration Surgery

Trabeculectomy may obviate the need for medications. Adjunctive use of antimetabolites during surgery may aid in the effectiveness of the surgery.

FOLLOW-UP

1. Patients are reexamined after starting a new medication to evaluate its efficacy; for beta-blockers, prostaglandin analogs, and after ALT/SLT, it is usually best to recheck the patient in 3 to 6 weeks. With topical carbonic anhydrase inhibitors, alpha-agonists, and miotics, a steady state is achieved much more quickly, and recheck any time after 3 days is appropriate.

2. When damage is severe, or IOP high, it may be necessary to see the patient within 1 to 3 days to ensure that the desired effect has occurred.

3. Once the IOP has been reduced adequately, patients are reevaluated in 3- to 6-month intervals for IOP and optic nerve checks. A goal of therapy is to reduce the IOP to a target pressure approximately 30% beneath the range at which glaucomatous progression occurred. This target pressure depends on the severity of disease and speed of progression, and it must be updated often.

4. Gonioscopy is performed yearly and after starting a new-strength cholinergic agent (e.g., pilocarpine).

5. Formal visual fields of the same type (e.g., Humphrey, Octopus) are rechecked every 6 to 12 months. If loss is severe, or IOP reduction is not thought to be adequate, visual fields may need to be repeated more often, perhaps at 1- to 3-month intervals until the cause of the condition is defined. Once stabilized, repeated field examinations at yearly intervals usually suffice to monitor stability.

6. Dilated retinal examinations should be performed yearly. If glaucomatous damage progresses, check patient compliance with medications before initiating additional therapy.

7. Patients must be questioned about side effects. They often do not associate eye drops with impotence, weight loss, or lightheadedness, and will not necessarily volunteer these and other significant symptoms. Specific questions appropriate for the agents used should be asked.

See the Drug Glossary for additional drug information.

9.2 OCULAR HYPERTENSION

SIGNS

Critical. Asymptomatic increased IOP, usually more than 21 mm Hg. Apparently normal anterior chamber angle anatomy on gonioscopic evaluation. Apparently normal optic nerve and visual field.

DIFFERENTIAL DIAGNOSIS

• POAG (see 9.1, Primary Open-Angle Glaucoma).

• Secondary open-angle glaucoma [e.g., lens-induced, inflammatory, exfoliative, pigmentary, steroid-induced, developmental anterior segment abnormalities, angle recession, traumatic (as a result of direct injury, blood, or debris), ICE syndrome, glaucoma related to increased episcleral venous pressure (e.g., Sturge–Weber syndrome, carotid–cavernous fistula), glaucoma related to intraocular tumors].

• CACG (Findings of POAG except PAS are present on gonioscopy. Patients with CACG typically have an insidious onset, but may also be the result of acute angle closure glaucoma or uveitis.).

WORKUP

1. History and complete examination as with POAG. See 9.1, Primary Open-Angle Glaucoma.

2. We recommend obtaining baseline stereoscopic disc photos, image analysis (e.g., HRT or GDx), and automated visual field testing (Humphrey, Octopus) or kinetic visual field (e.g., Goldmann). The purpose is to be able to detect changes over time. Visual fields must be normal. If any abnormalities are present, consider repeated testing in 2 to 4 weeks to exclude the possibility of learning curve artifacts. If the defects are judged to be real, the diagnosis is not ocular hypertension alone. Some additional entities are present.

3. CCT (The IOP should be adjusted based on corneal thickness algorithms.).

TREATMENT

1. If there are no suggestive optic nerve or visual field changes and IOP is less than 24 mm Hg, no treatment other than close observation is necessary.

2. In general, patients with an IOP greater than 24 to 32 mm Hg may be treated with medications even if no other optic nerve or visual field changes are present. A decision to treat a patient should be based on the patient's choice to elect therapy and baseline risk factors such as age, central corneal thickness, initial IOP, horizontal and vertical C/D ratio, and pattern standard deviation as

described in the OHTS. If treatment is elected, a therapeutic trial in one eye, as described for treatment of POAG, should be used. Some clinicians may elect to monitor these patients with close observation. See 9.1, Primary Open-Angle Glaucoma.

FOLLOW-UP

1. For patients not undergoing treatment, close follow-up for the first few years is absolutely necessary. Patients should be monitored every 3 to 6 months for pressure and optic nerve examinations. Formal visual field testing should be repeated every 6 to 12 months for the first 1 to 2 years to ensure no progression. After the first few years, patients should be checked every 6 to 12 months for IOP, and dilated fundus examination performed. Visual field testing should be repeated every 1 to 2 years. Five to 10% of patients with ocular hypertension progress over 5 years to development of POAG. Because it is not known whether the patient will ever experience symptoms due to glaucoma, therapy must be used with caution.

2. For patients undergoing treatment, follow-up is the same as for patients with POAG. See 9.1, Primary Open-Angle Glaucoma.

BIBLIOGRAPHY

Gordon MO, Beiser JA, Brandt JD, et al. The Ocular Hypertension Treatment Study: baseline factors that predict the onset of primary open-angle glaucoma. *Arch Ophthalmol* 2002;120: 714–720, discussion 829–830.

Kass MA, Heuer DK, Higginbotham EJ, et al. The Ocular Hypertension Treatment Study: a randomized trial determines that topical ocular hypotensive medication delays or prevents the onset of primary open-angle glaucoma. *Arch Ophthalmol* 2002;120:701–713.

9.3 ANGLE-RECESSION GLAUCOMA

SYMPTOMS

Usually asymptomatic until the late stages, at which point unilateral visual field or acuity loss may be noted. A history of hyphema or trauma to the glaucomatous eye can usually be elicited. Glaucoma due to the angle recession itself (not from the trauma that caused the angle recession) usually takes approximately 20 years to develop after the trauma. Typically unilateral.

SIGNS

Critical. Glaucoma (see 9.1, Primary Open-Angle Glaucoma) in an eye with characteristic gonioscopic findings. These findings include an uneven iris insertion with an area of torn or absent iris processes and posteriorly recessed iris to reveal a widened ciliary band. In some cases, these abnormalities and the angle recession extend for 360 degrees. Comparison with corresponding angle structures of the normal contralateral eye help in identification of recessed areas.

Other. The scleral spur may appear abnormally white on gonioscopy because of the recessed angle; other signs of previous trauma may be present (e.g., cataract, iris sphincter tears).

DIFFERENTIAL DIAGNOSIS

See 9.1, Primary Open-Angle Glaucoma.

WORKUP

1. History: Trauma? Family history of glaucoma?

2. Complete ocular examination including measurement of IOP and slit-lamp, gonioscopic, and dilated examination with special attention to the optic nerve.

3. Baseline documentation of the optic discs (e.g., stereoscopic disc photos, red-free photographs, image analysis, or meticulous drawings).

4. Formal visual field examination, preferably automated (e.g., Humphrey, Octopus) in cases suspect for or with definite glaucoma.

TREATMENT

Similar to that for POAG (see 9.1, Primary Open-Angle Glaucoma), except miotics (e.g., pilocarpine) may be ineffective or even cause increased IOP as a result of a reduction of uveoscleral outflow. ALT is rarely effective in this condition.

FOLLOW-UP

Patients with angle recession without glaucoma are examined yearly. Those with glaucoma are examined according to the guidelines of 9.1, Primary Open-Angle Glaucoma. Follow-up should carefully monitor both eyes because there is a high incidence of delayed open-angle glaucoma and steroid-responsive IOP in the uninvolved as well as the traumatized eye.

9.4 INFLAMMATORY OPEN-ANGLE GLAUCOMA

SYMPTOMS

Pain, photophobia, decreased vision; symptoms may be minimal.

SIGNS

Critical. IOP above the patient's baseline, often unilateral with a significant amount of aqueous white blood cells and flare, open angle on gonioscopy. Early in the course, there may not be the characteristic optic nerve and visual field findings, but these may develop with time. See the critical signs of POAG (see 9.1, Primary Open-Angle Glaucoma) for specific optic nerve and visual field changes.

Other. Miotic pupil, PAS, inflammatory precipitates on the posterior corneal surface or trabecular meshwork, conjunctival injection, ciliary flush.

Note: *Acute IOP increase is distinguished from chronic IOP increase by the presence of corneal edema, pain, and the perception of halos around light.*

DIFFERENTIAL DIAGNOSIS

• Glaucomatocyclitic crisis (Posner–Schlossman syndrome). [Markedly increased IOP (usu-

ally 40 to 60 mm Hg), open angle and absence of synechiae on gonioscopy, mild anterior chamber reaction with few fine keratic precipitates, and minimal to no conjunctival injection. Unilateral with recurrent attacks. See 9.13, Glaucomatocyclitic Crisis.].

• Acute angle-closure glaucoma (Angle closed in the involved eye and usually narrow in the contralateral eye, mid-dilated pupil that reacts poorly to light, iris bombé, corneal edema, mild anterior chamber reaction without keratic precipitates. See 9.10, Acute Angle-Closure Glaucoma.).

• Pigmentary glaucoma (Acute increase in IOP, often after exercise or pupillary dilatation; pigment cells in the anterior chamber, on the trabecular meshwork, and along the posterior corneal surface. The angle is open, and radial iris transillumination (TI) defects are often present. See 9.6, Pigmentary Glaucoma.).

• Neovascular glaucoma (Iris and anterior chamber angle neovascularization are present. See 9.14, Neovascular Glaucoma.).

• Fuchs heterochromic iridocyclitis (Asymmetry of the iris color, mild iritis in the eye with the lighter-colored iris, usually unilateral, often associated with cataract, glaucoma, or both.

Conjunctival injection and ciliary flush are minimal. See 12.1, Anterior Uveitis.).

ETIOLOGY

- Anterior uveitis.

- Intermediate and posterior uveitis.

- Panuveitis.

- Keratouveitis. (Corneal disease present in addition to uveitis.)

- After trauma or intraocular surgery.

WORKUP

1. History: Previous attacks? Systemic disease [e.g., juvenile rheumatoid arthritis, ankylosing spondylitis, sarcoidosis, acquired immunodeficiency syndrome (AIDS)]? Previous corneal disease, especially herpetic keratitis? Recent dilating drops or a systemic anticholinergic agent (suggests angle-closure glaucoma)?

2. Slit-lamp examination: Assess the degree of conjunctival injection and aqueous cell and flare.

3. Measure IOP.

4. Gonioscopy of the anterior chamber angle: Is the angle open? Synechiae present? Neovascular membrane present?

5. Evaluate the optic nerve.

TREATMENT

1. Topical steroid (e.g., prednisolone acetate, 1%) q1–6h, depending on the severity of the anterior chamber cellular reaction.

   Note: Topical steroids are not used, or are used with extreme caution, in patients with an infectious process, particularly a fungal or herpes simplex infection.

2. Mydriatic/cycloplegic (e.g., cyclopentolate, 2%, scopolamine, 0.25% or atropine, 1% t.i.d.).

3. Topical beta-blocker (e.g., timolol or levobunolol, 0.5%, b.i.d.) if not contraindicated (e.g., asthma, COPD).

One or more of the following pressure-reducing agents can be used in addition to the other treatments, depending on the IOP and the status of the optic nerve:

4. Topical alpha-agonist (e.g., apraclonidine, 0.5%, or brimonidine, 0.15% or 0.2%, b.i.d. to t.i.d.).

5. Carbonic anhydrase inhibitor (e.g., methazolamide, 25 to 50 mg p.o., b.i.d. to t.i.d., or acetazolamide, 250 mg p.o., q.i.d., or 500 mg sequel p.o., b.i.d., or dorzolamide, 2%, or brinzolamide, 1%, t.i.d.).

6. Hyperosmotic agent when IOP is acutely increased (e.g., mannitol, 20%, 1 to 2 g/kg intravenously (i.v.) over 45 minutes; a 500-mL bag of mannitol, 20% contains 100 g of mannitol).

7. Manage the underlying problem.

8. When IOP remains dangerously increased despite maximal medical therapy (a rare event), glaucoma filtering surgery with adjunct antifibrosis therapy may be indicated.

   Note: Miotics (e.g., pilocarpine) and prostaglandin agonists (e.g., latanoprost, bimatoprost, travoprost, unoprostone) are contraindicated in inflammatory glaucoma.

FOLLOW-UP

1. Patients are seen every 1 to 7 days at first. The higher the IOP and the greater the amount of glaucomatous damage already present (e.g., the larger the optic nerve cup), the more frequent the follow-up.

2. Steroids are tapered as the inflammation subsides.

3. Antiglaucoma medications are discontinued as IOP returns to normal. Steroid-response glaucoma should always be considered in unresponsive cases (see 9.5, Steroid-Response Glaucoma).

9.5 STEROID-RESPONSE GLAUCOMA

SIGNS

Critical. Increased IOP with use of corticosteroids. Usually takes 2 to 4 weeks after starting topical steroids. May be seen after prolonged use of large doses of steroids in other forms (e.g., skin creams, nasal inhalers) or with subconjunctival depot or intravitreal injection of steroids. With systemic (oral or i.v.) steroid use, IOP may increase within a few days. On cessation of steroids, the IOP typically decreases to the level before the use of steroids. The rate of decrease relates to the duration of topical use and the severity of the pressure increase. The IOP increase is due to reduced outflow facility of the pigmented trabecular meshwork, and when this is severe, the IOP may remain increased for months after steroids are stopped. When systemic steroids are stopped, the IOP usually decreases to pretreatment levels within a few days.

Other. Signs of POAG may develop, including optic nerve cupping and field loss in an eye with an open anterior chamber angle.

Note: *Patients with POAG or a predisposition to development of glaucoma (i.e., family history, diabetes, black race, and high myopia) are more likely to experience a steroid response and subsequent glaucoma.*

DIFFERENTIAL DIAGNOSIS

Inflammatory open-angle glaucoma. (Increased IOP as a result of anterior chamber inflammation. Because steroids are used to treat ocular inflammation, it may be difficult to determine the cause of the increased IOP. See 9.4, Inflammatory Open-Angle Glaucoma.)

WORKUP

1. History: Duration of steroid use? Previous steroid use or an eye problem from steroid use? Glaucoma or family history of glaucoma? Diabetes?

2. Complete ocular examination: Evaluate the degree of ocular inflammation and determine presence of iris or angle neovascularization (by gonioscopy), pigment suggestive of pigment dispersion syndrome or pseudoexfoliation, blood in Schlemm canal, PAS, and so forth. Measure IOP and inspect the optic nerve.

3. Optic disc photographs and image analysis are obtained, and formal visual field (e.g., Humphrey, Octopus) examination performed when the optic nerve appears damaged or when the duration of IOP increase is prolonged or unknown.

4. If using topical steroids, may attempt discontinuation of steroid in one eye to see if IOP improves.

TREATMENT

Any or all of the following may be necessary to reduce IOP.

1. Discontinue the steroid or reduce the frequency of its administration (steroids should not be discontinued abruptly, but rather tapered).

2. Reduce the concentration or dosage of the steroid (e.g., topical prednisolone acetate, 1%, can be changed to topical prednisolone acetate, 0.12%).

3. Switch from a potent steroid with a greater propensity to produce a steroid response (e.g., prednisolone acetate) to one with a lesser propensity (e.g., fluorometholone or loteprednol).

4. Switch to a topical nonsteroidal antiinflammatory drug (NSAID; e.g., diclofenac, 0.1%).

5. Start antiglaucoma therapy. See 9.4, Inflammatory Open-Angle Glaucoma, for medical therapy options.

Notes

1. When a high IOP is found in a patient taking topical steroids for inflammatory glaucoma, it may be difficult to determine the cause of the increased IOP (i.e., whether it is the result of the inflammatory reaction or the steroids). If the inflammation is moderate to severe, we usually increase the steroids initially to reduce the inflammation while initi-ating antiglaucoma (e.g., topical beta-blocker) therapy. If the inflammation subsides, but IOP remains increased, the glaucoma is assumed to be steroid induced, and the outlined treatment regimen is followed.

2. When a dangerously high IOP that is uncontrollable with medication develops after a depot steroid injection, the steroid may need to be excised.

9.6 PIGMENT DISPERSION/PIGMENTARY GLAUCOMA

DEFINITION

Pigment dispersion refers to a pathologic increase in the trabecular meshwork pigment, associated with characteristic mid-peripheral, spokelike iris TI defects. Normally, the amount of pigment in the trabecular meshwork increases with aging, but does not exceed grade 2. Abnormal pigment dispersion is grade 3 to 4 trabecular pigmentation with increasing radial TI defects or increasing corneal endothelial pigmentation with time.

SYMPTOMS

May be asymptomatic or the patient may experience episodes of blurred vision, eye pain, and colored halos around lights after exercise or pupillary dilatation. More common in young adult, myopic men (age 20 to 45 years). Usually bilateral, but asymmetric.

SIGNS

Critical. Mid-peripheral, spokelike iris TI defects corresponding to iridozonular contact; dense homogeneous pigmentation of the trabecular meshwork for 360 degrees (seen on gonioscopy).

Other. A vertical pigment band on the corneal endothelium typically just inferior to the visual axis (Krukenberg spindle); pigment deposition on the equatorial lens surface, on Schwalbe line, and sometimes along the iris (which can produce iris heterochromia). The angle often shows a wide ciliary body band and is graded D or E 30 r or q (Spaeth classification; see Appendix 11), with 3+ to 4+ pigmentation of the posterior trabecular meshwork at the 12-o'clock position. Pigmentary glaucoma is characterized by the pigment dispersion syndrome plus glaucoma (optic nerve cupping, characteristic glaucomatous visual field changes, or increased IOP). Typically, large fluctuations in IOP can occur, during which pigment cells may be seen floating in the anterior chamber.

DIFFERENTIAL DIAGNOSIS

• Exfoliative glaucoma (Trabecular meshwork pigmentation is black, less homogeneous, and more prominent inferiorly. Iris TI defects may be present, but they are near the pupillary margin and are usually less prominent. White, flaky material may be seen on the pupillary border and anterior lens capsule. The angle is narrower than in pigment dispersion syndrome. A Sampaolesi line in the angle at 6 o'clock is pathognomonic. See 9.7, Exfoliative Glaucoma.).

• Inflammatory open-angle glaucoma (White blood cells and flare in the anterior chamber; typically no iris TI defects. Central corneal endothelial pigment deposits sometimes appear. Absence of grade 3 to 4 pigmentation of trabecular meshwork. Pigmentation is greater inferiorly. The presence of PAS inferiorly is characteristic. See 9.4, Inflammatory Open-Angle Glaucoma.).

• Iris melanoma (Pigmentation of the angular structures accompanied by either a raised, pigmented lesion on the iris or a diffusely darkened iris. No iris TI defects. See 5.13, Malignant Melanoma of the Iris.).

• After irradiation (History of radiation; induces atrophy and depigmentation of the ciliary processes, with increased pigment deposition in outflow channels.).

WORKUP

1. History: Previous episodes of decreased vision or halos?

2. Slit-lamp examination, particularly checking for iris TI defects. Large defects may be seen by shining a small slit beam directly into the pupil to obtain a red reflex, but scleral TI is required if the defects are not extremely marked. Look for a Krukenberg spindle on the corneal endothelium. Look for pigment on lens equator by angling the slit beam nasally and having the patient look temporally (pathognomonic for pigmentary glaucoma).

3. Measure IOP.

4. Gonioscopy of the anterior chamber angle.

5. Evaluate the optic nerve.

6. Dilated retinal examination, with special attention to the periphery because of increased lattice degeneration in pigment dispersion.

7. Stereoscopic disc photographs or image analysis.

8. Visual field examination, preferably automated (e.g., Humphrey, Octopus).

TREATMENT

Depends on the IOP, status of the optic nerve, visual field changes, and extent of the symptoms. Often patients with pigment dispersion without glaucoma or symptoms are observed carefully. A stepwise approach to control IOP is usually taken when mild to moderate glaucomatous changes are present. When advanced glaucoma is discovered on initial examination, maximal medical therapy may be instituted initially (see 9.1, Primary Open-Angle Glaucoma).

1. Decreasing mechanical iridozonular contact. Two methods have been proposed.

—Miotic agents (a theoretic first line of therapy because they minimize iridozonular contact, which produces pigmentary release into the anterior chamber): However, because most patients are young and myopic, miotic drops, with resultant fluctuation in myopia, may not be practical. In addition, approximately 14% of patients have lattice retinal degeneration and are thus predisposed to retinal detachment from the use of miotics. In some cases, pilocarpine inserts (e.g., Ocuserts) used once per week or pilocarpine 4% gel, q.h.s., are tolerated.

—Peripheral laser iridotomy: Laser peripheral iridotomy has been recommended to reduce pigment dispersion by decreasing iridozonular contact, but it is still controversial.

Note: Miotics should be used cautiously because of the risk of retinal detachment in myopic patients.

2. Other antiglaucoma medications may be appropriate (see 9.1, Primary Open-Angle Glaucoma).

3. Consider ALT; these patients usually respond well. Younger patients respond better than older patients, in contrast to POAG.

4. Consider guarded filtration procedure when medical and laser therapy fail. These young myopic patients are at a greater risk for development of hypotony maculopathy.

FOLLOW-UP

Every 1 to 6 months, with a formal visual field test every 6 to 12 months, depending on the severity of the symptoms and the glaucoma.

9.7 EXFOLIATIVE GLAUCOMA (PSEUDOEXFOLIATION GLAUCOMA)

DEFINITION

A systemic disease in which grayish-white material is deposited on the lens, iris, ciliary epithelium, and trabecular meshwork. Presence of exfoliative material increases the risk of glaucoma sixfold. Currently, the most common identifiable entity causing glaucoma in white people.

SYMPTOMS

Usually asymptomatic in its early stages.

SIGNS

Critical. White, flaky material on the pupillary margin; anterior lens capsular changes (central zone of exfoliation material, often with rolled-up edges, middle clear zone, and a peripheral cloudy zone); peripupillary iris TI defects; and glaucoma (optic nerve cupping, glaucomatous visual field loss, or increased IOP). All of these signs are often asymmetric.

Other. Irregular black pigment deposition on the trabecular meshwork more marked inferiorly than superiorly; pigment anterior to Schwalbe line (Sampaolesi line) seen on gonioscopy, especially inferiorly. Bilateral, but often asymmetric. Poor response to dilation (with more advanced cases, believed to be secondary to iris dilator muscle atrophy). Incidence increases with age. These patients are more prone to having narrow angles.

DIFFERENTIAL DIAGNOSIS

• Pigmentary glaucoma [Pigmented trabecular meshwork accompanied by mid-peripheral iris TI defects. There may be a vertical pigment band on the corneal endothelium (Krukenberg spindle or Zentmyer line). Pigment on lens capsule anterior to the equator. See 9.6, Pigmentary Glaucoma.].

• Capsular delamination (true exfoliation) [Trauma, exposure to intense heat (e.g., glass blower), or severe uveitis can cause a thin membrane to peel off the anterior lens capsule. Glaucoma uncommon.].

• Primary amyloidosis (Amyloid material can deposit along the pupillary margin or anterior lens capsule. Glaucoma can occur.).

WORKUP

1. History: Occupational exposure to heat?

2. Slit-lamp examination with IOP measurement; often need to dilate the pupil to see the anterior lens capsular changes. Pupil usually dilates poorly.

3. Gonioscopy of the anterior chamber angle.

4. Optic nerve evaluation.

5. Stereo disc photographs or image analysis.

6. Visual field test, preferably automated (e.g., Humphrey, Octopus).

TREATMENT

1. For medical therapy, see 9.1, Primary Open-Angle Glaucoma.

2. Consider ALT, which has a higher initial success rate in exfoliative glaucoma than in POAG.

3. Consider guarded filtration procedure when medical or laser therapy fails.

4. The course of exfoliative glaucoma is usually not linear. Early, the condition may be relatively benign. However, the condition is associated with highly unstable IOP. When control starts to become increasingly difficult, the glaucoma may progress rapidly to cause advanced optic nerve damage, sometimes within a few months.

Note: Cataract extraction does not eradicate the glaucoma. Cataract extraction may be complicated by weakened zonular fibers and synechiae between the iris and peripheral anterior lens capsule. The posterior capsule is easily ruptured.

Every 1 to 3 months as with POAG, but with the awareness that damage in exfoliation syndrome can progress very rapidly, depending on the severity of the glaucoma.

Note: Many patients have exfoliation syndrome without glaucoma. These patients are re-examined every 6 to 12 months because they are at risk for glaucoma, but they are not treated unless glaucoma develops.

9.8 PHACOLYTIC GLAUCOMA

DEFINITION

Leakage of lens material from a cataract through an intact lens capsule leads to trabecular meshwork outflow obstruction.

SYMPTOMS

Unilateral pain, decreased vision, tearing, photophobia.

SIGNS

Critical. Markedly increased IOP, accompanied by iridescent particles and white material in the anterior chamber or on the anterior surface of the lens capsule. A hypermature (liquefied) or mature cataract is typical.

Other. Corneal edema, anterior chamber cells and significant flare, pseudohypopyon, and severe conjunctival injection. Gonioscopy reveals an open anterior chamber angle. Clumps of macrophages may be seen in inferior angle.

DIFFERENTIAL DIAGNOSIS

All of the following can produce an acute increase in IOP to high levels, but none displays iridescent particles and white material in the anterior chamber.

• Inflammatory glaucoma (Acute increased IOP as a result of severe anterior uveitis. See 9.4, Inflammatory Open-Angle Glaucoma.).

• Glaucomatocyclitic crisis (Recurrent idiopathic attacks of increased IOP with an open anterior chamber angle and mild iritis. See 9.13, Glaucomatocyclitic Crisis.).

• Acute angle-closure glaucoma (Increased IOP as a result of sudden closure of the anterior chamber angle, confirmed by gonioscopy. See 9.10, Acute Angle-Closure Glaucoma.).

• Lens-particle glaucoma ("Fluffed-up" lens material is seen in the anterior chamber; a history of traumatic lens damage or cataract extraction in the involved eye is characteristic. See 9.9, Lens-Particle Glaucoma.).

• Endophthalmitis (History of recent surgery or trauma; pain can be severe. See 12.10, Postoperative Endophthalmitis.).

• Glaucoma secondary to intraocular tumor (Unilateral cataract.).

• Others (e.g., traumatic glaucoma, ghost cell glaucoma, phacomorphic glaucoma, neovascular glaucoma).

WORKUP

1. History: Recent trauma or ocular surgery? Recurrent episodes? Uveitis in the past?

2. Slit-lamp examination: Look for iridescent or white particles as well as cells and flare in the anterior chamber. Evaluate for cataract and increased IOP producing corneal edema.

3. Gonioscopy of the anterior chamber angles of both eyes: Topical glycerin may be placed on the cornea after topical anesthesia to clear it temporarily if it is edematous.

4. Retinal and optic disc examination if possible. Otherwise, B-scan ultrasonography be-

fore cataract extraction to rule out an intraocular tumor or retinal detachment.

5. If the diagnosis is in doubt, a paracentesis can be performed to detect macrophages bloated with lens material on microscopic examination.

TREATMENT

The immediate goal of therapy is to reduce the IOP and to reduce the inflammation. The cataract should be removed promptly (within several days).

1. Topical beta-blocker (e.g., levobunolol or timolol, 0.25% to 0.5%, in one dose initially, and then b.i.d.), alpha-agonist (e.g., brimonidine, 0.15% or 0.2%, b.i.d. to t.i.d., apraclonidine, 0.5%, t.i.d.), or topical carbonic anhydrase inhibitor (e.g., dorzolamide, 2%, or brinzolamide, 1% t.i.d.).

2. Carbonic anhydrase inhibitor (e.g., acetazolamide, two 250-mg tablets p.o. in one dose, then 250 mg p.o., q.i.d.). Benefit of maintaining topical carbonic anhydrase inhibitor in addition to a systemic agent is controversial.

3. Topical cycloplegic (e.g., scopolamine, 0.25%, t.i.d.).

4. Topical steroid (e.g., prednisolone acetate, 1% every 15 minutes for four doses, then q1h).

5. Hyperosmotic agent if necessary and no contraindications are present (e.g., mannitol, 1 to 2 g/kg i.v. over 45 minutes; a 500-mL bag of mannitol, 20% contains 100 g of mannitol).

6. The IOP usually does not respond adequately to medical therapy. Although it is preferable to reduce IOP before cataract extraction, adequate IOP control may not be possible. Cataract removal is usually performed within 24 to 36 hours. If the IOP cannot be controlled medically, the patient may need hospitalization and urgent cataract extraction. Glaucoma surgery is usually not necessary at the same time as cataract surgery.

FOLLOW-UP

1. If patients are not hospitalized, they should be reexamined the day after surgery. Patients are usually hospitalized after their cataract surgery so that their IOP can be monitored over the ensuing 24 hours.

2. If the IOP returns to normal after the procedure, the patient should be rechecked within 1 week.

9.9 LENS-PARTICLE GLAUCOMA

DEFINITION

Lens material, liberated by trauma or surgery, that obstructs aqueous outflow channels.

SYMPTOMS

Pain, blurred vision, red eye, tearing, photophobia. History of recent ocular trauma or cataract surgery.

SIGNS

Critical. White, fluffy pieces of lens cortical material in the anterior chamber, combined with increased IOP. A break in the lens capsule may be observed in posttraumatic cases.

Other. Anterior chamber cell and flare, conjunctival injection, or corneal edema. The anterior chamber angle is open on gonioscopy.

DIFFERENTIAL DIAGNOSIS

See 9.8, Phacolytic Glaucoma. In phacolytic glaucoma, the cataractous lens has not been extracted or traumatized.

• Infectious endophthalmitis (Unless lens cortical material can be unequivocally identified in the anterior chamber, and there is nothing atypical about the presentation, endophthalmitis must be excluded. See 12.10, Postoperative Endophthalmitis, and 12.12, Traumatic Endophthalmitis.).

- Phacoanaphylactic endophthalmitis (Follows trauma or intraocular surgery, producing anterior chamber inflammation and sometimes a high IOP. The inflammation is often granulomatous, and fluffy lens material is not present in the anterior chamber.).

- Phacomorphic glaucoma (A cataractous lens becomes intumescent and physically closes the anterior chamber angle.).

WORKUP

1. History: Recent trauma or ocular surgery?

2. Slit-lamp examination: Search the anterior chamber for lens cortical material and measure the IOP.

3. Gonioscopy of the anterior chamber angle.

4. Optic nerve evaluation: The degree of optic nerve cupping helps determine how long the increased IOP can be tolerated.

TREATMENT

1. Topical beta-blocker (e.g., levobunolol or timolol, 0.25% to 0.5%, b.i.d.), topical alpha-agonist (e.g., brimonidine, 0.15% or 0.2%, b.i.d. to t.i.d., or apraclonidine, 0.5%, t.i.d.), topical carbonic anhydrase inhibitor (e.g., dorzolamide, 2%, or brinzolamide, 1%, b.i.d. to t.i.d.).

2. Carbonic anhydrase inhibitor (e.g., methazolamide, 25 to 50 mg p.o., b.i.d. to t.i.d., or acetazolamide, 250 mg p.o., q.i.d., or 500 mg sequel p.o., b.i.d.). Benefit of maintaining topical carbonic anhydrase inhibitor in addition to a systemic agent is controversial.

3. Topical cycloplegic (e.g., scopolamine, 0.25%, t.i.d.).

4. Topical steroid (e.g., prednisolone acetate, 1%, q.i.d.).

—If IOP is markedly increased (e.g., more than 45 mm Hg in a previously healthy eye or less in a patient with previous optic nerve damage), a hyperosmotic agent is added to reduce the pressure acutely (e.g., mannitol, 1 to 2 g/kg i.v. over 45 minutes; a 500-mL bag of mannitol, 20% contains 100 g of mannitol).

—If medical therapy fails to control the IOP, the residual lens material must be removed surgically.

FOLLOW-UP

Depending on the IOP and the health of the optic nerve, patients are reexamined in 1 to 7 days.

9.10 ACUTE ANGLE-CLOSURE GLAUCOMA

SYMPTOMS

Pain, blurred vision, colored halos around lights, frontal headache, nausea and vomiting.

SIGNS

Critical. Closed angle in the involved eye, acutely increased IOP, corneal microcystic edema. Shallow anterior chamber in both eyes.

Other. Conjunctival injection; fixed, mid-dilated pupil.

ETIOLOGY

- Pupillary block [Anatomically predisposed in eyes with narrow anterior chamber angle recess, anterior iris insertion of the iris root, or both; common in Asians, Eskimos, and hyperopes. May be precipitated by topical mydriatics or, rarely, miotics, systemic anticholinergics (e.g., antihistamines or antipsychotics), accommodation (e.g., reading), or dim illumination (e.g., movie theater). The angle is narrow or occludable in the contralateral eye.].

• Angle crowding as a result of an abnormal iris configuration [e.g., high peripheral iris roll or plateau iris syndrome angle closure occurs despite a patent peripheral iridectomy (PI). See 9.12, Plateau Iris.].

Note: A secondary mechanical cause of angle-closure glaucoma should be suspected when the anterior chamber angles are asymmetric (i.e., one angle is narrow but the other is deep).

DIFFERENTIAL DIAGNOSIS

Other causes of acute IOP increase, but with an open angle.

• Glaucomatocyclitic crisis (Posner–Schlossman syndrome) (Recurrent IOP spikes in one eye, mild cell and flare with or without fine keratic precipitates; the eye is usually not inflamed and not painful. See 9.13, Glaucomatocyclitic Crisis.).

• Inflammatory open-angle glaucoma (Moderate to severe anterior chamber reaction. See 9.4, Inflammatory Open-Angle Glaucoma.).

• Retrobulbar hemorrhage or inflammation (Proptosis and restriction of ocular motility. See 3.9, Traumatic Retrobulbar Hemorrhage.).

• Traumatic (hemolytic) glaucoma (History of trauma, red blood cells in the anterior chamber. See 3.4, Hyphema and Microhyphema.).

• Pigmentary glaucoma (Deep anterior chamber. Pigment cells floating in the anterior chamber, often after exercise or pupillary dilatation; radial iris TI defects. See 9.6, Pigmentary Glaucoma.).

Other causes of acute IOP increase, with closed angle: Secondary angle-closure glaucomas.

• Neovascular or inflammatory membrane pulling the angle closed (Abnormal misdirected blood vessels along the pupillary margin, the trabecular meshwork, or both are seen. See 9.14, Neovascular Glaucoma.).

• Mechanical closure of the angle secondary to anterior displacement of the lens–iris diaphragm:

—Lens-induced [Pupillary block as a result of a large lens (phacomorphic) or small lens (nanophthalmos), or zonular loss/weakness (e.g., traumatic, advanced pseudoexfoliation).].

—Choroidal detachment (serous or hemorrhagic) (Usually follows surgery; diagnose by indirect ophthalmoscopy, B-scan ultrasonography, or both.) .

—Medication-induced [Usually bilateral with possible serous choroidal detachment and often accompanied by a myopic shift. A history of oral topiramate, topical carbonic anhydrase inhibitors, and sulfa derivatives (note that acetazolamide/methazolamide are sulfa derivatives) should be explored. Ultrasonographic biomicroscopy (or high-frequency B-scan ultrasonography of the anterior segment) is often helpful in establishing the diagnosis.].

—Choroidal swelling after extensive retinal laser surgery or after placement of a tight encircling band in retinal detachment surgery.

—Posterior segment tumor (e.g., choroidal or ciliary body melanoma; see 11.32, Malignant Melanoma of the Choroid).

—Aqueous misdirection syndrome (see 9.17, Malignant Glaucoma).

• PAS (IOP increase is not acute; caused by uveitis, laser trabeculoplasty, ICE syndrome, others.).

WORKUP

1. History: Family history? Retinal problem? Recent laser treatment or surgery? Medications?

2. Slit-lamp examination: Look for keratic precipitates, posterior synechiae, iris neovascularization, a swollen lens, anterior chamber cells and flare or iridescent particles, and a

shallow anterior chamber. Glaukomflecken (small anterior subcapsular lens opacities) indicate prior attacks.

3. Measure IOP.

4. Gonioscopy of both anterior chamber angles: Corneal edema can usually be cleared by using topical hyperosmolar agents (e.g., glycerin). Compression gonioscopy may help determine if the trabecular blockage is reversible and may break an acute attack. Gonioscopy of the involved eye after IOP is reduced is essential in determining whether the angle has opened and whether neovascularization is present.

5. Careful examination of the fundus looking for signs of central retinal vein occlusion, hemorrhage, and optic nerve cupping. If cupping is pronounced, treatment is more urgent.

TREATMENT

Depends on etiology of angle-closure, severity, and duration of attack. Severe, permanent damage may occur within several hours. If visual acuity is hand movements or worse, IOP reduction is truly urgent, and medications should include all topical glaucoma medications not contraindicated, i.v. acetazolamide, and i.v. osmotics. If IOP is less than 50 mm Hg, and vision loss is less severe, parenteral/oral agents may not be needed. See 9.14, Neovascular Glaucoma, 9.16, Postoperative Glaucoma, and 9.17, Malignant Glaucoma (Aqueous Misdirection Syndrome) for specific treatment of these conditions.

1. Topical beta-blocker (e.g., levobunolol or timolol, 0.5%) in one dose (use with caution with concurrent asthma or COPD).

2. Topical steroid (e.g., prednisolone acetate, 1%) every 15 to 30 minutes for four doses, then hourly.

3. Topical apraclonidine, 1%, or brimonidine, 0.15% or 0.2%, for one dose.

4. Carbonic anhydrase inhibitor (e.g., acetazolamide, 250 to 500 mg i.v., or two 250-mg tablets p.o., in one dose) if IOP decrease is considered urgent.

5. When acute angle-closure glaucoma is the result of:

   a. Phakic pupillary block or angle crowding: Pilocarpine, 1% to 2%, every 15 minutes for two doses, and pilocarpine, 0.5%, in the contralateral eye for one dose.

   b. Aphakic or pseudophakic pupillary block or mechanical closure of the angle: Do not use pilocarpine. A mydriatic and cycloplegic agent (e.g., cyclopentolate, 2%, and phenylephrine, 2.5%, every 15 minutes for four doses) is used when laser or surgery is not initially used because of corneal edema, inflammation, or both.

6. In cases of phacomorphic glaucoma, the lens should be removed as soon as the eye is quieted with steroids and the IOP maximally controlled.

7. In cases of medication-induced secondary angle-closure glaucoma, the IOP should be managed medically and the inciting medication should be discontinued immediately. The angle closure resolves a few days to weeks after discontinuation of the medication and IOP returns to normal range.

8. Address systemic problems such as pain and vomiting.

9. Recheck the IOP and visual acuity in 1 hour.

   a. If IOP does not decrease and vision does not improve, repeat topical medications and give i.v. mannitol, 1 to 2 g/kg i.v. over 45 minutes (a 500-mL bag of mannitol, 20% contains 100 g of mannitol). Oral isosorbide is usually not tolerated and should be used only if patient is not nauseated.

   b. If IOP does not decrease after two courses of maximal medical therapy, a laser PI should be considered if there is an adequate view of the iris.

c. If IOP still does not decrease after the second round of medication and a second attempt at a laser PI, then a surgical PI is needed and, in some cases, a guarded filtration procedure.

d. If the IOP decreases significantly and the angle is determined to be open by gonioscopy, definitive treatment is performed once the cornea is clear and the anterior chamber is quiet (see the following). In most cases, this requires waiting 1 to 5 days or more for the inflammation to resolve. The attack cannot be considered broken unless the IOP decreases to a level lower than that of the fellow eye. Patients are discharged on the following medications and followed daily:

—Prednisolone acetate, 1%, four to eight times per day to quiet the eye. This should not be continued longer than necessary.

—Acetazolamide, 500 mg sequel p.o., b.i.d.

—Topical beta-blocker (e.g., levobunolol or timolol, 0.5%, b.i.d.) or alpha-agonist (e.g., brimonidine 0.15% or 0.20% b.i.d.).

—Pilocarpine, 1% to 2%, q.i.d. (in cases of phakic pupillary block or angle crowding).

Note: Some believe that once the attack is broken, only pilocarpine and prednisolone acetate are necessary if normal outflow is reestablished (i.e., the angle is open again).

10. If IOP is still increased or the angle is still closed, surgery is needed.
    If indicated by gonioscopy, PI to the fellow eye should be performed within 1 or 2 weeks.

DEFINITIVE TREATMENT

Pupillary block (all forms) or angle crowding

1. Laser (YAG) PI to the involved eye.

2. Laser PI to the contralateral eye if it is occludable. If corneal edema prohibits laser in the involved eye at the time of initial treatment, the contralateral eye can be lasered first. An untreated fellow eye has a 40% to 80% chance of development of acute angle closure in 5 to 10 years.

3. Surgical iridectomy if a laser PI is not possible.

4. Consider a guarded filtration procedure (trabeculectomy), with a tightly sutured scleral flap, when the IOP remains high despite an iridectomy and maximal medical treatment, especially in presence of significant optic nerve cupping.

Secondary or mechanical angle closure

1. Consider argon laser gonioplasty to open the angle, particularly in cases that are the result of extensive retinal laser surgery, a tight encircling band from retinal detachment surgery, or nanophthalmos.

2. Consider goniosynechialysis for chronic angle closure of less than 6 months' duration.

3. Treat the underlying problem. Systemic steroids may be required to treat serous choroidal detachments secondary to AIDS or other choroidal inflammation.

FOLLOW-UP

After definitive treatment of one or both eyes, patients are reevaluated in weeks to months initially, and then less frequently. Visual fields (e.g., Humphrey, Octopus) and stereo disc photographs or image analysis are obtained for baseline purposes.

*Notes

1. *The patient's cardiovascular status and electrolyte balance must be considered when contemplating osmotic agents, carbonic anhydrase inhibitors, and beta-blockers.*

2. *When mechanical angle-closure glaucoma is suspected, B-scan ultrasonography or ultrasonographic biomicroscopy may be helpful in diagnosis.*

3. *If a repeated attack of angle closure occurs despite a patent iridectomy, a plateau iris syndrome may be present (see 9.12, Plateau Iris).*

4. *The appearance of the cornea may worsen when the IOP decreases, with increasing thickness and folds.*

5. *Vision needs to be monitored carefully. Worsening sight is a sign of increasing urgency for pressure reduction.*

6. *The patient should be instructed to alert relatives about the occurrence of angle-closure attacks. Primary angle-closure glaucoma is a highly inheritable condition and one third to one half of first-degree relatives will be expected to have occludable anterior chamber angles.*

7. *Angle-closure glaucoma may be seen without an increased IOP. The diagnosis should*

be suspected in a patient who had pain and reduced acuity and is noted to have

—*An edematous, thickened cornea in one eye.*

—*Normal or markedly asymmetric pressure in both eyes.*

—*Shallow anterior chambers in both eyes.*

—*Occludable anterior chamber angle in the fellow eye (gonioscopy may not be helpful in an eye with corneal haziness due to stromal thickening).*

8. *In cases of bilateral angle closure secondary to sulfonamide-induced ciliary body edema/anterior choroidal effusion, care is primarily supportive. Acetazolamide and methazolamide should not be used because they are sulfa-containing medications.*

9.11 CHRONIC ANGLE-CLOSURE GLAUCOMA

SYMPTOMS

Usually asymptomatic, although patients with advanced disease may present with decreased vision or visual field loss.

SIGNS

Critical. Gonioscopy reveals broad bands of PAS in portions of the anterior chamber angle. The PAS block visualization of the underlying structures of the angle. The IOP may be elevated.

Other. The optic nerve may demonstrate a glaucomatous loss of nerve tissue, and visual field testing may reveal a scotoma.

DIFFERENTIAL DIAGNOSIS

• Prolonged acute angle-closure glaucoma or multiple episodes of subclinical attacks of acute angle closure resulting in development of PAS.

• Previous uveitic glaucoma with development of PAS.

• Regressed neovascularization of the anterior chamber angle from ischemic vascular occlusions, ocular ischemic syndrome, or proliferative diabetic retinopathy resulting in development of PAS.

• Previous laser to the trabecular meshwork, although the PAS associated with these treatments often appear as small peaks of PAS rather than broad bands.

• Previous flat anterior chamber from surgery, trauma, or hypotony for a period that resulted in the development of PAS before anterior chamber reformation.

WORKUP

1. History: Presence of symptoms of previous episodes of acute angle closure. Previous history of proliferative diabetic retinopathy, retinal vascular occlusion, or ocular ischemic syndrome. Previous history of trauma, hypotony, uveitis, or laser treatment.

2. Complete ocular examination including slit lamp, gonioscopy, measurement of the IOP, and dilated fundus examination and evaluation of the optic nerve.

3. Baseline documentation of the optic nerves (stereoscopic disc photos, image analysis, or optic disc drawing). Formal visual field testing (e.g., Humphrey, Octopus, or Goldmann perimetry) should be performed in all patients.

TREATMENT

See 9.1, Primary Open-Angle Glaucoma.

*Notes

1. *Laser trabeculoplasty usually is not effective in patients with chronic angle-closure glaucoma and can induce greater scarring of the angle.*

2. *Laser iridoplasty may be performed to attempt to decrease the formation of new PAS. This may not be effective, or may serve as a temporary measure, and if successful may be repeated. If iridoplasty fails and other medical therapy has been maximized, the patient may need surgery (see 9.1, Primary Open-Angle Glaucoma).*

9.12 PLATEAU IRIS

SYMPTOMS

Usually asymptomatic, unless acute angle-closure glaucoma develops (decreased vision, throbbing pain, nausea, and vomiting; see 9.10, Acute Angle-Closure Glaucoma).

SIGNS

Critical. Flat iris plane and normal anterior chamber depth centrally, convex peripheral iris with an anterior iris apposition seen on gonioscopy. With acute angle closure associated with a plateau iris, the axial anterior chamber depth may be normal, but the peripheral iris bunches up to occlude the angle (see 9.10, Acute Angle-Closure Glaucoma).

DIFFERENTIAL DIAGNOSIS

• Acute angle-closure glaucoma associated with pupillary block (The central anterior chamber depth is decreased, and the entire iris has a convex appearance. See 9.10, Acute Angle-Closure Glaucoma.)

• Aqueous misdirection syndrome [Marked diffuse shallowing of the anterior chamber, often after cataract extraction or glaucoma surgery. See 9.17, Malignant Glaucoma (Aqueous Misdirection Syndrome).].

• For other disorders, see 9.10, Acute Angle-Closure Glaucoma.

TYPES

1. Plateau iris configuration: Because of the anatomic configuration of the angle, acute angle-closure glaucoma may develop in these patients from only a mild degree of pupillary block. These angle-closure attacks may be cured by PI because it relieves the pupillary block.

2. Plateau iris syndrome: The peripheral iris can bunch up in the anterior chamber angle and obstruct aqueous outflow without any element of pupillary block. The diagnosis can be by gonioscopy or ultrasonographic biomicroscopy when angle-closure glaucoma occurs despite a patent PI.

WORKUP

1. Slit-lamp examination: Specifically check for the presence of a patent PI and the critical signs listed previously.

2. Measure IOP.

3. Gonioscopy of both anterior chamber angles.

4. Undilated optic nerve evaluation.

5. Can be confirmed with ultrasonographic biomicroscopy.

   Note: If dilation must be performed in a patient suspected of having a plateau iris, warn the patient that this may provoke an acute angle-closure attack. May use phenylephrine (Neo-Synephrine), 2.5% to dilate if dapiprazole, 0.5% is available for reversal. If an anticholinergic agent is needed to dilate, then use only tropicamide, 0.5%. Recheck the IOP every few hours until the pupil returns to normal size. Have the patient notify you immediately if symptoms of acute angle closure develop.

TREATMENT

If acute angle closure is present:

1. Treat acute angle-closure glaucoma medically, if present (see 9.10, Acute Angle-Closure Glaucoma).

2. A laser PI is performed within 1 to 3 days if the angle-closure attack can be broken medically. If the attack cannot be controlled, a laser or surgical PI may need to be done as an emergency procedure.

3. One week after the laser PI, the eye should be dilated with a weak mydriatic (e.g., tropicamide, 0.5%). If the IOP increases, plateau iris syndrome is diagnosed and should be treated with a weak miotic (e.g., pilocarpine, 0.5% to 1%, t.i.d. to q.i.d., long term) or with an iridoplasty.

4. If angle-closure glaucoma develops spontaneously despite a patent PI, then the plateau iris syndrome exists and should be treated as described previously.

5. Consider a laser iridoplasty to break an acute attack not responsive to medical treatment and PI.

6. If the patient's IOP does respond to a laser PI (i.e., with plateau iris configuration, not syndrome by definition), then a prophylactic laser PI may be indicated in the contralateral eye within 1 to 2 weeks.

If acute angle closure is not present:

1. Laser PI to relieve the pupillary block component.

2. Check gonioscopy every 4 to 6 months to evaluate the angle.

   —Perform iridoplasty if new PAS or further narrowing of the angle develop.

   —If the angle continues to develop new PAS or becomes narrower despite iridoplasty, then treat as CACG (see 9.11, Chronic Angle-Closure Glaucoma).

FOLLOW-UP

1. Subsequent to a PI for an attack of acute angle-closure glaucoma, patients are reevaluated in 1 week, 1 month, and 3 months, and then yearly if no problems have developed. Examination should include IOP and gonioscopy at each visit; look for a narrowing angle recess or increasing angle closure. The PI should be examined for patency.

2. Patients with a plateau iris configuration who have never had an acute angle-closure attack are examined every 6 months. At each visit, IOP is measured and gonioscopy is performed; look for PAS formation and further narrowing of the anterior chamber angle. Dilation should cautiously be performed periodically (approximately every 2 years) to ensure that the PI remains adequate to prevent angle closure.

9.13 GLAUCOMATOCYCLITIC CRISIS

(POSNER–SCHLOSSMAN SYNDROME)

SYMPTOMS

Mild pain, decreased vision, observation of rainbows around lights. Often, a history of similar episodes is obtained. Usually unilateral in young to middle-aged patients.

SIGNS

Critical. Markedly increased IOP (usually 40 to 60 mm Hg), open angle without synechiae on gonioscopy, minimal conjunctival injection (white eye), very mild anterior chamber reaction (few aqueous cells and little flare).

Other. Corneal epithelial edema, ciliary flush, pupillary constriction, iris hypochromia, few fine keratic precipitates on the corneal endothelium or trabecular meshwork.

DIFFERENTIAL DIAGNOSIS

• Inflammatory open-angle glaucoma (Significant amount of aqueous cells and flare, conjunctival injection, and pain. Synechiae may be present. May be bilateral. See 9.4, Inflammatory Open-Angle Glaucoma.).

• Acute angle-closure glaucoma (Closed angle in the involved eye and usually a narrow angle in the contralateral eye; painful conjunctival injection; corneal edema; patient may have history of recent dilatation with drops or use of systemic anticholinergic medication. See 9.10, Acute Angle-Closure Glaucoma.).

• Pigmentary glaucoma [Acute increase in IOP, often after exercise or pupillary dilatation, pigment cells in the anterior chamber, open angle, radial iris TI defects, vertical base-down triangle of pigmented cells on the posterior corneal surface (Krukenberg spindle), and pigment in the trabecular meshwork seen on gonioscopy. See 9.6, Pigmentary Glaucoma.].

• Neovascular glaucoma (Iris or angle neovascularization is present. See 9.14, Neovascular Glaucoma.).

• Fuchs heterochromic iridocyclitis (Asymmetry of iris color, mild iritis in the eye with the lighter-colored iris, usually unilateral, often associated with cataract, glaucoma, or both. The increase in IOP is rarely as acute. See 12.1, Anterior Uveitis.).

• Others (e.g., herpes simplex and herpes zoster keratouveitis).

WORKUP

1. History: Recent dilating drops, systemic anticholinergic agents, or exercise? Previous attacks? Corneal or systemic disease?

2. Slit-lamp examination: Assess the degree of conjunctival injection and aqueous cell and flare. Measure IOP.

3. Gonioscopy of the anterior chamber angle: Angle open? Synechiae, neovascular membrane, or keratic precipitates present?

4. Optic nerve evaluation.

5. Stereo optic disc photos or image analysis and formal visual field testing (e.g., Humphrey or Octopus).

6. Retinal examination: Vasculitis? Snowbanking of pars planitis?

TREATMENT

1. Topical beta-blocker (e.g., timolol or levobunolol, 0.5%, b.i.d.), topical alpha-agonist (e.g., brimonidine, 0.15% or 0.2%, b.i.d. to t.i.d., or apraclonidine, 0.5%, t.i.d.), topical carbonic anhydrase inhibitor (e.g., dorzolamide, 2%, or brinzolamide, 1%, b.i.d. to t.i.d.).

2. Topical steroid (e.g., prednisolone acetate, 1%, q.i.d.).

3. Substitute a systemic carbonic anhydrase inhibitor (e.g., methazolamide, 25 to 50 mg p.o., b.i.d. to t.i.d., or acetazolamide, 500 mg sequel p.o., b.i.d.) for a topical carbonic an-

hydrase inhibitor if IOP is significantly increased.

4. Hyperosmotic agents (e.g., mannitol, 20%, 1 to 2 g/kg i.v. over 45 minutes) are used acutely when the IOP is determined to be dangerously high for the involved optic nerve. A 500-mL bag of mannitol, 20% contains 100 g of mannitol.

5. Consider a cycloplegic agent (e.g., cyclopentolate, 1%, t.i.d.) if the patient is symptomatic.

FOLLOW-UP

1. Patients are seen every few days at first, and then weekly until the episode resolves. At-

tacks usually subside within a few hours to a few weeks.

2. Medical or surgical therapy may be required, depending on the baseline level of IOP between attacks.

3. If the IOP decreases to levels that are not associated with disc or visual field damage, no treatment is necessary.

4. Steroids are tapered rapidly if they are used for 1 week or less, and slowly if they are used for longer.

5. Note that both eyes are at risk for development of chronic open-angle glaucoma.

9.14 NEOVASCULAR GLAUCOMA

DEFINITION

Glaucoma caused by a fibrovascular membrane, overgrowing the anterior chamber angle structures. Initially, the angle may appear open, but blocked by the membrane. The fibrovascular membrane eventually contracts, causing PAS formation and secondary angle-closure glaucoma. Rarely, may have neovascularization of the angle without neovascularization of the iris at the pupillary margin. The etiology of the fibrovascular membrane is ischemia from a variety of causes.

SYMPTOMS

May be asymptomatic or patient may complain of pain, red eye, photophobia, and decreased vision.

SIGNS

Critical

• Stage 1: Abnormal, nonradial, misdirected blood vessels along the pupillary margin, the trabecular meshwork, or both. No signs of glaucoma.

• Stage 2: Stage 1 plus increased IOP (open-angle neovascular glaucoma).

• Stage 3: Partial or complete angle-closure glaucoma caused by a fibrovascular membrane covering the trabecular meshwork. PAS and florid iris neovascularization are common.

Other. Mild anterior chamber cells and flare, conjunctival injection, corneal edema when an acute increase in IOP occurs, hyphema, eversion of the pupillary margin allowing visualization of the iris pigment epithelium (ectropion uvea), optic nerve cupping, visual field loss.

DIFFERENTIAL DIAGNOSIS

• Inflammatory glaucoma (Increased IOP, abundant anterior chamber cells and marked flare, and dilated normal iris blood vessels may be seen. No neovascular vessels. Normal iris blood vessels run radially, have a sense of direction, and are usually symmetric 360 degrees around the pupillary margin. The angle is open. See 9.4, Inflammatory Open-Angle Glaucoma.).

• Primary acute angle-closure glaucoma (No signs of new iris blood vessels. Usually a shallow anterior chamber with a closed or narrow angle in both eyes. See 9.10, Acute Angle-Closure Glaucoma.).

ETIOLOGY

- Diabetic retinopathy.
- Central retinal vein occlusion, particularly the ischemic type.
- Central retinal artery occlusion.
- Ocular ischemic syndrome (carotid occlusive disease).
- Others (e.g., branch retinal vein occlusion, chronic uveitis, chronic retinal detachment, intraocular tumors, trauma, other ocular vascular disorders, radiation therapy, chronic long-standing increased IOP).

WORKUP

1. History: Determine the underlying etiology.
2. Complete ocular examination, including IOP measurement and gonioscopic evaluation of the anterior chamber angle to determine what degree of the angle is closed, if any. A dilated retinal evaluation is essential in determining the cause of the iris neovascularization.
3. Fluorescein angiography as needed to identify an underlying retinal abnormality or in preparation for retinal laser treatment [panretinal photocoagulation (PRP)].
4. Carotid noninvasive studies to rule out carotid disease when no retinal lesion can be found accountable for the neovascularization.
5. B-scan ultrasonography is indicated when the retina cannot be visualized to rule out an intraocular tumor or retinal detachment.

TREATMENT

1. Reduce inflammation and pain: Topical steroid (e.g., prednisolone acetate, 1%, q1–6h) and a cycloplegic (e.g., atropine, 1%, t.i.d.). Atropine may reduce IOP when the angle is closed by increasing uveoscleral outflow.
2. Reduce the IOP if it is increased. Any or all of the following medications are used:

   —Topical beta-blocker (e.g., levobunolol or timolol, 0.5%, b.i.d.).

   —Topical alpha-agonists (e.g., apraclonidine, 0.5%, or brimonidine, 0.15% or 0.2%, b.i.d. to t.i.d.).

   —Systemic or topical carbonic anhydrase inhibitor (e.g., methazolamide, 25 to 50 mg p.o., b.i.d. to t.i.d., or acetazolamide, 500 mg p.o., b.i.d., dorzolamide, 2%, or brinzolamide, 1%, b.i.d. to t.i.d.).

   Note: Miotics (e.g., pilocarpine) are contraindicated because of their effects on the blood–aqueous barrier. Epinephrine compounds (e.g., dipivefrin) are usually ineffective and are not often used.

3. If retinal ischemia is thought to be responsible for the iris neovascularization, then treat with PRP. If the retina cannot be visualized, lower the IOP and treat the retina once the cornea clears. Treatment with cryoablation can also be considered in cases where the cornea does not clear and the retina cannot be visualized adequately to perform PRP. These procedures are used if the angle is open or if filtration surgery (regardless of whether the angle is open or closed) is going to be performed.
4. Glaucoma filtration surgery may be performed when the neovascularization is inactive and the IOP cannot be controlled with medical therapy. Tube-shunt procedures or YAG laser cyclophotocoagulation may be helpful to control IOP in some patients with active neovascularization. It is often best to perform PRP before attempting filtration surgery.
5. Goniophotocoagulation (laser photocoagulation of new vessels in the angle) may be used in addition to the previously described treatment in patients with significant angle neovascularization, but minimal

to no angle closure. This procedure may reduce the risk of angle closure during the interval required for the PRP to take effect (often several weeks), but this is not well established.

6. In eyes without useful vision, topical steroids and cycloplegics may be adequate therapy. The pain in neovascular glaucoma is not primarily a function of the IOP, and reducing IOP may not be needed if the goal is pain control only. Beta-blockers, retrobulbar alcohol injection, or enucleation may be required to reduce pain (see 13.16, The Blind, Painful Eye).

7. Treat the underlying disorder; see the appropriate section.

FOLLOW-UP

The presence of iris neovascularization, especially when accompanied by high IOP, requires urgent therapeutic intervention, usually within 1 to 2 days. Angle closure can proceed relatively rapidly (within days to weeks).

Note: Iris neovascularization without glaucoma is managed in a manner similar to that described; however, there is no need for antiglaucomatous therapy unless IOP increases.

9.15   IRIDOCORNEAL ENDOTHELIAL SYNDROME

DEFINITION

Three overlapping syndromes—essential iris atrophy, Chandler, and iris nevus (Cogan–Reese)—that share an abnormal corneal endothelial cell layer, which can grow across the anterior chamber angle. Secondary angle closure can result from contraction of this tissue.

SYMPTOMS

Asymptomatic in its early stages. Later, the patient notes an irregular iris appearance, blurred vision, or pain in one eye. Patients are typically young to middle-aged adults. Familial cases are extremely rare.

SIGNS

Critical. Corneal endothelial changes (fine, hammered-metal appearance) localized, irregular PAS that often extend beyond Schwalbe line, deep central anterior chamber, unilaterality, and iris alterations as follows:

• Essential iris atrophy: Marked iris thinning often leading to iris holes and displacement and distortion of the pupil.

• Chandler syndrome: Mild iris thinning and pupil distortion. The corneal changes are most marked in this variant. Patients often have corneal edema even at normal IOP.

• Cogan–Reese syndrome: Pigmented nodules on the iris surface, variable iris atrophy. The iris changes may also be seen in Chandler syndrome and essential iris atrophy.

Other. Corneal edema, elevated IOP, optic nerve cupping, or visual field loss. Typically unilateral, although mild corneal changes consistent with this syndrome are sometimes found in the contralateral eye. However, the glaucoma is nearly always unilateral.

DIFFERENTIAL DIAGNOSIS

• Axenfeld–Rieger syndrome [Prominent, anteriorly displaced Schwalbe line (posterior embryotoxon), peripheral iris strands extending to Schwalbe line, iris thinning with atrophic holes, may have dental, craniofacial, and skeletal abnormalities. Bilateral and congenital. See 8.12, Developmental Anterior Segment and Lens Anomalies.].

- Posterior polymorphous dystrophy (Bilateral. Endothelial vesicles or bandlike lesions, occasionally associated with iridocorneal adhesions, corneal edema, and glaucoma. See 4.24, Corneal Dystrophies.).

- Fuchs endothelial dystrophy (Bilateral corneal edema and endothelial guttata. The iris and anterior chamber angle are normal. See 4.25, Fuchs Endothelial Dystrophy.).

- Iris melanoma (Pigmented iris lesion or lesions noted to enlarge over time. See 5.13, Malignant Melanoma of the Iris.).

- Prior uveitis (Pigmented keratic precipitates, posterior synechiae, cataract.).

WORKUP

1. Family history: ICE syndrome is not inherited; Axenfeld–Rieger syndrome and posterior polymorphous dystrophy are often autosomal dominant.

2. Slit-lamp examination: Assess the cornea and iris and measure IOP.

3. Gonioscopy of the anterior chamber angle.

4. Optic nerve examination.

5. Slit-lamp photos and stereoscopic disc photographs or image analysis.

6. Visual field test, preferably automated (e.g., Humphrey, Octopus).

7. Consider obtaining corneal endothelial specular microscopy.

TREATMENT

No treatment is needed unless glaucoma or corneal edema is present, at which point one or more of the following treatments is used:

1. Antiglaucomatous medications for corneal edema or glaucoma (see 9.1, Primary Open-Angle Glaucoma). The IOP may need to be reduced beneath a critical level to rid the cornea of edema. This critical level may become lower as the patient ages.

2. Hypertonic saline solutions (e.g., sodium chloride, 5% drops, q.i.d., and ointment, q.h.s.) may help to reduce corneal edema.

3. Consider filtering procedure (tube shunt or trabeculectomy) when medical therapy fails to maintain the IOP low enough to prevent corneal edema or progression of optic nerve damage. Laser trabeculoplasty and laser PI are ineffective.

4. Consider a corneal transplant in cases of advanced chronic corneal edema in the presence of good IOP control.

FOLLOW-UP

Depends on the level of IOP and state of the nerve. If asymptomatic with healthy optic nerve, may see every 12 months. If glaucoma is present, then every 1 to 3 months, depending on the severity of the glaucoma.

9.16 POSTOPERATIVE GLAUCOMA

EARLY POSTOPERATIVE GLAUCOMA

IOP tends to start to increase approximately 1 hour after cataract extraction and usually returns to normal within 1 week. Etiologies include retained viscoelastic material, pupillary block, hyphema, pigment dispersion, and generalized inflammation. Most normal eyes can tolerate an IOP up to 30 mm Hg for this duration. However, eyes with preexisting optic nerve damage require antiglaucoma medications (e.g., levobunolol, 0.5%, b.i.d., timolol, 0.5%, b.i.d., brimonidine, 0.15% or 0.2%, b.i.d.

to t.i.d., dorzolamide, 2%, t.i.d., brinzolamide, 1%, t.i.d., or methazolamide, 25 to 50 mg p.o., b.i.d. to t.i.d.) for any significant pressure increase. Most eyes with an IOP greater than 30 mm Hg should likewise be treated. If inflammation is excessive, increase the topical steroid dose to every 30 to 60 minutes while awake and consider a topical NSAID (e.g., diclofenac or ketorolac, q.i.d.; see 9.4, Inflammatory Open-Angle Glaucoma).

PUPILLARY BLOCK

DIFFERENTIAL DIAGNOSIS OF PUPILLARY BLOCK

Early postoperative period (within 2 weeks)

• Inflammation secondary to prostaglandin release, blood, fibrin, and the like.

• Hyphema.

• Failure to filter after filtration surgery due to tight scleral flap, blocked sclerostomy (e.g., iris, vitreous, blood, fibrin).

• Malignant glaucoma (aqueous misdirection).

• Suprachoroidal hemorrhage.

• Anterior chamber lens with vitreous loss: Vitreous plugs the pupil if iridectomy is not performed.

Late postoperative period (after 2 weeks)

• Pupillary block glaucoma.

• Failing bleb (after filtering surgery).

• Suprachoroidal hemorrhage.

• Uveitis, glaucoma, hyphema syndrome.

• Malignant glaucoma (when cycloplegics are stopped).

• Steroid-induced glaucoma.

SIGNS

Increased IOP, shallow or partially flat anterior chamber, absence of a patent PI. Iris typically has marked anterior bowing (iris bombé). Evidence of iris adhesions to lens or intraocular lens.

TREATMENT OF PUPILLARY BLOCK

1. If the cornea is clear and the eye is not significantly inflamed, then a PI is performed, usually by YAG laser. Because the PI tends to close, it is often necessary to perform two or more iridectomies. They need to be larger than in the eye with primary angle-closure glaucoma.

2. If the cornea is hazy, the eye is inflamed, or a PI cannot be performed immediately, then:

—Mydriatic agent (e.g., cyclopentolate, 2%, and phenylephrine, 2.5%, every 15 minutes for four doses).

—Carbonic anhydrase inhibitor (e.g., acetazolamide, two 250-mg tablets p.o. or 500 mg i.v.).

—Topical beta-blocker (e.g., timolol or levobunolol, 0.5%), one dose.

—Topical alpha-agonist (e.g., brimonidine, 0.15% or 0.2%, or apraclonidine, 1.0%), one dose.

—Topical steroid (e.g., prednisolone acetate, 1%, every 15 to 30 minutes for four doses). If the IOP is too high, some clinicians recommend dosing the steroid every 30 to 60 minutes while awake for 1 day with the return the next day.

—PI, preferably YAG laser, as soon as available and when the eye is less inflamed. If the cornea is edematous and cloudy, topical glycerin may be used to clear it temporarily.

—A surgical PI may be needed.

—If angle has become closed, a guarded filtration procedure or tube shunt may be needed.

UVEITIS, GLAUCOMA, HYPHEMA SYNDROME

SIGNS

Anterior chamber cells and flare and increased IOP, often with a hyphema. Usually secondary to irritation from a malpositioned anterior or posterior chamber intraocular lens; often with a vitreous wick.

TREATMENT OF UVEITIS, GLAUCOMA, HYPHEMA SYNDROME

1. Atropine, 1%, t.i.d.

2. Topical steroid (e.g., prednisolone acetate, 1%, q.i.d. or more often if the uveitis is severe), and consider topical NSAID (e.g., diclofenac, q.i.d.).

3. Systemic carbonic anhydrase inhibitor (e.g., acetazolamide, 250 mg p.o., q.i.d., or 500 mg sequel p.o., b.i.d., or methazolamide, 25 to 50 mg p.o., b.i.d. to t.i.d.) or may consider topical carbonic anhydrase inhibitor (e.g., dorzolamide, 2%, or brinzolamide, 1%, t.i.d.).

4. Topical beta-blocker (e.g., timolol or levobunolol, 0.5%, b.i.d.), alpha-agonist (e.g., brimonidine, 0.15% or 0.2%, b.i.d. to t.i.d., or apraclonidine, 0.5%, t.i.d.).

5. Consider argon laser treatment to control the hemorrhage if a bleeding site can be identified.

6. Consider surgical repositioning, replacement, or removal of the intraocular lens, especially if PAS are forming or CME persists.

7. Consider YAG vitreolysis if discrete strands can be seen.

   Note: Functional patency of iridectomy is difficult to determine. A helpful way to distinguish uveitis, glaucoma, hyphema syndrome from malignant glaucoma is injection of fluorescein (as for a retinal angiogram) into the antecubital vein with pupillary block glaucoma; fluorescein is not seen entering the anterior chamber or structures except after approximately 30 seconds as it diffuses through the blood vessels. In malignant glaucoma, the fluorescein streams into the retrolental space.

GHOST CELL GLAUCOMA

Degenerated red blood cells pass from the vitreous into the anterior chamber and obstruct the trabecular meshwork. These cells are tan. Often occurs after a large vitreous hemorrhage with a posterior capsular opening, allowing easy access of the red blood cells into the anterior chamber. Usually occurs 1 to 4 weeks after the vitreous hemorrhage.

TREATMENT OF GHOST CELL GLAUCOMA

1. Medical treatment: see 9.1, Primary Open-Angle Glaucoma.

2. Anterior chamber irrigation.

3. Posterior vitrectomy to clear the blood, if medical management fails.

MALIGNANT GLAUCOMA

See 9.17, Malignant Glaucoma.

STEROID-RESPONSE GLAUCOMA

See 9.5, Steroid-Response Glaucoma.

FOLLOW-UP FOR POSTOPERATIVE GLAUCOMA

Patients should usually not be sent out of the office or emergency department with an IOP greater than 35 to 40 mm Hg. If the patient is monocular or has significant optic nerve damage, then the IOP should be even lower. For aphakic/pseudophakic pupillary block, be certain that the angle is open and the block is relieved (by using gonioscopy). If these criteria are met, the patient must be reevaluated in 1 to 7 days, depending on the particular situation.

9.17 MALIGNANT GLAUCOMA

(AQUEOUS MISDIRECTION SYNDROME)

SYMPTOMS

May be very mild in the early stages. Later, moderate pain, red eye, photophobia may develop; often occurs after surgical treatment of angle-closure glaucoma; also occurs in association with shallow anterior chamber after surgery without a patent PI, as with tube-shunt operations, and may be induced by miotics (even without surgery).

SIGNS

Critical. Shallow or flat anterior chamber and increased IOP in the presence of a patent PI and in the absence of a choroidal detachment. Absence of iris bombé.

DIFFERENTIAL DIAGNOSIS (TABLE 9.1)

• Pupillary block glaucoma (Iris bombé, adhesions of iris to other anterior chamber structures. See 9.16, Postoperative Glaucoma.).

• Acute angle-closure glaucoma (No history of surgery; other eye has shallow anterior chamber and narrow angle. See 9.10, Acute Angle-Closure Glaucoma.).

• Choroidal detachment (Shallow or flat anterior chamber, but the IOP is typically low. A choroidal detachment is seen on funduscopic examination or by B-scan ultrasonography in most cases. See 11.21, Choroidal Detachment.).

• Suprachoroidal hemorrhage (Sudden onset of shallow or flat anterior chamber, excruciat-

TABLE 9.1 POSTOPERATIVE COMPLICATIONS OF GLAUCOMA SURGERY

Diagnosis	Intraocular Pressure	Anterior Chamber	Iris Bombé	Pain	Bleb
Inflammation	Mildly elevated	Deep	No	Possible	Varies
Hyphema	Mild–moderately elevated	Varies	Not early	Possible	Varies
Failure to filter	Moderately elevated	Deep	No	Moderate	Falling
Malignant glaucoma	Early: moderately elevated Late: moderately–markedly elevated	Shallow everywhere Grade 2 or 3	No	Moderate	Falling or absent
Suprachoroidal hemorrhage	Early: markedly elevated, later falling to mild or moderately elevated	Grade 1 and 2 flat	No	Excruciating	Varies
Pupillary block	Early, moderately elevated, may become markedly elevated	Grade 1–3 flat	Yes	None or mild	None
Serous choroidal detachment	Low	Grade 1–3 flat	No	Ache	Frequently present

ing pain, increased IOP early. Dark, nonserous choroidal detachment seen on funduscopic examination or B-scan ultrasonography.).

ETIOLOGY

It is believed that aqueous is misdirected and accumulates in the vitreous, displacing the vitreous forward, pushing the ciliary processes, the crystalline lens, the intraocular implant, or the anterior vitreous face anteriorly, causing secondary angle closure.

WORKUP

1. History: Previous eye surgery?

2. Slit-lamp examination: Determine if a patent PI is present. Pupillary block is unlikely in the presence of a patent PI unless it is plugged or bound down, or plateau iris syndrome is present. Is iris bombé present?

3. Gonioscopy of the anterior chamber angle.

4. Dilated retinal examination unless a phakic angle closure is likely.

5. Consider B-scan ultrasonography to rule out a choroidal detachment and suprachoroidal hemorrhage if they cannot be ruled out by ophthalmoscopy.

TREATMENT

1. If an iridectomy is not present or it is not certain whether an existing one is patent, pupillary block cannot be ruled out, and a PI should be performed (see 9.10, Acute Angle-Closure Glaucoma).

   If signs of malignant glaucoma are still present with a patent PI, attempt medical therapy directed at controlling the IOP and possibly return aqueous flow to the normal pathway.

2. Atropine, 1%, and phenylephrine, 2.5%, q.i.d. topically.

3. Carbonic anhydrase inhibitor (e.g., acetazolamide, 500 mg i.v. or two 250-mg tablets p.o., then 250 mg p.o., q.i.d.).

4. Hyperosmotic agent (e.g., mannitol, 20%, 1 to 2 g/kg i.v. over 45 minutes; a 500-mL bag of mannitol, 20% contains 100 g of mannitol).

5. Topical beta-blocker (e.g., timolol or levobunolol, 0.5%, b.i.d.).

6. Topical apraclonidine, 1.0%, or brimonidine, 0.15% or 0.2%, b.i.d.

If the attack is broken (the anterior chamber deepens and the IOP returns to normal), maintain atropine, 1% once per day, indefinitely.

If steps 1 through 6 are unsuccessful, consider one or more of the following surgical interventions to disrupt the anterior hyaloid face in an attempt to restore the normal anatomic flow of aqueous and alleviate the misdirection syndrome:

7. YAG laser disruption of the anterior hyaloid face and posterior capsule if the patient is aphakic or pseudophakic. May attempt through a preexisting large PI if phakic.

8. Vitrectomy and reformation of the anterior chamber and rupture of the anterior hyaloid face.

9. Lensectomy with disruption of the anterior hyaloid or vitrectomy.

10. Argon laser treatment of the ciliary processes.

    Note: A choroidal detachment may be present, yet undetectable. Therefore, a sclerotomy to drain a choroidal detachment may be advisable before vitrectomy.

11. PI in the contralateral eye if the angle appears occludable; usually performed at a later date.

FOLLOW-UP

Variable, depending on the therapeutic modality used. PI is usually performed in an occludable contralateral eye 1 week after treatment of the involved eye.

9.18 POSTOPERATIVE COMPLICATIONS OF GLAUCOMA SURGERY

BLEB INFECTION (BLEBITIS)

See 9.19, Blebitis.

INCREASED POSTOPERATIVE INTRAOCULAR PRESSURE AFTER FILTERING PROCEDURE

GRADE OF SHALLOWING OF ANTERIOR CHAMBER

I. Peripheral iris–cornea contact.

II. Entire iris in contact with cornea.

III. Lens (or pseudophakia or vitreous face)–corneal contact.

DIFFERENTIAL DIAGNOSIS (TABLE 9.1)

If the anterior chamber is deep (formed), consider the following:

• Occlusion of the filtration opening *internally:* By an iris plug, hemorrhage, fibrin, vitreous or viscoelastic material.

• Occlusion of filtration *externally:* By a tight trabeculectomy flap (sutured tightly or scarred).

Note: Diagnosis is made by careful slit-lamp examination and gonioscopy.

If the anterior chamber is flat or shallow and IOP is increased, consider the following:

• Suprachoroidal hemorrhage [Sudden onset of severe pain, commonly 1 to 5 days after surgery, with injection, variable IOPs (15 to 45 mm Hg), hazy cornea, shallow chamber. Diagnosis confirmed by indirect ophthalmoscopy or B-scan ultrasonography.].

• Malignant glaucoma [see 9.17, Malignant Glaucoma (Aqueous Misdirection Syndrome)].

• Pupillary block (see 9.16, Postoperative Glaucoma).

TREATMENT

1. If the bleb is not formed and the anterior chamber is deep, point pressure with an applicator on the edge of the bleb should be used to try to determine if the sclerostomy will drain.

2. If the trabeculectomy flap is too tight, suture lysis may be indicated.

3. If sclerostomy is blocked with iris, pressure on the globe of any sort is contraindicated. Intracameral injection of acetylcholine, slowly, can pull the iris out of the sclerostomy if used before 12 to 24 hours after surgery. If this fails, and sclerostomy is completely blocked by iris, and acetylcholine fails, transcorneal mechanical retraction of the iris may work. If sclerostomy is blocked with vitreous, it may occasionally be possible to photodisrupt the sclerostomy with a YAG laser. If blood or fibrin plugs the sclerostomy, time may clear the problem.

4. For suprachoroidal hemorrhage, if the IOP is mildly increased and the chamber is formed, observation with medical management is indicated. If the flat chamber persists, the IOP remains increased, there is corneal–lenticular touch, or the pain is intolerable, surgical drainage of the choroidal hemorrhage is necessary.

5. Medical therapy may be needed if these measures are not successful (see 9.1, Primary Open-Angle Glaucoma).

6. If all of these fail, reoperation may be necessary.

LOW POSTOPERATIVE INTRAOCULAR PRESSURE AFTER FILTERING PROCEDURE

Low pressures (5 to 9 mm Hg) are not desirable. An IOP less than 8 mm Hg is associated with increased incidence of flat anterior chamber, choroidal detachment, and suprachoroidal hemorrhage. An IOP less than 4 mm Hg is even more likely to be associated with problems, including macular hypotony and corneal edema.

DIFFERENTIAL DIAGNOSIS AND TREATMENT (TABLE 9.1)

1. Very large filtering bleb with a formed (deep) chamber (overfiltration): It is desirable to have a large bleb in the first few weeks after trabeculectomy. However, if it is still present 6 to 8 weeks after surgery, the patient is symptomatic, IOP is decreasing, or anterior chamber is shallowing, consider shell tamponade or autologous blood injections into the bleb. If IOP is stable and anterior chamber is deep, leave alone.

2. Large bleb with a flat chamber: Treatment is indicated when recognized and includes cycloplegics (atropine, 1%, t.i.d.) and careful observation. If the anterior chamber becomes more shallow (e.g., grade I becoming grade II), IOP decreases as bleb flattens, or there is development of choroidal detachment, the anterior chamber should be reformed with a viscoelastic material.

3. No bleb with flat chamber: Check carefully for a wound leak by Seidel testing (see Appendix 4). If positive, aqueous suppressants, patching, or surgical closure may be necessary. If Seidel test is negative, look for a cyclodialysis cleft by gonioscopy or for serous choroidal detachments. Cyclodialysis clefts are managed by cycloplegics, laser or cryotherapy closure, or surgical closure. Serous choroidal detachments are often observed and are not frequently drained, unless associated with recurrent flat anterior chamber and persistent hypotony.

MISCELLANEOUS COMPLICATIONS OF FILTERING PROCEDURE

Cataracts, corneal edema, corneal dellen, endophthalmitis, uveitis, hyphema.

COMPLICATIONS OF ANTIMETABOLITES (5-FLUOROURACIL, MITOMYCIN C)

Corneal epithelial defects, corneal edema, conjunctival wound leaks, bleb overfiltration, bleb rupture, scleral thinning.

COMPLICATIONS OF CYCLODESTRUCTIVE PROCEDURES

Pain, uveitis, decreased vision, cataract, hypotony, scleral thinning, suprachoroidal effusion, suprachoroidal hemorrhage, sympathetic ophthalmia.

9.19   BLEBITIS

DESCRIPTION

Infection of the filtering bleb. May occur any time after glaucoma filtering procedures (days to years).

- Mild: Bleb infection but NO anterior chamber or vitreal involvement.

- Moderate: Bleb infection with anterior chamber inflammation but NO vitreal involvement.

- Severe: Bleb infection with anterior chamber and vitreal involvement. See 12.10, Postoperative Endophthalmitis.

SYMPTOMS

Red eye and discharge early. Later, aching pain, photophobia, decreased vision, mucous discharge.

SIGNS

- Mild: Bleb appears milky, with loss of translucency. Microhypopyon in loculations of the bleb, IOP rising. Turbid fluid in bleb possibly with frank purulent material in or leaking from the bleb, intense conjunctival injection.

- Moderate: Findings of *Mild* with anterior chamber cell and flare, possibly an anterior chamber hypopyon, with no vitreal inflammation.

- Severe: Findings of *Moderate* with vitreal involvement. Same appearance of endophthalmitis except with bleb involvement.

DIFFERENTIAL DIAGNOSIS

- Episcleritis [Sectoral inflammation (rarely superior) but no inflammation of bleb. See 5.6, Episcleritis.].

- Conjunctivitis (Little to no decrease in vision, no pain or photophobia. Bacterial conjunctivitis can progress to blebitis if not promptly treated. See 5.1, Acute Conjunctivitis.).

- Anterior uveitis (Anterior segment findings similar except there is no inflammation of the bleb. See 12.1, Anterior Uveitis.).

- Endophthalmitis (Similar anterior segment findings as blebitis, except with vitreous cells and inflammation. May have more intense pain, eyelid edema, chemosis, greater decrease in vision, hypopyon, and fibrinous reaction than blebitis. See 12.10, Postoperative Endophthalmitis.).

- Ischemic bleb (In immediate postoperative period after the use of antimetabolites. Conjunctiva is opaque with sectorial conjunctival injection. The view of the fluid in the bleb may be obscured.).

WORKUP

1. Slit-lamp examination with close examination of the bleb, anterior chamber, and vitreous. Search for hole in the bleb. Look for microhypopyon by using gonioscopy.

2. Culture bleb or perform anterior chamber tap for *Moderate*; for *Severe*, see 12.10, Postoperative Endophthalmitis.

Note: Commonly isolated organisms have *been* Staphylococcus epidermidis, Staphylococcus aureus, *and other gram-positive organisms in the first days to weeks after surgery. If blebitis occurs months to years later,* Streptococcus, Haemophilus influenzae, S. aureus, Moraxella, Pseudomonas, *and* Serratia *are more common.*

3. B-scan ultrasonography of the vitreous may reveal inflammation if visualization is difficult.

TREATMENT

1. Mild: intensive topical antibiotics with either of two regimens:

   —Fortified cefazolin or vancomycin *and* fortified gentamicin, amikacin, or tobramycin alternating every half hour for the first 24 hours. A loading dose of one drop of each every 5 minutes, repeated four times, is often given.

   or

   —Fluoroquinolones q1h after a loading dose.

   —Reevaluate in 6 to 12 hours and again at 12 to 24 hours. Must not be getting worse.

   —Start steroids 24 hours after antibiotics started and blebitis resolving.

2. Moderate: Same approach as mild blebitis, plus cycloplegics and more careful monitoring.

3. Severe: Admit and treat as endophthalmitis (see 12.10, Postoperative Endophthalmitis).

FOLLOW-UP

Daily until infection is resolving. Admission to the hospital is indicated for noncompliance or worsening of infection.

CHAPTER 10

NEURO-OPHTHALMOLOGY

10.1 ANISOCORIA

See Figure 10.1.

CLASSIFICATION

1. The abnormal pupil is constricted.

—Unilateral use of a miotic (green-top) eye drop (e.g., pilocarpine).

—Iritis (Eye pain, redness, and anterior-chamber cells and flare.).

—Horner syndrome (Mild ptosis is usually present on the side of the small pupil; positive cocaine test.).

—Argyll Robertson (syphilitic) pupil [The pupil is irregular in shape, reacts poorly or not at all to light, but constricts normally during convergence. Although the disease is typically bilateral, a mild degree of anisocoria is often present. Should have positive syphilis serology (fluorescent treponemal antibody, absorbed [FTA-ABS] or microhemagglutination–*Treponema pallidum* [MHA-TP]).].

—Long-standing Adie pupil (The pupil is initially dilated, but over time may constrict. At the slit lamp, it can be seen to react slowly and irregularly to a bright light. It is supersensitive to pilocarpine 0.125%.).

2. The abnormal pupil is dilated.

—Iris sphincter muscle damage from trauma (Torn pupillary margin or iris transillumination defects seen on slit-lamp examination.).

—Adie tonic pupil (The pupil is irregular, reacts minimally to light and slowly to convergence, but is supersensitive to weak cholinergic agents such as pilocarpine, 0.125%, or methacholine, 2.5%.).

—Third nerve palsy [Associated ptosis and extraocular muscle palsies. The pupil will not react to weak cholinergic agents, but will constrict to regular-strength miotic drops (e.g., pilocarpine, 1%).].

—Unilateral use of a mydriatic (red-top, dilating) eye drop (e.g., atropine) or scopolamine patch for motion sickness [If the drop has been instilled recently, the pupil will not react to pilocarpine, 1%, drops. If the effect of the drop is wearing off (e.g., atropine was used 1 to 2 weeks previously), the eye may be dilated and partly reactive to pilocarpine.].

3. Physiologic anisocoria (Pupil size disparity is the same in light as in dark, and the pupils react normally to light. The size difference is usually, but not always less than 1 mm in diameter.).

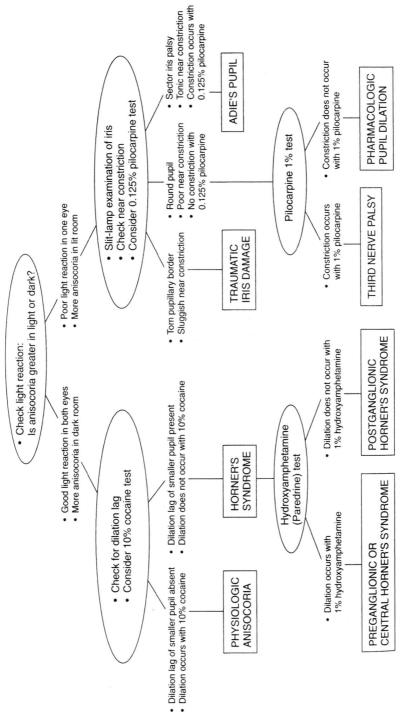

FIGURE 10.1 Flow diagram for the workup of anisocoria. (Modified from Thompson HS, Pilley SF. Unequal pupils. A flow chart for sorting out the anisocorias. *Surv Ophthalmol* 1976;21:45–48, with permission.)

WORKUP

1. History: When was the anisocoria first noted? Any associated symptoms or signs? History of ocular trauma? Use of any eye drops or ointments? History of syphilis? History of decreased vision? Old photographs?

2. Ocular examination: Try to determine which is the abnormal pupil by observing the pupillary size. If it is uncertain which is the abnormal pupil, compare pupil sizes in light and in dark. Anisocoria greater in light suggests the abnormal pupil is the larger pupil; anisocoria greater in dark suggests the abnormal pupil is the smaller pupil. Test the pupillary reaction to light. Evaluate for the presence of a relative afferent pupillary defect. Evaluate pupillary near response (abnormal in Adie pupil, Argyll Robertson pupils, and dorsal midbrain syndrome). Look for ptosis, evaluate ocular motility, and examine the pupillary margin with a slit lamp.

—If the abnormal pupil is small, a diagnosis of Horner syndrome may be confirmed by a cocaine test (see 10.2, Horner Syndrome). In the presence of ptosis and an unequivocal increase in anisocoria in dim illumination, a cocaine test is unnecessary because the diagnosis is made clinically.

—If the abnormal pupil is large and there is no sphincter muscle damage or signs of third nerve palsy (extraocular motility deficit, ptosis), the pupils are tested with one drop of pilocarpine, 0.125%. Within 10 to 15 minutes, an Adie pupil will usually have constricted significantly more than the fellow pupil (see 10.4, Adie Tonic Pupil).

Note: Soon after the development of an Adie pupil, the pupil may not react to a weak cholinergic agent.

—If the pupil does not constrict with pilocarpine, 0.125%, or pharmacologic dilatation is suspected, pilocarpine, 1%, is instilled in both eyes. A normal pupil constricts sooner and to a greater extent than the pharmacologically dilated pupil. An eye that recently received a strong mydriatic agent such as atropine usually will not constrict at all.

See 10.2, Horner Syndrome, 10.3, Argyll Robertson Pupils, 10.4, Adie Tonic Pupils, and 10.5, Isolated Third Nerve Palsy, for more information regarding diagnosis and treatment of the specific entity causing anisocoria.

10.2 HORNER SYNDROME

SYMPTOMS

Droopy eyelid, pupil size disparity; often asymptomatic.

SIGNS

Critical. Anisocoria that is greater in dim illumination (especially during the first few seconds after the room light is dimmed) because of a small pupil that does not dilate as well as the normal, larger pupil. Mild ptosis and lower eyelid elevation ("reverse ptosis") occur on the same side as the small pupil.

Other. All of the following may occur on the side affected by Horner syndrome: Lower intraocular pressure, lighter iris color in congenital cases (iris heterochromia), loss of sweating ability (anhidrosis, distribution depends on the site of the lesion), increase in accommodation due to decreased pupil size (older patients can be noted to hold their reading card closer in the Horner eye). Light and near reactions are intact.

DIFFERENTIAL DIAGNOSIS

See 10.1, Anisocoria.

ETIOLOGY

• First-order neuron disorder: Stroke (e.g., vertebrobasilar artery insufficiency or infarct); tumor; multiple sclerosis (MS), and, rarely, severe osteoarthritis of the neck with bony spurs.

• Second-order neuron disorder: Tumor (e.g., lung carcinoma, metastasis, thyroid adenoma, neurofibroma). Patients with arm pain should be suspected of having a Pancoast tumor. In children, consider neuroblastoma, lymphoma, or metastasis.

• Third-order neuron disorder: Headache syndrome (e.g., cluster, migraine, Raeder paratrigeminal syndrome), internal carotid dissection, herpes zoster virus, otitis media, Tolosa–Hunt syndrome, neck trauma/tumor/inflammation.

• Congenital Horner syndrome: Trauma (e.g., during delivery).

WORKUP

1. If the diagnosis is uncertain, it may be confirmed with a cocaine test: One drop of cocaine, 10%, is placed into each eye and then repeated 1 minute later. Check the pupils in 15 minutes. If no change in pupillary size is noted, repeat one set of drops and recheck the pupils in another 15 minutes. A Horner pupil dilates less than the normal pupil.

2. Hydroxyamphetamine, 1% (e.g., Paredrine), is used to distinguish a third-order neuron disorder from a first- and second-order neuron disorder: Place one drop of hydroxyamphetamine, 1%, into each eye, repeating the drop 1 minute later. Check the pupils in 30 minutes. Failure of the Horner pupil to dilate to an equivalent degree as the fellow eye indicates a third-order neuron lesion.

Notes: Hydroxyamphetamine should not be administered within 24 hours of cocaine or they will interfere with each other's action. Both tests are thought to require an intact corneal epithelium and no prior eye drop administration for accurate results.

3. Determine the duration of the Horner syndrome from the patient's history and an examination of old photographs. New-onset Horner syndrome requires a more extensive diagnostic workup. An old Horner syndrome is more likely to be benign.

4. History: Headaches? Arm pain? Previous stroke? Previous surgery that may have damaged the sympathetic chain, including cardiac, thoracic, thyroid or neck surgery? History of head or neck trauma? Ipsilateral neck pain?

5. Physical examination (especially check for supraclavicular nodes, thyroid enlargement, or a neck mass).

Because the hydroxyamphetamine test is only 40% to 97% sensitive in determining the location of the lesion, a patient with new-onset Horner syndrome requires a workup based on other clinical signs and symptoms. In the absence of any clues to etiology, imaging of the entire sympathetic pathway is recommended. The following studies focus on paraspinal, mediastinal, cervical carotid, and skull base regions.

6. Computed tomography (CT) scan of the chest to evaluate lung apex for possible mass (e.g., Pancoast tumor).

7. Magnetic resonance imaging (MRI) of the brain and neck.

8. Complete blood count (CBC) with differential.

9. Magnetic resonance angiography (MRA) of head/neck or carotid Doppler ultrasonography if carotid artery dissection possible (especially with neck pain). Carotid angiography if MRA or Doppler equivocal.

10. Lymph node biopsy when lymphadenopathy is present.

TREATMENT

1. Treat the underlying disorder if possible (Carotid dissection usually requires urgent anticoagulation to prevent thrombosis: Consider neurovascular surgical consultation.).

2. Ptosis surgery may be performed as needed.

FOLLOW-UP

1. Acute Horner syndromes should be worked up as soon as possible to rule out life-threatening causes.

2. Chronic Horner syndromes can be evaluated with less urgency. With the exception of possible amblyopia in children, which occurs only when the eyelid covers the visual axis, there are no ocular complications that necessitate close follow-up.

10.3 ARGYLL ROBERTSON PUPILS

SYMPTOMS

Usually asymptomatic.

SIGNS

Critical. Small, irregular pupils that exhibit "light-near" dissociation (react poorly or not at all to light but constrict normally during convergence). By definition, vision is normal.

Other. The pupils do not dilate well. May initially be unilateral, but always becomes bilateral, although possibly asymmetric.

DIFFERENTIAL DIAGNOSIS

See 10.1, Anisocoria.
   Other causes of "light-near" dissociation:

• Bilateral optic neuropathy or severe retinopathy (Visual acuity is reduced, pupil size is normal.).

• Adie tonic pupil (Unilateral or bilateral irregularly dilated pupil that constricts slowly and unevenly to light. Normal vision. See 10.4, Adie Tonic Pupil.).

• Dorsal midbrain (Parinaud) syndrome (Bilateral, normal to large pupils. Accompanied by convergence–retraction nystagmus and supranuclear upgaze palsy. See 10.4, Adie Tonic Pupil, and 10.19, Nystagmus.).

ETIOLOGY

Tertiary syphilis.

WORKUP

1. Test the pupillary reaction to light and convergence: To test the reaction of the pupil to convergence, patients are asked to look first at a distant target and then at their own finger, which the examiner holds in front of them and slowly brings in toward their face.

2. Slit-lamp examination: Look for interstitial keratitis.

3. Dilated fundus examination: Search for chorioretinitis, papillitis, and uveitis.

4. FTA-ABS or MHA-TP, rapid plasma reagin (RPR) or Venereal Disease Research Laboratories test (VDRL).

5. Consider a lumbar puncture if the diagnosis of syphilis is established (see 13.5, Acquired Syphilis).

TREATMENT

1. The decision to treat is based on whether active disease is present and whether the patient has been treated appropriately in the past.

2. See 13.5, Acquired Syphilis, for treatment indications and specific antibiotic therapy.

FOLLOW-UP

This is not an emergency, but a diagnostic workup and determination of syphilitic activity should be undertaken within a few days of detecting Argyll Robertson pupils.

10.4   ADIE TONIC PUPIL

SYMPTOMS

Difference in the size of the pupils, blurred near vision; photophobia; may be asymptomatic.

SIGNS

Critical. An irregularly dilated pupil exhibiting minimal or no reaction to light, slow constriction to convergence, and slow redilation. It is typically unilateral at first and is found most often in young women. The pupil demonstrates supersensitivity to weak cholinergic agents (e.g., pilocarpine, 0.125%). Slit-lamp evaluation reveals sectorial papillary paralysis (vermiform movements).

Other. It may develop acutely and may become bilateral. The pupil dilates normally to mydriatic agents. Deep tendon reflexes (knees and ankles) are often absent (Adie syndrome). The involved pupil may become smaller than the normal pupil over time.

Note: Supersensitivity may not be present soon after the development of an Adie pupil and may need to be tested a few weeks later.

DIFFERENTIAL DIAGNOSIS

See 10.1, Anisocoria.

Note: Parinaud syndrome may produce bilateral mid-dilated pupils that react poorly to light but constrict normally during convergence (i.e., not tonic). Eyelid retraction and a supranuclear paralysis of upgaze with retraction nystagmus may also be present. A pinealoma or other midbrain abnormality must be ruled out by MRI.

ETIOLOGY

Idiopathic (most), orbital trauma or infection, herpes zoster infection, autonomic neuropathies, Guillain–Barré syndrome, others.

WORKUP

See 10.1, Anisocoria, for a general workup when the diagnosis is uncertain.

1. Observe the suspect pupil with the slit lamp, shining a bright light on it. The Adie pupil will contract slowly and irregularly.

2. Test for a supersensitive pupil. Have the patient fixate at a distance, and measure the pupil size of each eye. Instill one drop of pilocarpine, 0.125%, in each eye, and recheck the pupil size in 10 to 15 minutes. The tonic pupil constricts significantly more than the contralateral pupil in Adie syndrome.

   Note: The dilute pilocarpine test may occasionally be positive in familial dysautonomia.

3. If Adie pupil or supersensitivity or both are present and the patient is younger than 1 year, refer him or her to a pediatric neurologist to rule out familial dysautonomia (Riley–Day syndrome).

TREATMENT

Pilocarpine, 0.125%, b.i.d. to q.i.d., for cosmesis and to aid in accommodation, if desired.

FOLLOW-UP

If the diagnosis is established with certainty, follow-up is routine.

10.5 ISOLATED THIRD NERVE PALSY

SYMPTOMS

Double vision that disappears when one eye is closed; droopy eyelid, with or without pain.

Note: Pain does not distinguish between microvascular infarction and compression.

SIGNS

Critical

• External ophthalmoplegia (i.e., motility impaired).

—Complete palsy: Limitation of ocular movement in all fields of gaze except temporally.

—Incomplete palsy: Partial limitation of ocular movement.

—Superior division palsy: Ptosis and an inability to look up.

—Inferior division palsy: Inability to look nasally or inferiorly; pupil may be involved.

• Internal ophthalmoplegia (i.e., pupil reaction impaired)

—Pupil-involving: A fixed, dilated or minimally reactive pupil.

—Pupil-sparing: Pupil not dilated and normally reactive to light.

—Relative pupil-sparing: Pupil partially dilated and sluggishly reactive to light.

Other. An exotropia or hypotropia. Aberrant regeneration [elevation of the upper eyelid with gaze down or nasally; sometimes pupil constriction (usually segmental) when looking up, down, or nasally].

Note: Aberrant regeneration may occur spontaneously (primary regeneration) without a preceding acute third nerve palsy. This is usually caused by a cavernous sinus tumor or aneurysm.

DIFFERENTIAL DIAGNOSIS

• Myasthenia gravis [Diurnal variation of symptoms and signs, pupil never involved, increased eyelid droop after sustained upgaze, weak orbicularis oculi muscle, positive edrophonium chloride (i.e., Tensilon) test, ice-pack test, or sleep test. See 10.10, Myasthenia Gravis.].

• Thyroid eye disease (Eyelid lag, stare, injection over the rectus muscles, proptosis, resistance on forced duction testing, abnormal CT scan of the orbits, no ptosis. See 7.2, Thyroid-Related Orbitopathy.).

• Chronic progressive external ophthalmoplegia (CPEO) (Bilateral, slowly progressive ptosis and limitation of ocular motility, pupil spared, often no double vision. See 10.11, Chronic Progressive External Ophthalmoplegia.).

• Orbital inflammatory pseudotumor (Pain and proptosis are usually present. See 7.3, Orbital Inflammatory Pseudotumor.).

• Internuclear ophthalmoplegia (INO) (Unilateral or bilateral adduction deficit with horizontal nystagmus of opposite abducting eye. No ptosis. Lesion in ipsilateral brainstem medial longitudinal fasciculus. See 10.12, Internuclear Ophthalmoplegia.).

• Skew deviation (Supranuclear brainstem lesion producing asymmetric, mainly vertical ocular deviation not consistent with single cranial nerve defect. See 10.12, Internuclear Ophthalmoplegia.).

• Parinaud syndrome/dorsal midbrain lesion (Inability to look up; pupils react slowly to light and briskly to convergence; no ptosis; eyelid-retraction and convergence-retraction nystagmus may be present. Bilateral.).

• Giant cell arteritis (GCA) (Extraocular muscle ischemia causing nonspecific motility deficits. Pupil not involved. Age older than 50 years, associated systemic symptoms. See 10.16, Arteritic Ischemic Optic Neuropathy.).

ETIOLOGY

- Pupil-involving:

  —*More common:* Aneurysm (particularly a posterior communicating artery aneurysm).

  —*Less common:* Tumor, trauma, congenital, uncal herniation, cavernous sinus mass lesion, pituitary apoplexy, orbital disease, herpes zoster, leukemia. In children, ophthalmoplegic migraine.

- Pupil-sparing: Ischemic microvascular disease; rarely cavernous sinus syndrome, GCA.

- Relative pupil-sparing: Ischemic microvascular disease; less likely aneurysm.

- Aberrant regeneration present: Trauma, aneurysm, tumor, congenital. Not microvascular. (Signs of aberrant regeneration include eyelid retraction on downgaze, eyelid elevation or pupillary constriction on attempted adduction, or globe retraction on upgaze/downgaze.)

WORKUP

1. History: Onset and duration of diplopia? Recent trauma? Pertinent medical history [e.g., diabetes, hypertension, known cancer or central nervous system (CNS) mass, recent infections]. Specifically ask about risk factors for GCA.

2. Complete ocular examination: Check for pupillary involvement, the directions of motility restriction (in both eyes), ptosis, a visual field defect (visual fields by confrontation), proptosis, resistance to retropulsion, orbicularis muscle weakness and eyelid fatigue with sustained upgaze. Look carefully for signs of aberrant regeneration (discussed previously).

3. Full neurologic examination: Carefully assess the other cranial nerves on both sides. (The ipsilateral fourth nerve can be assessed by focusing with the slit lamp on a superior conjunctival blood vessel and asking the pa-

tient to look down and nasally. The eye should intort, and the blood vessel should turn down and toward the nose.)

4. Immediate imaging study of the brain (preferably gadolinium-enhanced MRI and MRA) to rule out mass/aneurysm is indicated for

   a. Pupil-involving (relatively or completely involved) third nerve palsies.

   b. Pupil-sparing third nerve palsies only in the following groups of patients:

      —Patients younger than 50 years of age (unless there is known long-standing diabetes or hypertension).

      —Patients with incomplete third nerve palsies (i.e., with sparing of some muscle function) because this condition may be evolving into a pupil-involving third nerve palsy. (These patients may alternatively be monitored closely over 5 to 7 days for development of pupil involvement.)

      —Patients whose third nerve palsy is over 3 months in duration, but has not improved.

      —Patients with an additional cranial nerve or neurologic abnormalities.

   c. All patients in whom aberrant regeneration develops, with the exception of regeneration after traumatic third nerve palsies.

   d. Children younger than 10 years, regardless of the state of the pupil.

      Note: Imaging is usually not required in pupil-sparing third nerve palsies that do not fit these criteria, especially when patients have known vasculopathic risk factors such as diabetes or hypertension.

5. Cerebral angiography is indicated for all patients older than 10 years with pupil-involving third nerve palsies and whose imaging study is negative or shows a mass consistent with an aneurysm.

6. CBC with differential in children.

7. Edrophonium chloride (i.e., Tensilon) test when myasthenia gravis is suspected and the pupil is not involved (see 10.10, Myasthenia Gravis).

8. For suspected ischemic disease: Check blood pressure, fasting blood sugar, glycosylated hemoglobin.

9. Immediate erythrocyte sedimentation rate (ESR) if GCA is possible (see 10.16, Arteritic Ischemic Optic Neuropathy).

TREATMENT

1. Treat the underlying abnormality.

2. If the third nerve palsy is causing symptomatic diplopia, an occlusion patch may be placed over the involved eye. Patching is usually not performed in children younger than 9 to 11 years because of the risk of amblyopia. Children should be monitored closely for the development of amblyopia in the deviated eye.

FOLLOW-UP

1. **Pupil-sparing:** Observe daily for 5 to 7 days from onset of symptoms for delayed pupil involvement, and then recheck every 4 to 6 weeks. Patients should regain the function lost from their third nerve palsy within 3 months. If the palsy does not reverse by 3 months, the pupil dilates, additional neurologic abnormalities develop, aberrant regeneration appears, or an incomplete third nerve palsy progresses, then an immediate MRI is obtained. Refer to internist for management of vasculopathic disease risk factors.

2. **Pupil-involving:** If imaging and angiography are negative, a lumbar puncture should be considered and the patient should be followed as in pupil-sparing case, earlier.

10.6   ISOLATED FOURTH NERVE PALSY

SYMPTOMS

Binocular vertical diplopia (double vision that disappears when one eye is occluded; one image appears on top of or up and to the side of the second image with both eyes open), difficulty reading, sensation that objects appear tilted; may be asymptomatic.

SIGNS

Critical. Deficient inferior movement of an eye when attempting to look down and in. The three-step test isolates a palsy of the superior oblique muscle (see the following discussion).

Other. The involved eye is higher (hypertropic) when patient looks straight ahead. The hypertropia increases when looking in the direction of the uninvolved eye or tilting the head toward the ipsilateral shoulder. The patient often maintains a head tilt toward the contralateral shoulder to eliminate double vision.

DIFFERENTIAL DIAGNOSIS

All of the following may produce binocular vertical diplopia, hypertropia, or both.

• Myasthenia gravis [Double vision worse toward the end of the day when fatigued, usually accompanied by ptosis, positive edrophonium chloride (i.e., Tensilon) test. See 10.10, Myasthenia Gravis.].

• Thyroid eye disease (May have proptosis, eyelid lag, stare, or injection over the involved rectus muscles. Positive forced duction test. See 7.2, Thyroid-Related Orbitopathy.).

• Orbital inflammatory disease (pseudotumor) (Pain and proptosis are common. See 7.3, Orbital Inflammatory Pseudotumor.).

• Orbital fracture (History of trauma. Can cause entrapment or fibrosis of the inferior rectus muscle. Positive forced duction test. See 3.8, Orbital Blow-out Fracture.).

• Skew deviation (The three-step test does not isolate a particular muscle. Rule out a posterior fossa or brainstem lesion by MRI of the brain. See 10.12, Internuclear Ophthalmoplegia.).

• Incomplete third nerve palsy (Inability to look down and out, usually with adduction weakness. Intorsion on attempted downgaze. Three-step test does not isolate superior oblique. See 10.5, Isolated Third Nerve Palsy.).

• Brown syndrome [Limitation of elevation in adduction due to restriction of superior oblique tendon. May be congenital or acquired (e.g., trauma, inflammation). Positive forced duction test. See 8.5, Strabismus Syndromes.].

• GCA (Extraocular muscle ischemia causing nonspecific motility deficits or neural ischemia mimicking cranial nerve palsy. Age older than 50 years, associated systemic symptoms. See 10.16, Arteritic Ischemic Optic Neuropathy.).

ETIOLOGY

• More common: Trauma; vascular infarct (often the result of underlying diabetes or hypertension); congenital, idiopathic, or demyelinating disease.

• Rare: Tumor, hydrocephalus, aneurysm, GCA.

WORKUP

1. History: Onset and duration of the diplopia? Misaligned eyes or head tilt since early childhood? Trauma? Stroke?

2. Examine old photographs to determine whether the head tilt is of long standing, indicating an old or congenital fourth nerve palsy.

Note: A congenital fourth nerve palsy can be distinguished from an acquired fourth nerve palsy by measuring the vertical fusional amplitudes. A patient with an acquired fourth nerve palsy has a normal vertical fusional amplitude of 1 to 3 prism diopters. On the other hand, a patient with a congenital fourth nerve palsy has greater than 1 to 3 prism diopters (often up to 10 to 15 prism diopters) of fusional amplitude. This is detected by using vertical prism bars. If a patient can fuse greater than 1 to 3 prism diopters, then the fourth nerve palsy is congenital.

3. Three-step test:

—**Step 1:** Determine which eye is deviated upward in primary gaze (looking straight ahead). This is best seen with the cover–uncover test (see Appendix 2). The higher eye comes down after being uncovered.

—**Step 2:** Determine whether the upward deviation is greater when the patient looks to the left or to the right.

—**Step 3:** Determine whether the upward deviation is greater when tilting the head to the left shoulder or right shoulder.

As mentioned previously, patients with a superior oblique muscle paresis have a hyperdeviation that is worse when turning the elevated eye nasally and when tilting the head toward the shoulder ipsilateral to the elevated eye.

Patients with a bilateral fourth nerve palsy demonstrate hypertropia of the right eye when looking left, hypertropia of the left eye when looking right, and a "V"-pattern esotropia (the eyes cross more when looking down).

4. Perform the double Maddox rod test[1] if a bilateral fourth nerve palsy is suspected.

5. Vertical fusional amplitudes greater than 1 to 3 prism diopters are suggestive of congenital fourth nerve palsy.

6. Edrophonium chloride (i.e., Tensilon) test, ice-pack test, or sleep test if myasthenia gravis is suspected (see 10.10, Myasthenia Gravis).

7. CT scan head and orbits (axial and coronal views) for suspected orbital disease.

8. Blood pressure measurement, fasting blood sugar, and glycosylated hemoglobin. Immediate ESR if GCA is possible.

9. MRI of the brain for:

   —A fourth nerve palsy accompanied by other cranial nerve or neurologic abnormalities (i.e., not an isolated palsy).

   —All patients younger than 45 years with no definite history of significant head

trauma, and patients aged 45 to 55 years with no vasculopathic risk factors or trauma.

TREATMENT

1. Treat the underlying disorder.

2. An occlusion patch may be placed over one eye or fogging plastic tape can be applied to one lens of patient's spectacles to relieve symptomatic double vision. Patching is usually not performed in children younger than 9 to 11 years because of the risk of amblyopia.

3. Prisms in spectacles may be prescribed for small, stable hyperdeviations.

4. Strabismus surgery may be indicated for bothersome double vision in primary or reading position, for a manifest head tilt, or to improve appearance. We usually wait at least 6 months after the onset of the palsy for the deviation to stabilize and because many palsies resolve spontaneously.

FOLLOW-UP

1. **Congenital fourth nerve palsy** (i.e., head tilt in old photographs, enlarged vertical fusion amplitude): Routine.

2. **Acquired fourth nerve palsy:** As per the underlying disorder identified in the workup. If the workup is negative (the lesion is presumed vascular or idiopathic), then reexamine the patient in 1 to 3 months. If the palsy does not resolve in 3 months or if an additional neurologic abnormality develops, appropriate imaging studies of the brain are indicated. Patients are instructed to return immediately if they notice any changes (e.g., ptosis, worsening diplopia, sensory abnormality).

---

[1]A white Maddox rod is placed before one eye and a red Maddox rod is placed before the other eye in a trial frame, aligning the axes of each rod along the 90-degree vertical mark. While looking at a white light in the distance, the patient is asked if both the white and red lines seen through the Maddox rods are horizontal and parallel to each other (sometimes placing a 6-prism diopter base-down in front of one eye helps the patient determine if the lines are parallel, but this should not be performed in the presence of hypertropia). When the lines are not horizontal and parallel, the patient is asked to rotate the Maddox rod(s) until they are parallel. If he or she rotates the top of this vertical axis outward (away from the nose) for more than 10 degrees total for the two eyes, then a bilateral superior oblique muscle paresis exists.

10.7 ISOLATED SIXTH NERVE PALSY

SYMPTOMS

Binocular horizontal diplopia (double vision producing side-by-side images; single vision is restored when one eye is closed or covered), worse for distance than near, most pronounced in the direction of the paretic lateral rectus muscle.

SIGNS

Critical. One eye does not turn outward (temporally).

Other. Lack of restriction on forced-duction testing. (See Appendix 5 for forced-duction test description.) No proptosis.

DIFFERENTIAL DIAGNOSIS

All of the following may produce limitation of abduction.

• Thyroid eye disease (Proptosis, injection of blood vessels over the restricted muscle, restriction on forced-duction testing. See 7.2, Thyroid-Related Orbitopathy.).

• Myasthenia gravis [Symptoms worse toward the end of day with fatigue, orbicularis oculi weakness and ptosis may or may not be present, positive edrophonium chloride (i.e., Tensilon) test. See 10.10, Myasthenia Gravis.].

• Orbital inflammatory disease (pseudotumor) (Proptosis, pain, restriction on forced-duction testing. See 7.3, Orbital Inflammatory Pseudotumor.).

• Orbital trauma (Medial wall fracture causing entrapment of the ipsilateral medial rectus muscle, restriction on forced-duction testing. See 3.8, Orbital Blow-out Fracture.).

• Duane syndrome, type 1 (Congenital; narrowing of the palpebral fissure and retraction of the globe on adduction. See 8.5, Strabismus Syndromes.).

• Möbius syndrome (Congenital; bilateral facial paralysis present. See 8.5, Strabismus Syndromes.).

• Convergence spasm (The pupils constrict on attempted abduction.).

• GCA (Extraocular muscle ischemia, age older than 50 years, associated systemic symptoms. See 10.16, Arteritic Ischemic Optic Neuropathy.).

ETIOLOGY

Adults

• More common: Vasculopathic (diabetes, hypertension, atherosclerosis), trauma, idiopathic.

• Less common: Increased intracranial pressure, cavernous sinus mass (e.g., meningioma, aneurysm, metastasis), MS, sarcoidosis/vasculitis, after myelography or lumbar puncture, stroke (usually with other neurologic deficits), meningeal inflammation/infection (e.g., Lyme disease, tertiary syphilis), GCA.

Children

Benign postviral or postvaccination condition, trauma, increased intracranial pressure (multiple causes; e.g., obstructive hydrocephalus), pontine glioma, Gradenigo syndrome (petrositis causing sixth and often seventh nerve involvement, with or without eighth and fifth nerve involvement on the same side; associated with complicated otitis media).

WORKUP

Adults

1. History: Do the symptoms fluctuate during the day? History of cancer, diabetes, or thyroid disease?

2. Complete neurologic and ophthalmic examinations; pay careful attention to the function of the other cranial nerves and the appearance of the optic disc. It is especially important to evaluate the fifth cranial nerve; corneal sensation (supplied by the first division) can be tested by touching a wisp of cotton or a tissue to the corneas *before* ap-

plying topical anesthetic. Ophthalmoscopy looking for papilledema is required because increased intracranial pressure can result in unilateral or bilateral sixth nerve palsy.

3. Check blood pressure, fasting blood sugar, and glycosylated hemoglobin.

4. MRI of the brain is indicated for the following patients:

   —Younger than 45 years (if MRI is negative, consider lumbar puncture).

   —Sixth nerve palsy accompanied by severe pain or any other neurologic or neuro-ophthalmic sign.

   —Any history of cancer. Consider MRI for patients aged 45 to 55 years with no history of vasculopathic disease.

   —Bilateral sixth nerve palsy.

   —Papilledema is present.

5. Immediate ESR if GCA is possible (see 10.16, Arteritic Ischemic Optic Neuropathy.).

6. Consider RPR, FTA-ABS, Lyme titer.

Children

1. History: Recent illness or trauma? Neurologic symptoms, lethargy, or behavioral changes? Chronic ear infections?

2. Complete neurologic and ophthalmic examinations as described for adults.

3. Otoscopic examination to rule out complicated otitis media.

4. MRI of the brain in all children.

TREATMENT

1. Any underlying problem revealed by the workup is treated.

2. An occlusion patch may be placed over one eye or fogging plastic tape applied to one spectacle lens to relieve symptomatic diplopia. In patients younger than 9 to 11 years, patching is avoided, and these patients are monitored closely for the development of amblyopia (see 8.6, Amblyopia).

3. Prisms in glasses may be fit for chronic stable deviations (e.g., after stroke). Consider strabismus surgery for stable deviation that persists more than 6 months.

FOLLOW-UP

Reexamine every 6 weeks after the onset of the palsy until it resolves. MRI of the head is indicated if any neurologic signs or symptoms develop during the follow-up period, the abduction deficit increases, or the isolated sixth nerve palsy does not resolve in 3 to 6 months.

10.8   ISOLATED SEVENTH NERVE PALSY

SYMPTOMS

Weakness or paralysis of one side of the face, inability to close one eye, excessive drooling.

SIGNS

Critical. Weakness or paralysis of the facial musculature on one side.

• Central lesion: Weakness or paralysis of lower facial musculature only. (Upper eyelid closure and forehead wrinkling intact.)

• Peripheral lesion: Weakness or paralysis of upper and lower facial musculature.

Other. Flattened nasolabial fold, droop of corner of the mouth, ectropion, or lagophthalmos. May have ipsilateral decreased taste on anterior two thirds of tongue, decreased basic tear production, or hyperacusis. May have an injected eye with a corneal epithelial defect. Synkinesis. [Simultaneous movement of muscles supplied by different branches of the facial nerve or simultaneous stimulation of visceral efferent fibers of facial nerve (e.g., corner of mouth contracts when eye closes, excessive lacrimation when eating ["crocodile" tears]). Due to aberrant regeneration and therefore implies chronicity.]

ETIOLOGY

Central Lesions

• Cortical: Lesion of contralateral motor cortex or internal capsule (e.g., stroke, tumor). (Loss of voluntary facial movement; emotional facial movement sometimes intact. May also have ipsilateral hemiparesis.)

• Extrapyramidal: Lesion of basal ganglia (e.g., parkinsonism, tumor, vascular lesion of basal ganglia). (Loss of emotional facial movement; volitional facial movement intact. Not a true facial paralysis.)

• Brainstem: Lesion of ipsilateral pons (e.g., MS, stroke, tumor). (Often with ipsilateral sixth nerve palsy, contralateral hemiparesis. Occasionally with cerebellar signs.)

Peripheral Lesions

• Cerebellopontine angle (CPA) masses (e.g., acoustic neuroma, facial neuroma, meningioma, cholesteatoma, metastasis). (Gradually progressive onset, although sometimes acute. May have facial pain or twitching. May have eighth nerve dysfunction, including hearing loss, vertigo, or dysequilibrium.)

• Trauma

—Temporal bone fracture [History of head trauma. May have Battle sign (ecchymoses over mastoid region), cerebrospinal fluid otorrhea, hearing loss, vertigo, or vestibular nystagmus.].

—Other [Accidental or iatrogenic (e.g., facial laceration, local anesthetic block, parotid or mastoid surgery).].

• Otitis

—Acute otitis media.

—Chronic suppurative otitis media.

—Malignant otitis externa (*Pseudomonas* infection in diabetic or elderly patients. Begins in external auditory canal but may progress to osteomyelitis, meningitis, or abscess.).

• Ramsay–Hunt syndrome (herpes zoster oticus) (Viral prodrome followed by ear pain; vesicles on pinna, external auditory canal, tongue, face, or neck. Progresses over 10 days. May have sensorineural hearing loss, tinnitus, or vertigo.).

• Guillain–Barré syndrome (Viral syndrome followed by progressive motor weakness or paralysis or cranial nerve palsies, or both. Loss of deep tendon reflexes. May have bilateral facial palsies.).

• Lyme disease (May have rash, fever, fatigue, arthralgias, myalgias, or nausea. There may or may not be a history of tick bite. See 13.6, Lyme Disease.).

• Sarcoidosis (May have uveitis, parotitis, skin lesions, or lymphadenopathy. May have bilateral facial palsies. See 12.6, Sarcoidosis.).

• Parotid neoplasm (Slowly progressive paralysis of all or portion of facial musculature. Parotid mass with facial pain.)

• Metastasis [History of primary tumor (e.g., breast, lung, prostate) with multiple cranial nerve palsies in rapid succession. Can be the result of basilar skull metastasis or carcinomatous meningitis.].

• Bell palsy (Idiopathic seventh nerve palsy. Most common, but other etiologies must be ruled out. May have viral prodrome followed by ear pain, facial numbness, decreased tearing or taste. Facial palsy may be complete or incomplete and progress over 10 days. May be recurrent, rarely bilateral. Possible familial predisposition.).

• Others [e.g., diabetes mellitus, botulism, human immunodeficiency virus (HIV), syphilis, Epstein–Barr virus, acute porphyrias, nasopharyngeal carcinoma, collagen–vascular disease.].

WORKUP

1. History: Onset and duration of facial weakness? First bout or recurrence? Facial or ear pain? Trauma? Stroke? Recent infec-

tion? Hearing loss, tinnitus, dizziness, or vertigo? History of sarcoidosis or cancer?

2. Thorough neurologic examination: Determine if facial palsy is central or peripheral, complete or incomplete. Assess taste with bitter or sweet solution on anterior two thirds of tongue on affected side. Carefully assess other cranial nerves, especially the fifth, sixth, and seventh. Look for motor weakness, cerebellar signs.

3. Complete ocular examination: Check ocular motility and look for nystagmus. Assess orbicularis strength bilaterally, degree of ectropion, and Bell phenomenon. Examine cornea carefully for signs of exposure (superficial punctate keratitis, abrasion, or ulcer). Perform Schirmer test to assess basic tear production (see 4.3, Dry-Eye Syndrome, for explanation of Schirmer test). Check for signs of uveitis.

4. Otolaryngologic examination: Examine ear and oropharynx for vesicles, masses, or other lesions. Palpate parotid for mass or lymphadenopathy. Check hearing.

5. CT scan if history of trauma to rule out basilar skull fracture: Axial and coronal cuts with attention to temporal bone.

6. MRI or CT scan of brain if any other associated neurologic signs or with history of cancer: If sixth nerve involvement, pay attention to brainstem. If eighth nerve involvement, pay attention to CPA. If multiple cranial nerves involved, pay attention to base of skull.

7. Chest radiograph and angiotensin-converting enzyme level if sarcoidosis suspected.

8. Lyme titer, Epstein–Barr virus titer, RPR, HIV test, CBC with differential, as needed, depending on suspected etiology.

9. Rheumatoid factor, ESR, anti-nuclear antibody (ANA), anti-neutrophil cytoplasmic antibody if collagen–vascular disease suspected.

10. Echocardiogram, Holter monitor, carotid noninvasive studies in patients with a history of stroke.

11. Lumbar puncture in patients with history of primary neoplasm to rule out carcinomatous meningitis (repeat up to three times if negative to increase sensitivity).

TREATMENT

1. Treat the underlying disease as follows:

—**Stroke:** Refer to neurologist.

—**CPA masses, temporal bone fracture, nerve laceration:** Refer to neurosurgeon.

—**Otitis:** Refer to otolaryngologist.

—**Ramsay–Hunt syndrome:** If seen within 72 hours of onset, start acyclovir, 800 mg, five times per day for 7 to 10 days (contraindicated in pregnancy and renal failure; see Drug Glossary). Refer to otolaryngologist.

—**Guillain–Barré syndrome:** Refer to neurologist. May require urgent hospitalization for rapidly progressive motor weakness or respiratory distress.

—**Lyme disease:** Refer to infectious disease specialist. May need lumbar puncture. Treated with oral doxycycline, penicillin, or intravenous (i.v.) ceftriaxone.

—**Sarcoidosis:** Treat uveitis if present (see 12.6, Sarcoidosis). Consider brain MRI or lumbar puncture or both to rule out CNS involvement; if present, refer to neurologist. Refer to internist for systemic evaluation. May require oral prednisone for systemic or CNS disease.

—**Metastatic disease:** Refer to oncologist. Systemic chemotherapy, radiation, or both may be required.

2. In idiopathic/Bell palsy, 86% of patients recover completely with observation only within 2 months. Options for treatment (controversial) include:

—Facial massage or electrical stimulation of facial musculature.

—Oral steroids [e.g., prednisone, 60 mg orally (p.o.), q.d., for 4 days, tapering to 5 mg q.d., over 10 days]. Consider in patients with complete palsy.

—Surgical decompression of facial nerve by otolaryngologist. If not resolved after 3 months, order MRI of brain to rule out mass lesion.

3. The primary ocular complication of facial palsy is corneal exposure, which is managed as follows (see also 4.5, Exposure Keratopathy):

—Mild exposure keratitis: Artificial tears, q.i.d., with lubricating ointment, q.h.s.

—Moderate exposure keratitis: Preservative-free artificial tears q1–2h, moisture chamber during the day with lubricating ointment, or tape tarsorrhaphy, q.h.s. Consider a temporary tarsorrhaphy.

—Severe exposure keratitis: Temporary or permanent tarsorrhaphy. For expected chronic facial palsy, consider eyelid gold weight or spring implants to facilitate eyelid closure.

FOLLOW-UP

1. Recheck all patients at 1 and 3 months and more frequently if corneal complications arise.

2. In nonresolving facial palsy with repeatedly negative workup, consider referral to neurosurgeon or plastic surgeon for facial nerve graft, cranial nerve reanastomosis, or temporalis muscle transposition for patients who strongly desire facial reanimation.

10.9   CAVERNOUS SINUS AND ASSOCIATED SYNDROMES

(MULTIPLE OCULAR MOTOR NERVE PALSIES)

SYMPTOMS

Double vision, eyelid droop, facial pain or numbness.

SIGNS

Critical. Limitation of eye movement corresponding to any combination of a third, fourth, or sixth nerve palsy on one side; facial pain or numbness or both corresponding to one or more branches of the fifth cranial nerve; a droopy eyelid and a small pupil (Horner syndrome); the pupil also may be dilated if the third cranial nerve is involved. All signs involve the same side of the face when one cavernous sinus/superior orbital fissure is involved. Consider orbital apex syndrome when proptosis and optic neuropathy are present.

Other. Proptosis may be present when the superior orbital fissure is involved.

DIFFERENTIAL DIAGNOSIS

• Myasthenia gravis [Eyelid droop and limitation of eye movements, especially with fatigue; weakness of the orbicularis oculi muscle; positive edrophonium chloride (i.e., Tensilon) test. No pupillary abnormality, no pain, no proptosis.].

• CPEO (Slowly progressive, painless, bilateral limitation of eye movements with ptosis. The pupils are normal, and the orbicularis oculi muscles are usually weak.).

• Orbital lesions (e.g., tumor, thyroid disease, pseudotumor). [Proptosis and resistance to retropulsion are usually present, in addition to motility restriction. Results of forced-duction tests are abnormal (see Appendix 5). May have an afferent pupillary defect if the optic nerve is involved.]

*Note: Orbital apex syndrome combines the superior orbital fissure syndrome with optic nerve

dysfunction, and most commonly results from an orbital lesion.

• Brainstem disease (Tumors and vascular lesions of the brainstem can produce multiple ocular motor nerve palsies. MRI of the brain is best for making this diagnosis.).

• Carcinomatous meningitis (Diffuse seeding of the leptomeninges by metastatic tumor cells can produce a rapidly sequential bilateral cranial nerve disorder. Diagnosis is made by serial lumbar punctures.).

• Skull base tumors, especially nasopharyngeal carcinoma (Most commonly affects the sixth cranial nerve, but the second, third, fourth, and fifth cranial nerves may be involved as well. Typically, one cranial nerve after another is affected by invasion of the base of the skull. The patient may have cervical lymphadenopathy, nasal obstruction, ear pain or popping caused by serous otitis media or blockage of the eustachian tube, weight loss, or proptosis.).

• Progressive supranuclear palsy (Vertical limitation of eye movements; initially, downward gaze restriction, dementia, and rigidity of the neck and trunk. All eye movements are eventually lost.).

• Rare [Myotonic dystrophy, the bulbar variant of the Guillain–Barré syndrome (Miller–Fisher variant), intracranial sarcoidosis, others.].

ETIOLOGY

• Arteriovenous fistula [carotid–cavernous ("high-flow") or dural–cavernous ("low-flow")]. [Proptosis, chemosis, dilated and tortuous ("corkscrew") episcleral and conjunctival blood vessels. Intraocular pressure is often increased. Enhanced ocular pulsation ("pulsatile proptosis") may be present, sometimes discernible on slit-lamp examination during applanation. A bruit may be heard by the patient, and sometimes by the physician if the globe or temple region is auscultated. Reversed, arterialized flow in the superior ophthalmic vein is detectable with orbital color Doppler ultrasonography; orbital CT scan or MRI may show an enlarged superior ophthalmic vein. High-flow fistulas have an abrupt onset and are most commonly caused by trauma or rupture of an intracavernous aneurysm, whereas low-flow fistulas have a more insidious presentation, most commonly in hypertensive women older than 50 years.]

• Tumors within the cavernous sinus [May be primary intracranial neoplasms with direct involvement (e.g., meningioma, pituitary adenoma, craniopharyngioma); or metastatic tumors to the cavernous sinus, either local (e.g., nasopharyngeal carcinoma, perineural spread of a periocular squamous cell carcinoma) or distant metastasis (e.g., breast, lung, lymphoma).].

Note: Previously resected tumors may invade the cavernous sinus years after resection.

• Intracavernous aneurysm (Usually not ruptured. If aneurysm does rupture, the signs of a carotid–cavernous fistula develop.).

• Mucormycosis (Must be suspected in all diabetic patients, particularly those in ketoacidosis, and any debilitated or immunocompromised individual with multiple cranial nerve palsies, with or without proptosis. Onset is typically acute. Nasal discharge of blood may be present, and nasal examination may reveal a black, crusty material. This condition is life-threatening.).

• Pituitary apoplexy (Acute onset of the critical signs listed previously; often bilateral with severe headache, decreased vision, and possibly bitemporal hemianopsia or blindness. An enlarged sella turcica or an intrasellar mass, usually with acute hemorrhage, is seen on CT scan or MRI of the brain.).

• Herpes zoster (Patients with the typical zoster rash may develop ocular motor nerve palsies as well as a mid-dilated pupil that reacts better to convergence than to light.).

• Cavernous sinus thrombosis (Proptosis, chemosis, and eyelid edema. Usually bilateral. Fever, nausea, vomiting, and an altered level of consciousness often develop. May result from spread of infection from the face, mouth, throat, sinus, or orbit. Less commonly noninfectious, resulting from trauma or surgery.).

• Tolosa–Hunt syndrome (Acute idiopathic inflammation of the superior orbital fissure or anterior cavernous sinus. Orbital pain often precedes restriction of eye movements. Recurrent episodes are common. This is a diagnosis of exclusion.).

- Others (e.g., sarcoidosis, Wegener granulomatosis, mucocele, tuberculosis, and other infections).

WORKUP

1. History: Diabetes? Hypertension? Recent trauma? Prior cancer (including skin cancer)? Weight loss? Ocular bruit? Recent infection? Severe headache? Diurnal variation of symptoms? History of previously removed skin cancer?

2. Ophthalmic examination: Pay special attention to pupils, extraocular motility, Hertel exophthalmometry, and resistance to retropulsion.

3. Examine the periocular skin for malignant lesions.

4. CT scan (axial and coronal views) or MRI of the sinuses, orbit, and brain, or both.

5. Consider color Doppler imaging if arteriovenous fistula is suspected.

If the CT scan and MRI are negative, consider any or all of the following:

6. Serial lumbar puncture (three times if first two are negative to increase sensitivity) to rule out carcinomatous meningitis in patients with a history of primary carcinoma.

7. Nasopharyngeal examination with or without a biopsy to rule out nasopharyngeal carcinoma.

8. Lymph node biopsy when lymphadenopathy is present.

9. CBC with differential, ESR, ANA, rheumatoid factor to rule out infection, malignancy, and systemic vasculitis. Antineutrophilic cytoplasmic antibody if Wegener granulomatosis is suspected.

10. Cerebral arteriography is rarely required to rule out an aneurysm or arteriovenous fistula because most of these are seen by noninvasive imaging studies.

11. If cavernous sinus thrombosis is being considered, obtain two to three sets of peripheral blood cultures, and also culture the presumed primary source of the infection.

TREATMENT/FOLLOW-UP

Arteriovenous Fistula

1. Many dural fistulas close spontaneously, with intermittent ipsilateral carotid massage, or after arteriography. Others may require neurosurgical or interventional neuroradiologic techniques.

2. Treat secondary glaucoma with aqueous suppressants [i.e., topical beta-blocker (e.g., timolol or levobunolol, 0.25% to 0.5%, b.i.d.) or topical α_2-agonist (e.g., brimonidine, 0.2%, or apraclonidine, 0.5%, t.i.d.), or both, with or without a carbonic anhydrase inhibitor (e.g., topical dorzolamide, 2%, t.i.d., or methazolamide, 50 mg p.o., b.i.d.)]. Drugs that increase outflow facility (e.g., epinephrine, latanoprost, and pilocarpine) are usually not so effective because the intraocular pressure is increased as a result of increased episcleral venous pressure. (See 9.1, Primary Open-Angle Glaucoma.)

Metastatic Disease to the Cavernous Sinus

Often requires systemic chemotherapy (if a primary is found) with or without radiation therapy to the metastasis. Refer to an oncologist.

Intracavernous Aneurysm

Refer to a neurosurgeon for workup and possible treatment.

Mucormycosis

1. Immediate hospitalization because this is a rapidly progressive and possibly life-threatening disease.

2. Consult an infectious disease specialist and an otolaryngologist as required.

3. Begin amphotericin B, 0.25 to 0.30 mg/kg i.v., in D_5W slowly over 3 to 6 hours on the first day, 0.5 mg/kg i.v., on the second day, and then up to 0.8 to 1.0 mg/kg i.v., q.d. The duration of treatment is determined by the clinical condition.

Note: Renal status and electrolytes must be checked before initiating therapy with amphotericin B, and then monitored closely during treatment (see Drug Glossary).

4. Early surgical debridement of all necrotic tissue (possibly including orbital exenteration), plus irrigation of the involved areas with amphotericin B, is often necessary to eradicate the infection.

5. Treat the underlying medical condition, with appropriate consultation as required.

Pituitary Apoplexy

Refer immediately to neurosurgeon for surgical consideration. These patients are often quite ill.

Herpes Zoster

See 4.15, Herpes Zoster Virus.

Cavernous Sinus Thrombosis

1. For possible infectious cases (usually caused by *Staphylococcus aureus*), hospitalize the patient and treat with i.v. antibiotics for several weeks. One possible regimen:

   Nafcillin, 1 to 2 g i.v., q4h, or cefazolin, 1 g i.v., q8h (or vancomycin 1 g i.v., q12h if the patient is penicillin allergic);

   plus

   Ceftazidime, 1 to 2 g i.v., q8h.

Modify therapy based on blood culture and antibiotic sensitivity results.

2. Intravenous fluid replacement is usually required.

3. For aseptic cavernous sinus thrombosis, consider systemic anticoagulation (heparin followed by warfarin) or aspirin, 325 mg p.o., q.d. Systemic anticoagulation therapy may require collaboration with a medical internist.

4. Exposure keratopathy is treated with lubricating ointment (e.g., Refresh PM, q.h.s.). (See 4.5, Exposure Keratopathy.)

5. Treat secondary glaucoma as described previously for arteriovenous fistulas.

Tolosa–Hunt Syndrome

Prednisone, 60 to 100 mg p.o. q.d., for 2 to 3 days, and then a short taper (e.g., over 5 to 10 days) as the pain subsides. If pain persists after 72 hours, stop steroids and initiate reinvestigation to rule out other disorders.

Note: Other infectious or inflammatory disorders also may respond to steroids initially, so these patients need to be monitored closely. (See Drug Glossary for systemic steroid guidelines.)

10.10 MYASTHENIA GRAVIS

SYMPTOMS

Droopy eyelid or double vision that is worse toward the end of the day or when the individual is fatigued; may have weakness of facial muscles, proximal limb muscles, and difficulty swallowing or breathing.

SIGNS

Critical. Worsening of eyelid droop with sustained upgaze or double vision with continued eye movements, weakness of the orbicularis muscle on the affected side (cannot close the eyelid as forcefully as on the unaffected side), no pupillary abnormalities.

Other. Upward twitch of ptotic eyelid when shifting gaze from inferior to primary position (Cogan lid twitch). Can have complete limitation of ocular movements.

DIFFERENTIAL DIAGNOSIS

- Eaton–Lambert syndrome (A myasthenia-like paraneoplastic condition associated with carcinoma, especially lung cancer. Isolated eye signs do not occur, although eye signs may accompany systemic signs of weakness. Unlike myasthenia, muscle strength increases after exercise. Electromyography distinguishes between the two conditions.).

• Myasthenia-like syndrome due to medication (e.g., penicillamine, aminoglycosides).

• CPEO [No diurnal variation of symptoms or relation to fatigue; usually a negative intravenous edrophonium chloride (i.e., Tensilon) test. See 10.11, Chronic Progressive External Ophthalmoplegia.].

• Kearns–Sayre syndrome (CPEO and retinal pigmentary degeneration in a young person; heart block develops a few years later. See 10.11, Chronic Progressive External Ophthalmoplegia.).

• Third nerve palsy (Pupil may be involved, no orbicularis weakness, no fatigability, no diurnal variation. See 10.5, Isolated Third-Nerve Palsy.).

Note: Myasthenia does not respect the boundaries of specific cranial nerves, and the pupil is never involved.

• Horner syndrome (Miosis accompanies the ptosis. Pupil does not dilate well in darkness. See 10.2, Horner Syndrome.).

• Levator muscle dehiscence or disinsertion (High eyelid crease on the side of the droopy eyelid, no variability of eyelid droop, no orbicularis weakness.).

• Thyroid eye disease (No ptosis. May have eyelid retraction or eyelid lag, may or may not have exophthalmos, no diurnal variation of double vision. Graves disease occurs in 5% of patients with myasthenia gravis. See 7.2, Thyroid-Related Orbitopathy.).

• Orbital inflammatory disease (pseudotumor) (Proptosis, pain with ocular movements, inflammation. See 7.3, Orbital Inflammatory Pseudotumor.).

• Myotonic dystrophy (May have ptosis and rarely, gaze restriction. After a handshake, these patients are often unable to release their grip. May have a Christmas tree cataract.).

ETIOLOGY

Autoimmune disease; sometimes associated with underlying thyroid dysfunction. May be associated with occult thymoma or antecedent infection. Increased incidence of other autoimmune disease (e.g., lupus, MS, rheumatoid arthritis). All age groups can be affected.

WORKUP

1. History: Do the signs fluctuate with the time of the day and fatigue? Any systemic weakness? Difficulty swallowing, chewing, or breathing? Medications?

2. Have the patient focus on your finger in upgaze for 1 minute. Observe whether the eyelid droops more than expected.

3. Assess orbicularis strength by asking the patient to squeeze the eyelids shut while you attempt to force them open.

4. Test pupillary function.

5. Blood test for acetylcholine receptor antibodies (positive in 60% to 88% of patients with myasthenia, but less likely to be positive in ocular myasthenia gravis).

6. In adults, edrophonium chloride (i.e., Tensilon) test, ice-pack test (see later), or sleep test (see later) may confirm the diagnosis. Tensilon test is performed as follows:

—Identify one prominent feature (e.g., ptosis, diplopia) to observe during test. Have a cardiac monitor (not portable) and injectable atropine readily available.

—Inject Tensilon, 0.2 mL (2 mg) i.v. Observe for 1 minute. If an improvement in the selected feature is noted, the test is positive and may be stopped at this point. If no improvement or untoward reaction to the medication develops, continue.

—Tensilon, 0.4 mL (4 mg) i.v. Observe for 30 seconds for a response or side effect. If neither develops, proceed.

—Tensilon, 0.4 mL (4 mg) i.v. If no improvement is noted within 2 additional minutes, the test is negative.

Note: Cholinergic crisis, syncopal episode, and respiratory arrest, although rare, may be precipitated by a Tensilon test. Treatment includes atropine, 0.4 mg i.v., while monitoring vital signs.

—Improvement within the stated time period is diagnostic of myasthenia gravis (rarely a patient with CPEO, an intracavernous tumor, or some other rare disorder will have a false-positive result). A negative test does not exclude myasthenia.

7. For the ice-pack test, an ice pack is placed over closed eyes for 2 minutes. Improvement of ptosis is a positive test.

8. In children, observation for improvement immediately after a 1- to 2-hour nap (sleep test) is a safe alternative.

9. Check swallowing function and proximal limb muscle strength to rule out systemic involvement.

10. Thyroid function tests [thyroid-stimulating hormone (TSH)].

11. CT scan of the chest to rule out thymoma.

12. Consider ANA, rheumatoid factor, and other tests to rule out other autoimmune disease.

13. Order single-fiber electromyography of orbicularis muscle if Tensilon test is negative or contraindicated.

TREATMENT

Refer to a neurologist familiar with this disease.

1. If the patient is having difficulty swallowing or breathing, urgent hospitalization with consideration for plasmapheresis or ventilatory support, or both may be indicated.

2. If the condition is mild and not disturbing to the patient, therapy need not be instituted (the patient may patch one eye as needed).

3. If the condition is disturbing or more than mild, an oral anticholinesterase agent such as pyridostigmine (e.g., Mestinon, 60 mg p.o., q.i.d., for an adult) should be given. The dosage must be adjusted according to the response. (Patients rarely benefit from greater than 120 mg p.o., q3h, of pyridostigmine.) Overdosage may produce cholinergic crisis.

4. If symptoms persist, consider systemic steroids. (There is no uniform agreement concerning the dosage. One way is to start with prednisone, 20 mg p.o., q.d., increasing the dose slowly until the patient is receiving 100 mg/day. These patients may require hospitalization for several days when the steroids are started if they have systemic myasthenia.)

5. Azathioprine (e.g., Imuran, 1 to 2 mg/kg/day) may be helpful in older patients.

6. Treat any underlying thyroid disease or infection.

7. Surgical removal of the thymus can be performed. Thymectomy on patients without a thymoma occasionally helps.

FOLLOW-UP

1. If systemic symptoms are present, patients need to be monitored closely at first (every 1 to 4 days) until improvement is demonstrated.

2. Patients who have had their isolated ocular abnormality for an extended time (e.g., months) need not be seen again for weeks (assuming no worsening of the condition develops).

3. Patients should always be warned to return immediately if swallowing or breathing difficulties arise. After isolated ocular myasthenia has been present for approximately 2 years, progression to systemic involvement is unlikely.

Note: Newborn infants of myasthenic mothers should be observed carefully for signs of myasthenia. Poor sucking reflex, ptosis, or decreased muscle tone may be seen.

10.11 CHRONIC PROGRESSIVE EXTERNAL OPHTHALMOPLEGIA

SYMPTOMS

Gradual onset of a droopy eyelid, ocular misalignment, and other muscle weakness may or may not be present; ocular involvement is usually bilateral; there is no diurnal variation; there may be a family history. Diplopia is rare.

SIGNS

Critical. Ptosis, limitation of ocular motility (sometimes complete limitation), normal pupils.

Other. Weak orbicularis oculi muscles, weakness of limb and facial muscles, exposure keratopathy.

DIFFERENTIAL DIAGNOSIS

See 10.10, Myasthenia Gravis, for a complete list. The following are four syndromes that must be ruled out when CPEO is diagnosed. All of them may have CPEO as part of their clinical picture:

• Kearns–Sayre syndrome (Onset before age 20 years, retinal pigmentary degeneration with a salt-and-pepper appearance, heart block that usually occurs years after the ocular signs and may cause sudden death. There is usually no double vision. Other signs may include hearing loss, mental retardation, cerebellar signs, short stature, delayed puberty, nephropathy, vestibular abnormalities, increased cerebrospinal fluid protein, and characteristic findings on muscle biopsy. Inheritance pattern is maternal through mitochondrial DNA.).

• Abetalipoproteinemia (Bassen–Kornzweig syndrome) (Retinal pigmentary degeneration similar to retinitis pigmentosa, diarrhea, ataxia, and other neurologic signs, acanthocytosis of red blood cells seen on peripheral blood smear, increased cerebrospinal fluid protein. See 11.24, Retinitis Pigmentosa, for treatment.).

• Refsum disease (Retinitis pigmentosa and increased blood phytanic acid level. May have polyneuropathy, ataxia, hearing loss, anosmia, others. See 11.24, Retinitis Pigmentosa, for treatment.).

• Ocular pharyngeal dystrophy (Difficulty swallowing, sometimes leading to aspiration of food; may have autosomal dominant inheritance.).

• Mitochondrial myopathy and encephalopathy, lactic acidosis, and strokelike episodes (MELAS) (Occurs in children and young adults. May have headache, transient hemianopia, hemiparesis, nausea, vomiting. Elevated serum and cerebrospinal fluid lactate levels and may have abnormalities on MRI.).

WORKUP

1. Careful history: Determine the rate of onset (gradual versus sudden, as in cranial nerve disease).

2. Family history.

3. Examine the pupils and ocular motility carefully.

4. Test orbicularis oculi strength.

5. Fundus examination: Look for diffuse pigmentary changes.

6. Check swallowing function.

7. Edrophonium chloride (i.e., Tensilon) test, ice-pack test, or sleep test to check for myasthenia gravis (see 10.10, Myasthenia Gravis).

   Note: Sometimes patients with CPEO are supersensitive to Tensilon.

8. Consider a lumbar puncture if Kearns–Sayre syndrome is a possibility.

9. Yearly electrocardiograms by a cardiologist if Kearns–Sayre syndrome is a possibility.

10. Lipoprotein electrophoresis and peripheral blood smear if abetalipoproteinemia is suspected.

11. Serum phytanic acid level if Refsum disease is suspected.

TREATMENT

There is no cure for CPEO, but associated abnormalities are managed as follows:

1. Treat exposure keratopathy with lubricants at night (e.g., Refresh PM ointment) and artificial tears during the day (e.g., Refresh tears four to eight times per day). (See 4.5, Exposure Keratopathy.)

2. Single vision reading glasses or base-down prisms within reading glasses may help reading when downward gaze is restricted.

3. In Kearns–Sayre syndrome, a pacemaker may be required.

4. In ocular pharyngeal dystrophy, dysphagia and aspirations may require cricopharyngeal surgery.

5. In severe ptosis, consider ptosis crutches or surgical repair, but watch for worsening exposure keratopathy.

6. Genetic counseling.

FOLLOW-UP

Depends on ocular and systemic findings.

10.12   INTERNUCLEAR OPHTHALMOPLEGIA

SYMPTOMS

Blurry vision, double vision, or vague visual complaints.

SIGNS

Critical. Weakness or paralysis of adduction, with horizontal jerk nystagmus of the abducting eye.

Other. A skew deviation (either eye is turned upward, but the three-step test cannot isolate a specific muscle; see 10.6, Isolated Fourth Nerve Palsy), and upbeat nystagmus in upgaze when INO is bilateral. The involved eye can sometimes turn in when attempting to read (intact convergence). Unilateral or bilateral. Bilateral disease can give an exotropia. (WEBINO— "wall-eyed," bilateral INO.)

DIFFERENTIAL DIAGNOSIS

Other entities that may cause weakness of inward eye movement.

• Myasthenia gravis [May closely mimic INO; however, ptosis and orbicularis oculi weakness are common. Nystagmus of INO is faster; myasthenia gravis is more gaze paretic. Symptoms worsen toward the end of the day when the patient is fatigued. An edrophonium chloride (i.e., Tensilon) test, ice-pack test, or sleep test is usually positive. See 10.10, Myasthenia Gravis.].

• Orbital disease (e.g., tumor, thyroid disease, inflammatory pseudotumor) (Proptosis, globe displacement, or pain may also be present. Nystagmus is usually not present. Results of orbital CT scan are abnormal. See 7.1, Orbital Disease.).

ETIOLOGY

• MS (more common in young patients, usually bilateral).

• Ischemic vascular disease of the brainstem (more common in elderly patients, usually unilateral).

- Brainstem mass lesion (e.g., tumor).

WORKUP

1. History: Age? Are symptoms always present or do they occur only toward the end of the day with fatigue? Previous episode of optic neuritis, urinary incontinence, numbness or paralysis of an extremity, or another unexplained neurologic event (MS)?

2. Complete evaluation of eye movement to rule out other eye movement disorders (e.g., sixth nerve palsy, skew deviation).

   Note: Ocular motility can appear to be full, but a muscular weakness can be detected by observing slower saccadic eye movement in the involved eye compared with the contralateral eye. The adducting saccade is assessed by having the patient fix on the examiner's finger held laterally and then asking the patient to make a rapid eye movement from lateral to primary gaze. If an INO is present, the involved eye will show a slower adducting saccade than the uninvolved eye. The contralateral eye may be tested in a similar fashion.

3. Edrophonium chloride (i.e., Tensilon) test, ice-pack test, or sleep test when the diagnosis of myasthenia gravis cannot be ruled out (see 10.10, Myasthenia Gravis).

4. MRI of the brainstem and midbrain.

TREATMENT/FOLLOW-UP

1. Patients with the diagnosis of stroke are admitted to the hospital for neurologic evaluation and observation.

2. Otherwise, patients are managed by physicians familiar with the underlying disease.

10.13 OPTIC NEURITIS

SYMPTOMS

Loss of vision deteriorating over hours (rarely) to days (most commonly), with the nadir approximately 1 week after onset. Visual loss may be subtle or profound. Usually unilateral, but may be bilateral. Age typically 18 to 45 years. Orbital pain, especially with eye movement. Acquired loss of color vision. Reduced perception of light intensity. May have other focal neurologic symptoms (e.g., weakness, numbness, tingling in extremities). May have antecedent flulike viral syndrome. Occasionally altered perception of moving objects (Pulfrich phenomenon), or a worsening of symptoms with exercise or increase in body temperature (Uhthoff sign).

SIGNS

Critical. Relative afferent pupillary defect in unilateral or asymmetric cases; decreased color vision; central, cecocentral, arcuate, or altitudinal visual field defects.

Other. Swollen disc (one-third) with or without peripapillary flame-shaped hemorrhages (papillitis most commonly seen in children and young adults) or a normal disc (two-thirds, retrobulbar optic neuritis more common in adults). Posterior vitreous cells may be observed.

DIFFERENTIAL DIAGNOSIS

- Ischemic optic neuropathy [Visual loss is sudden, no pain with ocular motility, optic nerve swelling tends to be pale. Visual field defects are most commonly inferior altitudinal. In ischemic optic neuropathy caused by GCA, patients are older than 50 years. In nonarteritic ischemic optic neuropathy (NAION), patients are typically 40 to 60 years of age. See 10.16, Arteritic Ischemic Optic Neuropathy, and 10.17, Nonarteritic Ischemic Optic Neuropathy.].

• Acute papilledema (Bilateral disc edema, no decreased color vision, no decreased visual acuity, no pain with ocular motility, no vitreous cells. Spontaneous venous pulsations are almost always absent. An enlarged blind spot is often noted on visual field testing. See 10.14, Papilledema.).

• Severe systemic hypertension (Bilateral disc edema, increased blood pressure, flame-shaped retinal hemorrhages, and cotton-wool spots. See 11.9, Hypertensive Retinopathy.).

• Orbital tumor compressing the optic nerve (Unilateral, often proptosis or restriction of extraocular motility is evident; there are no vitreous cells even when disc swelling is present. See 7.1, Orbital Tumor.).

• Intracranial mass compressing the afferent visual pathway (Normal disc, positive afferent pupillary defect, decreased color vision, mass evident on CT scan or MRI of the brain.).

• Leber's optic neuropathy (Usually occurs in men in the second or third decade of life, may or may not have family history, rapid visual loss of one and then the other eye within days to months, may have peripapillary telangiectases. Disc swelling is followed by optic atrophy. See 10.18, Miscellaneous Optic Neuropathies.).

• Toxic or metabolic optic neuropathy [Progressive painless bilateral visual loss, may be secondary to alcohol, malnutrition, various toxins (e.g., ethambutol, chloroquine, isoniazid, chlorpropamide, heavy metals), anemia, and others. See 10.18, Miscellaneous Optic Neuropathies.].

ETIOLOGY

• Idiopathic

• MS (frequently optic neuritis is the initial manifestation of MS).

• Childhood infections (e.g., measles, mumps, chickenpox).

• Other viral infections (e.g., mononucleosis, herpes zoster, encephalitis).

• Contiguous inflammation of the meninges, orbit, or sinuses.

• Granulomatous inflammations (e.g., tuberculosis, syphilis, sarcoidosis, cryptococcus).

• Intraocular inflammations.

WORKUP

1. For first episode or atypical case, MRI of the brain and orbits with gadolinium.

2. History: Determine the patient's age and the rapidity of onset of the visual loss. Previous episode? Pain with eye movement?

3. Complete ophthalmic and neurologic examinations, including pupillary assessment, color vision evaluation with color plates, evaluation of the vitreous for cells, and dilated retinal examination with optic nerve assessment.

4. Check blood pressure.

5. Visual field test, preferably automated (e.g., Octopus, Humphrey).

6. For atypical cases (e.g., out of typical age range, no pain with eye movement), consider the following: CBC, RPR, FTA-ABS, ANA, ESR.

TREATMENT

If patient seen acutely with no prior history of MS or optic neuritis:

1. If MRI reveals at least one area of demyelination, offer pulsed i.v. steroid in the following regimen within 14 days of decreased vision:

   —methylprednisolone 1 g/day i.v. for 3 days, then

   —prednisone 1 mg/kg/day p.o. for 11 days, then

   —a 4-day taper of prednisone p.o. (20 mg, then 10 mg, then 0 mg, then 10 mg).

   This treatment decreases recurrence of optic neuritis and shortens the duration of visual impairment. However, the long-term visual outcome is no different from that with observation alone because spontaneous recovery is the natural course in most cases.

2. If MRI shows two or more characteristic demyelinating lesions, refer to neurologist

for possible treatment with interferon-β-1a within 28 days. This has been shown to decrease the development of clinically definite MS and new brain MRI lesions.

3. With a negative MRI, the risk of MS is low but pulsed i.v. steroid may still be used to hasten visual recovery. Consider repeating MRI in 1 year.

4. Do not use oral prednisone as a primary treatment because of increased risk of recurrences.

In a patient with diagnosis of prior MS or optic neuritis, observation.

Notes:

1. See Drug Glossary for systemic steroid evaluation.

2. An antiulcer medication (e.g., ranitidine, 150 mg p.o., b.i.d.) is given along with systemic steroids.

FOLLOW-UP

1. In general, examine the patient every 1 to 3 months. Patients being treated with steroids must be followed more closely because of the risk of intraocular pressure increase.

2. Patients with CNS demyelination on MRI or a positive neurologic examination should be referred to a neurologist for evaluation and management of possible MS.

BIBLIOGRAPHY

Beck RW, Cleary PA, Anderson MM Jr, et al. A randomized, controlled trial of corticosteroids in the treatment of acute optic neuritis. The Optic Neuritis Study Group. *N Engl J Med* 1992; 326:581–588.

Beck RW, Cleary PA, Trobe JD, et al. The effect of corticosteroids for acute optic neuritis on the subsequent development of multiple sclerosis. The Optic Neuritis Study Group. *N Engl J Med* 1993;329:1764–1769.

Jacobs LD, Beck RW, Simon JH, et al. Intramuscular interferon beta-1a therapy initiated during a first demyelinating event in multiple sclerosis. CHAMPS Study Group. *N Engl J Med* 2000;343:898–904.

10.14   PAPILLEDEMA

DEFINITION

Optic disc swelling produced by increased intracranial pressure.

SYMPTOMS

Episodes of transient, often bilateral visual loss (lasting seconds), often precipitated by changes in posture; headache; double vision; nausea; vomiting; and, rarely, a decrease in visual acuity (a mild decrease in visual acuity can occur in the acute setting if associated with a macular disturbance). Visual field defects and severe loss of central visual acuity can occur with chronic papilledema.

SIGNS

Critical. Bilaterally swollen, hyperemic discs (in early papilledema, disc swelling may be asymmetric) with blurring of the disc margin, often obscuring the blood vessels. The nerve fiber layer is opacified.

Other. Papillary or peripapillary retinal hemorrhages (often flame shaped); loss of venous pulsations (20% of the normal population do not have venous pulsations); dilated, tortuous retinal veins; normal pupillary response and color vision; an enlarged physiologic blind spot by formal visual field testing.

As chronic papilledema ensues, the hemorrhages and cotton-wool spots resolve, peripapillary gliosis and narrowing of the peripapillary retinal vessels occur, and optociliary shunt vessels may develop on the disc. Loss of color vision, central visual acuity, and peripheral visual field, especially inferonasally, also occur.

Note: A unilateral or bilateral sixth nerve palsy also may result from increased intracranial pressure.

DIFFERENTIAL DIAGNOSIS

Other causes of disc swelling.

• Pseudopapilledema (e.g., optic disc drusen or congenitally anomalous disc). (Not true disc swelling. Vessels overlying the disc are not obscured, the disc is not hyperemic, and the surrounding nerve fiber layer is normal. Spontaneous venous pulsations are often present. Buried drusen may be seen, especially with B-scan ultrasonography.).

• Papillitis (An afferent pupillary defect and decreased color vision are often present, white blood cells are seen in the posterior vitreous, pain occurs with eye movement, and decreased visual acuity occurs in most cases, usually unilateral. See 10.13, Optic Neuritis.).

• Hypertensive optic neuropathy (Blood pressure extremely high, narrowed arterioles. May have arteriovenous crossing changes. Hemorrhages with or without cotton-wool spots extend to the peripheral retina. See 11.9, Hypertensive Retinopathy.).

• Central retinal vein occlusion (Hemorrhages extend far beyond the peripapillary area, dilated and tortuous veins, generally unilateral, acute loss of vision in most cases. See 11.7, Central Retinal Vein Occlusion.).

• Ischemic optic neuropathy (Disc swelling is pale, not hyperemic; initially unilateral with sudden, sometimes severe, visual loss. See 10.16, Arteritic Ischemic Optic Neuropathy, and 10.17, Nonarteritic Ischemic Optic Neuropathy.).

• Optic disc vasculitis (Unilateral disc swelling in a young patient. There may be flame-shaped hemorrhages in the periphery.).

• Infiltration of the optic disc (e.g., sarcoid or tuberculous granuloma, leukemia, metastasis, other inflammatory disease or tumor). (Other ocular or systemic abnormalities may be present. The disc may have an irregular outline. Usually unilateral.)

• Leber optic neuropathy (Usually occurs in men in the second to third decades of life; initially unilateral but rapidly bilateral; rapid, progressive visual loss; disc swelling associated with peripapillary telangiectases. Optic atrophy later develops. See 10.18, Miscellaneous Optic Neuropathies.).

• Orbital optic nerve tumors (Unilateral disc swelling, may or may not have proptosis. See 10.18, Miscellaneous Optic Neuropathies.).

• Diabetic papillitis (Disc edema in a young, type 1 diabetic patient; usually bilateral. May have moderate to severe retinopathy. See 13.2, Diabetes Mellitus.).

• Graves ophthalmopathy (May have a history of thyroid dysfunction. May have eyelid lag or retraction, ocular misalignment, proptosis, increased intraocular pressure, and resistance to retropulsion. See 7.2, Thyroid-Related Orbitopathy.).

• Uveitis (e.g., syphilis or sarcoidosis) (May produce pain or photophobia. May have injection, keratic precipitates, anterior chamber cell and flare, posterior synechiae and vitreous cells. See 12.3, Posterior Uveitis.).

• Amiodarone toxicity (May present with subacute visual loss and disc edema.).

Note: Optic disc swelling in a patient with a history of leukemia is often a visually threatening sign of leukemic infiltration of the optic nerve. Immediate radiation therapy is usually required to preserve vision.

ETIOLOGY

• Primary and metastatic intracranial tumors.

• Aqueductal stenosis producing hydrocephalus.

• Pseudotumor cerebri (Often occurs in young, overweight females. See 10.15, Pseudotumor Cerebri.).

- Subdural and epidural hematomas (From trauma.).

- Subarachnoid hemorrhage [Severe headache, may have preretinal hemorrhages (Terson syndrome).].

- Arteriovenous malformation.

- Brain abscess (Often produces high fever.).

- Meningitis [Fever, stiff neck, headache (e.g., syphilis, tuberculosis, Lyme disease, bacterial).].

- Encephalitis (Often produces mental status abnormalities.).

- Intracranial venous sinus thrombosis.

WORKUP

1. History and physical examination, including blood pressure measurement.

2. Ocular examination, including a pupillary and color vision (using color plates) assessment, posterior vitreous evaluation to check for white blood cells, and a dilated fundus examination by using indirect ophthalmoscopy. The optic disc is best examined with a slit lamp and Hruby, fundus contact, or 60-diopter lens.

3. Emergency CT scan (axial and coronal views) or MRI and magnetic resonance venography (MRV) of the head/orbit.

4. Lumbar puncture if the CT or MRI/MRV or both do not reveal the cause of the papilledema. Consider blood tests for thyroid disease, diabetes, and anemia.

TREATMENT

Treatment should be directed at the underlying cause of the increased intracranial pressure.

10.15   PSEUDOTUMOR CEREBRI

(IDIOPATHIC INTRACRANIAL HYPERTENSION)

SYMPTOMS

Headache (usually worse in the morning), transient episodes of visual loss (typically lasting seconds) often precipitated by changes in posture, double vision (objects appear side by side; the double vision resolves when one eye is covered), tinnitus, dizziness, nausea, or vomiting. Occurs predominantly in obese women.

SIGNS

Critical. By definition, a patient with pseudotumor cerebri displays the following findings:

- Increased intracranial pressure with papilledema.

- Negative MRI of the brain.

- Increased opening pressure on lumbar puncture with normal cerebrospinal fluid composition.

Other. See 10.14, Papilledema. As with other causes of papilledema, may have a unilateral or bilateral sixth nerve palsy. No other lateralizing signs on neurologic examination besides sixth nerve palsy.

DIFFERENTIAL DIAGNOSIS

See 10.14, Papilledema.

ASSOCIATED FACTORS

Obesity, pregnancy, and various medications, including oral contraceptives, tetracycline, nalidixic acid, cyclosporine, and vitamin A (more than 100,000 U/day). Systemic steroid withdrawal may also be causative.

WORKUP

1. History: Inquire specifically about medications.

2. Ocular examination, including pupillary examination, ocular motility, color vision testing (color plates), and optic nerve evaluation.

3. Systemic examination, including blood pressure and temperature.

4. MRI/MRV of the orbit and brain. Any patient with papilledema needs to be imaged immediately. If results are normal, the patient should have a thorough neuroophthalmologic evaluation, including a lumbar puncture, to rule out other causes of papilledema and to determine the opening pressure (see 10.14, Papilledema).

5. Visual field test is the most important method for following these patients (e.g., Octopus, Humphrey, Goldmann).

TREATMENT

Pseudotumor cerebri may be a self-limited process. Treatment is indicated in the following situations:

Severe, intractable headache.

Evidence of progressive decrease in visual acuity or visual field loss.

Some ophthalmologists suggest treating all patients with papilledema.

Methods of treatment include the following.

1. Weight loss if overweight.

2. Acetazolamide (e.g., Diamox 250 mg p.o., q.i.d., initially, building up to 500 mg, q.i.d., if tolerated). Use with caution in sulfa-allergic patients. Other diuretics (e.g., furosemide) have no proven efficacy.

3. Discontinuation of any causative medication.

If treatment by these methods is unsuccessful, one of the following may be tried.

4. A short course of systemic steroids preparatory to surgery.

5. Optic nerve sheath decompression surgery is often effective if vision is threatened (our choice).

6. Lumboperitoneal shunt if intractable headache is primary problem.

SPECIAL CIRCUMSTANCES

1. Pregnancy: No increased risk of fetal loss. Acetazolamide may be used after 20 weeks' gestation. Consider steroids if vision is threatened.

2. Children/adolescents: A secondary cause is identifiable in 50%.

Note: Any increase in intraocular pressure needs to be treated aggressively to avoid further injury to the optic nerve.

FOLLOW-UP

1. Every 2 to 3 weeks initially, monitor for visual loss, especially visual field loss, and then every 4 to 6 weeks, depending on the response to treatment.

2. In general, the frequency of follow-up depends on the chronicity of the papilledema. The more chronic, the more frequent the follow-up.

10.16   ARTERITIC ISCHEMIC OPTIC NEUROPATHY

(GIANT CELL ARTERITIS)

SYMPTOMS

Sudden, painless, nonprogressive visual loss; initially unilateral, but may rapidly become bilateral; occurs in patients older than 50 years of age; antecedent or simultaneous headache, jaw claudication (pain with chewing), scalp tenderness especially over the superficial temporal arteries (tenderness with hair combing), proximal muscle and joint aches (polymyalgia rheumatica), anorexia, weight loss, or fever may occur.

SIGNS

Critical. Afferent pupillary defect; devastating visual loss (often counting fingers or worse); pale, swollen disc, often with flame-shaped hemorrhages. Later, optic atrophy and cupping occurs as the edema resolves. The ESR, C-reactive protein (CRP), and platelets may be markedly increased.

Other. Visual field defect (commonly altitudinal or involving the central field); a palpable, tender, and often nonpulsatile temporal artery; a central retinal artery occlusion or a cranial nerve palsy (especially a sixth nerve palsy) may occur.

DIFFERENTIAL DIAGNOSIS

• NAION (Patients may be younger, usually have less severe visual loss, do not have the accompanying symptoms of GCA listed previously, and usually have a normal ESR. See 10.17, Nonarteritic Ischemic Optic Neuropathy.).

• Inflammatory optic neuritis (papillitis) (Affects a younger age group, typically less severe and less sudden onset of visual loss, pain with eye movements, optic disc swelling is more hemorrhagic, posterior vitreous cells are often present, no symptoms of GCA. See 10.13, Optic Neuritis.).

• Compressive optic nerve tumor (Slowly progressive visual loss, few to no symptoms in common with GCA. See 10.18, Miscellaneous Optic Neuropathies.).

• Central retinal vein occlusion (Severe visual loss may be accompanied by an afferent pupillary defect and disc swelling, but the retina shows diffuse retinal hemorrhages extending out to the periphery. See 11.7, Central Retinal Vein Occlusion.).

• Central retinal artery occlusion (Sudden, painless, severe visual loss with an afferent pupillary defect, but the disc is not swollen, and retinal edema with a cherry-red spot is frequently observed. See 11.5, Central Retinal Artery Occlusion.).

WORKUP

1. History: Attempt to elicit the symptoms. Age is critical.

2. Complete ocular examination, particularly pupillary assessment, color plates, dilated retinal examination to rule out retinal causes of severe visual loss, and optic nerve evaluation.

3. Immediate ESR (Westergren is the most reliable method) and CRP (does not rise with age). A guideline for top normal ESR: men, age/2; women (age + 10)/2.

4. Perform a temporal artery biopsy if GCA is suspected from the symptoms, signs, or ESR. The ESR may not be increased.

   Note: The biopsy should be performed within 1 week after starting systemic steroids, but a positive result may be seen up to 1 month later. Biopsy is especially important in patients in whom steroids are relatively contraindicated (e.g., those with diabetes).

5. Consider an i.v. fluorescein angiogram (IVFA), which may show delayed choroidal filling.

TREATMENT

1. Systemic steroids should be given immediately once GCA is suspected. We give methylprednisolone, 250 mg i.v., q6h, for 12 doses in the hospital, and then switch to prednisone, 80 to 100 mg p.o., q.d. A temporal artery biopsy specimen is obtained while the patient is in the hospital.

2. If the temporal artery biopsy is positive for GCA, the patient must be maintained on prednisone, 80 to 100 mg p.o., q.d.

3. If the biopsy is negative on an adequate (2-cm) section, the likelihood of GCA is small. However, in highly suggestive cases, biopsy of the contralateral artery is performed.

4. Steroids are usually discontinued when the disease is not found in adequate biopsy specimens, unless the clinical presentation is classic and a response to treatment has occurred.

   Notes:

   1. *Without steroids (and occasionally on adequate steroids), the contralateral eye can become involved within 24 hours.*

2. *A histamine type 2 receptor blocker (e.g., ranitidine, 150 mg p.o., b.i.d.) or another antiulcer medication is given along with systemic steroids.*

3. *See Medical Glossary for systemic steroid workup.*

FOLLOW-UP

1. Patients suspected of having GCA must be evaluated and treated immediately.

2. After the diagnosis is confirmed by biopsy, the initial oral steroid dosage is maintained for 2 to 4 weeks until the symptoms resolve and ESR normalizes. The dosage is then tapered slowly, repeating the ESR with each dosage change or monthly to ensure that the new steroid dosage is enough to suppress the disease.

3. If the ESR increases or symptoms return, the dosage must be increased.

4. Treatment should last at least 6 to 12 months or more. The smallest dose that suppresses the disease is used.

10.17 NONARTERITIC ISCHEMIC OPTIC NEUROPATHY

SYMPTOMS

Sudden, painless, nonprogressive visual loss of moderate degree, initially unilateral, but may become bilateral. Typically occurs in patients older than 50 years of age.

SIGNS

Critical. Afferent pupillary defect, pale disc swelling often involving only a segment of the disc, flame-shaped hemorrhages, normal ESR.

• Nonprogressive NAION: Sudden initial decrease in visual acuity and visual field, which stabilizes.

• Progressive NAION: Sudden initial decrease in visual acuity and visual field followed by a

second decrease in acuity or visual field days to weeks later.

Other. Reduced color vision proportional to decrease in acuity, altitudinal or central visual field defect, optic atrophy (segmental or diffuse) after the edema resolves. Congenitally anomalous disc in fellow eye.

DIFFERENTIAL DIAGNOSIS

See 10.16, Arteritic Ischemic Optic Neuropathy.

ETIOLOGY

Idiopathic: Arteriosclerosis, diabetes, hypertension, hyperlipidemia, hyperhomocystinemia, anemia, and sleep apnea are associated risk factors, but causation has never been proven. Also, relative nocturnal hypotension is thought by some to play a role, especially in patients taking antihypertensive medication.

WORKUP

1. Same as 10.16, Arteritic Ischemic Optic Neuropathy.

2. A medical evaluation by an internist is obtained to rule out cardiovascular disease, diabetes, and hypertension.

TREATMENT

1. Observation.

2. Consider aspirin, 80 to 325 mg p.o., q.d., in conjunction with patient's primary medical doctor, although benefit in NAION has not been proven.

3. Patients should avoid taking blood pressure medication at bedtime if possible to help avoid nocturnal hypotension.

FOLLOW-UP

1. One month.

2. Up to 40% of patients have shown mild improvement in vision over 3 to 6 months in some studies. Optic nerve edema resolves in 4 to 8 weeks.

10.18   MISCELLANEOUS OPTIC NEUROPATHIES

TOXIC/METABOLIC OPTIC NEUROPATHY

SYMPTOMS

Painless, progressive, bilateral loss of vision.

SIGNS

Critical. Bilateral cecocentral or central visual field defects, signs of alcoholism or poor nutrition.

Other. Visual acuity of 20/50 to 20/200, reduced color vision, temporal disc pallor, optic atrophy, or normal-appearing disc initially.

ETIOLOGY

• Tobacco/alcohol abuse.

• Severe malnutrition with thiamine (vitamin B$_1$) deficiency.

• Pernicious anemia (Usually due to a problem with vitamin B$_{12}$ absorption.).

• Toxic [Often from chloramphenicol, ethambutol, isoniazid, digitalis, chloroquine, streptomycin, chlorpropamide, ethchlorvynol (e.g., Placidyl), disulfiram (e.g., Antabuse), and lead.].

WORKUP

1. History: Drug or substance abuse? Medications? Diet?

2. Complete ocular examination, including pupillary evaluation, color testing with color plates, and optic nerve examination.

3. Formal visual field test.

4. CBC.

5. Serum vitamin B$_1$, B$_{12}$, and folate levels.

6. Consider a heavy metal (i.e., lead, thallium) screen.

7. If disc is swollen, consider blood test for Leber hereditary optic neuropathy (clinical presentation of Leber neuropathy may mimic toxic/metabolic optic neuropathy).

TREATMENT

1. Thiamine, 100 mg p.o., b.i.d.

2. Folate, 1.0 mg p.o., q.d.

3. Multivitamin tablet, q.d.

4. Eliminate any causative agent (e.g., alcohol, medication).

5. Vitamin B_{12}, 1,000 mg intramuscularly (i.m.) every month for pernicious anemia (usually coordinated by the patient's internist).

FOLLOW-UP

Every month at first, and then every 6 to 12 months.

COMPRESSIVE OPTIC NEUROPATHY

SYMPTOMS

Slowly progressive visual loss, although occasionally acute or noticed acutely.

SIGNS

Critical. Central visual field defect, relative afferent pupillary defect.

Other. The optic nerve can be normal, pale, or, occasionally, swollen; proptosis; optociliary shunt vessels (small vessels around the disc that shunt blood from the retinal to the choroidal venous circulation).

ETIOLOGY

• Optic nerve glioma (Patients usually younger than 20 years, often associated with neurofibromatosis.).

• Optic nerve meningioma [Usually affects adult women. Orbital imaging may show an optic nerve mass, diffuse optic nerve thickening, or a railroad-track sign (increased contrast of the periphery of the nerve).].

• Any intraorbital mass (e.g., hemangioma, schwannoma).

WORKUP

All patients with progressive visual loss and optic nerve dysfunction should have MRI of the orbit and brain.

TREATMENT

1. Depends on the etiology.

2. Treatments of optic nerve glioma and meningioma are controversial. These lesions are often monitored unless there is evidence of intracranial involvement, at which point surgical excision may be indicated.

LEBER OPTIC NEUROPATHY

SYMPTOMS

Rapidly progressive visual loss of one and then the other eye within days to months of each other, painless.

SIGNS

Critical. Mild swelling of optic disc progressing over weeks to optic atrophy; small, telangiectatic blood vessels near the disc that do not leak on IVFA, usually occurs in young men aged 15 to 30 years, and less commonly in women in their second to third decade of life.

Other. Visual acuity 20/200 to counting fingers, cecocentral visual field defect.

TRANSMISSION

By mitochondrial DNA, so it is transmitted by women to all offspring. However, 50% to 70% of sons and 10% to 15% of daughters manifest the disease. All daughters are carriers, and none of the sons can transmit the disease.

WORKUP

Send blood for known Leber mutations.

TREATMENT

1. No effective treatment is available.

2. Genetic counseling should be offered.

3. A cardiology consult may be indicated because patients have an increased incidence of cardiac conduction defects.

DOMINANT OPTIC NEUROPATHY

Mild to moderate bilateral visual loss (20/40 to 20/200) usually presenting at approximately age 4 years, slow progression, temporal disc pallor, cecocentral visual field defect, tritanopic (blue–yellow) color defect on Farnsworth–Munsell 100-hue test, strong family history, no nystagmus.

COMPLICATED HEREDITARY OPTIC ATROPHY

Bilateral optic atrophy with spinocerebellar degenerations (e.g., Friedreich, Marie, Behr), polyneuropathy (e.g., Charcot–Marie–Tooth), or inborn errors of metabolism.

RADIATION OPTIC NEUROPATHY

Delayed effect (usually 1 to 5 years) after radiation therapy to the eye, orbit, sinus, nasopharynx, and occasionally brain with acute or gradual stepwise visual loss, often severe. Disc swelling, radiation retinopathy, or both may or may not be present. Enhancement of optic nerve or chiasm on MRI.

10.19 NYSTAGMUS

Nystagmus is divided into congenital or acquired forms.

SYMPTOMS

Asymptomatic unless acquired after 8 years of age, at which point the environment may be noted to oscillate horizontally, vertically, or torsionally, or vision may seem blurred or unstable.

SIGNS

Critical. Repetitive oscillations of the eye horizontally, vertically, or torsionally.

• Jerk nystagmus: The eye slowly drifts in one direction (slow phase) and then abruptly returns to its original position (fast phase), only to drift again and repeat the cycle.

• Pendular nystagmus: Drift occurs in two phases of equal speed, giving a smooth back-and-forth movement of the eye.

CONGENITAL FORMS OF NYSTAGMUS

INFANTILE NYSTAGMUS

Onset at age 2 to 3 months, with wide, swinging eye movements. At age 4 to 6 months, small pendular eye movements are added, and at age 6 to 12 months, jerk nystagmus and a null point (a position of gaze where the nystagmus is minimized) develop. Compensatory head nodding develops at any point up to 20 years of age. Infantile nystagmus is usually horizontal and uniplanar (same direction in all gazes), and typically dampens with convergence. May have a latent component.

DIFFERENTIAL DIAGNOSIS

• Opsoclonus (Repetitive, irregular, multidirectional eye movements associated with cerebellar or brainstem disease, postviral encephalitis, visceral carcinoma, or neuroblastoma.).

• Spasmus nutans (Head nodding and head turn with vertical, horizontal, or torsional nystagmus appearing between 6 months and 3 years of age and resolving between 2 and 8 years of age. Unilateral or bilateral. Glioma of the optic chiasm may produce an identical clinical picture and needs to be ruled out with MRI.).

• Latent nystagmus (see the following).

• Nystagmus blockage syndrome (see the following).

ETIOLOGY

• Idiopathic

- Albinism (Iris transillumination defects and foveal hypoplasia are common. See 13.12, Albinism.).

- Aniridia (Bilateral, near-total absence of iris from birth. See 8.12, Developmental Anterior Segment and Lens Anomalies.).

- Leber congenital amaurosis [Markedly abnormal or flat electroretinogram (ERG).].

- Others (e.g., bilateral optic nerve hypoplasia, bilateral congenital cataracts, rod monochromatism, optic nerve or macular disease).

WORKUP

1. History: Age of onset? Head nodding? Known ocular or systemic abnormalities? Medications? Family history?

2. Complete ocular examination: Carefully observe the eye movements, check for iris transillumination, and inspect the optic disc and macula for disease.

3. Consider obtaining an eye movement recording if the diagnosis of infantile nystagmus is uncertain.

4. When opsoclonus cannot be ruled out, obtain a urinary vanillylmandelic acid and consider an abdominal CT scan to rule out neuroblastoma and visceral carcinoma.

5. In selected cases and in all cases of suspected spasmus nutans, an MRI of the brain (axial and coronal views) may be obtained to rule out an organic lesion.

TREATMENT

1. Maximize vision by refraction.

2. Treat amblyopia if indicated.

3. If small face turn: Prescribe prism in glasses with base in direction of face turn.

4. If large face turn: Consider muscle surgery.

LATENT NYSTAGMUS

Occurs only when one eye is viewing. Fast phase of nystagmus beats toward viewing eye.

Manifest latent nystagmus: Occurs in children with strabismus or decreased vision in one eye, in whom the nonfixating or poorly seeing eye behaves as an occluded eye.

*Note: When testing visual acuity in one eye, fog (i.e., add plus lenses in front of) rather than occluding the opposite eye to minimize induction of latent nystagmus.

TREATMENT

1. Maximize vision by refraction.

2. Treat amblyopia if indicated.

3. Consider muscle surgery if symptomatic strabismus exists.

NYSTAGMUS BLOCKAGE SYNDROME

Any nystagmus that decreases when the fixating eye is in adduction and demonstrates an esotropia to dampen the nystagmus.

TREATMENT

For large face turn, consider muscle surgery.

ACQUIRED FORMS OF NYSTAGMUS

ETIOLOGY

- Visual loss (e.g., dense cataract, trauma, cone dystrophy) (Usually monocular and vertical nystagmus.).

- Toxic/metabolic (e.g., alcohol intoxication, lithium, barbiturates, phenytoin, salicylates, benzodiazepines, phencyclidine, other anticonvulsants or sedatives, Wernicke encephalopathy, thiamine deficiency).

- CNS disorders (e.g., thalamic hemorrhage, tumor, stroke, trauma, MS).

- Nonphysiologic (Voluntary, rapid, horizontal, small oscillatory movements of the eyes that usually cannot be sustained more than 30 seconds without fatigue.)

TYPES OF NYSTAGMUS WITH LOCALIZING NEUROANATOMIC SIGNIFICANCE

- See-saw (One eye rises and intorts while the other descends and extorts. Most commonly, the lesion involves the chiasm or third ventricle, or both. May have a bitemporal hemianopia resulting from a parasellar mass. Rarely congenital.).

• Convergence retraction (Convergence-like eye movements are accompanied by retraction of the globe into the orbit when the patient attempts to look up. There is limitation of upward gaze and eyelid retraction. Pupils are large and unreactive to light but do constrict with convergence. Papilledema may be present. Usually, a pineal gland tumor or other midbrain abnormality is responsible.).

• Upbeat (The fast phase of the nystagmus is up. Most commonly, the lesion involves the brainstem or vermis of the cerebellum when the nystagmus is present in primary position. If the nystagmus is present only in upgaze, the most likely etiology is drug effect.).

• Rebound (Triggered by changing directions of gaze. The fast phase is in the direction of gaze, but fatigue occurs with sustained gaze, and the fast phase then changes direction. When gaze is returned to primary position, the fast phase increases in the direction the eye takes in returning to the primary position. Most commonly, the lesion involves the cerebellum.).

• Gaze-evoked (Not present when the individual looks straight, but appears as the eyes look to the side. Nystagmus increases when looking in direction of fast phase. Slow frequency. Most commonly the result of alcohol intoxication, sedatives, cerebellar or brainstem disease.).

• Downbeat [The fast phase of nystagmus is down. Most commonly, the lesion is at the cervicomedullary junction (e.g., Arnold–Chiari malformation).].

• Periodic alternating [Fast eye movements are in one direction (with head turn) for 60 to 90 seconds, and then reverse direction for 60 to 90 seconds. The cycle repeats continuously. May be congenital or, rarely, the result of blindness. Acquired forms not caused by blindness are most commonly the result of lesions of the cervicomedullary junction.].

• Vestibular [Horizontal or horizontal rotary nystagmus. May be accompanied by vertigo, tinnitus, or deafness. May be due to dysfunction of vestibular end organ (inner ear disease), eighth cranial nerve, or eighth nerve nucleus in brainstem. Destructive lesions produce fast phases opposite to affected end organ or nerve. Irritative lesions produce fast phase in the same direction as the affected end organ. Vestibular nystagmus associated with interstitial keratitis is called Cogan syndrome.].

• Spasmus nutans (Develops between 18 months and 3 years of age. Triad: head turn, head nodding, pendular nystagmus. May be caused by optic chiasmal glioma.).

DIFFERENTIAL DIAGNOSIS

• Superior oblique myokymia (Small, unilateral, vertical, and torsional movements of one eye can be seen with a slit lamp or ophthalmoscope. Symptoms and signs are more pronounced when the involved eye looks inferonasally. Usually benign, resolving spontaneously. Can be treated with carbamazepine, 200 mg p.o., t.i.d. A medical consult for hematologic evaluation before carbamazepine use and periodic evaluation during therapy are recommended.).

• Opsoclonus (Rapid, chaotic conjugate saccades. Etiology in children is neuroblastoma or encephalitis. In adults, it can be seen with drug intoxication or following infarction.).

• Myoclonus [Pendular oscillation associated with contraction of nonocular muscles (e.g., palate, tongue, facial muscles). Involves olive nucleus in medulla.].

WORKUP

1. History: Nystagmus, strabismus, or amblyopia in infancy? Oscillopsia? Drug or alcohol use? Vertigo? Episodes of weakness, numbness, or decreased vision in the past (MS)?

2. Family history: Nystagmus? Albinism? Eye disorder?

3. Complete ocular examination: Pay close attention to the eye movements. Slit-lamp or optic disc observation may be helpful in subtle cases. Iris transillumination should be performed to rule out albinism.

4. Obtain an eye movement recording when congenital nystagmus is being considered.

5. Visual field examination, particularly with see-saw nystagmus.

6. Consider a drug/toxin/dietary screen of the urine, serum, or both.

7. CT scan or MRI as needed. (Make sure the scan carefully evaluates the area that most commonly causes the particular nystagmus.)

   Note: The cervicomedullary junction and cerebellum are best evaluated with sagittal MRI.

TREATMENT

1. The underlying etiology must be treated.

2. The nystagmus of periodic alternating nystagmus may respond to baclofen. (Baclofen is given in three divided doses, starting with a total daily dose of 15 mg p.o., and increasing by 15 mg every 3 days until a desired therapeutic effect is obtained. Do not exceed 80 mg/day. If there is no improvement with the maximal tolerated dose, the dosage should be tapered slowly. Baclofen is not recommended for use in children.)

3. Severe, disabling nystagmus can be treated with retrobulbar injections of botulinum toxin.

FOLLOW-UP

A workup should be instituted as soon as possible to rule out a CNS abnormality.

10.20 AMAUROSIS FUGAX

SYMPTOMS

Monocular visual loss that usually lasts seconds to minutes, but may last up to 1 to 2 hours. Vision returns to normal.

SIGNS

Critical. May see an embolus within an arteriole or the ocular examination may be negative.

Other. Signs of the ocular ischemic syndrome (dilated but not tortuous retinal veins; midperipheral dot and blot hemorrhages; neovascularization of the iris, disc, or retina), an old branch retinal artery occlusion (sheathed arteriole), or neurologic signs caused by ischemia of a cerebral hemisphere [transient ischemic attacks (TIA); e.g., contralateral arm or leg weakness].

DIFFERENTIAL DIAGNOSIS

All of the following conditions may produce transient visual loss:

• Papilledema (Optic disc swelling is evident. Visual loss lasts seconds, is usually bilateral and is often associated with postural change or Valsalva maneuver. See 10.14, Papilledema.).

• GCA (Patients are typically older than 55 years of age and have an elevated ESR, temporal headache, scalp tenderness, jaw claudication, or muscle pains. Transient visual loss may precede an ischemic optic neuropathy or central retinal artery occlusion. See 10.16, Arteritic Ischemic Optic Neuropathy.).

• Impending central retinal vein occlusion (Dilated, tortuous retinal veins are observed on funduscopic examination. See 11.7, Central Retinal Vein Occlusion.).

• Retinal migraine (Usually a diagnosis of exclusion. Typically occurs in patients younger than 40 years of age. May have recurrent episodes. Focal retinal arteriolar narrowing is sometimes observed. See 10.25, Migraine.).

• Intermittent intraocular hemorrhage (e.g., vitreous hemorrhage).

• Others (e.g., optic nerve head drusen).

ETIOLOGY

• Embolus from the carotid artery (most common), heart, or aorta.

• Vascular insufficiency as a result of arteriosclerotic disease of vessels anywhere along the path from the aorta to the globe causing hypoperfusion precipitated by a postural change or cardiac arrhythmia.

• Hypercoagulable/hyperviscosity state.

• Rarely, an intraorbital tumor may compress the optic nerve or a nourishing vessel in certain gaze positions, causing transient visual loss.

WORKUP

1. *Immediate ESR when GCA is suspected.*

2. History: Monocular visual loss or homonymous hemianopsia? (Did the patient cover one eye to test vision?) Duration of visual loss? Previous episodes of amaurosis fugax or TIA? Cardiovascular disease factors? Use of oral contraceptives? Heart disease or operations?

3. Ocular examination, including a confrontational visual field examination and a dilated retinal evaluation: Look for an embolus or signs of other disorders mentioned previously.

4. Medical examination (cardiac and carotid auscultation).

5. Consider an IVFA (focal arterial staining at the site of the embolus may be seen).

6. Ophthalmic color Doppler ultrasonography may reveal a retrolaminar central retinal artery stenosis or embolus proximal to the lamina cribrosa.

7. CBC with differential and platelet count, fasting blood sugar, glycosylated hemoglobin, and lipid profile (to rule out polycythemia, thrombocytosis, diabetes, and hyperlipidemia).

8. Noninvasive carotid artery evaluation (e.g., duplex Doppler ultrasonography).

9. Cardiac evaluation (including an echocardiogram).

TREATMENT

1. Carotid disease.

   —Consider aspirin 325 mg p.o., q.d.

   —Consider referral for carotid endarterectomy in the presence of a surgically accessible, high-grade carotid stenosis or occlusion if the potential benefit of the procedure outweighs the risks.

   —Control hypertension and diabetes (follow-up with a medical internist).

   —Stop smoking.

2. Cardiac disease.

   —Consider aspirin 325 mg p.o., q.d. (e.g., for mitral valve prolapse).

   —Consider hospitalization and anticoagulation (e.g., heparin therapy) in the presence of a mural thrombus.

   —Consider referral for cardiac surgery as needed.

   —Control arteriosclerotic risk factors as described previously (follow-up with medical internist).

3. If carotid and cardiac disease are ruled out, a vasospastic etiology can be considered. Treatment with a calcium channel blocker may be beneficial.

FOLLOW-UP

Patients with recurrent episodes of amaurosis fugax (especially if accompanied by signs of cerebral TIA) require immediate diagnostic and sometimes therapeutic attention.

10.21 VERTEBROBASILAR ARTERY INSUFFICIENCY

SYMPTOMS

Transient, bilateral blurred vision lasting from a few seconds to a few minutes, sometimes accompanied by flashing lights. Ataxia, vertigo, dysarthria or dysphasia, and hemiparesis or hemisensory loss may accompany the visual symptoms. History of drop attacks (the patient suddenly falls to the ground without warning or loss of consciousness). Recurrent attacks are common.

SIGNS

Normal ocular examination.

DIFFERENTIAL DIAGNOSIS

Causes of transient visual loss.

• Papilledema (Bilateral visual loss lasts 5 to 15 seconds. See 10.14, Papilledema.).

• Migraine (Visual loss from 10 to 45 minutes, often with history of migraine headache or carsickness, or a family history of migraine. May or may not be followed by a headache. See 10.25, Migraine.).

• Amaurosis fugax (Monocular, usually lasts minutes, appears as if a curtain drops down in front of the eye. See 10.20, Amaurosis Fugax.).

• GCA (Can cause transient visual loss in patients older than 50 years. Usually associated with temporal headache, scalp tenderness, pain with chewing, weight loss, fever, and anorexia. See 10.16, Arteritic Ischemic Optic Neuropathy.).

• Vertebral artery dissection (After trauma or resulting from atherosclerotic disease.).

WORKUP

1. History: Associated symptoms of vertebrobasilar insufficiency? History of carsickness or migraine? Symptoms of GCA?

2. Dilated fundus examination: Look for retinal emboli or papilledema.

3. Blood pressure in each arm: Look for the subclavian steal syndrome.

4. Cardiac auscultation to rule out arrhythmia.

5. Electrocardiography and Holter monitor for 24 hours: Look for sick sinus syndrome, ventricular ectopy.

6. Consider carotid noninvasive flow studies.

7. MRA or transcranial/vertebral artery Doppler ultrasonography to evaluate posterior cerebral blood flow.

8. CBC to rule out anemia and polycythemia, with immediate ESR if GCA is possible.

9. Consider cervical spine radiographs to rule out compressive cervical spine disease if arthritis of the neck is present.

TREATMENT

1. Aspirin, 81 mg p.o., q.d.

2. Control hypertension, diabetes, and hyperlipidemia if present, as per medical internist.

3. Reduce fat and cholesterol intake; stop smoking.

4. Correct any underlying problem revealed by the workup.

FOLLOW-UP

One week to check test results.

10.22 CORTICAL BLINDNESS

SYMPTOMS

Bilateral complete or severe loss of vision. Patients may deny they are blind (Anton syndrome).

SIGNS

Critical. Markedly decreased vision and visual field in both eyes (sometimes no light perception) with normal pupillary responses.

ETIOLOGY

• Most common: Bilateral occipital lobe infarctions.

• Other: Toxic, postpartum (amniotic embolus).

• Rare: Neoplasm (e.g., metastasis, meningioma).

WORKUP

1. Test vision with a near card (sometimes patients with bilateral occipital lobe infarcts appear completely blind, but actually have a very small residual visual field and are unable to locate a distant eye chart).

2. Complete ocular and neurologic examinations.

3. MRI of the brain.

4. Rule out functional visual loss by appropriate testing (see 10.23, Nonphysiologic Visual Loss).

5. Cardiac auscultation to rule out arrhythmia.

6. Check blood pressure.

7. CBC to rule out polycythemia in cases of stroke.

8. Refer to a neurologist or internist for evaluation of stroke risk factors.

TREATMENT

1. Patients diagnosed with a stroke within 72 hours of the onset of symptoms are admitted to the hospital for neurologic evaluation and observation.

2. If possible, treat the underlying condition.

3. Arrange for services to help the patient function at home and in the environment.

FOLLOW-UP

As per the internist or neurologist.

10.23 NONPHYSIOLOGIC VISUAL LOSS

SYMPTOMS

Loss of vision. Malingerers frequently are involved with an insurance claim or are looking for some other form of financial gain. Hysterics truly believe they have lost vision.

SIGNS

Critical. No ocular or neuroophthalmic findings that would account for the decreased vision. Normal pupillary light reaction.

DIFFERENTIAL DIAGNOSIS

• Amblyopia [Poor vision in one eye since childhood, rarely both eyes. Patient often has strabismus (eye misalignment best seen with a cover test) or anisometropia (one eye is usually more far-sighted, astigmatic, or very near-sighted). May have a history of eye patching as a child. Vision is no worse than counting fingers, especially in the temporal periphery of an amblyopic eye. See 8.6, Amblyopia.].

- Cortical blindness (Bilateral complete or severe visual loss with normal pupils. MRI of the brain shows bilateral occipital lobe infarcts in most cases. See 10.22, Cortical Blindness.).

- Retrobulbar optic neuritis (Afferent pupillary defect may be present. See 10.13, Optic Neuritis.).

- Cone–rod dystrophy (Positive family history, decreased color vision, abnormal results on dark adaptation studies and ERG. See 11.27, Cone Dystrophies.).

- Chiasmal tumor (Visual loss may precede optic atrophy. Pupils usually react sluggishly to light, and an afferent pupillary defect is usually present. Visual fields are abnormal.).

WORKUP

The following tests may be used to deceive a patient with nonphysiologic visual loss (i.e., to fool the malingerer or hysteric into seeing better than he or she admits to seeing).

Two codes are used in the list below:

U: This test may be used in patients feigning unilateral decreased vision;

B: This test may be used in patients feigning bilateral vision loss.

Patients Claiming No Light Perception

Determine whether each pupil reacts to light (U): When one eye has no light perception, its pupil will not react to light. The pupil should not appear dilated unless the patient has bilateral lack of light perception or third nerve involvement.

Patients Claiming Hand-Motion to No Light Perception

1. **Test for an afferent pupillary defect (U):** A defect should be present in unilateral visual loss to this degree. If not, the diagnosis of nonphysiologic visual loss is made.

2. **Mirror test (U or B):** If the patient claims unilateral visual loss, cover the better-seeing eye with a patch; otherwise leave both uncovered. Ask the patient to hold eyes still and slowly tilt a large mirror from side to side in front of the eyes, holding it beyond the patient's range of hand-motion vision. If the eyes move, the patient can see better than hand motion.

3. **Optokinetic test (U or B):** Patch the uninvolved eye when unilateral visual loss is claimed. Ask the patient to look straight ahead, and slowly move an optokinetic tape in front of the eyes (or rotate an optokinetic drum). If nystagmus can be elicited, vision is better than hand motion.

4. **Worth four-dot test (U):** Place red–green glasses on patient, and quickly turn on four-dot pattern and ask patient how many dots are seen. If patient closes one eye (cheating), try reversing the glasses and repeating test. If all four dots are seen, vision is better than hand-motion.

Patients Claiming 20/40 to 20/400 Vision

1. **Visual acuity testing (U or B):** Start with the 20/10 line and ask the patient to read it. When the patient claims incompetence, look amazed and then offer reassurance. Inform the patient you will go to a larger line and show the 20/15 line. Again, force the patient to work to see this line. Slowly proceed up the chart, asking the patient to read each line as you pass it (including the three or four 20/20 lines). Make the patient feel incompetent. By the time the 20/30 or 20/40 lines are reached, the patient may in fact read one or two letters correctly. The visual acuity can then be recorded.

2. **Fog test (U):** For example, in a patient feigning visual loss on the right. If patient wears glasses, dial patient's correction into phoropter, if not dial in plano. Add +4.00 to the left. Put patient in phoropter with both eyes open. Tell patient to use both eyes to read each line, starting at the 20/15 line and working up the chart slowly, as described previously. Record visual acuity (this should be visual acuity of the right eye). Close phoropter over the right eye. Ask patient to read the same line as before; work up the chart until patient is able to read line. Record visual acuity (this should be visual acuity of the left eye with +4.00 fog).

3. **Retest visual acuity in the supposedly "poorly seeing eye" at 10 feet from the chart (U or B):** Vision should be twice as good (e.g., a patient with 20/100 vision at 20 feet should read 20/50 at 10 feet). If it is better than expected, record the better vision. If it worse, the patient has nonphysiologic visual loss.

4. **Test near vision (U or B):** If normal near vision can be documented, nonphysiologic visual loss or myopia has been documented.

5. **Visual field testing (U or B):** Goldmann visual field tests often reveal inconsistent responses and nonphysiologic field losses.

Children

1. Tell the child that there is an eye abnormality, but the strong drops about to be administered will cure it. Dilate the child's eyes (e.g., tropicamide, 1%), and retest the visual acuity in 40 minutes. Children, as well as adults, sometimes need a "way out."

2. Test as described previously.

TREATMENT

1. Patients are usually told that no ocular abnormality can be found that accounts for their decreased vision.

2. Hysterical patients often benefit from being told that everything is going to be all right and that their vision can be expected to return to normal by their next visit. Psychiatric referral is sometimes indicated.

FOLLOW-UP

1. If nonphysiologic visual loss is highly suspected but cannot be proven, reexamine in 1 to 2 weeks.

2. Consider obtaining an ERG, IVFA, or a CT scan or MRI of the brain, or a combination of these.

3. If functional visual loss can be documented, have the patient return as needed.

   Note: *Always try to determine the patient's actual visual acuity if possible, and carefully document your findings.*

10.24 HEADACHE

Most headaches are not dangerous or ominous symptoms; however, they can be symptoms of a life- or vision-threatening problem. We list accompanying signs and symptoms that may indicate a life- or vision-threatening headache and some of the specific signs and symptoms of various headaches.

WARNING SYMPTOMS AND SIGNS OF A SERIOUS DISORDER

• Scalp tenderness, weight loss, pain with chewing, muscle pains, or malaise in patients at least 55 years of age (GCA).

• Optic nerve swelling.

• Fever.

• Altered mentation or behavior.

• Stiff neck.

• Decreased vision.

• Neurologic signs.

• Subhyaloid (preretinal) hemorrhages on fundus examination.

LESS ALARMING BUT SUGGESTIVE SYMPTOMS AND SIGNS

• Onset in a previously headache-free individual.

• A different, more severe headache than the usual headache.

• A headache that is always in the same location.

• A headache that awakens the person from sleep.

- A headache that does not respond to pain medications that previously relieved it.

- Nausea and vomiting, particularly projectile vomiting.

- A headache followed by migraine visual symptoms (abnormal time course of events).

ETIOLOGY

Life- or Vision-Threatening

- GCA (Age older than 55 years, weight loss, fever, malaise, anorexia, muscle aches, scalp tenderness, pain on chewing, palpable tender nodule or cordlike pulseless area along the temporal artery, or decreased vision. May have high ESR. See 10.16, Arteritic Ischemic Optic Neuropathy.).

- Acute angle-closure glaucoma (Decreased vision, red and painful eye, cloudy cornea, fixed mid-dilated pupil, high intraocular pressure. See 9.10, Acute Angle-Closure Glaucoma.).

- Ocular ischemic syndrome (Periorbital eye pain, mid-peripheral retinal hemorrhages, dilated retinal veins, neovascularization of the iris, disc, or retina, spontaneous or easily inducible retinal arterial pulsations, light-induced amaurosis fugax. See 11.10, Ocular Ischemic Syndrome.).

- Malignant hypertension (Marked increase of blood pressure, often accompanied by retinal cotton-wool spots, hemorrhages, and, when severe, optic nerve swelling. Headaches typically are occipital in location. See 11.9, Hypertensive Retinopathy.).

- Increased intracranial pressure (May have papilledema, loss of venous pulsations[2] in the disc vessels, or a sixth cranial nerve palsy. Headaches usually worse in the morning and worsened with Valsalva. See 10.14, Papilledema.).

---

[2]The presence of spontaneous venous pulsations indicates normal intracranial pressure at that moment; however, the absence of pulsations has little significance. A significant number of normal individuals do not have spontaneous venous pulsations. If there are spontaneous venous pulsations, at that moment, the intracranial pressure is less than 180 mm Hg.

- Infectious CNS disorder (meningitis or brain abscess). (Fever, stiff neck, mental status changes, photophobia, neurologic signs.).

- Structural abnormality of the brain (e.g., tumor, aneurysm, arteriovenous malformation). (Mental status change, signs of increased intracranial pressure, or neurologic signs during, and often after, the headache episode.).

- Subarachnoid hemorrhage (Extremely severe headache, stiff neck, mental status change; rarely, subhyaloid hemorrhages seen on fundus examination, usually from a ruptured aneurysm.).

- Epidural or subdural hematoma (Follows head trauma; altered level of consciousness; may produce anisocoria.).

Others

- Migraine (see 10.25, Migraine).

- Cluster (see 10.26, Cluster Headaches).

- Tension.

- Herpes zoster virus [Headache or pain may precede the herpetic vesicles (see 4.15, Herpes Zoster Virus).].

- Sinus disease.

Note: A "sinus" headache can be a serious headache in diabetic patients and immunocompromised hosts because mucormycosis may be responsible (see 10.9, Cavernous Sinus and Associated Syndromes).

- Tolosa–Hunt syndrome (see 10.9, Cavernous Sinus and Associated Syndromes).

- Cervical spine disease.

- Temporomandibular joint syndrome.

- Dental disease.

- Trigeminal neuralgia (tic douloureux).

- Anterior uveitis (see 12.1, Anterior Uveitis).

- After spinal tap.

- Paget disease.

- Depression/psychogenic.

- Convergence insufficiency (see 13.8, Convergence Insufficiency).

- Accommodative spasm (see 13.9, Accommodative Spasm).

WORKUP

1. History: Ask about the location, intensity, frequency, possible precipitating factors, and time of day of the headaches. Determine the patient's age of onset, what relieves the headaches, and whether there are any associated signs or symptoms. Specifically, ask about the serious or suggestive symptoms and signs listed: trauma, medications and birth control pills, family history of migraine, and whether the patient experienced motion sickness or cyclic vomiting as a child.

2. Complete ocular examination, including pupillary, motility, and visual field evaluation; intraocular pressure measurement, optic disc and venous pulsation assessment, and a dilated retinal examination. Manifest and cycloplegic refractions may be helpful.

   *Note: The presence of spontaneous venous pulsations indicates normal intracranial pressure at that moment; however, the absence of pulsations has little significance. A significant number of normal individuals do not have spontaneous venous pulsations. If spontaneous venous pulsa-tions, at that moment, intracranial pressure is less than 180 mm Hg.

3. Neurologic examination (check neck flexibility and other meningeal signs).

4. Palpate the temporal arteries in potential GCA cases (to see if they are swollen, hard, and tender). Ask specifically about jaw claudication, scalp tenderness, temporal headaches, and unexpected weight loss.

5. Temperature and blood pressure.

6. Immediate ESR with or without temporal artery biopsy when GCA is suspected (see 10.16, Arteritic Ischemic Optic Neuropathy).

7. CT scan (axial and coronal views) or MRI of the brain when an intracranial abnormality is suspected.

8. Carotid noninvasive flow studies when ocular ischemic syndrome is suspected.

9. Lumbar puncture (in the hospital) is obtained in suspected cases of meningitis or subarachnoid hemorrhage, after CT scan or MRI of the brain.

10. Refer the patient to a neurologist; ear, nose, and throat specialist; internist; or family physician, as indicated.

TREATMENT/FOLLOW-UP

See individual sections.

10.25 MIGRAINE

SYMPTOMS

Typically unilateral (although it may occur behind both eyes or across the entire front of the head), throbbing or boring head pain accompanied by nausea, vomiting, mood changes, fatigue, or photophobia. Visual disturbances, including flashing (zigzagging) lights, blurred vision, or a visual field defect lasting 15 to 50 minutes, may precede the migraine and is called the *aura*. Neurologic deficits may occur. A family history is common, as is a history of car sickness or cyclic vomiting as a child. Migraine in children may be seen as recurrent abdominal pain and malaise. Of these patients, 60% to 70% are girls.

*Note: Most unilateral migraine headaches at some point change sides of the head. Patients who always have a headache on the same side of the head may have a more serious headache disorder.

Note: Pay close attention to temporal order of symptoms: Determine if headache precedes visual symptoms. This order of events is more common with arteriovenous malformations, mass lesions with cerebral edema, or seizure focus.

SIGNS

Usually none. Complicated migraines may have a permanent neurologic or ocular deficit (see the following discussion).

DIFFERENTIAL DIAGNOSIS

See 10.24, Headache.

CLASSIFICATION

Definitions and classifications vary.

1. Migraine without aura (common migraine; 80%): Nausea, vomiting, fatigue, and mood changes are associated with this variant.

2. Migraine with aura (classic migraine; 10%): The headache is preceded by a 15- to 50-minute visual disturbance or transient focal neurologic change. See Complicated Migraine (later) for specific types of visual and neurologic defects.

3. Acephalic migraine (visual migraine without headache): The patient experiences the visual aura of a classic migraine without the subsequent headache. Some of these patients have and some have not had migraine headaches in the past.

4. Complicated migraine: A subset of migraine in which neurologic deficits outlast the headache. Rarely, a deficit may be permanent.

—Cerebral: A neurologic deficit involving the motor, sensory, or visual systems. Onset can be at the height of a migraine headache, but more commonly it follows the headache. Examples include focal motor deficits, speech disorders, and paresthesias of the extremities, face, tongue, or lips. "Hemiplegic migraine" consists of total paralysis or weakness on one side of the body.

—Ophthalmoplegic: Ipsilateral paralysis of one or more extraocular muscles, usually occurring during a migraine attack in childhood. The ophthalmoplegia usually occurs as the headache is resolving.

—Retinal: Sudden monocular visual loss in a migraine patient. Light flashes and headache do not usually occur.

—Basilar artery migraine: Mimics vertebrobasilar artery insufficiency with bilateral blurring or blindness, vertigo, gait disturbances, formed hallucinations, and dysarthria in a patient with migraine.

ASSOCIATIONS OR PRECIPITATING FACTORS

Birth control or other hormonal pills, puberty, pregnancy, menopause, foods containing tyramine or phenylalanine (e.g., aged cheeses, wines, chocolate, cashew nuts), nitrates or nitrites, monosodium glutamate, alcohol, fatigue, emotional stress, or bright lights.

WORKUP

See 10.24, Headache for a general headache workup.

1. History: May establish the diagnosis.

2. Ocular and neurologic examinations, including refraction.

3. CT scan or MRI of the head is indicated for:

   —Atypical migraines (e.g., migraines that are always on the same side of the head, those with an unusual sequence, such as visual disturbances persisting into or occurring after the headache phase).

   —Complicated migraines.

4. Consider checking for uncontrolled blood pressure or low blood sugar (hypoglycemic headaches are almost always precipitated by stress or fatigue).

TREATMENT

1. Avoid agents that precipitate the headaches (e.g., stop using birth control pills; avoid al-

cohol and any foods that may precipitate attacks; reduce stress).

2. Correct any significant refractive error.

3. Medications to be used at the onset of the headache (the earlier the better) in patients with infrequent headaches:

 a. Initial therapy: Aspirin or nonsteroidal antiinflammatory agents (e.g., tolfenamic acid, 200 mg, q3h, naproxen sodium, 750 mg, in one dose).

 b. More potent therapy (when initial therapy fails):

 —Ergotamine,[3] 2 mg in one dose, and then every 30 minute for two extra doses if no relief (maximum dose is three tablets or 6 mg total per attack, no more than 10 mg per week).

 —Ergotamine,[3] 1 mg with caffeine, 100 mg, in one tablet. Two tablets at the onset of symptoms followed by one tablet every 30 minutes (maximum dose, 6 mg of ergotamine per attack, and no more than 10 mg per week).

 —Dihydroergotamine, 4.0 mg p.o., in one dose.

 —Butorphanol nasal spray, one spray in one nostril.

 —Sumatriptan, 6 mg, subcutaneous single dose. Maximum dose is two injections in 24 hours. Do not give second dose if first is ineffective. Do not use if any ergotamine-containing drug (e.g., ergotamine, dihydroergotamine) has been given in the past 24 hours (because vasoconstriction could be additive).

 —Sumatriptan, 25 mg p.o., single dose; if no relief after 2 hours, a second dose of up to 100 mg may be taken. If headache returns, may repeat after 2 hours have passed from previous dose. Maximum oral dose is 300 mg in a 24-hour period.

 —Sumatriptan, 20 mg, nasal spray, single dose.

 —For prolonged attacks lasting longer than 24 hours, some physicians recommend systemic steroids.

 Note: Opioid drugs should be avoided.

4. Prophylactic medication to be used in patients with frequent or severe headache attacks (e.g., two or more headaches per month) or those with neurologic changes:

 a. Propranolol (e.g., Inderal),[4] 10 to 80 mg p.o., q.d., in divided doses initially; slowly increase the dose by 10 to 20 mg every 2 to 3 days until the desired effect is obtained (can go up to 160 to 240 mg/day). May also use timolol p.o., 10 to 15 mg, b.i.d. Metoprolol may have fewer side effects for asthmatic and diabetic patients (100 mg in one slow-release tablet per day).

 b. Amitriptyline (e.g., Elavil),[5] 25 to 200 mg p.o., q.h.s. (start at a low dose and increase the dose by 25 mg every 1 to 2 weeks if needed).

 c. Calcium channel blockers (e.g., flunarizine, 5 to 10 mg q.d.); we rarely use these.

 d. Methylsergide, 2 to 4 mg p.o., b.i.d. (ergot-containing medication).

5. Antinausea medication as needed for an acute episode (e.g., prochlorperazine, 25 mg rectally, b.i.d.).

FOLLOW-UP

Patients are usually reevaluated in 4 to 6 weeks to assess the efficacy of the therapy.

---

[3]Contraindicated in elderly patients or those with cardiovascular, cerebrovascular, renal, or hepatic disease, and pregnant patients. Muscle weakness and pain or even cardiac ischemic pain can occur.

[4]Do not give to patients with asthma, congestive heart failure, bradycardia, or hypotension. Do not discontinue this drug suddenly; it must be tapered slowly.

[5]Do not give to patients taking a monoamine oxidase inhibitor or patients with narrow anterior chamber angles or benign prostatic hypertrophy.

10.26 CLUSTER HEADACHE

SYMPTOMS

Typically unilateral, very painful, periorbital, frontal, or temporal headache associated with ipsilateral tearing, rhinorrhea, sweating, nasal stuffiness, or a droopy eyelid or a combination of these. Usually lasts for minutes to hours. Typically recurs once or twice daily for several weeks, followed by a headache-free interval of months to years. The cycle can then repeat itself. Predominantly affects men. The headache awakens patients, whereas migraine does not.

SIGNS

Ipsilateral conjunctival injection, facial flush, or Horner syndrome (third-order neuron etiology) may be present. Ptosis may become permanent.

PRECIPITATING FACTORS

Alcohol, nitroglycerin.

DIFFERENTIAL DIAGNOSIS

• Migraine headache (Family history of migraines or a history of car sickness or cyclic vomiting in many cases. The associated symptoms listed previously are typically absent. See 10.25, Migraine.).

• Chronic paroxysmal hemicrania (Several attacks per day with a dramatic response to oral indomethacin.).

• Others (see 10.24, Headache).

WORKUP

1. History and complete ocular examination.

2. Neurologic examination, particularly a cranial nerve evaluation.

3. Consider a hydroxyamphetamine (e.g., Paredrine) test if Horner syndrome accompanies a suspected cluster headache to confirm a third-order neuron etiology (see 10.2, Horner Syndrome).

4. Obtain an MRI of the brain when the history is atypical or a neurologic abnormality other than a third-order neuron Horner syndrome is found.

TREATMENT

1. No treatment is necessary if the headache is mild.

2. No alcoholic beverages or cigarette smoking during a cluster cycle.

3. Abortive therapy for acute attack:

   —Oxygen, 5 to 8 L/min by face mask for 10 minutes at onset of attack. Relieves pain in 70% of adults.

   —Ergotamine inhalation is the fastest way to reach therapeutic blood levels (e.g, Medihaler, three puffs, 5 minutes apart).

   —Dihydroergotamine, i.m. or i.v. (1.0 mg i.m. in one dose).

   —Corticosteroids (e.g., dexamethasone, 8.0 mg i.v. in one dose).

4. When headaches are moderate to severe and are unrelieved by nonprescription medication, one of the following drugs may be an effective prophylactic agent during cluster periods:

   —Calcium channel blockers (e.g., verapamil, 360 to 480 mg/day p.o., in divided doses).

   —Ergotamine, 1 to 2 mg p.o., q.d.

   —Methysergide, 2 mg p.o., b.i.d., with meals. Do not use for longer than 3 to 4 months because of the significant risk of retroperitoneal fibrosis. Methysergide is not recommended in patients with coronary artery or peripheral vascular disease, thrombophlebitis, hypertension, pregnancy, or hepatic or renal disease.

   —Oral steroids (e.g., prednisone, 40 to 80 mg p.o., for 1 week, tapering rapidly over an additional week if possible) and an antiulcer agent (e.g., ranitidine, 150 mg p.o., b.i.d.).

—Lithium, 600 to 900 mg p.o., q.d., is administered in conjunction with the patient's medical doctor. Baseline renal (blood urea nitrogen, creatinine, urine electrolytes) and thyroid function tests (triiodothyronine, thyroxine, TSH) are obtained. Lithium intoxication may occur in patients using indomethacin, tetracycline, or methyldopa.

5. Some physicians administer an ergotamine inhaler (9 mg/mL, containing 0.36 mg per inhalation), one inhalation every 5 minutes for three inhalations (maximum every 12 to 24 hours) or ergotamine, 2 mg sublingual, every 30 minutes for three times (maximum in 24 hours) to be started at the onset of an attack. Ergotamine pills may be used in prophylaxis. Ergotamine has the same contraindications as methysergide. We do not use ergotamine as a first-line agent.

6. If necessary, an acute, severe attack can be treated with i.v. diazepam.

FOLLOW-UP

1. Patients started on systemic steroids are seen within a few days and then every several weeks to evaluate the effects of treatment and monitor intraocular pressure.

2. Patients taking methysergide or lithium are reevaluated in 7 to 10 days. Plasma lithium levels are monitored in patients taking this agent.

CHAPTER 11

RETINA

11.1 POSTERIOR VITREOUS DETACHMENT

SYMPTOMS

Floaters ("cobwebs," "bugs," "tadpole," or comma-shaped objects that change position with eye movement), blurred vision, flashes of light, which are more common in dim illumination and are temporally located.

SIGNS

Critical. One or more discrete light gray to black vitreous opacities, often in the shape of a ring ("Weiss ring"), suspended over the optic disc. The opacities float within the vitreous as the eye moves from side to side.

Other. Vitreous hemorrhage, peripheral retinal and disc margin hemorrhages, pigmented cells in the anterior vitreous, retinal break or detachment.

Note: *The presence of pigmented cells [released retinal pigment epithelial (RPE) cells] in the anterior vitreous or vitreous hemorrhage in association with acute posterior vitreous detachment (PVD) indicates a high probability of a coexisting retinal break (see 11.2, Retinal Break).*

DIFFERENTIAL DIAGNOSIS

• Vitritis (It may be difficult to distinguish PVD with pigmented anterior vitreous cells from vitreous inflammatory cells. In vitritis, the vitreous cells may be found in both the posterior and anterior vitreous, the condition may be bilateral, and the cells are not typically pigmented. A history of uveitis may be elicited. See 12.3, Posterior Uveitis.).

• Migraine (Patients complain of flashing lights in a zig-zag pattern that obstruct vision, last approximately 20 minutes, and are sometimes multicolored. A headache may or may not follow. No vitreous or retinal abnormalities are found on examination. See 10.24, Headache.).

The following may occur with or without PVD, producing similar symptoms:

• Retinal break.

• Vitreous hemorrhage.

• Retinal detachment (RD).

WORKUP

1. History: Distinguish between the visual distortion of migraine, from the light sparks of PVD, which are commonly accompanied by new floaters. Determine the duration of the symptoms.

2. Complete ocular examination, particularly a dilated retinal examination by using indirect ophthalmoscopy and scleral depression to

rule out a retinal break and detachment. A slit-lamp examination of the anterior vitreous, looking for pigmented cells, should be performed (see Appendix 8).

3. PVD may be visualized by focusing in the vitreous, anterior to the disc, by using

—Indirect ophthalmoscopy.

—Direct ophthalmoscopy. (The ophthalmoscope is initially focused on the cornea, and the lens wheel is moved from higher toward lower plus lenses while the patient is asked to move his or her eye from left to right. The Weiss ring is seen to float by.).

—A slit-lamp and a 60- or 90-diopter, or contact lens examination. (Pull the slit lamp back once focus on the disc is obtained. A gray-to-black strand may be seen suspended in the vitreous.).

TREATMENT

No treatment is indicated for PVD. If an acute retinal break is found, the patient should receive laser or cryotherapy promptly to prevent the development of an RD (see 11.2, Retinal Break).

Note: A retinal break surrounded by pigment is old and usually does not require treatment.

FOLLOW-UP

1. The patient should be given a list of RD symptoms (an increase in floaters or flashing lights, or the appearance of a persistent curtain or shadow anywhere in the field of vision) and told to return immediately if these symptoms develop.

2. If no retinal break or hemorrhage is found, the patient should be scheduled for repeated examination with scleral depression in 2 to 4 weeks, 2 to 3 months, and 6 months after the symptoms first develop.

3. If no retinal break is found, but mild vitreous hemorrhage or peripheral punctate retinal hemorrhages are present, repeated examinations are performed 1 to 2 weeks, 4 weeks, 3 months, and 6 months after the event.

4. If a vitreous hemorrhage dense enough to obscure visualization of the retina is found, ultrasonography is indicated to rule out an RD, tumor, or hemorrhagic macular degeneration. Occasionally the flap of a tear can be identified. Bed rest, with the head of the bed elevated, may be used for 24 to 48 hours to hasten settling of the blood (see 11.22, Vitreous Hemorrhage).

11.2   RETINAL BREAK

SYMPTOMS

Acute retinal break: Flashes of light, floaters ("cobwebs" or "flies" that move with eye movement), and sometimes blurred vision.

Chronic retinal breaks or atrophic retinal holes: Usually asymptomatic.

SIGNS

Critical. A full-thickness retinal defect, usually seen in the periphery.

Other

• Acute retinal break: Pigmented cells in the anterior vitreous, vitreous hemorrhage, PVD, retinal flap, an operculum (a free-floating piece of retina) suspended in the vitreous cavity above the retinal hole.

• Chronic retinal break: A ring of pigmentation surrounding the break, demarcation line between attached and detached retina, signs (but not symptoms) of an acute retinal break.

PREDISPOSING LESIONS

Lattice degeneration, high myopia, aphakia, pseudophakia, age-related retinoschisis, vitreoretinal tufts, meridional folds, history of previous retinal break or detachment in the fellow eye, trauma.

DIFFERENTIAL DIAGNOSIS

• Meridional fold (Small radial fold of retina perpendicular to the ora serrata and overlying an oral tooth; may have small retinal hole at the base.).

• Meridional complex (Meridional fold that extends to a ciliary process.).

• Vitreoretinal tuft (Focal area of vitreous traction causing elevation of the retina.).

• Paving stone degeneration.

• Lattice degeneration.

WORKUP

1. Complete ocular examination, particularly a dilated fundus examination of both eyes by using indirect ophthalmoscopy and scleral depression.

2. Scleral depression is usually not performed until 2 to 4 weeks after a traumatic hyphema or microhyphema.

3. A slit-lamp examination with a fundus contact lens is often quite helpful in evaluating retinal breaks.

TREATMENT

In general, laser therapy, cryotherapy, or scleral buckling surgery is required within 24 to 72 hours for acute retinal breaks, and only rarely for chronic breaks. Each case must be individualized; however, we follow these general guidelines:

1. Treatment recommended

—Acute symptomatic break (e.g., a horseshoe or operculated tear).

—Acute traumatic break (including a dialysis).

2. Treatment to be considered

—Asymptomatic retinal break that is large (e.g., greater than 1.5 mm) or above the horizontal meridian or both, particularly if there is no PVD.

—Asymptomatic retinal break in an aphakic or pseudophakic eye, an eye in which the involved or the contralateral eye has had an RD, or in a highly myopic eye.

FOLLOW-UP

1. Patients with predisposing lesions or retinal breaks that do not require treatment are followed every 6 to 12 months.

2. Patients treated for a retinal break are reexamined in 1 week, 1 month, 3 months, and then every 6 to 12 months.

3. RD symptoms (an increase in floaters or flashing lights or the appearance of a curtain, shadow, or bubble anywhere in the field of vision) are explained to all patients, and patients are told to return immediately if these symptoms develop.

11.3 RETINAL DETACHMENT

There are three distinct types of RD. All three forms show an elevation of the retina.

RHEGMATOGENOUS RETINAL DETACHMENT (RRD)

SYMPTOMS

Flashes of light, floaters, a curtain or shadow moving over the field of vision, peripheral or central visual loss, or both.

SIGNS

Critical. Elevation of the retina from the RPE by fluid in the subretinal space due to an accompanying full-thickness retinal break or breaks (see 11.2, Retinal Break).

Other. Pigmented cells in the anterior vitreous, vitreous hemorrhage, PVD, usually lower intraocular pressure (IOP) in the affected eye than the contralateral eye, clear subretinal fluid that does not shift with body position, sometimes fixed retinal folds. The detached retina is often corrugated and partially opaque in appearance. An afferent pupillary defect (APD) may be present.

Note: A chronic RRD often shows a pigmented demarcation line at the posterior extent of the RD, intraretinal cysts, fixed folds, or white dots underneath the retina (subretinal precipitates) or a combination of these. It should be differentiated from retinoschisis, which produces an absolute visual field defect.

ETIOLOGY

A break in the retina allows syneretic fluid to move through and separate the overlying retina from the RPE.

WORKUP

1. Indirect ophthalmoscopy with scleral depression. Slit-lamp examination with contact lens may help in finding small breaks.

2. B-scan ultrasonography may be helpful if media opacities impede a clear view.

EXUDATIVE RETINAL DETACHMENT (ERD)

SYMPTOMS

Minimal to severe visual loss or a visual field defect; visual changes may vary with changes in head position.

SIGNS

Critical. Serous elevation of the retina with shifting subretinal fluid. (The area of detached retina changes when the patient changes position: While sitting, the subretinal fluid accumulates inferiorly, detaching the retina inferiorly; while in the supine position, the fluid accumulates in the posterior pole, detaching the macula.) There is no retinal break; fluid accumulation is due to breakdown of the normal inner or outer blood–retinal barrier. The detachment does not extend to the ora serrata.

Other. The detached retina is smooth and may become quite bullous. A mild APD may be present.

ETIOLOGY

• Neoplastic [e.g., choroidal malignant melanoma (MM), metastasis, choroidal hemangioma, multiple myeloma, capillary retinal hemangioma]. [Intravenous fluorescein angiography (IVFA) and ultrasound may be helpful in making a differential diagnosis.].

• Inflammatory disease [e.g., Vogt–Koyanagi–Harada (VKH) syndrome, posterior scleritis, other chronic inflammatory processes].

• Congenital abnormalities (e.g., optic pit, morning-glory syndrome and choroidal coloboma—although these almost always have a retinal break).

• Vascular (Coats disease, malignant hypertension.).

• Nanophthalmos (Small eyes with a small cornea and a shallow anterior chamber but a large lens and a thick sclera.).

- Idiopathic central serous chorioretinopathy (CSCR) (May be seen with bullous RD from multiple, large RPE detachments.).

- Uveal effusion syndrome [Bilateral detachments of the peripheral choroid, ciliary body, and retina; leopard-spot RPE changes (when retina is reattached); cells in the vitreous; dilated episcleral vessels.].

WORKUP

1. IVFA may show source of subretinal fluid.

2. B-scan ultrasonography may help delineate the underlying cause.

TRACTIONAL RETINAL DETACHMENT (TRD)

SYMPTOMS

Visual loss or visual field defect; may be asymptomatic.

SIGNS

Critical. The detached retina appears concave with a smooth surface; cellular and vitreous membranes exerting traction on the retina are present; retinal striae extending from these areas may also be seen. (Detachment may become a convex RRD if a tractional retinal tear develops.).

Other. The retina is immobile, and the detachment rarely extends to the ora serrata. A mild APD may be present.

ETIOLOGY

Fibrocellular bands in the vitreous (e.g., resulting from proliferative diabetic retinopathy, sickle cell retinopathy, retinopathy of prematurity, toxocariasis, trauma, previous giant retinal tear) contract and detach the retina.

WORKUP

1. Indirect ophthalmoscopy with scleral depression. Slit-lamp examination with contact lens may help in finding small breaks.

2. B-scan ultrasonography may be helpful if media opacities impede a clear view.

DIFFERENTIAL DIAGNOSIS FOR ALL THREE TYPES OF RETINAL DETACHMENT

- Acquired/age-related degenerative retinoschisis (Commonly bilateral, usually inferotemporal, no pigmented cells or hemorrhage are present in the vitreous, the retinal vessels in the inner retinal layers are often sheathed peripherally, white "snowflakes" are often seen on the inner retinal layers; the patient is asymptomatic. An absolute scotoma, as opposed to a relative scotoma as seen with an RRD, is found on visual field testing. A demarcation line is usually not present. When a demarcation line is present, we must look for a retinal break because long-standing detachments may simulate schisis and may even demonstrate an absolute field defect.).

- X-linked retinoschisis (Petaloid foveal changes are present over 90% of the time. Dehiscences occur in the nerve fiber layer 50% of the time.).

- Choroidal detachment (Orange–brown, more solid in appearance than an RD, the ora serrata can usually be seen without scleral depression, the detachment often extends 360 degrees around the globe. Hypotony is usually present.).

TREATMENT

1. Patients with acute RRD or TRD that threatens the fovea should be placed on bed rest until surgical repair is performed urgently. (Surgical options include laser photocoagulation, cryotherapy, pneumatic retinopexy, vitrectomy, and scleral buckle.)

2. All RRDs that do not threaten fixation or with macula-off detachments or TRDs that involve the macula are repaired at the earliest convenience, preferably within a few days.

3. Chronic RDs are treated within 1 week.

4. For ERD, successful treatment of the underlying condition often leads to resolution of the detachment.

FOLLOW-UP

Patients treated for RD may be reexamined at 1 day, 1 week, 2 weeks, 1 month, 2 to 3 months, then every 6 to 12 months.

11.4 RETINOSCHISIS

Retinoschisis, a splitting of the retina, occurs in X-linked (juvenile) and age-related degenerative forms.

X-LINKED (JUVENILE) RETINOSCHISIS

SYMPTOMS

Decreased vision [often due to vitreous hemorrhage (25%) and macular changes] or asymptomatic. The condition is congenital, but may not be detected at birth if an examination is not performed. A family history may or may not be elicited.

SIGNS

Critical. Foveal schisis seen as stellate maculopathy: cystoid foveal changes with retinal folds that radiate from the center of the foveal configuration (petaloid pattern). Unlike the cysts of cystoid macular edema (CME), they do not stain on IVFA. The macular appearance changes in adulthood.

Other. Separation of the nerve fiber layer from the outer retinal layers in the retinal periphery with the development of nerve fiber layer breaks; this peripheral retinoschisis occurs in 50% of patients, most commonly in the inferotemporal quadrant of the fundus, and is bilateral. RD, vitreous hemorrhage, and pigmentary changes also may occur. Pigmented demarcation lines may be seen even though the retina is not detached at the time. This is not the case for acquired age-related degeneration.

INHERITANCE

X-linked recessive.

DIFFERENTIAL DIAGNOSIS

• Age-related degenerative retinoschisis (see the following).

• RRD (Usually unilateral and acquired. It extends to the ora serrata and lacks the foveal changes described previously. Anterior chamber cells and flare and pigment in the vitreous are often seen. See 11.3, Retinal Detachment.).

WORKUP

1. Family history.

2. Dilated retinal examination with scleral depression to rule out an outer layer retinal break or detachment.

TREATMENT

1. No treatment for stellate maculopathy.

2. For unresolved vitreous hemorrhage, consider vitrectomy.

3. Surgical repair of an RD should be performed.

4. Superimposed amblyopia should always be considered in children younger than 9 to 11 years when one eye is more severely affected, and a trial of patching should be considered (see 8.6, Amblyopia).

FOLLOW-UP

Every 6 months; sooner if treating amblyopia.

AGE-RELATED (SENILE) DEGENERATIVE RETINOSCHISIS

SYMPTOMS

Usually asymptomatic, may have decreased vision.

SIGNS

Critical. The schisis cavity is dome shaped with a smooth surface and is usually located temporally, especially inferotemporally. The retinal split is usually bilateral and may show sheathing of retinal vessels and "snowflakes," or "frosting" (persistent Mueller fibers) on the elevated inner wall of the schisis cavity. (In contrast to X-linked juvenile retinoschisis, splitting usually occurs at the level of the outer plexiform layer.) The area of schisis is not mobile, and there is no associated RPE or vitreous pigmentation.

Other. Prominent cystoid degeneration near the ora serrata, an absolute scotoma corresponding to the area of schisis is found on visual field testing, hyperopia is common, and there are no pigment cells or hemorrhage in the vitreous. An RRD may occasionally develop.

DIFFERENTIAL DIAGNOSIS

• RRD (The surface is not smooth but corrugated in appearance and can be seen to move more with eye movements. In contrast, schisis does not, retinal vessels are not sheathed, no "snowflakes" or "frosting" can be seen on the retinal elevation, one or more full-thickness holes are present, and pigmented cells or hemorrhage may be present in the vitreous. A longstanding RD may resemble retinoschisis, but intraretinal cysts, demarcation lines between attached and detached retina, and white retroretinal dots may be seen. A relative scotoma is found on visual field testing. See 11.3, Retinal Detachment,).

• X-linked juvenile retinoschisis (see previous).

WORKUP

1. Slit-lamp evaluation to rule out the presence of anterior chamber inflammation or pigmented anterior vitreous cells, both of which should not be present in isolated retinoschisis.

2. Dilated retinal examination with scleral depression to rule out a concomitant RD or an outer layer retinal hole, which may lead to an RD.

3. A fundus contact lens evaluation of the retina as needed to aid in recognizing outer layer retinal breaks.

TREATMENT

1. Surgery is indicated when a clinically significant RD develops.

2. A small RD walled off by a demarcation line is usually not treated. This may take the form of pigmentation at the posterior border of outer layer breaks.

FOLLOW-UP

Every 6 months. RD symptoms (an increase in floaters or flashing lights or the appearance of a curtain or shadow anywhere in the field of vision) are explained to all patients, and patients are told to return immediately if these symptoms develop.

11.5 CENTRAL RETINAL ARTERY OCCLUSION

SYMPTOMS

Unilateral, painless, acute vision loss (counting fingers to light perception in 94% of eyes) occurring over seconds; may have a history of amaurosis fugax, and may be noted on arising in the morning.

SIGNS

Critical. Superficial opacification or whitening of the retina in the posterior pole and a cherry-red spot in the center of the macula.

Other. A marked APD; narrowed retinal arterioles; box-carring or segmentation of the blood column in the arterioles. Occasionally, retinal arteriolar emboli or cilioretinal artery sparing of the foveola is evident. If visual acuity is light perception or worse, strongly suspect ophthalmic artery occlusion.

DIFFERENTIAL DIAGNOSIS

• Acute ophthalmic artery occlusion [Usually no cherry-red spot in the foveola; the entire retina appears whitened. The treatment is the same as for central retinal artery occlusion (CRAO).].

- Inadvertent intraocular injection of gentamicin.

- Other causes of a cherry-red spot (e.g., Tay–Sachs or other storage diseases) (Present in early life, other systemic manifestations, usually bilateral.).

ETIOLOGY

- Embolus (especially carotid or cardiac).

- Thrombosis.

- Giant cell arteritis (GCA) (May produce CRAO or an ischemic optic neuropathy. See later for concomitant symptoms.).

- Collagen–vascular disease other than GCA (e.g., systemic lupus erythematosus, polyarteritis nodosa).

- Hypercoagulation disorders (e.g., oral contraceptives, polycythemia, anti-phospholipid syndrome).

- Rare causes (e.g., migraine, Behçet disease, syphilis, sickle cell disease).

- Trauma

WORKUP

1. Immediate erythrocyte sedimentation rate (ESR) to rule out GCA if the patient is 50 years of age or older. This is obtained immediately after the paracentesis. If the patient's history or ESR, or both, are consistent with GCA, high-dose systemic steroids are started. See 10.16, Arteritic Ischemic Optic Neuropathy, for additional details.

2. Check blood pressure.

3. Other blood tests: Fasting blood sugar, glycosylated hemoglobin, complete blood count (CBC) with differential, prothrombin time/activated partial thromboplastin time (PT/PTT). In patients younger than 50 years or with appropriate risk factors or positive review of systems, consider lipid profile, antinuclear antibody (ANA), rheumatoid factor, fluorescent treponemal antibody, absorbed

(FTA-ABS), serum protein electrophoresis, hemoglobin electrophoresis, and anti-phospholipid antibodies.

4. Carotid artery evaluation (duplex Doppler ultrasonography of the carotid arteries).

5. Cardiac evaluation [electrocardiography (ECG), echocardiography, and possibly Holter monitoring].

6. Consider IVFA, electroretinography (ERG), or both to confirm the diagnosis.

Note: It has been suggested that only patients with high-risk characteristics for cardioembolic disease merit echocardiography. These high-risk characteristics include the following: a history of subacute bacterial endocarditis, rheumatic heart disease, mitral valve prolapse, recent myocardial infarction, prosthetic valve, intravenous (i.v.) drug abuse, congenital heart disease, valvular heart disease, any detectable heart murmur, and ECG changes (atrial fibrillation, acute ST segment elevation or Q waves).

TREATMENT

No treatment modality has been proven effective in the treatment of CRAO. However, there are anecdotal reports of improvement after the following treatments, if instituted soon (within 90 to 120 minutes) after the occlusive event.

1. Immediate ocular massage (fundus contact lens or digital massage).

2. Anterior chamber paracentesis (Fig. 11.1): Place a drop of topical anesthetic (e.g., tetracaine or cocaine 2% to 4%) in the eye and anesthetize the base of the medial rectus muscle by holding a cotton-tipped applicator dipped in the topical anesthetic against the muscle for 1 minute. Retract the eyelid with an eyelid speculum, and with an operating microscope or slit lamp (a microscope is easier), grasp the base of the medial rectus muscle with fixation forceps at the anesthetized site. With a 30-gauge short needle on a tuberculin syringe, enter the eye temporally at the limbus with the bevel of the needle pointing up and away from the eye.

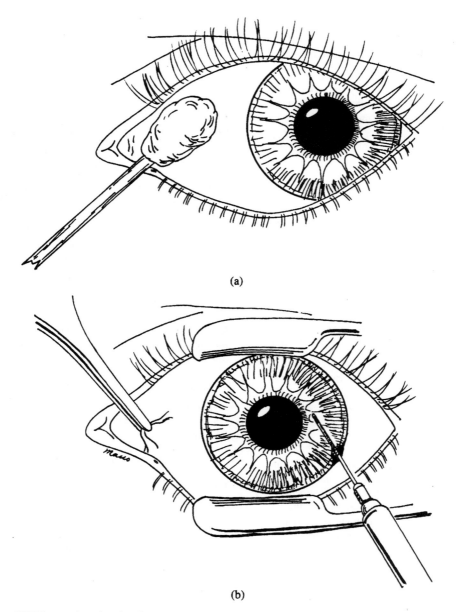

(a)

(b)

FIGURE 11.1 Anterior chamber paracentesis. **a:** The base of the medial rectus is anesthetized with a cotton-tipped applicator dipped in cocaine, 2% to 4%. **b:** While the globe is fixated with forceps, a 30-gauge needle is passed through the cornea into the anterior chamber. The needle should stay over the iris.

Be sure to keep the tip of the needle over the iris (not the lens) when entering the anterior chamber. Withdraw fluid until the chamber shallows slightly (usually 0.1 to 0.2 mL). Alternatively, the plunger may be left out of the syringe to allow passive egress of aqueous. Withdraw the needle and place a drop of antibiotic on the eye [e.g., levofloxacin (Quixin), gatifloxacin (Zymar), or moxifloxacin (Vigamox).].

3. Acetazolamide, 500 mg i.v., or two 250-mg tablets, orally (p.o.), or a topical beta-blocker (e.g., timolol, or levobunolol, 0.5% b.i.d.) is used to reduce the IOP.

FOLLOW-UP

1. Refer to an internist for a complete workup.

2. Repeat eye examination in 1 to 4 weeks, checking for neovascularization of the iris/disc, which develops in up to 20% of patients, at a mean of 4 weeks after onset. If neovascularization develops, panretinal photocoagulation (PRP) should be performed.

11.6 BRANCH RETINAL ARTERY OCCLUSION

SYMPTOMS

Unilateral, painless, abrupt loss of partial visual field; a history of transient visual loss (amaurosis fugax) may be elicited.

SIGNS

Critical. Superficial opacification or whitening along the distribution of a branch retinal artery. The affected retina becomes edematous.

Other. Narrowed branch retinal artery; box-carring, segmentation of the blood column, or emboli are sometimes seen in the affected branch retinal artery. Cotton-wool spots may appear in the involved area.

ETIOLOGY

See 11.5, Central Retinal Artery Occlusion.

WORKUP

See 11.5, Central Retinal Artery Occlusion. An ERG, however, is not helpful.

*Note: When a branch retinal artery occlusion is accompanied by optic nerve edema or retinitis, obtain appropriate serologic testing to rule out cat-scratch disease [Bartonella (Rochalimaea) henselae], syphilis, Lyme disease, and toxoplasmosis.

TREATMENT

1. No ocular therapy of proven value is available. Ocular massage (and, rarely, anterior chamber paracentesis) may dislodge a cholesterol embolus (cholesterol emboli appear as bright, reflective crystals, usually at a vessel bifurcation).

2. Treat any underlying medical problem.

FOLLOW-UP

1. Patients need to be evaluated immediately to treat any underlying disorders (especially GCA).

2. Reevaluate every 3 to 6 months initially to monitor progression. Ocular neovascularization after branch retinal artery occlusion is rare.

11.7 CENTRAL RETINAL VEIN OCCLUSION

SYMPTOMS

Painless loss of vision, usually unilateral.

SIGNS

Critical. Diffuse retinal hemorrhages in all 4 quadrants of the retina; dilated, tortuous retinal veins.

Other. Cotton-wool spots; disc edema and hemorrhages; retinal edema; optociliary shunt vessels on the disc; neovascularization of the optic disc, retina, or iris.

DIFFERENTIAL DIAGNOSIS

• Ocular ischemic syndrome (carotid occlusive disease) [Veins are usually dilated and irregular (but not tortuous). Although neovascularization of the disc is present in one third of cases, disc edema and hemorrhages are not characteristic. Retinal hemorrhages tend to be in the mid-periphery. Patients may have a history of amaurosis fugax, transient ischemic attacks, or orbital pain. IOP is often low. Central retinal artery perfusion pressure is low in this entity. See 11.10, Ocular Ischemic Syndrome.].

• Diabetic retinopathy [Hemorrhages and microaneurysms are usually concentrated in the posterior pole, exudate is more prominent, and the condition is typically bilateral. IVFA may be required to distinguish this condition from central retinal vein occlusion (CRVO). See 13.2, Diabetes Mellitus.].

• Papilledema (Bilateral disc swelling with flame-shaped hemorrhages surrounding the disc but not extending to the peripheral retina; results from increased intracranial pressure. See 10.14, Papilledema.).

• Radiation retinopathy (History of irradiation is critical in diagnosis. Disc swelling with radiation papillopathy, and retinal neovascularization may be present. Generally, cotton-wool spots are a more prominent feature than hemorrhages.).

ETIOLOGY

• Atherosclerosis of the adjacent central retinal artery (The artery compresses the central retinal vein in the region of the lamina cribrosa, secondarily inducing thrombosis in the lumen of the vein.).

• Hypertension.

• Optic disc edema.

• Glaucoma (The ocular disease most commonly associated with CRVO.).

• Optic disc drusen.

• Hypercoagulable state (e.g., polycythemia, lymphoma, leukemia, sickle cell disease, multiple myeloma, cryoglobulinemia, Waldenström macroglobulinemia, anti-phospholipid syndrome, activated protein C resistance, hyperhomocysteinemia).

• Vasculitis (e.g., sarcoid, syphilis, systemic lupus erythematosus).

• Drugs (e.g., oral contraceptives, diuretics).

• Abnormal platelet function.

• Retrobulbar external compression (e.g., thyroid disease, orbital tumor).

• Migraine (rare).

TYPES

Ischemic CRVO: Multiple cotton-wool spots (usually more than ten), extensive retinal hemorrhage, and widespread capillary nonperfusion on IVFA. Often a relative APD is present and acuity is 20/400 or worse.

Nonischemic CRVO: Mild fundus changes. No APD is present and often acuity is better than 20/400.

WORKUP

Ocular

1. Complete ocular examination, including IOP measurement, careful slit-lamp biomi-

croscopy and gonioscopy to rule out neovascularization of the iris or angle, and dilated fundus examination.

2. IVFA: The more retinal capillary nonperfusion noted on IVFA, the greater the risk of neovascularization.

3. If the diagnosis of CRVO is uncertain, oculopneumoplethysmography or ophthalmodynamometry may help to distinguish CRVO from carotid disease. Ophthalmic artery pressure is low in carotid disease but is normal to increased in CRVO.

Note: It is important to distinguish ischemic from nonischemic CRVO. The presence of a relative APD, decreased b-wave amplitude on ERG, visual field constriction, and visual acuity 20/400 or worse are the most reliable signs of an ischemic CRVO.

Systemic

1. History: Medical problems, medications, eye diseases?

2. Check blood pressure.

3. Blood tests: Fasting blood sugar, glycosylated hemoglobin, CBC with differential, platelets, PT/PTT, ESR, lipid profile, homocysteine, ANA, FTA-ABS.

4. If clinically indicated, consider hemoglobin electrophoresis, Venereal Disease Research Laboratories test (VDRL), cryoglobulins, anti-phospholipid antibodies, lupus anticoagulant, serum protein electrophoresis, and chest radiograph.

5. Complete medical evaluation, with careful attention to the possibility of cardiovascular disease or hypercoagulability.

TREATMENT

1. Discontinue oral contraceptives; change diuretics to other antihypertensive medications if possible.

2. Reduce IOP if increased (e.g., more than 20 mm Hg) in either eye (see 9.1, Primary Open-Angle Glaucoma).

3. Treat underlying medical disorders.

4. If neovascularization of the iris or angle is present, PRP must be performed promptly. PRP should also be considered if neovascularization of the optic nerve or retina are present. Prophylactic PRP is usually not recommended. However, if timely follow-up cannot be assured, prophylactic PRP is a reasonable consideration.

5. Aspirin, 81 to 325 mg p.o., q.d. is often recommended. Although in theory this treatment seems logical, no clinical trials demonstrated efficacy to date.

FOLLOW-UP

1. Visual acuity 20/40 or better. Every 1 to 2 months for the first 6 months, with a gradual tapering of the interval to annual follow-ups.

2. Visual acuity less than 20/200. Every month for the first 6 months, with a gradual taper based on the patient's condition.

3. Undilated gonioscopy looking for neovascularization of the iris, followed by careful dilated fundus examination looking for neovascularization of the disc or retina should be performed at each follow-up visit. Evidence of early neovascularization of the iris should prompt immediate PRP, and monthly follow-up until stabilized or regressed.

4. Patients should be informed that there is an 8% to 10% risk for development of a branch retinal vein occlusion (BRVO) or CRVO in the fellow eye.

BIBLIOGRAPHY

Central Vein Occlusion Study Group. Baseline and early natural history report. The Central Vein Occlusion Study. *Arch Ophthalmol* 1993; 111:1087.

11.8 BRANCH RETINAL VEIN OCCLUSION

SYMPTOMS

Blind spot in the visual field or loss of vision, usually unilateral.

SIGNS

Critical. Superficial hemorrhages in a sector of the retina along a retinal vein. The hemorrhages usually do not cross the horizontal raphe (midline).

Other. Cotton-wool spots, retinal edema, a dilated and tortuous retinal vein, narrowing and sheathing of the adjacent artery, retinal neovascularization, vitreous hemorrhage.

DIFFERENTIAL DIAGNOSIS

• Diabetic retinopathy (Dot-and-blot hemorrhages and microaneurysms extend across the horizontal raphe. Nearly always bilateral. See 13.2, Diabetes Mellitus.).

• Hypertensive retinopathy (Narrowed retinal arterioles. Hemorrhages are not confined to a sector of the retina and usually cross the horizontal raphe. Bilateral in most. See 11.9, Hypertensive Retinopathy.).

ETIOLOGY

Disease of the adjacent arterial wall (usually the result of hypertension, arteriosclerosis, or diabetes) compresses the venous wall at a crossing point.

WORKUP

1. History: Systemic disease, particularly hypertension or diabetes?

2. Complete ocular examination, including dilated retinal examination with indirect ophthalmoscopy to look for retinal neovascularization and a macular examination with a slit lamp and a 60- or 90-diopter lens, or fundus contact lens to detect macular edema.

3. Check blood pressure.

4. Blood tests: fasting blood sugar, CBC with differential and platelets, PT/PTT, and ESR. If clinically indicated, consider a more comprehensive workup (see 11.7, Central Retinal Vein Occlusion).

5. Medical examination (usually performed by an internist to check for cardiovascular disease).

6. An IVFA is obtained after the hemorrhages have cleared or sooner if neovascularization is suspected.

TREATMENT

1. Retinal laser photocoagulation is indicated for:

   —Chronic macular edema (3 to 6 months' duration) reducing vision below 20/40 in the absence of macular capillary nonperfusion. Grid treatment to the area of macular edema is used.

   —Retinal neovascularization: Sector PRP to the ischemic area, as delineated by IVFA evidence of capillary nonperfusion, is performed.

2. Underlying medical problems are treated appropriately.

FOLLOW-UP

Every 1 to 2 months at first, and then every 3 to 12 months, checking for neovascularization and macular edema.

BIBLIOGRAPHY

Branch Retinal Vein Occlusion Study Group. Argon laser photocoagulation for macular edema in branch vein occlusion. *Am J Ophthalmol* 1984;98:271.

Branch Retinal Vein Occlusion Study Group. Argon laser scatter photocoagulation for prevention of neovascularization and vitreous hemorrhage in branch vein occlusion. *Arch Ophthalmol* 1986;104:34.

11.9 HYPERTENSIVE RETINOPATHY

SYMPTOMS

Usually asymptomatic, although may have decreased vision.

SIGNS

Critical. Generalized or localized retinal arteriolar narrowing, almost always bilateral.

Other

• Chronic hypertension: Arteriovenous crossing changes, retinal arteriolar sclerosis ("copper" or "silver" wiring), cotton-wool spots, flame-shaped hemorrhages, arterial macroaneurysms, central or branch occlusion of an artery or vein. Rarely, neovascular complications can develop.

• Acute ("malignant") hypertension: Hard exudates often in a "macular star" configuration, retinal edema, cotton-wool spots, flame-shaped hemorrhages, swelling of the optic nerve head (papilledema). Rarely, RD, vitreous hemorrhage. Focal chorioretinal atrophy (Elschnig spots of choroidal nonperfusion) are a sign of past episodes of acute hypertension.

*Note: When hypertensive changes are found only in one eye, suspect carotid artery obstruction on the side of the normal-appearing eye, sparing the retina from the effects of the hypertension.

DIFFERENTIAL DIAGNOSIS

• Diabetic retinopathy (Hemorrhages are usually dot and blot, microaneurysms are common, vessel attenuation is less common. See 13.2, Diabetes Mellitus.).

• Collagen–vascular disease (May show multiple cotton-wool spots, but few to no other fundus findings characteristic of hypertension.).

• Anemia (Hemorrhage predominates without marked arterial changes.).

• Radiation retinopathy (Can appear similar to hypertension. A history of irradiation to the eye or an adnexal structure such as the brain, sinus, or nasopharynx can usually be elicited. It may develop any time after the radiation therapy, but it most commonly occurs within a few years.).

• CRVO or BRVO (Unilateral, multiple hemorrhages, venous dilatation and tortuosity, no arteriolar narrowing. May be the result of hypertension. See 11.7, Central Retinal Vein Occlusion, or 11.8, Branch Retinal Vein Occlusion.).

ETIOLOGY

• Primary hypertension (No known underlying cause.).

• Secondary hypertension (Typically the result of preeclampsia/eclampsia, pheochromocytoma, kidney disease, adrenal disease, or coarctation of the aorta.).

WORKUP

1. History: Known hypertension, diabetes, or adnexal radiation?

2. Complete ocular examination, particularly dilated fundus examination.

3. Check blood pressure.

4. Refer patient to a medical internist or the emergency department of a hospital. The urgency generally depends on the blood pressure reading and whether the patient is symptomatic. As a general rule, a diastolic blood pressure of 110 to 120 mm Hg or the presence of chest pain, difficulty breathing, headache, change in mental status, or blurred vision with optic disc swelling requires immediate medical attention.

TREATMENT

Control the hypertension (as per the internist).

FOLLOW-UP

Every 2 to 3 months at first, and then every 6 to 12 months.

11.10 OCULAR ISCHEMIC SYNDROME

(CAROTID OCCLUSIVE DISEASE)

SYMPTOMS

Decreased vision, ocular or periorbital pain, afterimages or prolonged recovery of vision after exposure to bright light, may have a history of transient monocular visual loss (amaurosis fugax). Usually unilateral. Typically occurs in patients who are aged 50 to 80 years. Men outnumber women by two to one.

SIGNS

Critical. Although retinal veins are dilated and irregular in caliber, they are typically not tortuous. The retinal arterioles are narrowed. Associated findings include mid-peripheral retinal hemorrhages (80% prevalence), iris neovascularization (66%), and posterior segment neovascularization (37%).

Other. Episcleral injection, corneal edema, mild anterior uveitis, neovascular glaucoma, iris atrophy, cataract, retinal microaneurysms, cotton-wool spots, spontaneous pulsations of the central retinal artery, and cherry-red spot. CRAO may occur.

DIFFERENTIAL DIAGNOSIS

• CRVO (Similar signs, but may have optociliary shunt vessels or edema of the disc and dilated retinal veins that are tortuous and regular in caliber. Decreased vision after exposure to light and orbital pain are not typically found. Ophthalmodynamometry may distinguish this condition from ocular ischemic syndrome. See 11.7, Central Retinal Vein Occlusion.).

• Diabetes (Bilateral, usually symmetric. Retinal hemorrhages usually concentrate in the posterior pole, but may occur first in the periphery; and hard exudates are often present. See 13.2, Diabetes Mellitus.).

• Aortic arch disease (Caused by atherosclerosis, syphilis, or Takayasu arteritis. Produces a clinical picture identical to ocular ischemic syndrome, which is usually bilateral. Examination reveals absent arm and neck pulses, cold hands, and spasm of the arm muscles with exercise.).

ETIOLOGY

• Carotid disease (Usually greater than 90% stenosis.).

• Ophthalmic artery disease (Less common.).

WORKUP

1. History: Previous episodes of transient monocular visual loss? Cold hands or spasm of arm muscles with exercise?

2. Complete ocular examination: Search carefully for neovascularization of the iris, disc, or retina.

3. Medical examination (arm pulses, cardiac and carotid auscultation). Evaluate for hypertension, diabetes, and atherosclerotic disease.

4. Consider IVFA for diagnostic or therapeutic purposes.

5. Noninvasive carotid artery evaluation (e.g., duplex Doppler ultrasonography, oculoplethysmography, magnetic resonance angiography).

6. Consider orbital color Doppler ultrasonography.

7. Consider ophthalmodynamometry if the diagnosis of CRVO cannot be excluded (ophthalmic artery pressure is low in carotid disease but is normal to increased in CRVO).

8. Carotid arteriography is reserved for patients in whom surgery is to be performed.

9. Consider a cardiology consultation, given the high association with cardiac disease.

TREATMENT

Often unsuccessful.

1. Carotid endarterectomy for significant stenosis (refer to neurovascular surgeon).

2. Consider PRP in the presence of neovascularization.

3. Manage glaucoma if present (see 9.14, Neovascular Glaucoma).

4. Control hypertension and diabetes, and reduce cholesterol level (refer to internist).

5. Stop smoking.

FOLLOW-UP

Depends on the age and general health of the patient and the symptoms and signs of disease. Surgical candidates should be evaluated urgently.

11.11 CENTRAL SEROUS CHORIORETINOPATHY

SYMPTOMS

Blurred or dim vision, objects appear distorted and miniature in size, colors appear washed-out, central scotoma. Usually unilateral, sometimes asymptomatic.

SIGNS

Critical. Localized serous detachment of the neurosensory retina in the region of the macula without subretinal blood or lipid exudates. The margins of the detachment are sloping and merge gradually into the attached retina. It is best seen with a fundus contact lens by using a slit lamp.

Other. Visual acuity usually ranges from 20/20 to 20/80, Amsler grid testing reveals distortion of straight lines often with scotoma; a small APD or a serous RPE detachment may be present. May see deposition of subretinal fibrin. Focal pigment epithelial irregularity may mark sites of previous episodes.

DIFFERENTIAL DIAGNOSIS

These entities may produce a serous detachment of the sensory retina in the macular area.

• Age-related macular degeneration (ARMD) [Patient usually older than 50 years, drusen, pigment epithelial alterations, may have a choroidal (subretinal) neovascular membrane (CNVM), of-

ten bilateral. See 11.13 and 11.14, Age-Related Macular Degeneration.].

• Optic pit (The optic disc has a small defect, a pit, in the nerve tissue. A serous RD may be present contiguous with the optic disc. See 11.12, Optic Pit.).

• Macular detachment as a result of an RRD (a hole in the retina can be found; see 11.3, Retinal Detachment) or macular hole.

• Choroidal tumor (A mass is visible by indirect ophthalmoscopy. See 11.32, Malignant Melanoma of the Choroid.).

• Pigment epithelial detachment (PED) [The margins of a PED are more distinct than those of central serous chorioretinopathy (CSCR). Occasionally, PED may accompany CSCR or ARMD.].

• Others (e.g., idiopathic choroidal effusion, inflammatory choroidal disorders).

ETIOLOGY

• Idiopathic (Usually occurs in men aged 25 to 50 years. Patients with lupus have an increased incidence of CSCR. In women, CSCR typically occurs at a slightly older age. There is also an association with pregnancy.).

• Increased endogenous cortisol levels may play a role in the pathogenesis of CSCR. (This helps explain a putative association with psychological or physiologic stress.).

• Exogenous cortisol (i.e., corticosteroid use, including nasal corticosteroid sprays) has also been associated with CSCR; such use should be stopped, if possible.

WORKUP

1. Amsler grid test to document the area of field involved (see Appendix 3).

2. Slit-lamp examination of the macula with a fundus contact, Hruby, or 60- or 90-diopter lens to rule out a concomitant CNVM. In addition, search for an optic pit of the disc.

3. Dilated fundus examination by using indirect ophthalmoscopy to rule out a choroidal tumor or RRD.

4. Consider an IVFA if the diagnosis is uncertain or presentation atypical, a CNVM is suspected, or laser treatment is to be considered.

TREATMENT

The prognosis for spontaneous recovery of visual acuity to at least 20/30 is excellent. The prognosis is worse for patients with recurrent disease, multiple areas of detachment, or prolonged course. Laser therapy has been shown to accelerate visual recovery, but does not improve final visual outcome.

FOLLOW-UP

1. Examine most patients every 6 to 8 weeks until the condition spontaneously resolves or, if no resolution occurs, for 4 to 6 months.

2. Laser photocoagulation may be considered under the following circumstances:

   —Persistence of a serous detachment beyond 4 to 6 months.

   —Recurrence of the condition in an eye that sustained a permanent visual deficit from a previous episode.

   —Occurrence in the contralateral eye after a permanent visual deficit resulted from a previous episode.

   —Patient absolutely requires prompt restoration of vision (e.g., occupational necessity).

3. If laser photocoagulation is to be performed, use low intensity to reduce the chance of iatrogenic CNVM.

11.12 OPTIC PIT

SYMPTOMS

Asymptomatic if isolated. May notice distortion of straight lines or edges, blurred vision, a blind spot, or micropsia if a serous macular detachment develops.

SIGNS

Critical. Small, round depression (usually hypopigmented or gray in appearance) in the nerve tissue of the optic disc. Most are temporal, but approximately one third are central.

Other. May develop a localized detachment of the sensory retina extending from the disc to the macula, usually unilateral.

DIFFERENTIAL DIAGNOSIS

• Acquired pit (pseudopit) (Sometimes seen in patients with low-tension glaucoma or primary open-angle glaucoma. May be accompanied by flame hemorrhages at the disc margin. See 9.1, Primary Open-Angle Glaucoma.).

• Other causes of a serous macular detachment (e.g., CSCR; see 11.11, Central Serous Chorioretinopathy).

WORKUP

1. Optic disc evaluation to detect the pit.

2. Slit-lamp examination of the macula with a fundus contact lens or 60- or 90-diopter lens

to evaluate for a serous macular detachment and to rule out a CNVM.

3. Measure IOP.

4. Consider an IVFA to rule out a CNVM in patients with a serous macular detachment.

TREATMENT

1. **Isolated optic pit:** No treatment required.

2. **Optic pit with a serous macular detachment:** Laser photocoagulation to the temporal margin of the optic disc is used in most cases. Surgery (vitrectomy) may be used in refractory cases.

FOLLOW-UP

1. **Isolated optic pits:** Yearly examination; sooner if symptomatic.

2. **Optic pits with serous macular detachment:** Reexamine every few weeks after treatment to check for resorption of subretinal fluid. Watch for amblyopia in children.

11.13 NONEXUDATIVE (DRY) AGE-RELATED MACULAR DEGENERATION

SYMPTOMS

Gradual loss of central vision, Amsler grid changes; may be asymptomatic.

SIGNS

Critical. Macular drusen, clumps of pigment in the outer retina, and RPE atrophy, almost always in both eyes.

Other. Confluent retinal and choriocapillaris atrophy (e.g., geographic atrophy), dystrophic calcification.

DIFFERENTIAL DIAGNOSIS

• Peripheral drusen (Drusen are located outside of the macular area, not within it.).

• Myopic degeneration (Typically, high myopia with characteristic peripapillary changes in addition to the macular degeneration. Drusen are not seen. See 11.16, High Myopia.).

• CSCR (Parafoveal serous retinal elevation, RPE detachments, and mottled RPE atrophy, without drusen, usually in patients younger than 50 years of age. See 11.11, Central Serous Chorioretinopathy.).

• Inherited central retinal dystrophies (e.g., Stargardt disease, pattern dystrophy, Best disease, others) (Variable macular pigmentary changes, atrophy, or accumulation of lipofuscin or a combination of these. Usually younger than 50 years, without drusen, familial occurrence. See specific entity.).

• Toxic retinopathies (e.g., chloroquine toxicity) [Mottled hypopigmentation with ring of hyperpigmentation (bull's-eye maculopathy) without drusen. History of drug ingestion.].

• Inflammatory maculopathies (e.g., multifocal choroiditis, rubella, serpiginous choroidopathy) (Variable chorioretinal atrophy, often with vitreous cells and without drusen. See specific entity.).

WORKUP

1. Amsler grid to document or detect a central or paracentral scotoma (see Appendix 3).

2. Macular examination with a 60- or 90-diopter or a fundus contact lens: Look for signs of the exudative form.

3. IVFA when exudative ARMD cannot be ruled out clinically, when RPE detachment is present, or when visual acuity has declined rapidly to rule out CNVM. Drusen and RPE atrophy are often more visible on IVFA.

TREATMENT

1. People with intermediate dry ARMD, or advanced dry or exudative ARMD in one eye but not the other eye, are at high risk for development of advanced stages of ARMD. Treatment with a high-dose combination of vitamin C (500 mg), vitamin E (400 IU), beta-carotene (15 mg), and zinc (80 mg) reduces the risk of progression to advanced ARMD by approximately 25%, and reduces the risk of vision loss caused by advanced ARMD by approximately 19% at 5 years. Beta-carotene and zinc supplementation should be withheld in smokers because of a potential increased risk of lung cancer.

2. Low-vision aids may benefit some patients with bilateral loss of macular function.

FOLLOW-UP

Every 6 to 12 months, watching for signs of the exudative form. Patients are given an Amsler grid to take home and use on a daily basis. They are instructed to return immediately if a change is noted on Amsler grid.

11.14   EXUDATIVE (WET) AGE-RELATED MACULAR DEGENERATION

SYMPTOMS

Distortion of straight lines or edges, rapid onset of visual loss, blind spot in the central or paracentral visual field.

SIGNS

Critical. Drusen accompanied by a choroidal (subretinal) neovascularization (CNVM; grayish-green membrane beneath the retina) or RPE detachment.

Other. Subretinal hemorrhages (minimal or extensive), subretinal lipid exudates, subretinal pigment ring, subretinal fibrosis (disciform scar), retinal or vitreous hemorrhage. Nonexudative signs may be present.

RISK FACTORS FOR LOSS OF VISION

Advanced age, hyperopia, blue eyes, family history, soft (larger, ill-defined) drusen, focal pigment clumping, focal hyperpigmentation, RPE detachments, systemic hypertension, smoking.

Note: In patients with wet ARMD in one eye, the risk of a CNVM in the contralateral eye is 10% to 12% per year. Eyes at highest risk are those with multiple or confluent soft drusen with RPE clumping.

DIFFERENTIAL DIAGNOSIS

All of the following are associated with CNVM:

• Ocular histoplasmosis syndrome (Small white–yellow chorioretinal scars are seen in the mid-periphery and posterior pole along with chorioretinal scarring adjacent to the optic disc. See 11.15, Ocular Histoplasmosis.).

• Angioid streaks (Bilateral subretinal red–brown or gray bands of irregular contour that radiate from the optic disc. See 11.17, Angioid Streaks.).

• High myopia (Significant myopic refractive error, lacquer cracks in the posterior pole, myopic disc changes. See 11.16, High Myopia.).

• Polypoidal choroidal vasculopathy [Typically elderly patients with hypertension in whom serosanguineous submacular exudation develops. Indocyanine green (ICG) angiography may highlight choroidal aneurysms. Prognosis is more favorable than exudative ARMD.].

• Traumatic choroidal rupture (History of trauma, usually unilateral; a choroidal tear concentric to the optic disc is often noted. See 3.12, Traumatic Choroidal Rupture.).

- Other conditions disrupting Bruch membrane (Drusen of the optic nerve, choroidal tumors, photocoagulation scars, inflammatory chorioretinal lesions, and idiopathic.).

WORKUP

1. IVFA is performed as soon as possible if CNVM is suspected on clinical examination. IVFA may show well-defined or poorly defined dye leakage. Classic CNVM demonstrates early, well-defined, typically lacy hyperfluorescence, that leaks throughout the study. Occult CNVM demonstrates mid- to late-phase hyperfluorescence, typically mottled, that often is not well defined. Combination lesions of classic and occult CNVM are often observed.

2. ICG angiography may be helpful in delineating the borders of some CNVM, especially in the presence of subretinal blood or exudate.

3. Amsler grid testing to detect and document the degree of central field involved (see Appendix 3).

4. Macular slit-lamp examination with a 60- or 90-diopter, Hruby, or fundus contact lens to detect CNVM. Must examine both eyes.

5. Blood pressure measurement. The presence of systemic hypertension in patients with CNVM appears to have a negative effect on the response to laser therapy.

TREATMENT

Laser photocoagulation should be applied within 72 hours of the IVFA to reduce the risk of severe visual loss in patients with treatable macular CNVM. Thermal laser photocoagulation is used to treat CNVM located greater than 200 μm from the center of the foveal avascular zone (FAZ)[1].

---

[1]The FAZ is an avascular area approximately 500 μm in diameter in the center of the fovea. It is easily observed with IVFA.

Photodynamic therapy with verteporfin has been shown to reduce the rate of moderate vision loss in patients with subfoveal, predominantly classic CNVM due to wet ARMD; visual improvement is uncommon.

FOLLOW-UP

Because of the high rate of neovascular activity after treatment (persistent and new CNVM), treated patients need to be monitored closely, especially during the first posttreatment year:

1. Amsler grid to be used at home daily. The patient is instructed to return immediately if a change is noted.

2. Scheduled examinations at approximately 2 weeks, 6 weeks, 3 months, and 6 months after treatment, and then every 6 months. Careful macular examination is performed as described previously.

3. IVFA is repeated 2 to 3 weeks after treatment and again when recurrent CNVM is suspected.

4. Retreatment with laser photocoagulation should be considered when recurrent CNVM is identified.

5. Risk factors for persistence of CNVM includes incomplete treatment of CNVM.

6. Risk factors for recurrence of CNVM include hypertension, cigarette smoking, contralateral eye with CNVM or disciform scar, or high-risk fundus features (soft drusen and pigment clumping).

BIBLIOGRAPHY

Age-Related Eye Disease Study Research Group. A randomized, placebo-controlled, clinical trial of high-dose supplementation with vitamins C and E, beta carotene, and zinc for age-related macular degeneration and vision loss: AREDS report no. 8. *Arch Ophthalmol* 2001; 119:1417–1736.

11.15 OCULAR HISTOPLASMOSIS

SYMPTOMS

Most often asymptomatic; can present with decreased or distorted vision. Patients often have lived in or visited the Ohio–Mississippi River Valley or areas where histoplasmosis is endemic and are usually in the 20- to 50-year age range.

SIGNS

Critical. Classic triad. Need two of the three to make the diagnosis:

• Yellow–white, punched-out round spots usually less than 1 mm in diameter, deep to the retina in any fundus location ("histo-spots"). Pigment clumps in or at the margin of the spots may be seen.

• A macular CNVM appearing as a gray–green patch beneath the retina, associated with detachment of the sensory retina, subretinal blood or exudate, or a pigment ring evolving into a disciform scar.

• Atrophy or scarring adjacent to the optic disc, sometimes with nodules or hemorrhage. There may be a rim of pigment separating the disc from the area of atrophy or scarring.

Other. Linear rows of small histo-spots in the peripheral fundus. The eye is uninflamed with minimal to no vitreous cells and no aqueous cells or flare.

DIFFERENTIAL DIAGNOSIS

• High myopia [May have atrophic spots in the posterior pole and a myopic crescent on the temporal side of the disc. A CNVM may develop. The atrophic spots are whiter than histo-spots and are not seen beyond the posterior pole. The myopic crescent has a rim of pigment on the outer (not inner) edge, separating the crescent from the retina. May have lacquer cracks. The disc is often tilted. See 11.16, High Myopia.].

• ARMD (The macular changes may appear similar, but typically there are macular drusen and patients are older than 50 years. There are no at-rophic round spots similar to histoplasmosis and no scarring or atrophy around the disc. See 11.13 and 11.14, Age-Related Macular Degeneration.).

• Old toxoplasmosis (White chorioretinal lesion associated with vitreous and sometimes aqueous cells. See 12.5, Toxoplasmosis).

• Angioid streaks (Histo-like spots may be seen in the mid-periphery, and macular degeneration may occur. Jagged red, brown, or gray lines appearing deep to the retinal vessels and radiating from the optic disc are typically seen. Often associated with pseudoxanthoma elasticum, sickle cell anemia, Paget disease, and other rarer systemic diseases. See 11.17, Angioid Streaks.).

• Multifocal choroiditis with panuveitis (Similar clinical findings, except anterior or vitreous inflammatory cells or both are also present. See 12.3, Posterior Uveitis.).

• Multiple evanescent white dot syndrome (Multiple, creamy white lesions at the level of the outer retina or the RPE with granular appearance to the fovea. There are a few vitreous cells and occasional sheathing of vessels. Vision typically returns to normal within weeks without treatment.).

ETIOLOGY

Fungal infection caused by *Histoplasma capsulatum*. Once acquired by inhalation, the organisms can pass to the choroid through the bloodstream.

WORKUP

1. History: Time spent in the Ohio–Mississippi River Valley or endemic area? Prior exposure to fowl?

2. Amsler grid test (see Appendix 3) to evaluate the central visual field of each eye.

3. Slit-lamp examination: Anterior chamber cells and flare should not be present.

4. Dilated fundus examination: Concentrate on the macular area with a slit lamp and fundus

contact, or 60- or 90-diopter lens. Look for signs of CNVM and vitreous cells.

5. IVFA (to help detect or treat a CNVM).

TREATMENT

1. Antifungal treatment is not helpful.

2. For well-defined CNVM seen on IVFA, focal laser photocoagulation is indicated.

3. Surgical removal of CNVM can also be considered when laser is likely to cause visual loss.

FOLLOW-UP

1. Treatment should be instituted within 72 hours of confirming the presence of CNVM by IVFA.

2. All patients (whether they will be, will not be, or have been treated) are to use an Amsler grid daily. Patients are instructed to return immediately if any sudden visual change is noted.

3. Treated patients are seen at 2 to 3 weeks, 4 to 6 weeks, 3 months, and 6 months after treatment and then every 6 months.

4. A careful macular examination is performed at each visit. IVFA is repeated at the 2- to 3-week posttreatment visit and whenever renewed neovascular activity is suspected.

5. Patients without CNVM are seen every 6 months when macular changes are present in one or both eyes and yearly when no macular disease is present in either eye.

11.16 HIGH MYOPIA

SYMPTOMS

Decreased vision (patients are usually beyond the fifth decade of life before progressive decrease in visual acuity occurs).

SIGNS

Critical. Myopic crescent (a crescent-shaped area of white sclera or choroidal vessels adjacent to the disc, separated from the normal-appearing fundus by a hyperpigmented line; this crescent may enlarge with time); an oblique (tilted) insertion of the optic disc, with or without vertical elongation; macular pigmentary abnormalities, a hyperpigmented spot in the macula (Fuchs spot); typically, but not always, a refractive correction of more than 6.00 to 8.00 diopters. Axial length greater than 26 to 27 mm.

Other. Temporal optic disc pallor, posterior staphyloma, entrance of the retinal vessels into the nasal part of the cup, the retina and choroid may be seen to extend over the nasal border of the disc, well-circumscribed areas of atrophy, spots of subretinal hemorrhage, choroidal scle-

rosis, yellow subretinal streaks (lacquer cracks), peripheral retinal thinning, lattice degeneration. A CNVM or RD may develop. Visual field defects may be present. Increased IOP with other evidence for primary open-angle glaucoma may be seen.

DIFFERENTIAL DIAGNOSIS

• ARMD (May develop CNVM and a similar macular appearance, but typically drusen are present, and the myopic features of the optic disc described previously are absent. See 11.13 and 11.14, Age-Related Macular Degeneration.).

• Ocular histoplasmosis [May develop CNVM and exhibit a peripapillary scar. A pigmented ring may separate the disc from the peripapillary atrophy, as opposed to pigmented ring separating the atrophic area from the adjacent retina. Round choroidal scars (punched-out lesions) are often seen scattered throughout the fundus. See 11.15, Ocular Histoplasmosis.].

• Tilted discs [Anomalous discs with a scleral crescent, most often inferonasally, an irregular vascular pattern as the vessels emerge from the disc (situs inversus), and an area of fundus ectasia in the direction of the tilt (inferonasally). Many patients have myopia and astigmatism. They do not have chorioretinal degeneration or lacquer cracks. Visual field defects corresponding to the areas of fundus ectasia are often seen. Most cases are bilateral.].

• Gyrate atrophy (Rare. Multiple, well-demarcated areas of chorioretinal atrophy beginning in the mid-periphery in childhood and then coalescing to involve a large portion of the fundus. Blood levels of ornithine are markedly increased. Patients are often highly myopic. Autosomal recessive. See 11.26, Gyrate Atrophy.).

• Toxoplasmosis (Well-circumscribed chorioretinal scar that does not typically develop CNVM; active disease shows retinitis and vitritis. See 12.5, Toxoplasmosis.).

WORKUP

1. Manifest or cycloplegic refraction, or both.

2. IOP measurement by applanation tonometry (Schiøtz tonometry may underestimate IOP in highly myopic eyes).

3. Dilated retinal examination, by using indirect ophthalmoscopy to search for retinal breaks or detachment. Scleral depression helps to reveal the far peripheral retina, but should not be performed over a staphyloma.

4. Slit-lamp and fundus contact, or 60- or 90-diopter lens examination of the macula, searching for CNVM (dirty gray or green lesion beneath the retina, subretinal blood or exudate, or subretinal fluid).

5. IVFA when a CNVM is suspected.

6. Formal visual field examinations (e.g., Humphrey, Octopus) to document field stability or change when glaucoma is suspected.

TREATMENT

1. Symptomatic retinal breaks are treated with laser photocoagulation, cryotherapy, or scleral buckling surgery. Treatment of asymptomatic retinal breaks may be considered when there is no surrounding pigmentation or demarcation line.

2. Extrafoveal or juxtafoveal CNVM may be considered for laser photocoagulation therapy within several days of obtaining an IVFA (see 11.13 and 11.14, Age-Related Macular Degeneration).

3. For glaucoma suspects, a single visual field often cannot distinguish myopic visual field loss from early glaucoma. Progression of visual field loss in the absence of progressive myopia, however, suggests the presence of glaucoma and the need for therapy (see 9.1, Primary Open-Angle Glaucoma).

4. Recommend wearing one-piece polycarbonate safety glasses for sports because there is an increased risk of choroidal rupture from minor trauma.

FOLLOW-UP

In the absence of complications, reexamine every 6 to 12 months, watching for the related disorders discussed earlier.

11.17 ANGIOID STREAKS

SYMPTOMS

Usually asymptomatic; decreased vision may result from CNVM.

SIGNS

Critical. Bilateral reddish brown or gray bands located deep to the retina, usually radiating in an irregular or spokelike pattern from the optic disc. CNVM leading to macular degeneration may occur.

Other. Mottled background fundus appearance (*peau d'orange*), most common in the temporal mid-periphery; subretinal hemorrhages after mild blunt trauma; reticular pigmentary changes in the macula; small, white, pinpoint chorioretinal scars (histo-like spots) in the mid-periphery; drusen of the optic disc (especially with pseudoxanthoma elasticum); granular pattern of hyperfluorescent lines on IVFA.

DIFFERENTIAL DIAGNOSIS

• Myopic chorioretinal degeneration (lacquer cracks) (High myopia, often with a tilted disc and peripapillary atrophy; may have macular degeneration. See 11.16, High Myopia.).

• Choroidal rupture (Subretinal streaks are usually concentric to the optic disc, yellow–white in color, and result from blunt ocular trauma. See 3.12, Traumatic Choroidal Rupture.).

ETIOLOGY

Fifty percent of cases are associated with systemic diseases; the remainder are idiopathic.

• Pseudoxanthoma elasticum (Most common. Loose skin folds in the neck, axillae, and on flexor aspects of joints, cardiovascular complications, increased risk of gastrointestinal bleeds.).

• Paget disease (Enlarged skull, bone pain, history of bone fractures, hearing loss, possible cardiovascular complications. May be asymptomatic. Increased serum alkaline phosphatase and urine calcium. Ten percent develop angioid streaks late; may develop visual loss due to optic nerve compression by enlarging bone.).

• Sickle cell disease [May be asymptomatic; may have decreased vision from fundus abnormalities (see 11.23, Sickle Cell Disease), or may have a history of recurrent infections or painless or painful crises. Positive sickle cell preparation and abnormal hemoglobin electrophoresis.].

• Ehlers–Danlos syndrome (Hyperelasticity of skin, loose joints.).

• Less common (Acromegaly, senile elastosis, lead poisoning, Marfan syndrome.).

WORKUP

1. History: Any known systemic disorders? Previous ocular trauma?

2. Complete ocular examination: Look carefully at the macula with a slit lamp and a 60- or 90-diopter, or a fundus contact lens to detect choroidal neovascularization.

3. IVFA if uncertain of the diagnosis or if CNVM is suspected.

4. Physical examination: Look for clinical signs of etiologic diseases.

5. Serum alkaline phosphatase and urine calcium levels if Paget disease is suspected.

6. Sickle cell preparation and hemoglobin electrophoresis in African-American patients.

7. Skin or scar biopsy if pseudoxanthoma elasticum is suspected.

TREATMENT

1. Focal laser photocoagulation for treatable choroidal neovascularization (see 11.13 and 11.14, Age-Related Macular Degeneration).

2. Management of any underlying systemic disease, if present, by a medical internist.

3. Recommend wearing one-piece polycarbonate safety glasses for sports because there is an increased risk of choroidal rupture from minor trauma.

FOLLOW-UP

1. Fundus examination every 6 months, observing for CNVM.

2. Amsler grid (see Appendix 3) is to be used at home on a daily basis. Patients are instructed to return immediately if a change is noted on Amsler grid.

11.18 CYSTOID MACULAR EDEMA

SYMPTOMS

Decreased vision.

SIGNS

Critical. Irregularity and blurring of the foveal light reflex, thickening with or without small intraretinal cysts in the foveal region.

Other. Loss of the choroidal vascular pattern underlying the macula. Vitreous cells, optic nerve swelling, and dot hemorrhage can appear in severe cases. A lamellar macular hole causing permanent visual loss can develop.

ETIOLOGY

• After any type of ocular surgery (including laser photocoagulation and cryotherapy) (The peak incidence after cataract surgery is approximately 6 to 10 weeks; the incidence increases with surgical complications including vitreous to the wound, iris prolapse, and vitreous loss.).

• Diabetic retinopathy.

• CRVOs and BRVOs.

• Uveitis (particularly pars planitis; see 12.2, Pars Planitis).

• Retinitis pigmentosa (RP).

• Topical drops (e.g., epinephrine, dipivefrin, and latanoprost) drops, especially in patients who have undergone cataract surgery (often reversed by discontinuing the drops).

• Retinal vasculitis (e.g., Eales disease, Behçet syndrome, sarcoidosis, necrotizing angiitis, multiple sclerosis, cytomegalovirus retinitis).

• Retinal telangiectases (e.g., Coats disease).

• ARMD.

• Associated with other conditions (occult inferior RRD or occult, foveal CNVM).

• Others (intraocular tumors, systemic hypertension, collagen–vascular disease, surface-wrinkling retinopathy, autosomal dominant CME, others).

• Pseudo-CME [No leakage on IVFA (e.g., nicotinic acid maculopathy [relatively high doses of nicotinic acid are used to treat hypercholesterolemia]), X-linked retinoschisis, Goldmann–Favre disease, pseudohole from an epiretinal membrane.].

WORKUP

1. History: Recent intraocular surgery? Diabetes? Previous uveitis or eye inflammation? Night blindness or family history of eye disease? Medications, including topical epinephrine, dipivefrin, or latanoprost?

2. Complete ocular examination, including a peripheral fundus evaluation (scleral depression inferiorly may be required to detect pars planitis). A macular examination is best performed with a slit lamp and a fundus contact lens, a Hruby lens, or a 60- or 90-diopter lens.

3. IVFA often shows early leakage of dye out of perifoveal capillaries and late macular staining, classically in a flower-petal or spoke-wheel pattern. Optic nerve head leakage is sometimes observed. Fluorescein leakage does not occur in nicotinic acid maculopathy.

4. Other diagnostic tests when indicated (e.g., fasting blood sugar or glucose tolerance test, ERG).

Note: Subclinical CME commonly develops after cataract extraction and is noted on IVFA. These cases are not treated.

TREATMENT

Seventy percent of postcataract CME cases resolve spontaneously within 6 months; treat if symptomatic with decreased vision.

1. Treat the underlying disorder if possible.

2. Topical nonsteroidal antiinflammatory drug (NSAID; e.g., ketorolac, q.i.d.) for 3 months (other topical NSAIDs not yet approved for CME).

3. Discontinue topical epinephrine, dipivefrin, or Xalatan drops and medications containing nicotinic acid.

4. Consider acetazolamide, 500 mg p.o., q.d., especially for postoperative patients, but also for those with RP and uveitis.

5. Other forms of therapy that have unproven efficacy but are occasionally used:

—Systemic NSAIDs (e.g., indomethacin, 25 mg p.o., t.i.d., for 6 weeks).

—Topical steroids (e.g., prednisolone acetate, 1%, q.i.d., for 3 weeks, and then taper over 3 weeks); may work best if used in combination with ketorolac.

—Systemic steroids (e.g., prednisone, 40 mg p.o., q.d., for 5 days, and then taper over 2 weeks).

—Subtenon steroid (e.g., methylprednisolone 80 mg/mL, in 0.5 mL).

—Diabetic macular edema may benefit from focal laser treatment (see 13.2, Diabetes Mellitus).

—Macular edema persisting for 3 to 6 months after a BRVO and reducing vision below 20/40 may improve with laser photocoagulation (see 11.8, Branch Retinal Vein Occlusion).

—Macular edema with or without vitreous incarceration in a surgical wound may be improved by vitrectomy or yttrium-aluminum garnet (YAG) laser lysis of the vitreous strand.

—Macular edema from pars planitis is often treated with steroids when vision is reduced below 20/40 (see 12.2, Pars Planitis).

FOLLOW-UP

Postsurgical CME is not an emergency condition. Other forms of macular edema may require an etiologic workup and may benefit from early treatment (e.g., elimination of nicotinic acid–containing medications).

11.19 MACULAR HOLE

SYMPTOMS

Decreased vision, typically around the 20/200 level for a full-thickness hole, better for a partial-thickness hole; sometimes distortion of vision or central scotoma. Three times more likely in women; usually occurs in sixth to eighth decade.

SIGNS

Critical. A round, red spot in the center of the macula, usually from one third to two thirds of a disc diameter in size, surrounded by a gray halo (marginal RD). A stage 1 idiopathic premacular hole demonstrates loss of the normal foveolar depression and often a yellow spot or ring in the center of the macula.

Other. Small, yellow precipitates in the hole, deep to the retina; retinal cysts at the margin of the hole or a small operculum above the hole, anterior to the retina (stage 4); or both.

Note: A partial-thickness (lamellar) hole is not so red and the surrounding gray halo is usually not present.

DIFFERENTIAL DIAGNOSIS

• Macular pucker with a pseudohole [An epiretinal membrane (surface wrinkling) on the surface of the retina may simulate a macular hole.].

• Solar retinopathy (Small, round, red or yellow lesion at the center of the fovea, with surrounding fine gray pigment in a sun-gazer or eclipse watcher.).

• Intraretinal cysts (e.g., chronic CME with prominent central cyst).

ETIOLOGY

May be caused by vitreous or epiretinal membrane traction on the macula, trauma, or CME; 10% bilateral.

WORKUP

1. History: Previous trauma? Previous eye surgery? Sun-gazer?

2. Complete ocular examination, including a macular examination with a slit lamp and 60- or 90-diopter lens, or fundus contact lens. Because many patients with macular hole have a PVD, examination of the peripheral fundus to rule out peripheral breaks is important.

3. A true macular hole can be differentiated from a pseudohole by directing a thin, vertical slit beam across the area in question by using a 60- or 90-diopter lens with the slit-lamp biomicroscope. The patient with a true hole will report a break in the line (Watzke–Allen test). A pseudohole may cause distortion of the line, but it should not be broken.

4. IVFA in stage 2 to 4 macular holes shows early foveal hyperfluorescence.

5. Optical coherence tomography helpful in ambiguous cases.

TREATMENT

1. Fifty percent of stage 1 premacular holes resolve spontaneously.

2. In selected cases of more advanced macular hole, vitrectomy may be beneficial. It is preferable to operate within the first 6 months of onset with the possibility of regaining half of the visual angle. The risk of RD is very small. However, symptoms of an RD (e.g., sudden increase in flashes and floaters, abundant "cobwebs" in the vision, or a curtain coming across the field of vision) are explained to patients, particularly those with high myopia. It is in the latter group that the macular hole sometimes leads to an RD, which requires surgical repair.

FOLLOW-UP

1. Patients with high myopia are seen every 6 months.

2. Other patients may be seen yearly.

3. All patients are seen sooner if RD symptoms develop.

4. Because there is a small risk that the condition may develop in the contralateral eye, patients are given an Amsler grid for periodic home monitoring.

11.20 EPIRETINAL MEMBRANE

(MACULAR PUCKER, SURFACE-WRINKLING RETINOPATHY)

SYMPTOMS

Most are asymptomatic; can have decreased or distorted vision or both. Typically occurs in middle-aged or elderly patients. Twenty percent bilateral. Development of epiretinal membrane in fellow eye unlikely if PVD already present in that eye.

SIGNS

Critical. Spectrum ranges from a fine, glistening membrane (cellophane maculopathy) to a thick, gray–white membrane (macular pucker) present on the surface of the retina in the macular area.

Note: When the epiretinal membrane is thin, it is often best appreciated with a 60- or 90-diopter lens. A glistening sparkle, much like cellophane, may be observed in the macular area.

Other. Retinal folds radiating out from the membrane, displacement or straightening of the macular retinal vessels, macular edema or detachment, signs of other ocular disease. A round, dark condensation of the epiretinal membrane in the macula may simulate a macular hole (termed *pseudohole*).

DIFFERENTIAL DIAGNOSIS

• Diabetic retinopathy (May produce preretinal fibrovascular tissue, which may displace retinal vessels or detach the macula. Macular edema may be present. Hemorrhages and microaneurysms are usually also found, and the changes are commonly bilateral.).

• CME.

ETIOLOGY

• Idiopathic.

• Retinal break, RRD.

• PVD.

• After retinal cryotherapy or photocoagulation.

• After intraocular surgery or trauma.

• Uveitis.

• Diabetic retinopathy.

• Other retinal vascular disease.

WORKUP

1. History: Previous eye surgery or eye disease? Diabetes?

2. Complete ocular examination, particularly a thorough dilated fundus evaluation. The macula is often best seen with a slit lamp and a 60- or 90-diopter, Hruby, or fundus contact lens.

TREATMENT

1. Treat the underlying disorder.

2. Surgical peeling of the membrane can be considered when it significantly reduces the vision.

FOLLOW-UP

This is not an emergency condition, and treatment may be instituted at any time. Infrequently, membranes separate from the retina, resulting in spontaneously improved vision. A small percentage of epiretinal membranes recur after surgical removal.

11.21 CHOROIDAL DETACHMENT

SYMPTOMS

Decreased vision or asymptomatic in a serous choroidal detachment. Moderate to severe pain, decreased vision may occur if the choroidal detachments are touching ("kissing choroidals"), or hemorrhagic. Red eye may also occur with a hemorrhagic choroidal detachment.

SIGNS

Critical. Smooth, bullous, orange–brown elevation of the retina and choroid that usually extends 360 degrees around the periphery in a lobular configuration. The ora serrata can be seen without scleral depression.

Other. Serous choroidal detachment: Low IOP (often less than 6 mm Hg), shallow anterior chamber with mild cell and flare, positive transillumination. Hemorrhagic choroidal detachment: High IOP (if detachment is large), shallow anterior chamber with mild cell and flare, no transillumination.

DIFFERENTIAL DIAGNOSIS

• Melanoma of the ciliary body (Not typically multilobular or symmetric in each quadrant of the globe. Pigmented melanomas do not transilluminate. B-scan ultrasonography may help to differentiate between the two. See 11.32, Malignant Melanoma of the Choroid.).

• RRD (Appears white and undulates with eye movements. A break is usually seen in the retina, and pigment cells are often present in the vitreous. See 11.3, Retinal Detachment.).

ETIOLOGY

Serous

• Intraoperative or postoperative (Wound leak, perforation of the sclera from a superior rectus bridle suture, iritis, cyclodialysis cleft, leakage or excess filtration from a filtering bleb, or after laser photocoagulation or cryotherapy. May occur days to weeks after the surgery.).

• Traumatic (Often associated with a ruptured globe.).

• RRD or after scleral buckling repair of a detachment.

• Rare (Nanophthalmos, uveal effusion syndrome, carotid–cavernous fistula, primary or metastatic tumor, scleritis, VKH syndrome.).

Hemorrhagic

• Intraoperative or postoperative (From anterior displacement of the ocular contents and rupture of the short posterior ciliary arteries.).

• Spontaneous (e.g., after perforation of a corneal ulcer).

WORKUP

1. History: Recent ocular surgery or trauma? Known eye or medical problem?

2. Slit-lamp examination: Check for the presence of a filtering bleb and perform Seidel test to rule out a wound leak (see Appendix 4).

3. Gonioscopy of the anterior chamber angle: Look for a cyclodialysis cleft.

4. Dilated retinal examination: Determine whether there is subretinal fluid, indicating a concomitant RD, and whether an underlying choroidal disease or tumor is present. Examination of the contralateral eye may be helpful in diagnosis.

5. In cases suggestive of melanoma, B-scan ultrasonography and transillumination of the globe are helpful in making a diagnosis. B-scan ultrasonography is also useful to distinguish between serous and hemorrhagic choroidal detachment.

6. Check the skin for vitiligo and the head for alopecia (VKH syndrome).

TREATMENT

General Treatment

1. Cycloplegic (e.g., atropine, 1%, t.i.d.).

2. Topical steroid (e.g., prednisolone acetate, 1%, four to six times per day).

3. Surgical drainage of the suprachoroidal fluid may be indicated for a flat or progressively shallow anterior chamber, particularly in the presence of inflammation (because of the risk of peripheral anterior synechiae), corneal decompensation resulting from lens–cornea touch, or "kissing" choroidals (apposition of two lobules of detached choroid).

Specific Treatment

Repair the underlying problem.

1. **Serous**

   —Wound leak or leaky filtering bleb: Patch for 24 hours, suture the site, use cyanoacry-

late glue, or place a bandage contact lens on the eye, or a combination of these.

   —Cyclodialysis cleft: Laser therapy, diathermy, cryotherapy, or suture the cleft to close it.

   —Uveitis: Topical cycloplegic and steroid as discussed previously.

   —Inflammatory disease: See the specific entity.

   —RD: Surgical repair. Proliferative vitreoretinopathy after repair is common.

2. **Hemorrhagic:** An anterior vitrectomy and drainage of the choroidal detachment is performed for severe cases with retina or vitreous to the wound. Otherwise use general treatment.

FOLLOW-UP

In accordance with the underlying problem.

11.22   VITREOUS HEMORRHAGE

SYMPTOMS

Sudden, painless loss of vision or sudden appearance of black spots with flashing lights.

SIGNS

Critical. In a severe vitreous hemorrhage, the red fundus reflex may be absent, and there may be no fundus view on ophthalmoscopy. Red blood cells can sometimes be appreciated when a slit lamp is focused posterior to the lens. In a mild vitreous hemorrhage, blood may be seen to obscure part of the retina and retinal vessels. Chronic vitreous hemorrhage has a yellow ochre appearance resulting from the breakdown of hemoglobin.

Other. A mild APD is possible. Depending on the etiology, there may be other fundus abnormalities.

DIFFERENTIAL DIAGNOSIS

• Vitritis (white blood cells in the vitreous) (The onset is rarely as sudden as in vitreous hemorrhage; anterior or posterior uveitis may also be present. No red blood cells are seen in the vitreous. See 12.3, Posterior Uveitis.).

• RD (May occur without a vitreous hemorrhage, yet the symptoms may be identical. The fundus view may be difficult in a highly elevated detachment; however, the retina can usually be viewed with an indirect ophthalmoscope. In cases of highly elevated detachments, slit-lamp examination may show the retina behind the lens. See 11.3, Retinal Detachment.).

ETIOLOGY

• Diabetic retinopathy (Almost always have a known history of diabetes and usually one of diabetic retinopathy. Diabetic retinopathy is usually evident in the contralateral eye. See 13.2, Diabetes Mellitus.).

- Retinal break (Commonly superior in cases of dense vitreous hemorrhage. This may be demonstrated by ultrasonography and scleral depression. See 11.2, Retinal Break.).

- RD (May be diagnosed by ultrasound if the retina cannot be viewed on clinical examination. See 11.3, Retinal Detachment.).

- Retinal vein occlusion (usually a BRVO) (Commonly occurs in older patients with a history of high blood pressure. May have a history of a vein occlusion or sudden visual loss in the eye months to years previously. See 11.8, Branch Retinal Vein Occlusion.).

- PVD (Common in middle-aged or elderly patients. Usually, patients note floaters and flashing lights. See 11.1, Posterior Vitreous Detachment.).

- ARMD, wet (Patients often acknowledge poor vision before the vitreous hemorrhage as a result of their underlying disease. Macular drusen or other findings of ARMD or both are found in the contralateral eye. May use B-scan ultrasonography to aid in the diagnosis. See 11.13 and 11.14, Age-Related Macular Degeneration.).

- Sickle cell disease (particularly SC disease) (African-American patients. May have peripheral retinal neovascularization in the contralateral eye, typically in a "sea-fan" configuration and salmon color. See 11.24, Sickle Cell Disease.).

- Trauma (by history).

- Intraocular tumor (May be visible on ophthalmoscopy or B-scan ultrasonography. See 5.13, Malignant Melanoma of the Iris, and 11.32, Malignant Melanoma of the Choroid.).

- Subarachnoid or subdural hemorrhage (Terson syndrome) (Frequently bilateral preretinal or vitreous hemorrhages may occur. A severe headache usually precedes the fundus findings. Coma may occur.).

- Eales disease (Usually occurs in men aged 20 to 30 years with peripheral retinal ischemia and neovascularization of unknown etiology. Decreased vision as a result of vitreous hemorrhage is frequently the presenting sign. The disease is often bilateral and is a diagnosis of exclusion.).

- Others (Coats disease, retinopathy of prematurity, retinal capillary angiomas of von Hippel–Lindau syndrome, congenital prepapillary vascular loop, retinal cavernous hemangioma, hypertension, radiation retinopathy, anterior segment hemorrhage because of an intraocular lens, bleeding diathesis, others.).

Note: In infancy and childhood consider birth trauma, shaken baby syndrome, traumatic child abuse, juvenile X-linked retinoschisis, pars planitis.

WORKUP

1. History: Any ocular or systemic diseases, specifically the ones mentioned previously? Trauma?

2. Complete ocular examination, including a slit-lamp examination to check for iris neovascularization, IOP measurement, and a dilated fundus examination of both eyes by using indirect ophthalmoscopy. In cases of spontaneous vitreous hemorrhage, scleral depression is performed if a retinal view can be obtained (we do not usually depress eyes until 2 weeks after traumatic hemorrhages.).

3. When no retinal view can be obtained, B-scan ultrasonography is performed to detect an associated RD or intraocular tumor. Flap retinal tears may be detected with scleral depression and sometimes seen on B-scan ultrasonography.

4. IVFA may aid in defining the etiology, although the quality of the angiogram may depend on the density of the hemorrhage.

TREATMENT

1. If the etiology of the vitreous hemorrhage is not known and a retinal break or a RD or both cannot be ruled out (e.g., there is no known history of one of the diseases mentioned previously, there are no changes in

the contralateral eye, and the fundus is obscured by a total vitreous hemorrhage), the patient is monitored closely as an outpatient.

2. Bed rest with the head of the bed elevated (and sometimes bilateral patching) for 2 to 3 days (this reduces the chance of recurrent bleeding and allows the blood to settle inferiorly, permitting a view of the superior peripheral fundus, a common site for responsible retinal breaks).

3. Eliminate aspirin, NSAIDs, and other anticlotting agents unless they are medically necessary.

4. The underlying etiology is treated as soon as possible (e.g., retinal breaks are sealed with cryotherapy or laser photocoagulation, detached retinas are repaired, and proliferative retinal vascular diseases are treated with laser photocoagulation or cryotherapy when there is no retinal view).

5. Surgical removal of the blood (vitrectomy) is usually performed for:

—Vitreous hemorrhage accompanied by RD or break seen on B-scan ultrasonography.

—Chronic vitreous hemorrhage (more than 3 to 6 months in duration).

—Vitreous hemorrhage with neovascularization of the iris.

—Hemolytic or ghost cell glaucoma.

Note: Vitrectomy for isolated vitreous hemorrhage (e.g., without RD) may be considered earlier than 6 months for diabetic patients or those with bilateral vitreous hemorrhage, depending on their visual needs.

FOLLOW-UP

The patient is evaluated daily for the first 2 to 3 days. If a total vitreous hemorrhage persists, and the etiology remains unknown, the patient is followed up with B-scan ultrasonography every 1 to 3 weeks to rule out an RD.

11.23   SICKLE CELL DISEASE

(INCLUDING SC, SICKLE TRAIT)

SYMPTOMS

Usually without ocular symptoms. May have floaters, flashing lights, or loss of vision with advanced disease. Systemically, patients with sickle cell anemia often have painful crises with severe abdominal or musculoskeletal discomfort. Patients are of African or Mediterranean extraction in most cases.

SIGNS

Critical. Peripheral retinal neovascularization in the shape of a fan ("sea-fan" sign), sclerosed peripheral retinal vessels, or an abnormal, dull gray peripheral fundus background color (as a result of peripheral arteriolar occlusions and ischemia).

Other. Tortuosity of retinal veins, black midperipheral fundus lesions with spiculated borders (black sunbursts), intraretinal and subretinal hemorrhages (salmon patch), refractile (iridescent) intraretinal deposits, angioid streaks, comma-shaped capillaries of the conjunctiva (especially along the inferior fornix). Vitreous hemorrhage and traction bands, RD, CRAO, and macular arteriolar occlusions may develop.

Note: Proliferative sickle cell retinopathy is thought to progress from peripheral arteriolar occlusions (stage 1) to peripheral arteriovenous anastomoses (stage 2) to retinal neovascularization (stage 3). The retinal neovascularization may spontaneously regress or may produce vitreous hemorrhage (stage 4) or TRD (stage 5).

DIFFERENTIAL DIAGNOSIS

(Other causes of peripheral retinal neovascularization.)

• Sarcoidosis (May also produce peripheral seafan neovascularization in young black individuals. However, granulomatous uveitis, vitritis with vitreous opacities, and sheathing of retinal veins are often present. See 12.6, Sarcoidosis.).

• Diabetes (Tends to have a more posterior location, dot/blot hemorrhages, and increased blood sugar. See 13.2, Diabetes Mellitus.).

• BRVO [Flame-shaped hemorrhages involving a sector or one half of the retina (the inferior or superior half); the hemorrhages do not cross the horizontal raphe. May see a sclerosed arteriole only in late stages. See 11.8, Branch Retinal Vein Occlusion.].

• Embolic (e.g., talc) retinopathy (History of intravenous drug abuse. May see refractile talc particles in the macular arterioles.).

• Eales' disease (Peripheral retinal vascular occlusion of unknown etiology; a diagnosis of exclusion.).

• Others (Retinopathy of prematurity, familial exudative vitreoretinopathy, chronic myelogenous leukemia, radiation retinopathy, pars planitis, carotid–cavernous fistula, ocular ischemic syndrome, collagen–vascular disease.).

WORKUP

1. Medical history and family history: Sickle cell disease, diabetes, or known medical problems? Intravenous drug abuse?

2. Dilated fundus examination by using indirect ophthalmoscopy.

3. Sickle cell preparation and hemoglobin electrophoresis (patients with sickle cell trait, as well as hemoglobin C disease, may have a negative Sickledex preparation).

4. Consider IVFA to aid in diagnostic and therapeutic considerations.

TREATMENT

There are no well-established indications or guidelines for treatment. The presence of retinal neovascularization, vitreous hemorrhage, or RD, however, typically warrants treatment. Laser photocoagulation or retinal surgery is typically performed.

FOLLOW-UP

1. No retinal disease present: Repeat dilated fundus examination yearly.

2. Retinal disease present: Repeat dilated fundus examination every 1 to 6 months, depending on severity.

11.24 RETINITIS PIGMENTOSA

SYMPTOMS

Difficulty with night vision (often night blindness) and loss of peripheral vision are most common. Poor central vision and color vision are late findings.

SIGNS

Critical. Classically, clumps of pigment dispersed throughout the peripheral retina in a perivascular pattern, often assuming a "bone spicule" arrangement, areas of depigmentation or atrophy of the RPE, narrowing of arterioles, vitreous cells, and, later, optic disc pallor. Vitreous opacities and cells are the most consistent sign in RP because certain subtypes of RP have little or no pigment deposition at all. Patients have progressive visual field loss, usually a ring scotoma, which progresses to a small central field. Results of ERG are usually moderately to markedly reduced.

Other. Focal or sectoral pigment clumping, CME, epiretinal membrane, posterior subcapsular cataract.

Inheritance Patterns

• Autosomal recessive (most common): Diminished vision and night blindness occur early in life. Visual loss is severe.

• Autosomal dominant: More gradual onset of RP, typically in adult life, variable penetrance, late onset of cataract. Visual loss less severe.

• X-linked recessive (most disabling): Onset similar to autosomal recessive. Female carriers often have salt-and-pepper fundus. Visual loss is severe.

SYSTEMIC DISEASES ASSOCIATED WITH HEREDITARY RETINAL DEGENERATION

Many systemic diseases and syndromes are associated with RP. The following is a short list of those syndromes for which treatment may be beneficial.

REFSUM DISEASE (PHYTANOYL-CoA HYDROXYLASE DEFICIENCY)

Autosomal recessive RP with increased serum phytanic acid level. May have cerebellar ataxia, progressive weakness of distal extremities, deafness, dry skin, anosmia, or progressive restriction of ocular motility.

TREATMENT

1. Give a low-phytanic acid, low-phytol diet (minimize the amount of milk products, animal fats, and green leafy vegetables in the patient's diet).

2. Examine serum phytanic acid levels every 6 months.

HEREDITARY ABETALIPOPROTEINEMIA (BASSEN–KORNZWEIG SYNDROME)

RP with fat intolerance, diarrhea, crenated erythrocytes (acanthocytes), ataxia, progressive restriction of ocular motility, and other neurologic symptoms as a result of deficiency in lipoproteins and malabsorption of the fat-soluble vitamins A, D, E, and K. Diagnosis based on serum apolipoprotein-B deficiency.

TREATMENT

1. Water-miscible vitamin A, 10,000 to 15,000 IU, p.o., q.d.

2. Vitamin E, 200 to 300 IU/kg, p.o., q.d.

3. Vitamin K, 5 mg, p.o., weekly.

4. Restrict dietary fat to 15% of caloric intake.

5. Biannual serum levels of vitamins A and E; yearly ERG, dark adaptometry, and PT; periodic nerve conduction studies.

6. Consider supplementing the patient's diet with zinc.

KEARNS–SAYRE SYNDROME

Pigmentary degeneration of the retina, often salt-and-pepper in appearance, with normal arterioles, progressive limitation of ocular movement, ptosis, and, later, heart block. Ocular signs usually appear before age 20 years. Transmitted by mitochondrial DNA. See 10.11, Chronic Progressive External Ophthalmoplegia.

TREATMENT

Refer the patient to a cardiologist for yearly ECGs. Patients may need a pacemaker.

DIFFERENTIAL DIAGNOSIS

Pseudoretinitis Pigmentosa

Disorders that produce a fundus picture similar to that of RP.

• Phenothiazine toxicity (Especially in patients taking more than 800 mg/day of thioridazine.).

• Syphilis (Positive FTA-ABS, asymmetric visual fields, abnormal fundus appearance, may have a history of recurrent uveitis, no family history of RP; the ERG is usually preserved to some degree.).

• Congenital rubella (A salt-and-pepper fundus appearance may be accompanied by microphthalmos, cataract, deafness, a congenital heart abnormality, or another systemic abnormality. The ERG is usually normal.).

• After resolution of a RD (e.g., toxemia of pregnancy or Harada disease) (The history is diagnostic.).

- Pigmented paravenous retinochoroidal atrophy [Paravenous localization of RPE degeneration and pigment deposition. No definite hereditary pattern. Variable visual fields and ERG (usually normal). May be nonprogressive, but long-term follow-up is not available.].

- After severe blunt trauma (Usually due to spontaneous resolution of RD.).

- After ophthalmic artery occlusion.

Note: The pigment abnormalities are at the level of the RPE with phenothiazine toxicity, syphilis, and congenital rubella. With resolved RD, the pigment is intraretinal.

Other Causes of Nyctalopia (Night Blindness)

- Gyrate atrophy [The fundus shows well-demarcated, scalloped areas of full-thickness atrophy, white–yellow in appearance, with thin margins of pigment outlining the areas of atrophy; the changes extend from the periphery toward the macula. Patients have high levels of ornithine in their blood (often ten times normal levels), urine, aqueous humor, and cerebrospinal fluid. Abnormal or nonrecordable ERG, visual field defects, high myopia, and cataracts are common. Autosomal recessive. See 11.26, Gyrate Atrophy.].

- Choroideremia (Choroidal atrophy accompanies scattered, small pigment granules, sparing the macula. Bone spicules are not seen. X-linked recessive. See 11.25, Choroideremia.).

- Vitamin A deficiency [Usually acquired from malnutrition or surgical resection of the bowel, but may be inherited (familial carotinemia). Marked night blindness; numerous small, yellow–white, well-demarcated spots deep in the retina seen peripherally; dry eye and/or Bitot spots (white lesions) on the conjunctiva. See 13.11, Vitamin A Deficiency.].

- Zinc deficiency [May cause abnormal dark adaptation (zinc is needed for vitamin A metabolism).].

- Congenital stationary night blindness [Night blindness from birth, normal visual fields, may have a normal or abnormal fundus, not progressive. Paradoxic pupillary response. One variant is Oguchi disease (Mizuo phenomenon).].

- Undercorrected myopia (May be the most common cause of poor night vision.).

WORKUP

1. Medical and ocular history pertaining to the diseases discussed previously.

2. Drug history.

3. Family history (for diagnostic and counseling purposes).

4. Ophthalmoscopic examination.

5. Formal visual field testing (e.g., Goldmann).

6. ERG (may help distinguish stationary rod–cone dysfunction from RP, a progressive disease) and dark adaptation studies.

7. Fundus photographs.

8. FTA-ABS if the diagnosis is uncertain.

9. If the patient is male and the type of inheritance is unknown, examine his mother and perform an ERG on her (women carriers of X-linked disease often have abnormal pigmentation in the mid-periphery and abnormal results on dark-adapted ERGs).

10. If neurologic abnormalities such as ataxia, polyneuropathy, deafness, or anosmia are present, obtain a fasting (at least 14 hours) serum phytanic acid level to rule out Refsum disease.

11. If hereditary abetalipoproteinemia is suspected, obtain serum cholesterol and triglyceride levels (levels are low), a serum protein and lipoprotein electrophoresis (lipoprotein deficiency is detected), and peripheral blood smears (acanthocytosis is seen).

12. If Kearns–Sayre syndrome is suspected, the patient must be examined by a cardiologist with sequential ECGs; patients can die of complete heart block.

TREATMENT

For the following conditions, consult
11.25, Choroideremia
11.26, Gyrate Atrophy
13.5, Acquired Syphilis
13.11, Vitamin A Deficiency

No definitive treatment for RP is currently known. However, vitamin A palmitate, 15,000 IU, was found in one study to slow ERG dysfunction. This very controversial treatment (which showed no visual benefits) is recommended only for nonpregnant patients older than 21 years of age. Monitor liver function test results and vitamin A levels.

Cataract surgery may improve central visual acuity. Oral acetazolamide may be effective for CME.

All patients benefit from genetic counseling and instruction on how to deal with their visual handicaps. In advanced cases, low-vision aids and vocational rehabilitation are helpful.

11.25 CHOROIDEREMIA

SYMPTOMS

Night blindness in male patients aged 4 to 30 years, followed by insidious loss of peripheral vision. Decreased central vision occurs late in the disease. Women, who are asymptomatic carriers, often have a salt-and-pepper fundus.

SIGNS

Critical

• Male: *Early:* Dispersed pigment granules throughout, sparing the macula. *Late:* Total absence of RPE and choriocapillaris.

• Female: Small, scattered, square intraretinal pigment granules overlying choroidal atrophy, most marked in the mid-periphery.

Other. Retinal arteriolar narrowing and optic atrophy can occur late in the process; constriction of visual fields, normal color vision, abnormal ERG. Late stages, near-total absence of choroid and RPE.

INHERITANCE

X-linked recessive.

DIFFERENTIAL DIAGNOSIS

• RP (No choroidal atrophy, may see bone spicules of pigment. See 11.24, Retinitis Pigmentosa.).

• Gyrate atrophy (Scalloped RPE and choriocapillaris atrophy, posterior subcapsular cataract, high myopia with astigmatism, hyperornithinemia. Autosomal recessive. See 11.26, Gyrate Atrophy.).

• Albinism (Blond fundus without RPE clumping; the choroidal vasculature is easily seen. Iris transillumination defects are present, and the foveal reflex is absent. ERG is normal. See 13.12, Albinism.).

• Thioridazine (e.g., Mellaril) retinopathy (Patients taking more than 800 mg/day of thioridazine. See 11.30, Phenothiazine Toxicity.).

WORKUP

1. History: Family history? Medications?

2. Dilated fundus examination of the patient's mother and other family members if possible.

3. Formal visual fields (e.g., Octopus, Humphrey).

4. ERG with or without dark adaptation studies.

5. IVFA may be diagnostic.

TREATMENT

No effective treatment for this condition is currently available. The following may be helpful in management.

1. Darkly tinted sunglasses may ameliorate symptoms.

2. Genetic counseling.

11.26 GYRATE ATROPHY

SYMPTOMS

Decreased vision, night blindness.

SIGNS

Critical. Multiple sharply defined areas of chorioretinal atrophy separated from each other by thin margins of pigment. The lesions begin in the mid-periphery in childhood and then coalesce to involve the entire fundus, sparing the fovea until late in the disease, usually in midlife. Ornithine levels are markedly increased in all body fluids.

Other. Posterior subcapsular cataract, high myopia, and astigmatism; optic disc pallor and narrowing of the retinal vessels appear later in the disease. Constriction of visual fields and abnormal to nonrecordable ERG, electrooculogram (EOG), and dark adaptation studies occur. Color vision typically remains relatively intact until late in the course of the disease. Carriers have normal fundi, but may have mild increase of ornithine levels.

INHERITANCE

Autosomal recessive.

DIFFERENTIAL DIAGNOSIS

All of the following can be distinguished by the presence of normal ornithine levels.

• Thioridazine retinopathy (Patient taking more than 800 mg/day of thioridazine. See 11.30, Phenothiazine Toxicity.).

• Paving stone degeneration (Patches of chorioretinal atrophy limited to the retinal periphery, usually inferiorly.).

• Choroideremia (Diffuse RPE and choroidal atrophy spread throughout the fundus. X-linked recessive. See 11.25, Choroideremia.).

• High myopia (Chorioretinal atrophy, most marked in the posterior pole, often with a staphyloma. See 11.16, High Myopia.).

WORKUP

1. Family history: Check for night blindness or severely decreased vision.

2. Dilated fundus examination.

3. Plasma ornithine and amino acid levels (expect ornithine to be six to ten times normal).

4. Consider ERG and IVFA if the ornithine level is not markedly increased.

TREATMENT

1. Supplemental vitamin B$_6$ (pyridoxine). The dose is not currently established; can try 20 mg/day p.o. initially and increase up to 500 mg/day p.o., if there is no response.

   Note: Only a small percentage of patients are vitamin B$_6$ responders.

2. Reduce dietary protein consumption and substitute artificially flavored solutions of essential amino acids without arginine (i.e., arginine-restricted diet).

FOLLOW-UP

1. Frequent serum ornithine levels are obtained initially to determine the amount of supplemental vitamin B$_6$ and the degree to which dietary protein needs to be restricted. Serum ornithine levels between 0.15 and 0.2 mmol/L are optimal. The frequency of blood tests may be reduced after the ornithine levels stabilize in this range.

2. Serum ammonia levels are monitored in patients restricting dietary arginine.

11.27 CONE DYSTROPHIES

SYMPTOMS

Slowly progressive bilateral visual loss, photophobia, and poor color vision. Vision is worse during the day than at night.

SIGNS

Critical

• *Early:* Essentially normal results on fundus examination, even with poor visual acuity. Abnormal cone function on the ERG (i.e., a reduced single-flash photopic response and a reduced flicker response).

• *Late:* Bull's-eye macular appearance or central geographic atrophy of the RPE and choriocapillaris.

Other. Nystagmus, temporal pallor of the optic disc, spotty pigment clumping in the macular area, tapetal-like retinal sheen. Rarely rod degeneration may ensue, leading to a RP-like picture (i.e., a cone–rod degeneration, which may have an autosomal dominant inheritance pattern).

INHERITANCE

Usually sporadic. Hereditary forms are usually autosomal dominant, but autosomal recessive and X-linked also occur.

DIFFERENTIAL DIAGNOSIS

• Stargardt disease (In early cases when the fundus flavimaculatus is absent. A normal ERG is usually present in the early stage. Primarily autosomal recessive. See 11.28, Stargardt Disease.).

• Chloroquine retinopathy (May produce a bull's-eye macular appearance and poor color vision. History of chloroquine or hydroxychloroquine use, no family history of cone degeneration, no nystagmus. See 11.31, Chloroquine/Hydroxychloroquine Toxicity.).

• Central areolar choroidal dystrophy (Geographic atrophy of the RPE with normal photopic ERG.).

• ARMD (Can have geographic atrophy of the RPE, but with normal color vision and photopic ERG. See 11.13 and 11.14, Age-Related Macular Degeneration.).

• Congenital color blindness (Normal visual acuity, onset at birth, not progressive.).

• RP (Night blindness and peripheral visual field loss are the first symptoms. Often peripheral retinal bone spicules are seen. Can be distinguished by dark-adaptation testing and ERG. See 11.24, Retinitis Pigmentosa.).

• Optic neuropathy or atrophy (Decreased acuity, impaired color vision, temporal or diffuse optic-disc pallor or both. May have a family history. See 10.16, Arteritic Ischemic Optic Neuropathy, 10.17, Nonarteritic Ischemic Optic Neuropathy, and 10.18, Miscellaneous Optic Neuropathies.).

• Nonphysiologic visual loss (Normal results on ophthalmoscopic examination, IVFA, ERG, and EOG. Patients can often be tricked into seeing better by special testing. See 10.23, Nonphysiologic Visual Loss.).

WORKUP

1. Family history.

2. Complete ophthalmic examination, including color plates and formal color testing (e.g., Farnsworth–Munsell 100-hue test, red test object for chloroquine).

3. Formal visual field test (e.g., Humphrey, Octopus).

4. ERG.

5. IVFA to help detect the bull's-eye macular pattern.

TREATMENT

There is no proven cure for this disease. The following measures may be palliative:

1. Heavily tinted glasses or contact lenses may help maximize vision.

2. Miotic drops (e.g., pilocarpine, 0.5% to 1%, q.i.d., during the day) are occasionally tried to improve vision and reduce photophobia.

3. Genetic counseling.

4. Low-vision aids as needed.

FOLLOW-UP

Yearly.

11.28 STARGARDT DISEASE

(FUNDUS FLAVIMACULATUS)

SYMPTOMS

Usually bilateral decreased vision in childhood or young adulthood. In the early stages, the decrease in vision is often out of proportion to the clinical ophthalmoscopic appearance; therefore we must be careful not to label the child a malingerer.

SIGNS

Critical
Any of the following may be present.

• A relatively normal-appearing fundus except for a heavily pigmented RPE.

• Yellow or yellow–white, flecklike deposits at the level of the RPE, usually in a pisciform (fish-tail) configuration, may be associated.

• Atrophic macular degeneration: May have a bull's-eye appearance as a result of atrophy of the RPE around a normal central core of RPE, a "beaten-metal" appearance, pigment clumping, or marked geographic atrophy.

• "Midnight" fundus on IVFA or autoreflectance due to lipofuscin.

Note: In early stages, vision drops before visible macular changes.

Other. Atrophy of the RPE just outside of the macula or in the mid-peripheral fundus, normal peripheral visual fields in most cases, and rarely an accompanying cone or rod dystrophy. The ERG is typically normal in the early stages, but may become abnormal late in the disease. The EOG is usually normal.

INHERITANCE

Usually autosomal recessive, but occasionally autosomal dominant.

DIFFERENTIAL DIAGNOSIS

• Fundus albipunctatus (Diffuse, small, white, discrete dots, most prominent in the mid-peripheral fundus and rarely present in the fovea; nonprogressive congenital night blindness; no atrophic macular degeneration or pigmentary changes. Visual acuity and visual fields remain normal.).

• Retinitis punctata albescens (Similar clinical appearance to fundus albipunctatus, but visual acuity, visual field, and night blindness progressively worsen. A markedly abnormal ERG develops.).

• Drusen [Small, yellow–white spots deep to the retina, sometimes calcified, usually developing later in life. IVFA helps distinguish (all drusen hyperfluoresce, whereas some lesions of fundus flavimaculatus do and some lesions do not hyperfluoresce, and some areas without flecks show hyperfluorescence).].

• Cone or cone–rod dystrophy (May have a bull's-eye macula, but have a significant color vision deficit and a characteristic ERG. See 11.27, Cone Dystrophies.).

• Batten disease and Spielmeyer–Vogt syndrome (May have bull's-eye maculopathy, autosomal recessive lysosomal storage disease, progressive dementia, seizures; may have variable degree of optic atrophy, attenuation of retinal vasculature, and peripheral RPE changes. Shows characteristic curvilinear or fingerprint inclusions on electron microscopy of peripheral blood or conjunctival biopsy.).

• Chloroquine/hydroxychloroquine maculopathy (History of use of this medication. Dose related. See 11.31, Chloroquine/Hydroxychloroquine Toxicity.).

• Nonphysiologic visual loss (Normal ophthalmoscopic examination, IVFA, ERG, and EOG. Patients can often be tricked into seeing better by special testing. See 10.23, Nonphysiologic Visual Loss.).

WORKUP

Indicated when the diagnosis is uncertain or must be confirmed.

1. History: Age at onset, medications, family history?

2. Dilated retinal examination.

3. IVFA often shows blockage of choroidal fluorescence producing a "silent choroid" or "midnight fundus" as a result of increased lipofuscin in the RPE cells.

4. ERG and EOG.

5. Formal visual field examination (e.g., Octopus, Humphrey).

TREATMENT

No known medical or surgical therapy is beneficial. The patient may benefit from low-vision aids, services dedicated to helping the visually handicapped, and genetic counseling.

11.29　BEST DISEASE

(VITELLIFORM MACULAR DYSTROPHY)

SYMPTOMS

Decreased vision or asymptomatic. Onset at birth, but may not be detected until years later if examination is not performed.

SIGNS

Critical. Yellow, round, subretinal lesion(s) likened to an egg yolk (lipofuscin) or in some cases to a pseudohypopyon. Typically bilateral and located in the fovea, measuring approximately one to two disc areas in size. Ten percent of lesions are multiple and extrafoveal. Normal ERG, abnormal EOG.

Other. The lesions may degenerate, and macular choroidal neovascularization, hemorrhage, and scarring may develop. In the scar stage, it may be indistinguishable from ARMD. May be hyperopic and have esophoria or esotropia.

INHERITANCE

Autosomal dominant with variable penetrance and expression. Carriers may have normal fundi but an abnormal EOG.

WORKUP

1. Family history (often helpful to examine family members).

2. Complete ocular examination, including a dilated retinal examination, carefully inspecting the macula with a slit lamp and a fundus contact, Hruby, or 60- or 90-diopter lens.

3. EOG to confirm the diagnosis or to detect the carrier state of the disease.

4. Consider IVFA to confirm the presence of or delineate a CNVM.

TREATMENT

There is no effective treatment for the underlying disease. Laser should be considered for well-defined CNVM outside the foveal center, but CNVMs are not as devastating as in ARMD.

FOLLOW-UP

Patients with treatable CNVM should be attended to promptly. Otherwise, there is no urgency in seeing patients with this disease. Patients are given an Amsler grid (see Appendix 3), instructed on its use, and told to return immediately if a change is noted.

Note: Pattern dystrophy can mimic Best disease. The egg-yolk lesions usually appear from ages 30 to 50 years, the disease is dominantly inherited, and the EOG may or may not be abnormal. Visual acuity is usually normal or slightly decreased until the sixth decade of life, when central vision may be compromised by geographic atrophy. There also is no effective treatment for this entity.

11.30 PHENOTHIAZINE TOXICITY

THIORIDAZINE (E.G., MELLARIL)

SYMPTOMS

Blurred vision, brownish vision, difficulty with night vision.

SIGNS

Pigment clumps between the posterior pole and the equator, areas of retinal depigmentation, retinal edema, visual field abnormalities (central scotoma and general constriction), depressed or extinguished ERG.

Note: Symptoms and signs may occur within weeks of starting phenothiazine therapy, particularly if very large doses (more than 2,000 mg/day) are taken.

DOSAGE USUALLY REQUIRED TO PRODUCE TOXICITY

800 mg/day chronically.

DIFFERENTIAL DIAGNOSIS

Pigment clumps in the retina.

• RP (Family history, pale optic disc, narrowed arterioles. See 11.24, Retinitis Pigmentosa.).

• Old syphilitic chorioretinopathy (Positive FTA-ABS, may have a history of an acute visual problem.).

• Viral chorioretinitis (Often associated with an anterior chamber reaction, vitreous cells, and other ocular signs.).

• Trauma (Usually unilateral, history of trauma.).

TREATMENT

Discontinue the medication.

BASELINE WORKUP

For patients in whom long-term treatment is anticipated.

1. Visual acuity.

2. Complete ophthalmoscopic examination.

3. Fundus photographs.

4. Visual field, preferably automated (e.g., Humphrey, Octopus, with or without a red test object).

5. Consider ERG.

6. Color vision testing, preferably with a Farnsworth–Munsell 100-hue test.

FOLLOW-UP

Every 6 months.

CHLORPROMAZINE (E.G., THORAZINE)

SYMPTOMS

Blurred vision or none.

SIGNS

Abnormal pigmentation of the eyelids, cornea, conjunctiva (especially within the palpebral fissure), and anterior lens capsule; anterior and posterior subcapsular cataract; rarely, a pigmentary retinopathy within the visual field and ERG changes described for thioridazine.

DOSAGE USUALLY REQUIRED TO PRODUCE TOXICITY

From 1,200 to 2,400 mg/day for longer than 12 months.

TREATMENT

Discontinue the medication if vision is affected.

BASELINE WORKUP

Same as for thioridazine.

FOLLOW-UP

Every 6 months.

11.31   CHLOROQUINE/HYDROXYCHLOROQUINE TOXICITY

SYMPTOMS

Decreased vision, abnormal color vision, difficulty adjusting to darkness.

SIGNS

Critical. Bull's-eye macula (a ring of depigmentation surrounded by a ring of increased pigmentation), loss of the foveal reflex.

Other. Increased pigmentation in the macula, arteriolar narrowing, vascular sheathing, peripheral pigmentation, decreased color vision, visual field abnormalities (central, paracentral, or peripheral scotoma), abnormal ERG and EOG, and normal dark adaptation. Whorl-like corneal changes also may be observed.

DOSAGE USUALLY REQUIRED TO PRODUCE TOXICITY

Chloroquine: More than 300 g total cumulative dose.

Hydroxychloroquine: More than 750 mg/day taken over months to years.

(Some believe that retinopathy will not develop if the daily dose is kept at less than 4.4 mg/kg/day of chloroquine and 7.7 mg/kg/day of hydroxychloroquine.).

DIFFERENTIAL DIAGNOSIS

The following can produce a bull's-eye macula.

• Cone dystrophy (Family history, usually younger than 30 years of age, severe photophobia, abnormal to nonrecordable photopic ERG. See 11.27, Cone Dystrophies.).

• Stargardt disease/fundus flavimaculatus (Family history, usually younger than 25 years of age, may have white–yellow flecks in the posterior pole and mid-periphery. See 11.28, Stargardt Disease.).

• ARMD (Drusen; pigment clumping and atrophy and detachment of the RPE or sensory retina may or may not occur. See 11.13 and 11.14, Age-Related Macular Degeneration.).

• Batten disease and Spielmeyer–Vogt syndrome (Pigmentary retinopathy, seizures, ataxia, and progressive dementia.).

TREATMENT

Discontinue the medication if signs of toxicity develop.

BASELINE WORKUP

For patients in whom long-term treatment is anticipated.

1. Visual acuity.

2. Ophthalmoscopic examination.

3. Posterior pole fundus photographs.

4. Visual field, preferably automated (e.g., Humphrey, Octopus, with or without red test object).

5. Color vision testing, preferably Farnsworth–Munsell 100-hue test.

FOLLOW-UP

Every 6 months.

Note: Once ocular toxicity develops, it usually does not regress even if the drug is withdrawn. In fact, new toxic effects may develop, and old ones may progress even after the chloroquine/hydroxychloroquine has been discontinued.

11.32   MALIGNANT MELANOMA OF THE CHOROID

SYMPTOMS

Decreased vision, a visual field defect, floaters, light flashes, pain; may be asymptomatic.

SIGNS

Critical. Gray–green or brown (melanotic) or yellow (amelanotic) choroidal mass that exhibits one or more of the following:

• Growth.

• Presence of subretinal fluid (i.e., RD).

• Height greater than 2 mm, especially with an abrupt elevation from the choroid.

• Ill-defined, large areas of orange pigment over the lesion.

• A mushroom shape with congested blood vessels in the dome of the tumor.

Note: A diffuse choroidal MM can appear as a minimally thickened dark choroid without a distinct mass.

Other. Overlying cystoid retinal degeneration, vitreous hemorrhage or vitreous pigment cells, drusen on the tumor surface, a CNVM, proptosis (from orbital invasion). Choroidal MM rarely occurs in blacks and more commonly occurs in light-skinned individuals.

DIFFERENTIAL DIAGNOSIS

Pigmented Lesions

• Nevi (Melanotic or amelanotic choroidal lesions that rarely exhibit significant growth, are not mushroom shaped, are usually less than 2 mm thick, and show gradual elevation from the choroid. They may have an associated shallow RD or well-defined small areas of orange pigment on their surface, but surface drusen are more typical. The main concern with nevi is evolution into melanoma. Factors that indicate possible growth of nevi into melanoma include thickness greater than 2 mm, presence of adjacent subretinal fluid, prominent orange pigment, less than 3 mm to the optic disc, and presence of symptoms.).

• Congenital hypertrophy of the RPE (Flat lesions that are often black, but may appear gray–green. The margins are often well delineated with a surrounding depigmented halo. Depigmented areas frequently appear as the lesion gets older.).

• Reactive hyperplasia of the RPE (Related to previous trauma or inflammation. Lesions are black, flat, have irregular margins, and may have associated white gliosis. Often multifocal.).

• ARMD (Subretinal blood can simulate a melanoma. This disease is typically bilateral in the posterior pole and associated with drusen and extensive exudate. Occasionally it can occur in the periphery. IVFA assists in differentiation.).

• Melanocytoma of the optic nerve (A black optic nerve lesion with fibrillated margins. It may grow slowly. IVFA may allow differentiation.).

• Choroidal detachment [Follows ocular surgery, trauma, or hypotony of another etiology. Dark peripheral multilobular fundus mass. (The ora serrata is often visible without scleral depression.). Localized suprachoroidal hemorrhage can be very difficult to differentiate from MM based on appearance alone because of its brown–black color. Transillumination allows differentiation between serous choroidal detachment and MM but is not helpful when there is a hemorrhagic component. In these situations, IVFA is the study of choice, usually allowing differentiation between the two entities.].

Nonpigmented Lesions

• Choroidal hemangioma (Red–orange, may be elevated, not mushroom shaped.).

• Metastatic carcinoma [Cream or light brown, flat or slightly elevated, extensive subretinal fluid, may be multifocal or bilateral. Patient may have a history of cancer (especially breast or lung cancer).].

• Choroidal osteoma (Yellow–orange, usually close to the optic disc, pseudopod-like projections of the margin, often bilateral, typically occurs in young women in their teens or twenties. Ultrasonography may show a calcified mass.).

• Posterior scleritis (Patients may have choroidal folds, pain, proptosis, uveitis, or anterior scleritis associated with an amelanotic mass. Look for the T-sign on ultrasonography.).

• Lymphoma.

WORKUP

1. History: Ocular surgery or trauma, cancer, anorexia, weight loss, or systemic illness?

2. Dilated fundus examination by using indirect ophthalmoscopy.

3. IVFA.

4. A- and B-scan ultrasonography: Documents thickness and confirms clinical impression. With choroidal melanoma, ultrasonography usually shows low to moderate reflectivity with choroidal excavation.

5. Consider a fine-needle aspiration biopsy in selected cases, and computed tomography scan or magnetic resonance imaging (MRI) of the orbit and brain.

6. If MM is confirmed:

   —Blood work: lactate dehydrogenase, gamma-glutamyl transferase, aspartate and alanine aminotransferases, and alkaline phosphatase. If liver enzymes are elevated, consider an MRI or liver scan to rule out a liver metastasis.

   —Chest radiograph.

   —Complete physical examination by a medical internist.

7. Referral to an internist for breast examination, chest radiograph, and consider a carcinoembryonic antigen assay if a choroidal metastasis is suspected.

TREATMENT

Depending on the results of the metastatic workup, the tumor characteristics, the status of the contralateral eye, and the age and general health of the patient, MM of the choroid may be managed by observation, photocoagulation, thermotherapy, radiation therapy, local resection, or enucleation.

CHAPTER 12

UVEITIS

12.1 ANTERIOR UVEITIS (IRITIS/IRIDOCYCLITIS)

SYMPTOMS

- Acute: Pain, red eye, photophobia, consensual photophobia (pain in the affected eye when a light is shone in the fellow eye).

- Chronic: Decreased vision. May have periods of exacerbations and remissions, with few or none of the acute symptoms [especially juvenile rheumatoid arthritis (JRA)].

SIGNS

Critical. Cells and flare in the anterior chamber, ciliary flush, keratic precipitates (KP):

- Fine ("stellate"; typically covers entire corneal endothelium): herpetic, Fuchs heterochromic iridocyclitis (FHIC), cytomegalovirus (CMV) retinitis, others.

- Large, greasy ("mutton-fat"; mostly on inferior cornea): sarcoidosis, syphilis, tuberculosis, lens induced, Vogt–Koyanagi–Harada (VKH) syndrome, herpetic, others.

Other. Low intraocular pressure (IOP; more commonly seen). Elevated IOP (especially herpetic, lens induced, FHIC, Posner–Schlossman syndrome), fibrin [human leukocyte antigen (HLA)-B27 or infectious endophthalmitis], hypopyon (HLA-B27, Behçet disease, infectious endophthalmitis, rifabutin, tumor), iris nodules (sarcoidosis, syphilis, tuberculosis), iris atro-

phy (herpetic), iris heterochromia (FHIC), iris synechiae (especially HLA-B27, sarcoidosis), band keratopathy (especially JRA in younger patients, any chronic uveitis in older), uveitis in a "quiet eye" (consider JRA, FHIC, masquerade syndromes), cystoid macular edema (CME).

DIFFERENTIAL DIAGNOSIS

- Posterior uveitis with spillover into the anterior chamber (Chief complaint will be floaters and decreased vision, positive findings on fundus examination. See 12.3, Posterior Uveitis.).

- Traumatic iritis (See 3.5, Traumatic Iritis.).

- Posner–Schlossman syndrome (Recurrent episodes of very high IOP and minimal inflammation. Also open angle on gonioscopy, corneal edema, fine KP, and fixed, mid-dilated pupil. See 9.13, Glaucomatocyclitic Crisis.).

- Drug-induced uveitis [e.g., rifabutin, cidofovir, sulfonamides, pamidronate (inhibits bone resorption)].

- Sclerouveitis (Uveitis secondary to scleritis; typically present with profound pain.).

- Tight contact lens (Red eye, corneal edema, epithelial defects, iritis ± hypopyon, no stromal infiltrates.).

- Infectious keratouveitis (History of corneal trauma or contact lens, corneal infiltrate is present.).

- Infectious endophthalmitis (History of recent surgery, pain, hypopyon, fibrin, vitritis, decreased vision, history of trauma, may have endogenous source with fever, elevated white count.).

- Schwartz syndrome (Glaucoma and anterior chamber reaction caused by a chronic low-lying retinal detachment, including retinal detachment with dialysis.).

- Tumor (Retinoblastoma in children, intraocular lymphoma in elderly, metastatic disease in all ages, others.).

ETIOLOGY

Acute

- Idiopathic.

- HLA-B27–associated uveitis. (Especially young men with low back pain.).

Note: Bilateral recurrent alternating anterior uveitis is very characteristic of HLA-B27 uveitis.

- Lens-induced uveitis (Often after incomplete extracapsular cataract extraction or trauma damaging the lens capsule; also may be secondary to a hypermature cataract or infection with *Propionibacterium acnes*.).

- Postoperative iritis (An anterior chamber reaction is expected after intraocular surgery. Severe reactions with excessive pain, however, must make the examiner consider endophthalmitis. See 12.11, Chronic Postoperative Uveitis.).

- Uveitis–glaucoma–hyphema (UGH) syndrome (Usually secondary to irritation from an intraocular lens (especially a closed-loop anterior chamber lens. See 9.16, Postoperative Glaucoma.).

- Behçet disease (Young adults, acute hypopyon, iritis, aphthous mouth ulcers, genital ulcerations, erythema nodosum, often retinal vasculitis and hemorrhages, may have recurrent episodes.).

- Lyme disease (Often a history of a tick bite. May have a skin rash or arthritis. See 13.6, Lyme Disease.).

- Anterior segment ischemia (Caused by carotid insufficiency or tight scleral buckle; flare out of proportion to the cellular reaction, pain.).

- Mumps, influenza, adenovirus, measles, chlamydia (Rare causes of transient anterior uveitis.).

- Other rare causes of anterior uveitis (Leptospirosis, Kawasaki disease, rickettsial disease.).

Chronic

- JRA [Usually young girls, eye may be white and without pain but flare may be present, often bilateral, iritis can occur before the arthritis, pauciarticular arthritis (fewer than five joints involved), positive anti-nuclear antibody (ANA), negative rheumatoid factor, increased erythrocyte sedimentation rate (ESR), glaucoma, cataracts, band keratopathy.].

- Chronic iridocyclitis of children (Usually young girls, similar to JRA except no arthritis.).

- FHIC (Usually unilateral, few symptoms, diffuse iris stromal atrophy often causing a lighter-colored iris, iris transillumination defects, blunting of the iris architecture, fine KP over the entire corneal endothelium, mild anterior chamber reaction, few if any posterior synechiae. Vitreous opacities, glaucoma, and cataracts are common.).

Chronic, Usually with Granulomatous Signs (Mutton-Fat Keratic Precipitates, Iris Nodules)

- Sarcoidosis [Usually African heritage, usually bilateral; may have dense posterior synechiae, conjunctival nodules, or signs of posterior uveitis (see 12.3, Posterior Uveitis). Mild to moderate anergy, abnormalities on chest radiography, positive gallium scan, and increased serum angiotensin-converting enzyme (ACE) are common. See 12.6, Sarcoidosis.].

- Herpes simplex/herpes zoster/varicella (Look for corneal scars, history of past unilateral recurrent red eye, occasionally history of skin vesicles, associated with increased IOP, followed by iris atrophy.).

- Syphilis [May have a maculopapular rash (often on the palms and soles), iris roseola (vascular papules on the iris), and interstitial keratitis with ghost vessels in late stages. Usually seen with uveitis in acquired syphilis versus interstitial keratitis in congenital syphilis. A positive Venereal Disease Research Laboratory (VDRL) or rapid plasma reagin (RPR) and positive fluorescent treponemal antibody, absorbed (FTA-ABS) are usually present. See 13.5, Acquired Syphilis.].

- Tuberculosis [Positive protein derivative of *tuberculin* (PPD), typical chest radiograph, occasionally phlyctenular keratitis, sometimes signs of posterior uveitis. See 12.3, Posterior Uveitis.].

- Others [Rare (e.g., leprosy, brucellosis).].

WORKUP

1. Obtain a history and review of systems (Tables 12.1 and 12.2).

   Note: Autoimmune diseases are uncommon in the very young or very old—consider masquerades.

   Note: Lyme disease is prevalent in many parts of the United States besides the Northeast.

Note: Inflammatory arthritis typically presents with stiffness in the morning that improves after activity.

2. Complete ocular examination, including an IOP check and a dilated fundus examination. The vitreous should be evaluated for cells (see Appendix 8).

3. A laboratory workup may be unnecessary in certain situations:

   —First-time occurrence of a mild, unilateral, nongranulomatous uveitis with a history and examination that are not suggestive of systemic disease.

   —Uveitis occurring in the setting of known systemic disease such as sarcoidosis or the patient is taking medicines known to cause uveitis (e.g., rifabutin).

   —Clinical findings are classic for a particular diagnosis (e.g., herpetic keratouveitis, FHIC, toxoplasmosis).

4. If the uveitis is bilateral, granulomatous, or recurrent, and the history and examination are unremarkable, then a nonspecific initial workup is conducted:

   —RPR or VDRL.

TABLE 12.1 EPIDEMIOLOGY

Age:	Infants	Children	Young Adults	Elderly
	TORCH infections, retinoblastoma	JRA, toxocariasis, toxoplasmosis	HLA-B27, Fuchs heterochromic iridocyclitis, pars planitis, idiopathic	Lymphoma and other masquerades, serpiginous, birdshot, acute retinal necrosis

Sex:	Female	Male		
	JRA, SLE	Ankylosing spondylitis, Reiter syndrome		

Race:	Caucasian	African American	Mediterranean, Middle Eastern	Asian
	HLA-B27, white dot syndromes, multiple sclerosis	Sarcoidosis, systemic lupus erythematosus	Behçet disease	Behçet disease, Vogt–Koyanagi–Harada syndrome

HLA, human leukocyte antigen; JRA, juvenile rheumatoid arthritis; TORCH, toxoplasmosis, rubella, cytomegalovirus, herpes simplex.

TABLE 12.2 REVIEW OF SYSTEMS

Musculoskeletal	
Arthritis	Behçet disease, Lyme disease, SLE, HLA-B27, relapsing polychondritis, juvenile rheumatoid arthritis
Heel pain	Reiter syndrome, HLA-B27
Pulmonary	
Asthma	Sarcoidosis, TB, Wegener
Pneumonia	Cytomegalovirus, AIDS, aspergillosis, SLE, sarcoidosis, Wegener
Neurologic/ear–nose–throat	
Auditory	VKH, sympathetic ophthalmia
Diet/hygiene	Poor handwashing—toxoplasmosis, toxocariasis
	Uncooked meat—toxoplasmosis, cysticercosis
	Unpasteurized milk—brucellosis, TB
Gatrointestinal	
Diarrhea	Whipple disease, ulcerative colitis, Crohn disease
Mouth ulcers	Behçet disease, Reiter syndrome, ulcerative colitis, herpes, sarcoidosis
Gastrourinary	
Genital ulcers	Reiter syndrome, Behçet disease, syphilis
Hematuria	Polyarteritis nodosa, SLE, Wegener granulomatosis
Urethral discharge	Urethral discharge—Reiter syndrome, syphilis, chlamydia
Skin	
Erythema nodosum	Behçet disease, sarcoidosis
Rash on palms and soles	Syphilis
Erythema chronicum migrans	Lyme disease
Lupus pernio (purple malar rash)	Sarcoidosis
Psoriasis	Psoriatic arthritis
Vitiligo and poliosis	VKH, sympathetic ophthalmia
Shingles	Varicella-zoster virus, acute retinal necrosis
Pets	
Puppy	Toxocariasis
Cat	Toxoplasmosis
Social History	
Drug abuse	Candida
Venereal disease	Syphilis, AIDS, Reiter syndrome

AIDS, acquired immunodeficiency syndrome; HLA, human leukocyte antigen; SLE, systemic lupus erythematosus; TB, tuberculosis; VKH, Vogt–Koyanagi–Harada syndrome.

—FTA-ABS or microhemagglutination–*Treponema pallidum* (MHA-TP).

—PPD and anergy panel.

—Chest radiograph to rule out sarcoidosis and tuberculosis.

5. If a specific diagnosis is suspected, perform the following workup (Table 12.3).

TREATMENT

1. Cycloplegic (scopolamine, 0.25% b.i.d., for mild to moderate inflammation; atropine, 1%, b.i.d. to q.i.d., for severe inflammation. Use atropine with caution in patients at risk for urinary retention.).

2. Topical steroid (prednisolone acetate, 1%, one drop q1–6h, depending on the severity). Most cases of moderate to severe acute uveitis require q1–2h dosing initially.

If the anterior uveitis is severe and is not responding well to frequent topical steroids, then consider periocular repository steroids (e.g., triamcinolone 20 to 40 mg subtenon injection). Before injecting depot steroids

TABLE 12.3 SUGGESTED DIAGNOSTIC WORKUP FOR ANTERIOR UVEITIS

Ankylosing spondylitis	HLA-B27, SI joint films, rheumatology consult
Reiter syndrome	HLA-B27, SI joint films (if symptomatic), cultures for *Chlamydia*
Psoriatic arthritis	HLA-B27, rheumatology and/or dermatology consult
Lyme disease	Lyme immunofluorescent assay or enzyme-linked immunosorbent assay
Juvenile rheumatoid arthritis or any suspect uveitis in children	Rheumatoid factor, antinuclear antibodies, rheumatology consult, radiographs of affected joints
Sarcoidosis	Chest radiograph, purified protein derivative + anergy panel, angiotensin-converting enzyme (see 12.6, Sarcoidosis)
Syphilis	(Rapid plasma reagin or Venereal Disease Research Laboratory) *and* (microhemagglutination–*Treponema pallidum* or fluorescent treponemal antibody, absorbed), human immunodeficiency virus
Ocular ischemic syndrome	Intravenous fluorescein angiography, carotid doppler studies

HLA, human leukocyte antigen; SI, sacroiliac.

periocularly, it is wise to use topical steroids at full strength for several weeks to make certain that the patient does not experience a significant IOP increase from steroids. See Appendix 7, which describes the technique of a subtenon injection.

3. If there is no improvement on maximal topical and repository steroids, or if the uveitis is bilateral and severe, consider systemic steroids, or referral to a rheumatologist for immunosuppressive therapy. Consider referral to a uveitis specialist.

4. Treat secondary glaucoma with aqueous suppressants (not with pilocarpine or prostaglandins). Glaucoma may result from:

—A severe inflammatory reaction with cellular blockage of the trabecular meshwork. See 9.4, Inflammatory Open-Angle Glaucoma.

—Synechiae formation giving rise to secondary angle closure. See 9.10, Acute Angle-Closure Glaucoma.

—Neovascularization of the iris, producing blockage of the trabecular meshwork or closure of the angle. See 9.14, Neovascular Glaucoma.

—A response to steroids. See 9.5, Steroid-Response Glaucoma.

5. If an exact etiology for the anterior uveitis is determined, then the specific management

outlined as follows should be added to these treatments.

—**Ankylosing spondylitis:** Often requires systemic antiinflammatory agents [e.g., aspirin, nonsteroidal antiinflammatory drugs (NSAIDs), naproxen (e.g., Naprosyn), or indomethacin]. Consider cardiology consult (there is a high incidence of heart block and aortic insufficiency), rheumatology consult, and physical therapy consult.

—**Inflammatory bowel disease:** Often benefits from systemic steroids or sulfadiazine or both and supplemental vitamin A. Needs a medical or gastrointestinal consult.

—**Reiter syndrome:** If urethritis is present, then the patient and sexual partners are treated for chlamydia (e.g., tetracycline, 250 to 500 mg, q.i.d., doxycycline, 100 mg, b.i.d., or erythromycin, 250 to 500 mg, q.i.d., for 3 to 6 weeks; can also use clarithromycin, azithromycin). Obtain medical, rheumatology, or physical therapy consult or a combination of these.

—**Psoriatic arthritis:** Consider a rheumatology or dermatology consult.

—**Glaucomatocyclitic crisis:** See 9.13, Glaucomatocyclitic Crisis.

—**Lens-induced uveitis:** Usually requires removal of lens material. See 9.8, Phacolytic Glaucoma and 9.9, Lens-Particle Glaucoma.

—**Herpes uveitis:** Herpes simplex requires prophylactic antivirals when atypical or taking steroids. May benefit from systemic antiviral medications (e.g., acyclovir). See 4.14, Herpes Simplex Virus; or 4.15, Herpes Zoster Virus.

—**UGH syndrome:** See 9.16, Postoperative Glaucoma.

—**Behçet disease:** Often needs systemic steroids or immunosuppressive agents (responds well to chlorambucil); consider a medical or rheumatology consult. Consider referral to a uveitis specialist for long-term management.

—**Lyme disease:** See 13.6, Lyme Disease.

—**JRA:** The steroid dosage is adjusted according to the degree of cells, not flare, present in the anterior chamber; prolonged cycloplegic therapy may be required. A rheumatology or pediatric consult is obtained for possible systemic steroid therapy or methotrexate.

Note: JRA has a high complication rate with cataract surgery.

—**Chronic iridocyclitis of children:** Same as JRA.

—**FHIC:** Usually does not respond to or require steroids (a trial of steroids may be attempted, but they should be tapered quickly if there is no response); cycloplegics are rarely necessary.

Note: Patients with FHIC usually do well with cataract surgery.

—**Sarcoidosis:** Often needs periocular and systemic steroids; a medicine or pulmonary consult is advisable for systemic evaluation (see 12.6, Sarcoidosis).

—**Syphilis:** See 13.5, Acquired Syphilis, and 8.8, Congenital Syphilis.

—**Tuberculosis:** Avoid systemic steroids. Refer the patient to an internist for consideration of systemic antituberculous treatment.

FOLLOW-UP

1. Every 1 to 7 days in the acute phase, depending on the severity; every 1 to 6 months when stable.

2. At each visit, the anterior chamber reaction and IOP should be evaluated.

3. A vitreous and fundus examination should be performed for all flareups, when vision is affected, or every 3 to 6 months.

4. If the anterior chamber reaction is improving, then the steroid drops can be slowly tapered [usually one drop per day every 3 to 7 days (e.g., q.i.d. for 1 week, then t.i.d. for 1 week, then b.i.d. for 1 week)]. Steroids are usually discontinued once all cells have disappeared from the anterior chamber (flare is often still present). Rarely, long-term low-dose steroids every day or every other day are required to keep the inflammation from recurring. Punctal occlusion techniques may increase potency of drug and decrease systemic absorption. The cycloplegic agents also can be tapered as the anterior chamber reaction improves. Cycloplegics should be used at least every evening until the anterior chamber is free of cells.

Note: As with most ocular and systemic diseases requiring steroid therapy, the steroid (be it topical or systemic) should never be discontinued abruptly. Sudden discontinuation of steroids can lead to severe rebound inflammation.

12.2 PARS PLANITIS/INTERMEDIATE UVEITIS

SYMPTOMS

Floaters and cloudy vision in the absence of pain, photophobia or external inflammation. Usually age 15 to 40 years and bilateral.

SIGNS

Critical. Vitreous cells, white exudative material over the inferior ora serrata and pars plana ("snowbank"), cellular aggregates floating in the inferior vitreous ("snowballs"). Vitreous hemorrhage may be the presenting sign in younger patients.

Note: Snowbanking can often be seen only with indirect ophthalmoscopy and scleral depression.

Other. Peripheral retinal vascular sheathing, peripheral neovascularization, mild anterior chamber inflammation, CME, posterior subcapsular cataract, secondary glaucoma, retinal gliosis, exudative retinal detachment.

DIFFERENTIAL DIAGNOSIS

• Idiopathic (50%).

• Most commonly associated systemic diseases are sarcoidosis and multiple sclerosis.

• Also may be associated with Lyme disease, JRA, *P. acnes*, or tubular interstitial nephritis and uveitis.

WORKUP

1. Chest radiograph, PPD, ACE level, RPR, FTA-ABS.

2. Consider intravenous fluorescein angiography (IVFA) to document CME or retinal vasculitis.

3. Consider enzyme-linked immunosorbent assay (ELISA) for Lyme disease, toxoplasmosis, cat-scratch disease.

4. Review of systems for focal neurologic deficits; refer to neurologist for multiple sclerosis workup if necessary.

TREATMENT

Treat all vision-threatening complications in symptomatic patients with active disease. Mild vitreous cell in the absence of symptoms or vision loss may be observed.

1. Topical prednisolone acetate, 1% (e.g., Pred Forte) q1–2h and simultaneous subtenon steroids (0.5 to 1.0 mL of subtenon triamcinolone 40 mg/mL). Repeat the injections every 1 to 2 months until the vision and CME are no longer improving, and then slowly taper the frequency of injections. Contraindicated in patients with steroid-responsive IOP. See Appendix 7 for the technique.

2. If there is no improvement after the first three subtenon injections, then consider systemic steroids (e.g., prednisone, 40 to 60 mg orally q.d., for 4 to 6 weeks), tapering gradually according to the patient's response.

Note: In bilateral cases, systemic steroid therapy is often preferred to bilateral periocular injections.

3. Transscleral cryotherapy to the area of snowbanking should be considered in patients who fail to respond to either oral or subtenon corticosteroids.

4. Finally, pars plana vitrectomy or the use of systemic immunosuppressive agents (e.g., methotrexate, cyclosporine) may be useful in refractory cases.

Notes:

1. *Some physicians delay periocular repository steroid therapy for several weeks to observe whether the patient is a steroid responder (i.e., a significant IOP in-*

crease caused by the topical steroids develops). If a steroid response is found, then the periocular steroid may need to be withheld.

2. Topical NSAIDs (e.g., ketorolac or diclofenac, q.i.d.) may be added in patients with CME.

3. Cataracts are a frequent complication of intermediate uveitis. If cataract extraction is performed, meticulous preoperative and postoperative control of inflammation is required. Consider a combined pars plana vitrectomy at the time of cataract surgery if significant vitreous opacification is present.

FOLLOW-UP

1. In the acute phase, patients are reevaluated every 1 to 4 weeks, depending on the severity of the condition.

2. In the chronic phase, reexamination is performed every 3 to 6 months.

12.3 POSTERIOR UVEITIS

SYMPTOMS

Blurred vision, floaters; occasionally redness, typically painless.

Note: Posterior uveitis with significant pain suggests acute retinal necrosis (ARN), syphilis, endogenous bacterial endophthalmitis, or posterior scleritis.

SIGNS

Critical. Cells in the anterior or posterior vitreous, or both, vitreous haze, retinal or choroidal inflammatory lesions, vasculitis (sheathing and exudates around vessels).

Other. Anterior segment inflammatory signs, CME.

DIFFERENTIAL DIAGNOSIS

(Masquerade syndromes)

Note: Always consider masquerade syndromes in the very old or very young patient.

• Large cell lymphoma (reticulum cell sarcoma) (Persistent vitreous cells in patients older than 50 years, which usually do not respond completely to systemic steroids. Yellow–white subretinal infiltrates, retinal edema and hemorrhage, anterior chamber inflammation, or neurologic signs may be present.).

• Malignant melanoma (A retinal detachment and associated vitritis may obscure the underlying tumor. B-scan ultrasonography usually detects the tumor in cases not detectable by indirect ophthalmoscopy. See 11.32, Malignant Melanoma of the Choroid.).

• Retinitis pigmentosa (Vitreous cells and macular edema may accompany "bone-spicule" pigmentary changes and attenuated retinal vessels. Drusen of the optic disc may be mistaken for disc swelling. Electroretinography aids in diagnosis. See 11.24, Retinitis Pigmentosa.).

• Rhegmatogenous retinal detachment (RRD) (A small number of pigmented anterior vitreous cells and an anterior uveitis frequently accompany a RRD. See 11.3, Retinal Detachment.).

• Retained intraocular foreign body [Persistent inflammation after a penetrating ocular injury. May have iris heterochromia. Diagnosed by indirect ophthalmoscopy, B-scan ultrasonography, ultrasonographic biomicroscopy, or computed tomography (CT) scan of the globe. See 3.15, Intraocular Foreign Body.].

- Posterior scleritis [May or may not have an accompanying anterior scleritis. Vitritis is accompanied by a subretinal mass or thickening and sometimes an exudative retinal detachment. Chorioretinal folds may be seen. IVFA and B-scan ultrasonography (showing T sign) are helpful in diagnosis.].

- Retinoblastoma (Almost always occurs in young children. May be seen with a pseudohypopyon and vitreous cells. One or more elevated white retinal lesions are usually, but not always, present. A retinal detachment, iris neovascularization, or both may be found. IVFA, CT scan, and B-scan ultrasonography may aid in diagnosis. See 8.1, Leukocoria.).

- Leukemia (Unilateral retinitis and vitritis may occur in patients already known to have leukemia.).

- Amyloidosis (Rare. Vitreous globules or membranes without any signs of anterior segment inflammation. A serum protein electrophoresis and diagnostic/therapeutic vitrectomy confirm the diagnosis.).

- Asteroid hyalosis [Small, white, refractile particles (calcium soaps) adherent to collagen fibers and floating in the vitreous. Usually asymptomatic and of no clinical significance.].

ETIOLOGY

More common

- Toxoplasmosis (A yellow–white retinal lesion adjacent to a pigmented chorioretinal scar. Usually with overlying focal dense vitritis. See 12.5, Toxoplasmosis.).

- Sarcoidosis (Mutton-fat KP, iris nodules, sheathing around retinal veins, snowbanks and vitreous snowballs may be present. See 12.6, Sarcoidosis.).

- Syphilis (Acute chorioretinitis and vitritis that may mimic almost any other condition. A skin rash on the palms, soles, or both may be present. Retinal pigment clumping, sometimes similar to retinitis pigmentosa, may later occur. May be associated with retinal vascular occlusive disease. Congenital syphilis typically produces a salt-and-pepper fundus. Positive FTA-ABS. See 13.5, Acquired Syphilis, and 8.8, Congenital Syphilis.).

- Pars planitis [Considered an intermediate uveitis. Usually a bilateral vitritis in patients 15 to 40 years of age with white exudative material covering the inferior ora serrata and pars plana. Cellular clumps in the vitreous (appearing as "snowballs") and peripheral vascular sheathing may be present. See 12.2, Pars Planitis.].

- Ocular histoplasmosis (Common in Ohio–Mississippi River Valley area. Yellow–white, punched-out chorioretinal scars, usually less than 1 mm in diameter, peripapillary atrophy, and often choroidal neovascularization. Vitreous cells absent. See 11.15, Ocular Histoplasmosis.).

After Surgery or Trauma

See 12.10, Postoperative Endophthalmitis; 12.11, Chronic Postoperative Uveitis; 12.12, Traumatic Endophthalmitis; and 12.15, Sympathetic Ophthalmia.

Immunocompromised Host

For example, patients with acquired immunodeficiency syndrome (AIDS) being treated with chemotherapy, or transplant recipients.

- CMV (Whitish patches of necrotic retina are mixed with retinal hemorrhage. Also seen in neonates. See 13.4, Acquired Immunodeficiency Syndrome.).

- *Candida.* [Seen also in hospitalized patients being treated with prolonged antibiotic therapy, intravenous (i.v.) drug abusers, and patients with long-standing catheters. Yellow–white, fluffy, retinal or preretinal lesions are found initially. Later, associated "cotton balls" develop in the vitreous. *Candida* may be cultured from the blood, urine, or an i.v. site.].

- Herpetic retinitis (Clinically similar to ARN, but may not have vitreous cells and may spare retinal vessels. May involve deep retina. Rapidly progressive. Treat like ARN. See 12.8, Acute Retinal Necrosis.).

- Endogenous endophthalmitis (Patients are typically septic, and many have an anterior chamber reaction or hypopyon in addition to the vitritis. See 12.13, Endogenous Bacterial Endophthalmitis.).

• Others (Herpes simplex, varicella-zoster, fungi, mycobacteria, others.).

Panuveitis

Describes a pattern of severe, diffuse inflammation of both anterior and posterior segments. Often bilateral.

• Sarcoidosis.

• VKH syndrome.

• Syphilis.

• Behçet disease.

• Toxoplasmosis.

• Lens-induced uveitis.

• Sympathetic ophthalmia.

• Tuberculosis.

Retinal Vasculitis

Retinal sheathing around vessels, branch retinal vein occlusion, branch retinal artery occlusion.

• Periphlebitis (predominantly veins).

—Sarcoidosis (sheathing and yellow "candlewax" exudates around veins).

—Syphilis.

—Pars planitis (vessel changes most prominent in the inferior periphery, NVE may be present).

—Sickle cell retinopathy (sea-fan neovascular changes in the periphery).

—Eales disease (peripheral neovascularization and/or avascular retina).

—Behçet disease.

• Arteritis (predominantly arteries).

—Giant cell arteritis.

—Polyarteritis nodosum.

—ARN.

—Behçet disease.

—Systemic lupus erythematosus.

—IRVAN (idiopathic retinal vasculitis, aneurysms and neuroretinitis).

Less Common

• Acute zonal occult outer retinopathy (Young women with an enlarged blind spot, visual field abnormalities, and photopsias. Initially have minimal fundus changes but later may develop RPE changes corresponding to the field defect.).

• Acute posterior multifocal placoid pigment epitheliopathy (AMPPE) (Acute visual loss in young adults, often after a viral illness. Multiple, yellow, puzzle-shaped subretinal lesions in both eyes. Lesions block early and stain late on IVFA.).

• ARN (Frequently seen as acute iridocyclitis. Unilateral or bilateral peripheral white patches of thickened retina with vascular sheathing. The patches of necrotic retina gradually enlarge and coalesce. Vitreous cells are abundant. Retinal detachment is common. See 12.8, Acute Retinal Necrosis.).

• Behçet disease [Usually a bilateral retinal vasculitis. Vitritis, anterior uveitis (often with a hypopyon), retinal vasculitis and occasionally hemorrhages or exudate. Recurrent oral or genital ulcers or both, erythema nodosum, or arthritis may be noted. See 12.1, Anterior Uveitis, and 12.7, Behçet Disease.].

• Birdshot retinochoroidopathy (Usually middle-aged, with bilateral, multiple, creamy yellow spots deep to the retina, approximately 1 mm in diameter, scattered around the equator of the fundus. Vitreous cells are more abundant than aqueous cells. Retinal or optic nerve edema or both may be present. Positive HLA-A29 in approximately 90% of patients. Visual loss may also occur from CME.).

• Cat-scratch disease (Unilateral, stellate macular exudates, optic nerve swelling, vitreous cells, positive *Bartonella* serology. See 5.3, Parinaud Oculoglandular Conjunctivitis.).

- Diffuse unilateral subacute neuroretinitis (Unilateral visual loss in children and young adults, thought to be caused by a nematode. Optic nerve swelling, vitreous cells, and deep gray–white retinal lesions are present initially. Later, optic atrophy, narrowing of retinal vessels, and atrophic pigment epithelial changes develop. May mimic retinitis pigmentosa. Vision and visual fields deteriorate with time.).

- Septic (embolic) retinitis [Sudden onset of decreased vision in a systemically ill patient. Retinal edema, vascular sheathing, and hemorrhages with white centers (Roth spots) may be accompanied by vitreous cells. Diseased heart valves are common sources.].

- Lyme disease (Produces varied forms of posterior uveitis. More common in New England and Mid-Atlantic states, particularly in patients who camp outdoors. A history of a tick bite, skin rash, Bell palsy, or arthritis may be elicited. See 13.6, Lyme Disease.).

- Multiple evanescent white-dot syndrome (Photopsia and acute unilateral visual loss, often after a viral illness, usually in young women. May be bilateral or sequential. Multiple, creamy white lesions at the level of the retinal pigment epithelium with foveal granularity and vitreous cells. There is often an enlarged blind spot on formal visual field testing. Vision typically returns to normal within weeks without treatment.).

- Multifocal choroiditis [Unilateral visual loss in myopic young women, typically bilateral. Multiple, small, round, pale inflammatory lesions (similar to histoplasmosis) are located at the level of the pigment epithelium and choriocapillaris. Vitreous cells and mild disc edema may be present. The lesions are predominantly in the macula and frequently respond to oral or periocular steroids, but typically recur. Laser photocoagulation may be considered in the presence of a choroidal neovascular membrane. Punctate inner choroidopathy may be a variant of multifocal choroiditis and is clinically similar. It is distinguished by fewer vitreous cells, lesions confined mostly to the posterior pole, and fewer recurrences than multifocal choroiditis.].

- Rubella (Usually seen in infants whose mothers contracted rubella during the pregnancy. Salt-and-pepper pigmentation of the retina is typical. Microphthalmos, cataract, or iris transillumination defects may be present. The optic nerve may be pale. An increased anti-rubella antibody titer can usually be demonstrated.).

- Serpiginous choroidopathy [Typically bilateral, recurrent chorioretinitis characterized by acute lesions (yellow–white subretinal patches with indistinct margins) bordering old atrophic scars; however, one third may begin peripherally. The chorioretinal changes usually extend from the optic disc outward. Patients are typically aged 30 to 60 years. A choroidal neovascular membrane may develop, requiring laser photocoagulation to prevent visual loss.].

- Toxocariasis (Usually occurs in children, affecting only one eye. The most common presentations are a macular granuloma with poor vision, unilateral pars planitis with peripheral granuloma, or endophthalmitis. A granuloma appears as an elevated, white retinal lesion. A peripheral lesion may be associated with a fibrous band extending to the optic disc, sometimes dragging the macular vessels away from their normal course. A severe vitritis and anterior uveitis may be present. A negative undiluted *Toxocara* titer in an immunocompetent host usually rules out this disease. See 8.1, Leukocoria.).

- Tuberculosis [Produces varied clinical manifestations. The diagnosis is usually made by ancillary laboratory tests. Miliary tuberculosis may produce multifocal, small, yellow–white choroidal lesions. Most patients have concomitant anterior granulomatous or nongranulomatous uveitis. A 2-week therapeutic trial of isoniazid, 300 mg p.o., q.d., and pyridoxine (vitamin B_6), 10 mg/day, may be given. If the uveitis is the result of tuberculosis, it should improve significantly in patients on this regimen.].

- VKH syndrome (Serous retinal detachment with vitreous cells, a swollen optic disc, or atrophic patches at the level of the retinal pigment epithelium may accompany an anterior chamber reaction. Patients are darkly pigmented, typically of Asian or Native American ancestry, and have or develop systemic signs including meningeal signs, vitiligo, alopecia, and poliosis. Harada disease implies posterior pole involvement with neurologic involvement. See 12.9, Vogt–Koyanagi–Harada Syndrome.).

• Whipple disease (Rare. Small, white vitreous opacities, retinal hemorrhages and exudates, or exudative material over the pars plana in a patient with diarrhea, arthralgia, and weight loss. The diagnosis is made by intestinal biopsy or, less commonly, by pars plana vitrectomy.).

• Others [*Nocardia, Coccidioides* species, *Aspergillus* species, *Cryptococcus* species, meningococcus, ophthalmomyiasis, onchocerciasis, and cysticercosis (seen in Africa and Central and South America), measles, Eales disease, Crohn disease, multiple sclerosis, subacute sclerosing panencephalitis, and age-related vitritis.].

WORKUP

1. History: Systemic disease or infection, skin rash, i.v. drug abuse, indwelling catheter, risk factors for AIDS? Recent eye trauma or surgery? Travel to the Ohio–Mississippi River Valley, Southwestern United States, New England, or Middle Atlantic area? Tick bite?

2. Complete ocular examination, including IOP measurement and careful ophthalmoscopic examination. Indirect ophthalmoscopy with scleral depression of the entire ora serrata is essential.

3. Consider IVFA to help in diagnosis or plan for therapy.

4. Blood tests (any of the following are obtained, depending on the suspected diagnosis): *Toxoplasma* titer, ACE level, FTA-ABS, RPR, ESR, ANA, HLA-B5 (Behçet disease), HLA-A29 (birdshot retinochoroidopathy), *Toxocara* titer, Lyme immunofluorescent assay or ELISA, and in neonates or immunocompromised patients, titers for CMV, herpes simplex, varicella-zoster, or rubella virus. Cultures of blood and i.v. sites may be helpful when infectious etiologies are suspected. Polymerase chain reaction (PCR) techniques are available for herpes zoster, herpes simplex, *Toxoplasma*, and other pathogens.

5. PPD with anergy panel.

6. Chest radiograph.

7. Urine for CMV in immunocompromised patients.

8. CT/magnetic resonance imaging (MRI) scan of the brain and lumbar puncture when reticulum cell sarcoma is suspected and when human immunodeficiency virus (HIV)–associated opportunistic infections indicate a potential for systemic, and in particular, central nervous system (CNS) involvement.

9. Diagnostic vitrectomy when appropriate (see individual sections).

See the individual sections for more specific guidelines for workup and treatment.

12.4 HUMAN LEUKOCYTE ANTIGEN (HLA)–B27–ASSOCIATED UVEITIS

SYMPTOMS

Acute pain, blurred vision, photophobia. Associated systemic complaints include inflammatory back pain, arthritis, oral ulcers (which are typically not as painful as those seen in Behçet disease), urethritis, psoriasis, inflammatory bowel disease.

SIGNS

Critical. Recurrent unilateral alternating anterior uveitis.

Other. Severe anterior chamber reaction with cell, flare, and fibrin. May have hypopyon. Tendency to form posterior synechiae early. Ciliary flush.

Three times more common in men than women.

DIFFERENTIAL DIAGNOSIS

• Hypopyon uveitis (HLA-B27, Behçet disease, infectious endophthalmitis, retinoblastoma, metastatic tumors, rifabutin.).

• Behçet disease (May also have hypopyon uveitis, arthritis, oral ulcers; but in Behçet disease, posterior involvement is much more common than in HLA-B27, and oral ulcers are much more painful.).

• Idiopathic anterior uveitis.

TYPES OF HLA-B27 DISEASE

• HLA-B27–associated uveitis without systemic disease.

• Ankylosing spondylitis (Young adult men, often with low back pain, abnormalities on sacroiliac spine radiographs, increased ESR, positive HLA-B27.).

• Inflammatory bowel disease (Chronic intermittent diarrhea, often alternating with constipation.).

• Reiter syndrome (Young adult men, conjunctivitis, urethritis, polyarthritis, occasionally keratitis, increased ESR, positive HLA-B27, may have recurrent episodes. Arthritis tends to involve the lower extremities.).

• Psoriatic arthritis (Characteristic skin findings and arthritis typically involves the upper extremities.).

WORKUP

1. HLA-B27 to confirm diagnosis.

2. Ankylosing spondylitis: Sacroiliac spine radiographs show sclerosis and narrowing of the joint spaces, ESR, HLA-B27.

3. Inflammatory bowel disease: Medical or gastrointestinal consult, HLA-B27.

4. Reiter syndrome: Conjunctival, urethral, and prostatic cultures (for *Chlamydia*) if indicated; joint radiographs if arthritis is present; a medical or rheumatology consult; consider an HLA-B27.

5. Psoriatic arthritis: A rheumatology or dermatology consult, HLA-B27.

TREATMENT

See 12.1, Anterior Uveitis. HLA-B27 uveitis often recurs.

12.5 TOXOPLASMOSIS

SYMPTOMS

Blurred vision, floaters, may have redness, photophobia. Pain is absent.

SIGNS

Critical. New, unilateral white–yellow retinal lesion often associated with an old pigmented chorioretinal scar. There is a moderate to severe focal vitreous inflammatory reaction directly over the lesion.

Other

• Anterior: Mild anterior chamber spillover may be present, increased IOP in 10% to 20%.

• Posterior: Vitreous debris, optic disc swelling, neuroretinitis, retinal vasculitis, retinal artery or vein occlusion in the area of the inflammation. Chorioretinal scars are occasionally found in the uninvolved eye. CME may be present.

• Optic nerve: Neuroretinitis with macular star, sectoral disc swelling that may extend further onto the retina than expected, neuritis with greater than expected vitritis.

*Note: Toxoplasmosis is the most common cause of posterior uveitis and accounts for approximately 90% of focal necrotizing retinitis.

*Note: Toxoplasmosis can also develop in the deep retina with few to no vitreous cells present. This is common in HIV-infected patients.

DIFFERENTIAL DIAGNOSIS

See 12.3, Posterior Uveitis, for a complete list. The following may closely simulate toxoplasmosis.

• Syphilis (Positive FTA-ABS. See 13.5, Acquired Syphilis.).

• Tuberculosis (Positive PPD with possible abnormalities on chest radiograph.).

• Toxocariasis (Usually affects children. A fibrous band may be seen radiating from a white retinal mass. Old chorioretinal scars are not typically seen. May have a history of exposure to puppies or eating dirt. Positive *Toxocara* ELISA.).

WORKUP

See 12.3, Posterior Uveitis, for a nonspecific workup when the diagnosis is in doubt.

1. History: Does the patient eat raw meat or has he or she been exposed to cats (sources of acquired infection)? Inquire about risk factors for AIDS in atypical cases (e.g., several active lesions without old chorioretinal scars).

2. Complete ocular examination, including a dilated fundus evaluation.

3. Serum anti-*Toxoplasma* antibody titer. Should have a positive titer from current or previous infection (the dilution is unimportant), but a negative titer on any dilution does not exclude the diagnosis. Immunoglobulin M (IgM) is found approximately 2 to 6 months after initial infection, after which only IgG remains.

   *Note: Ask the laboratory to do a 1:1 dilution because any titer of serum antibodies is significant in the setting of classic fundus findings.

4. Toxoplasmosis antibody titers may be performed on anterior chamber taps in equivocal cases.

5. FTA-ABS, PPD with anergy panel, chest radiograph, and a *Toxocara* ELISA when the diagnosis is uncertain.

6. IVFA if a choroidal neovascular membrane is suspected.

7. Consider an HIV test in atypical cases or when the patient is a high-risk candidate for AIDS.

8. Toxoplasmosis in HIV-infected patients may be multifocal, occur without vitritis, and has

a high incidence of toxoplasmosis encephalitis. Such patients should be referred to an experienced specialist.

TREATMENT

1. The disease is self-limited in an immunocompetent patient. Mild peripheral retinochoroiditis may not require treatment. If an anterior chamber reaction is present, a topical cycloplegic (e.g., cyclopentolate, 2%, t.i.d.) with or without a topical steroid (e.g., prednisolone acetate, 1%, q.i.d.), is given. No additional treatment is indicated. The drops are tapered as the anterior chamber reaction resolves. Antiglaucoma medications are used to control IOP.

2. Treatment should be considered in an immunocompetent patient if the lesion is present in the temporal arcade near the macula, is within 2 to 3 mm of the disc, is threatening a large retinal vessel, or is associated with a large hemorrhage, or if the vitritis is severe enough to cause a two-line decrease in vision. Immunocompromised patients should be treated because the disease does not resolve spontaneously. Dosing for the nonpregnant adult is as follows:

   a. Usual first-line therapy (for 3 to 6 weeks):

      —Pyrimethamine, 200 mg p.o. load (or two 100-mg doses p.o., 12 hours apart), and then 25 mg p.o., b.i.d.

      —Folinic acid, 10 mg p.o., twice weekly (to minimize bone marrow toxicity of pyrimethamine).

      —Sulfadiazine, 2 g p.o. load and then 1 g p.o., q.i.d.

   b. Prednisone may be added, after initiation of antibiotic therapy, at a dose of 20 to 40 mg p.o., q.d., beginning 12 to 24 hours after antimicrobial therapy has begun. Periocular steroids should not be given.

   c. Clindamycin, 450 to 600 mg p.o., q.i.d., may be used with pyrimethamine as alternative therapy (if the patient is sulfa allergic) or as an adjunct to previously discussed therapy.

   d. Other alternative therapies are used with success. Atovaquone (e.g., Mepron) has been used with good results and is able to kill *Toxoplasma* cysts *in vitro*. Its ability to prevent recurrences *in vivo* is not yet known. Another alternative treatment is trimethoprim/sulfamethoxazole (160 mg/800 mg) one tablet p.o., b.i.d., with or without clindamycin and prednisone.

   e. Anterior segment inflammation is treated with cycloplegia (e.g., cyclopentolate, 1% to 2%, t.i.d.) and topical steroid (e.g., prednisolone acetate, 1%, q.i.d.).

   Note: Systemic steroids should never be used without antimicrobial treatment and rarely used in immunocompromised patients. Before systemic steroid use, evaluation of fasting blood sugar and studies to rule out tuberculosis are prudent. Subtenon steroids should not be used if toxoplasmosis is suspected.

   If a patient is given pyrimethamine, a platelet count and complete blood count (CBC) must be obtained once or twice per week to check for a low platelet count and a low red or white blood cell count (pyrimethamine can depress the bone marrow). If the platelet count decreases below 100,000, then reduce the dosage of pyrimethamine and increase the folinic acid.

   Patients taking pyrimethamine should not take vitamins that contain folic acid. The medication should be given with meals to reduce anorexia. A small number of pyrimethamine pills should be given at each visit to ensure compliance.

   Patients on clindamycin should be warned about pseudomembranous colitis, and the medication should be stopped if diarrhea develops.

3. Laser photocoagulation, cryotherapy, and vitrectomy have been used as adjunctive treatment modalities.

4. Maintenance therapy (if patient is immunosuppressed)

   —Pyrimethamine, 25 to 50 mg p.o., q.d.

   —Sulfadiazine, 500 to 1,000 mg p.o., q.i.d.

   —Folinic acid, 10 mg p.o., q.d.

—If sulfa allergic, may use clindamycin, 300 mg p.o., q.i.d.

—Before cataract surgery in a patient with a history of toxoplasmosis, consider prophylaxis with trimethoprim/sulfamethoxazole, b.i.d. during the perioperative period.

FOLLOW-UP

In 3 to 7 days for blood tests or ocular assessment or both, and then every 1 to 2 weeks on therapy.

Notes:

1. *If a patient cannot use or must discontinue clindamycin, tetracycline, 2 g load p.o., followed by 250 mg p.o., q.i.d., is used alternatively. Do not give tetracycline to children or pregnant or breast-feeding women.*

2. *Pyrimethamine should not be given to pregnant or breast-feeding women.*

See 13.4, Acquired Immunodeficiency Syndrome, for additional information.

12.6 SARCOIDOSIS

SYMPTOMS

Bilateral ocular pain, photophobia, decreased vision. Systemic findings may include shortness of breath, parotid enlargement, fever, or arthralgias. Most common in 20- to 50-year age group. Ten times more common in those of African heritage than whites.

SIGNS

Critical. Iris nodules, large mutton-fat KP (especially in a triangular distribution on the inferior corneal endothelium), sheathing along peripheral retinal veins ("candle-wax dripping"), peripheral neovascularization.

Other. Conjunctival nodules, enlargement of lacrimal gland, dry eyes, posterior synechiae, glaucoma, cataract, intermediate uveitis, CME, vitritis, Dalen–Fuchs nodules (pale choroidal lesions that may simulate multifocal choroiditis).

Systemic signs. Shortness of breath, facial nerve palsy, enlargement of parotid, lacrimal or salivary glands, bilateral symmetric hilar adenopathy on chest radiograph, erythema nodosum (erythematous, tender nodules beneath the skin, often found on the shins), lupus pernio (a dusky purple rash on nose and cheeks), arthritis, lymphadenopathy, hepatosplenomegaly with elevated liver function test results.

Note: Uveitis, secondary glaucoma, cataracts, and macular edema are the most common as well as the most significant vision-threatening complications of ocular sarcoid.

DIFFERENTIAL DIAGNOSIS

• Other causes of mutton-fat KP and iris nodules include syphilis, tuberculosis, sympathetic ophthalmia, or lens-induced uveitis.

• Intermediate uveitis may be idiopathic or secondary to sarcoid, multiple sclerosis, or Lyme disease.

• Posterior uveitis with multiple chorioretinal lesions may be from birdshot chorioretinopathy, intraocular lymphoma, syphilis, sympathetic ophthalmia, multifocal choroiditis, or VKH syndrome.

• Others (see 12.1, Anterior Uveitis, and 12.3, Posterior Uveitis).

WORKUP

The following are the tests that are obtained when sarcoidosis is suspected clinically. See 12.1, Anterior Uveitis, and 12.3, Posterior Uveitis, for nonspecific uveitis workups.

Initial workup:

1. Chest radiography is the single most useful test. Sarcoidosis findings are almost always bilateral and symmetric and include hilar adenopathy and lung infiltrates indicative of pulmonary fibrosis. In cases of unilateral or

atypical lung disease, consider lymphoma or malignancy.

2. Serum ACE is elevated in 60% to 90% of patients with active sarcoidosis. A normal serum ACE level does not rule out sarcoidosis, and an elevated ACE is not specific for sarcoidosis. Leprosy, histoplasmosis, and tuberculosis may also present with uveitis and elevated ACE. Patients on oral steroids and ACE inhibitors (e.g., captopril for hypertension) may have falsely low ACE levels. Elevated ACE levels are most sensitive and specific when combined with positive findings on chest radiography or gallium scan. ACE levels in children are variable and less helpful in diagnosis.

3. PPD with anergy panel: Useful for differentiating tuberculosis from sarcoidosis. Up to 50% of sarcoidosis patients are anergic and have no response to PPD or controls.

4. Obtain biopsy of a conjunctival nodule or skin lesion. Sample at the edges of skin plaques or nodules. Sarcoid granulomas are not present in erythema nodosum and these lesions should not be sampled. An acid-fast stain and a methenamine–silver stain may be performed at the time of biopsy to rule out tuberculosis and fungal infection. A nondirected conjunctival biopsy in the absence of visible lesions has a low yield and is not recommended. Nondirected biopsies of minor salivary glands by an oral surgeon have a reported 58% true-positive rate.

5. Some authors recommend serum and urine calcium levels, liver function tests, and a serum lysozyme. A positive result on one of these tests in the absence of chest radiographic or other findings is usually not helpful in diagnosis. A serum lysozyme may be useful in children, when ACE levels are unreliable.

If laboratory and chest radiographic studies suggest sarcoidosis, or in the setting of a negative workup but a high clinical suspicion of sarcoidosis, the following tests should be considered:

1. Chest CT scan may be more sensitive than plain films because the mediastinum and the lung parenchyma can be better visualized.

2. Whole-body gallium scan is sensitive for sarcoidosis. A "panda sign" indicates involvement of lacrimal, parotid, and submandibular glands. A "lambda sign" indicates involvement of perihilar and paratracheal lymph nodes. A positive gallium scan *and* an elevated ACE level is 73% sensitive and 100% specific for sarcoidosis.

Difficult cases may be referred to a pulmonologist for pulmonary function tests and transbronchial lung biopsy.

TREATMENT

Consider referring patients to an internist or pulmonologist for systemic evaluation and medical management. Consider early referral to a uveitis specialist in complicated cases. A poor visual outcome has been reported with posterior uveitis, glaucoma, delay in definitive treatment, or presence of macula-threatening conditions such as CME.

1. **Anterior uveitis:**

   —Cycloplegic (e.g., cyclopentolate, 1% to 2%, or scopolamine, 0.25%, t.i.d.).

   —Topical steroid (e.g., prednisolone acetate, 1%, q1–6h, depending on the degree of inflammation).

2. **Posterior uveitis:**

   —Systemic steroids (e.g., prednisone, 20 to 100 mg p.o., q.d.) and a histamine type 2 receptor (H_2) blocker (e.g., ranitidine, 150 mg p.o., b.i.d.) are often required in the presence of posterior uveitis (including optic neuritis) or bilateral severe anterior disease. See Drug Glossary when considering systemic steroids.

   —Periocular steroids (e.g., triamcinolone, 40 mg/mL in 0.5 mL, subtenon injection every 3 to 4 weeks) may be considered instead of systemic steroids. See Appendix 7 for the technique.

—Methotrexate, azathioprine, cyclosporine, and cyclophosphamide have been used effectively as steroid-sparing agents.

Note: Topical steroids alone are inadequate for treatment of significant posterior uveitis

3. **CME:** See 11.18, Cystoid Macular Edema.

4. **Glaucoma:** See 9.4, Inflammatory Open-Angle Glaucoma; 9.5, Steroid-Response Glaucoma; 9.10, Acute Angle-Closure Glaucoma; or 9.14, Neovascular Glaucoma, depending on the origin of the glaucoma.

5. **Retinal neovascularization:** May require panretinal photocoagulation.

6. **Orbital disease** is managed with systemic steroids as described previously.

7. **Pulmonary disease**, seventh nerve palsy, CNS disease, and renal disease require systemic steroids and management by an internist. Hypercalcemia also may require medical treatment.

FOLLOW-UP

1. Patients are reexamined in 1 to 7 days, depending on the severity of inflammation. The steroid dosages are adjusted in accordance with the patient's response to treatment. As the inflammation subsides, the steroids and cycloplegic agent are tapered slowly. IOP is monitored, and fundus reevaluation is performed at each visit.

2. Asymptomatic patients with quiet eyes are seen every 3 to 6 months.

3. Patients being treated with steroids need to be monitored more closely (every 3 to 6 weeks).

4. Poor response to steroid treatment should prompt a workup for other causes of uveitis or referral to a subspecialist.

12.7 BEHÇET DISEASE

SYMPTOMS

Sudden onset of bilateral decreased vision, floaters, pain, photophobia.

SIGNS

Critical. Painful oral ulcers (98% to 100% of patients), genital ulcers, and uveitis.

Other

• Anterior: Fleeting hypopyon, anterior chamber reaction, scleritis.

Note: Patients with Behçet disease almost never have fibrin even if anterior chamber reaction is severe.

• Posterior: Vitritis, retinal vasculitis, branch retinal vein obstruction, focal necrotizing retinitis, waxy optic nerve pallor, arterial attenuation.

• Skin: Erythema nodosum, dermatographia, pathergy (formation of a local pustule in response to intradermal injection).

• Systemic: Arthritis, CNS disease.

EPIDEMIOLOGY

Age 20 to 40 years, especially Japanese, Turkish, or Middle Eastern descent.

DIFFERENTIAL DIAGNOSIS

• Sarcoidosis (Smoldering venous vasculitis, iris nodules, mutton-fat KP.).

Note: Sarcoidosis may sometimes present with oral ulcers.

• HLA-B27 (Severe fibrinous anterior segment reaction with fixed hypopyon, typically recurrent unilateral alternating rather than simultaneous bilateral onset.).

Note: The oral ulcers in Behçet disease are typically painful and make it difficult to eat or drink. The oral ulcers in HLA-B27 disease are not as severe.

- ARN (Large confluent areas of retinal whitening in periphery, typically more pain than in Behçet disease.).

- Wegener granulomatosis (Nephritis, orbital inflammation, sinus and pulmonary inflammation.).

- Syphilis.

- Systemic lupus erythematosus and other collagen vascular diseases.

WORKUP

- Chest radiograph, ACE level, PPD with anergy panel.

- RPR, FTA-ABS.

- Consider HLA-B27 in young men with positive review of systems.

- Granular-staining anti-neutrophil cytoplasmic antibody (c-ANCA) if Wegener granulomatosis suspected.

- Consider HLA-B5 testing.

TREATMENT

Note: Untreated, bilateral blindness develops in most patients with Behçet disease within 3 to 4 years. Death may result from CNS involvement. Therefore, all patients with Behçet disease and posterior uveitis should be referred to a specialist for consideration of immunosuppressive therapy.

1. Systemic corticosteroids should be started (prednisone 1 to 2 mg/kg p.o., q.d. with ranitidine 150 mg p.o., b.i.d.). Steroids have been shown to delay the onset of blindness but not to alter the long-term outcome.

2. All patients with Behçet disease and posterior uveitis should be referred to a specialist for consideration of early immunosuppressive therapy.

FOLLOW-UP

Daily during acute episode to monitor inflammation and IOP until patient can be seen by uveitis specialist.

12.8 ACUTE RETINAL NECROSIS

SYMPTOMS

Blurred vision (often with floaters), significant ocular pain, photophobia. Most patients are healthy and not immunocompromised.

SIGNS

Critical. Focal, well-demarcated areas of retinal necrosis located in the peripheral retina; rapid, circumferential progression of necrosis, evidence of occlusive vasculitis and prominent inflammatory reaction in the vitreous and anterior chamber. The posterior pole is typically spared.

Other. Anterior chamber reaction; increased IOP; sheathed retinal arterioles and sometimes venules, especially in the periphery; retinal hemorrhages (minor finding); optic disc edema; RRD occurs in approximately 70% of patients. (The RRD typically has multiple, large, irregular posterior breaks and is usually a late finding.) An optic neuropathy (disc edema or pallor with an afferent pupillary defect, decreased color vision, and a central scotoma) sometimes develops.

ETIOLOGY

ARN is a clinical syndrome caused by varicella-zoster virus (older patients), herpes simplex virus (younger patients), or, rarely, CMV.

TABLE 12.4 CYTOMEGALOVIRUS RETINITIS VERSUS ACUTE RETINAL NECROSIS VERSUS TOXOPLASMOSIS

	Cytomegalovirus	Acute Retinal Necrosis	Toxoplasmosis
Retinal hemorrhages:	Significant	Uncommon	Absent
Vitritis:	Minimal	Significant	Significant
Pain:	Absent	Significant	Moderate
Immune status:	Immunocompromised	Usually healthy	Either
Appearance:	"Brushfire" border with leading edge of active retinitis and necrotic retina and mottled retinal pigment epithelium in its wake	Sharply demarcated lesions with nearly homogeneous appearance and same age	"Headlight in fog" with dense vitritis and smooth edges

DIFFERENTIAL DIAGNOSIS

- Herpes virus family (varicella-zoster or herpes simplex).

- CMV retinitis (Table 12.4).

- Syphilis.

- Toxoplasmosis.

- Behçet disease.

- Fungal or bacterial endophthalmitis.

- Large cell lymphoma. (Elderly patient with unilateral vitritis, absence of pain, homogenous-appearing vitritis with preservation of underlying vitreous architecture.)

See 12.3, Posterior Uveitis.

WORKUP

See 12.3, Posterior Uveitis, for a nonspecific uveitis workup.

1. History: Risk factors for AIDS? Immunocompromised? If yes, the differential diagnosis includes CMV retinitis and syphilis.

2. Complete ocular examination: Evaluate the anterior chamber and the vitreous for cells, measure the IOP, and perform a dilated retinal examination by using indirect ophthalmoscopy and scleral depression.

3. Consider a CBC with differential, FTA-ABS, RPR, ESR, toxoplasmosis titers, PPD with anergy panel, and chest radiograph to rule out other etiologies.

4. Consider testing for HIV.

5. Consider anterior chamber paracentesis for herpes simplex and varicella-zoster virus PCR.

6. Consider IVFA.

7. An orbital CT scan or B-scan ultrasonography to look for an enlarged optic nerve in cases of suspected optic nerve dysfunction.

8. CT scan or MRI of the brain and lumbar puncture if large cell lymphoma, tertiary syphilis, or encephalitis is suspected.

TREATMENT

Note: All patients with ARN should be referred to a practitioner with experience in this disease.

1. Admit to the hospital. The goal of treatment is to decrease the incidence of the disease in the fellow eye. Treatment does not reduce the rate of retinal detachment in the first eye.

2. Acyclovir[1], 1,500 mg/m^2 of body surface area/day i.v., in three divided doses for 10 to 14 days. Then oral acyclovir (400 to 600 mg five times per day) for up to 6 weeks from

[1]The dosage of acyclovir needs to be reduced in patients with renal insufficiency. Blood urea nitrogen and creatinine levels are followed closely.

the onset of infection.[2] Regression of the retinitis is usually seen within 4 days. The lesions may progress during the first 48 hours of treatment. Famciclovir may be useful in cases that do not respond to acyclovir.

3. Topical cycloplegic (e.g., atropine, 1%, t.i.d.) and topical steroid (e.g., prednisolone acetate, 1%, q2–6h) in the presence of anterior segment inflammation.

4. Consider anticoagulation (e.g., heparin or warfarin for a total of 2 to 3 weeks) or antiplatelet therapy (aspirin, 125 to 650 mg, q.d.).

5. Systemic steroids (controversial): Some physicians administer steroids aggressively at the time of diagnosis (e.g., methylprednisolone, 250 mg i.v., q.i.d., for 3 days followed by prednisone, 60 mg p.o., b.i.d., for 1 to 2 weeks), particularly when the optic nerve is thought to be involved. Others delay steroid therapy for 1 or more weeks until the retinitis begins to clear. A typical oral corticosteroid regimen (initial or delayed therapy) is prednisone, 60 to 80 mg/day, for 1 to 2 weeks followed by a taper over 2 to 6 weeks. See Drug Glossary before starting systemic steroids.

6. See 9.4, Inflammatory Open-Angle Glaucoma, for treatment of increased IOP.

7. Consider prophylactic laser photocoagulation (confluent laser spots posterior to active retinitis) to wall off or prevent subsequent RRD.

8. Pars plana vitrectomy, with long-acting gas or silicone oil, is the best way to repair the associated complex RRD. Proliferative vitreoretinopathy is common.

FOLLOW-UP

1. Patients are seen daily in the hospital and are then examined every few weeks to months for the following year.

2. A careful fundus evaluation with scleral depression is performed at each visit to rule out retinal holes that may lead to a detachment. If the retinitis crosses the margin of prior laser treatment, consider applying additional laser therapy.

3. A pupillary examination should always be performed, and optic neuropathy should be considered if the retinopathy does not explain the amount of visual loss.

---

[2]Six weeks of treatment is based on the observation that occurrences in the second eye most often begin within 6 weeks of the onset in the first eye.

12.9 VOGT–KOYANAGI–HARADA SYNDROME

SYMPTOMS

Decreased vision, photophobia, pain, and red eyes, accompanied or preceded by a headache, stiff neck, nausea, vomiting, fever, and malaise. Hearing loss, dysacusia, and tinnitus frequently occur. Typically bilateral.

Note: Harada disease refers to inflammatory serous retinal detachments without associated systemic signs of VKH syndrome.

SIGNS

Critical
• Anterior: Anterior chamber flare and cells, granulomatous (mutton-fat) KP, perilimbal vitiligo.

• Posterior: Bilateral serous retinal detachments with underlying choroidal thickening, vitreous cells and opacities, optic disc edema (nerve may appear reddish with multiple striae).

- **Systemic:** (Early) loss of high-frequency hearing, meningismus and (late) alopecia, vitiligo, poliosis.

- **IVFA:** Multiple pinpoint leaking areas of hyperfluorescence at the level of the retinal pigment epithelium.

Other

- **Anterior:** Hyphema, iris nodules, peripheral anterior or posterior synechiae, scleritis, hypotony or increased IOP from forward rotation of ciliary processes.

- **Posterior:** Mottling and atrophy of the retinal pigment epithelium after the serous retinal detachment resolves (sunset fundus), retinal vasculitis, choroidal neovascularization, Dalen–Fuchs nodules.

- **Systemic:** Neurologic signs, including loss of consciousness, paralysis, and seizures, may occur.

- **Epidemiology:** Typically, patients are aged 20 to 50 years, female (77%), and have pigmented skin, especially Asian, Hispanic, or Native American.

DIFFERENTIAL DIAGNOSIS

See Table 12.5; also see 12.3, Posterior Uveitis, for a complete list. In particular, consider the following:

- Sympathetic ophthalmia (History of trauma or surgery to the uninvolved eye. Usually no

TABLE 12.5 DIFFERENTIAL DIAGNOSIS OF SEROUS RETINAL DETACHMENTS

Inflammatory signs usually present:
- Harada disease
- Malignant hypertension
- Toxemia of pregnancy
- Disseminated intravascular coagulopathy
- Idiopathic uveal effusion syndrome

Inflammatory signs usually absent:
- Central serous chorioretinopathy
- Choroidal tumors (especially metastases)
- Pigment epithelial detachment
- Congenital optic nerve pit
- Macular holes in high myopes

CNS, skin, or hair manifestations. See 12.15, Sympathetic Ophthalmia.)

- AMPPE (Ophthalmoscopic and IVFA features may be very similar, but there is less vitreous inflammation and no anterior segment involvement.)

- Other granulomatous panuveitides (e.g., syphilis, sarcoidosis, tuberculosis).

WORKUP

See 12.3, Posterior Uveitis, for a nonspecific uveitis workup.

1. **History:** Neurologic symptoms, hearing loss, or hair loss? Previous eye surgery or trauma?

2. Complete ocular examination, including a dilated retinal evaluation.

3. CBC, RPR, FTA-ABS, ACE, and PPD with anergy panel and possibly chest radiograph to rule out similar-appearing disorders.

4. Consider a CT scan with and without contrast or MRI of the brain during attacks with neurologic signs to rule out a CNS disorder.

5. Lumbar puncture during attacks with meningeal symptoms for cell count and differential, protein, glucose, VDRL, Gram and methenamine–silver stains, and culture. (Lymphocytosis is often seen in VKH and AMPPE.)

6. IVFA demonstrates multiple pinpoint leaking areas of hyperfluorescence at the level of the retinal pigment epithelium.

TREATMENT

Inflammation is controlled with steroids; the dose depends on the severity of the inflammation. In moderate to severe cases, the following regimen can be used initially. Steroids are tapered slowly as the condition improves.

1. Topical steroids (e.g., prednisolone acetate, 1%, q1h).

2. Systemic steroids (e.g., prednisone, 60 to 80 mg p.o., q.d.) and an H_2 blocker (e.g., raniti-

dine, 150 mg p.o., b.i.d.). See Drug Glossary for a systemic steroid workup.

3. Topical cycloplegic (e.g., scopolamine, 0.25%, t.i.d.).

4. Treatment of any specific neurologic disorders (e.g., seizures or coma).

5. Immunosuppressive agents (e.g., methotrexate, azathioprine, chlorambucil, cyclosporine) can be used under the supervision of a medical consultant in patients who cannot tolerate or are unresponsive to systemic steroids.

FOLLOW-UP

1. Initial management may require hospitalization.

2. Weekly, then monthly reexamination is performed, watching for recurrent inflammation and increased IOP.

3. The steroids are tapered slowly. Inflammation may recur up to 9 months after the steroids have been discontinued. If this occurs, the previously described treatment regimen should be reinstituted.

12.10 POSTOPERATIVE ENDOPHTHALMITIS

ACUTE (ONE TO SEVERAL DAYS AFTER SURGERY)

SYMPTOMS

Sudden onset of decreased vision and increasing eye pain.

SIGNS

Critical. Hypopyon, fibrin, severe anterior chamber reaction, vitreous cells and haze, decreased red reflex.

Other. Eyelid edema, intense conjunctival injection, chemosis.

ORGANISMS

• Most common: *Staphylococcus epidermidis.*

• Common: *Staphylococcus aureus,* streptococcal species (except *Pneumococcus,* which is not a common cause).

• Less common: Gram-negative bacteria (*Pseudomonas, Aerobacter,* and *Proteus* species, *Haemophilus influenzae, Klebsiella* species, *Escherichia coli, Bacillus* species, *Enterobacter* species) and anaerobes.

• Bleb associated: *Streptococcus* or gram-negative infections.

DIFFERENTIAL DIAGNOSIS

See 12.11, Chronic Postoperative Uveitis.

WORKUP

1. Complete ocular history and examination. Look for wound/bleb leak, exposed suture, vitreous to wound, dacryocystitis, blepharitis or other predisposing factors for endophthalmitis.

2. Consider B-scan ultrasonography, which may confirm the clinical suspicion by revealing marked vitreous cells and establishes a baseline against which the success of therapy can be measured. Also used to evaluate for retinal breaks if medium is too cloudy adequately to visualize the retina.

3. If vision is light perception or worse, a diagnostic (and therapeutic) vitrectomy is often performed. Cultures (blood, chocolate, Sabouraud, thioglycolate) and smears (Gram and Giemsa stains) are obtained, and intravitreal antibiotics are given as described in the following section. Otherwise, an anterior chamber paracentesis combined with vitreous aspiration of 0.2 mL is performed.

4. Consider CBC with differential and serum electrolytes.

TREATMENT

1. Vitreous tap for Gram stain, culture and sensitivities (use a 25-gauge needle on a tuberculin syringe 3.5 mm posterior to the limbus, withdraw 0.2 mL of fluid).

2. Intravitreal antibiotics (vancomycin 1 mg/0.1 mL and either ceftazidime 2.25 mg/0.1 mL or amikacin, 0.4 mg/0.1 mL) injected 3.5 mm posterior to the limbus.

3. Admit to hospital for observation and intensive topical steroids (e.g., prednisolone acetate, 1%, q1h around the clock).

4. Consider intensive topical fortified antibiotics (e.g., vancomycin and tobramycin, q1h around the clock for 24 to 48 hours). Intensive topical antibiotics are more important in the setting of filtering blebs, wound leaks, or exposed sutures.

5. Atropine, 1%, t.i.d. to q.i.d.

6. For postcataract endophthalmitis, immediate pars plana vitrectomy is beneficial if visual acuity on presentation is light perception or worse. Vitrectomy for other causes of endophthalmitis (bleb-related, posttraumatic, or endogenous) may be beneficial in selected cases.

7. Intravenous antibiotics are not routinely used. Consider i.v. levofloxacin, moxifloxacin, or gatifloxacin in special circumstances (e.g., bleb-related endophthalmitis or trauma). Third- and fourth-generation fluoroquinolones may penetrate the vitreous enough to reach therapeutic levels, especially in inflamed eyes.

Note: Vitrectomy offers the theoretical advantages of reducing bacterial load as well as providing material for diagnostic studies.

FOLLOW-UP

1. Monitor the clinical course q12h.

2. Relief of pain is a useful early sign of response to therapy.

3. Consider starting oral steroids (prednisone 60 mg p.o. each morning with ranitidine 150 mg p.o., b.i.d.) in patients who can tolerate steroids.

4. At 48 hours, patients should show response to treatment (relief of pain, decreased inflammation, decreased hypopyon). Consider reinjecting antibiotics if no improvement or if Gram stain shows an unusual organism. Consider vitrectomy if patient is deteriorating.

5. The antibiotic regimen is refined according to the patient's response to treatment and to the culture and sensitivity results.

6. If the patient is responding well to treatment, topical fortified antibiotics may be slowly tapered after 48 hours and then switched to regular strength or a fluoroquinolone. Close outpatient follow-up is warranted.

DELAYED ONSET (A WEEK TO A MONTH OR MORE AFTER SURGERY)

SYMPTOMS

Insidious decreased vision, increasing redness and pain.

SIGNS

Critical. Reduced visual acuity, anterior chamber and vitreous inflammation, vitreous abscesses, hypopyon; clumps of exudate in the anterior chamber, on the iris surface, or along the pupillary border.

Other. Corneal infiltrate and edema; may have a surgical bleb.

ORGANISMS

• Fungi (*Aspergillus, Candida, Cephalosporium, Penicillium* species; others).

• *P. acnes* (Recurrent, granulomatous anterior uveitis, often with a hypopyon, but with minimal conjunctival injection and pain. A white plaque or opacities on the posterior lens capsule may be evident. There is only a transient response to steroids.).

• Other bacteria [Related to a filtering bleb (often streptococci), vitreous wick, or partial suppression with antibiotics during or after surgery.].

DIFFERENTIAL DIAGNOSIS

See 12.11, Chronic Postoperative Uveitis.

WORKUP

1. Complete ocular history and examination.

2. Vitreous material for smears (Gram, Giemsa, and methenamine–silver) and cultures [blood, chocolate, Sabouraud, thioglycolate, and a solid medium for anaerobic culture (e.g., *Brucella* or blood agar); *P. acnes* will be missed unless proper anaerobic cultures are obtained]. Intravitreal antibiotics are given as described in the following section.

3. Consider CBC with differential, serum electrolytes, liver function studies.

TREATMENT

1. Initially treat as acute postoperative endophthalmitis, as described previously, but do not start steroids.

2. Immediate pars plana vitrectomy is beneficial if visual acuity on presentation is light perception or worse up to 6 weeks after surgery. Benefit beyond 6 weeks is not known.

3. If a fungal infection is suspected or an intraoperative smear is consistent with fungus, administer intravitreal amphotericin B, 5 to 10 µg at the time of vitrectomy. If fungus is identified on Gram stain, Giemsa stain, or calcofluor white, then use combination of topical and systemic antifungal medications. Use topical natamycin, 5%, q1h, and flucytosine, 37.5 mg/kg p.o., q6h, until specific organism is known. Role of systemic amphotericin B and fluconazole is unclear. Dosing information is provided later.

—Amphotericin B, 0.25 to 0.3 mg/kg/day i.v., initially (in test doses of 1 mg), and then increase the dose slowly to 0.75 to 1.0 mg/kg/day i.v. in divided doses.

—Consider miconazole, 10 mg in 1 mL, subconjunctivally.

—A therapeutic vitrectomy should be performed if it was not done with the initial cultures. Antifungal therapy is modified in accordance with sensitivity testing, clinical course, and tolerance to antifungal agents.

4. Removal of the lens and capsular remnants may be required for diagnosis and treatment of *P. acnes,* which may be sensitive to intravitreal penicillin, cefoxitin, clindamycin, or vancomycin.

5. If mild *S. epidermidis* is isolated, intraocular vancomycin alone may be sufficient.

FOLLOW-UP

1. Dependent on the organism.

2. In general, follow-up is as described previously for acute postoperative endophthalmitis.

3. Repeat CBC, serum electrolytes, and liver function tests two times per week during treatment for fungal endophthalmitis.

BIBLIOGRAPHY

Doft BH, Wisniewski SR, Kelsey SF, et al. Endophthalmitis Vitrectomy Study Group: Diabetes and postoperative endophthalmitis in the endophthalmitis vitrectomy study. *Arch Ophthalmol* 2001;119:650–656.

12.11 CHRONIC POSTOPERATIVE UVEITIS

Postoperative inflammation is typically mild in severity, responds promptly to steroids, and usually resolves within 6 weeks. This section presents several etiologies of postoperative uveitis and a workup that may be considered when postoperative inflammation is atypical.

ETIOLOGY

Severe intraocular inflammation in the early postoperative course

• Infectious endophthalmitis [Progressive and often severe ocular pain (but not always), deteriorating vision, fibrin in the anterior chamber, eyelid swelling, hypopyon, and vitreous inflammation and blunting of the red reflex. See 12.10, Postoperative Endophthalmitis.].

• Retained lens material (A severe granulomatous inflammation with mutton-fat KP, resulting from an autoimmune reaction to lens protein exposed during surgery.)

• Aseptic endophthalmitis (A severe sterile postoperative uveitis caused by excess tissue manipulation, especially vitreous manipulation, during surgery. A hypopyon and a mild vitreous cellular reaction may develop. Usually not characterized by profound or progressive pain or visual loss. Eyelid swelling and chemosis are atypical. Usually resolves with topical steroid therapy.)

• Inflammatory reaction to contaminants on the intraocular lens (e.g., polishing substances or substances used to sterilize the lens) or to the viscoelastic substance.

Persistent postoperative inflammation (e.g., beyond 6 weeks):

• Patient noncompliance with steroid drops (e.g., not taking the drops or not shaking them properly).

• Steroid drops tapered too abruptly.

• Iris or vitreous incarceration in the wound.

• UGH syndrome (Irritation of the iris or ciliary body by an intraocular lens. Increased IOP and red blood cells in the anterior chamber accompany the anterior segment inflammation.)

• Retinal detachment (Often produces a low-grade anterior chamber reaction. See 11.3, Retinal Detachment.)

• Low-grade endophthalmitis (e.g., *P. acnes*, fungal, or partially treated bacterial endophthalmitis).

• Epithelial downgrowth (Corneal or conjunctival epithelium grows into the eye through a corneal wound and may be seen on the posterior corneal surface. The iris may appear flattened because of the spread of the membrane over the anterior chamber angle onto the iris. Large cells may be seen in the anterior chamber, and glaucoma may be present. The diagnosis of epithelial downgrowth can be confirmed by observing the immediate appearance of white spots after medium-power argon laser treatment to the areas of iris covered by the membrane.)

• Preexisting uveitis (see 12.1, Anterior Uveitis).

Sympathetic ophthalmia

Diffuse granulomatous inflammation in both eyes, after trauma or surgery to one eye. See 12.15, Sympathetic Ophthalmia.

WORKUP

1. History: Is the patient taking and shaking the steroid drops properly? Did the patient stop the steroid drops abruptly? Was there a postoperative wound leak allowing epithelial downgrowth or fibrous ingrowth? Previous history of uveitis?

2. Complete ocular examination of both eyes, including a slit-lamp assessment of the anterior chamber reaction, a determination of

whether vitreous or residual lens material is present in the anterior chamber, and an inspection of the posterior lens capsule looking for posterior capsular opacities (as is seen in some cases of *P. acnes* infection). Gonioscopy (checking for iris or vitreous to the wound or small retained lens fragments in the inferior angle), an IOP measurement, a dilated indirect ophthalmoscopic examination (to rule out a retinal detachment or signs of chorioretinitis), and a posterior vitreous evaluation with a slit lamp and a 60-diopter, Hruby, or Goldmann contact lens looking for inflammatory cells should be performed.

3. Obtain B-scan ultrasonography when the fundus view is obscured.

4. A diagnostic surgical vitrectomy is usually performed for smears and cultures when nonpostoperative infectious endophthalmitis is suspected. For postoperative endophthalmitis, see 12.10, Postoperative Endophthalmitis. Anaerobic cultures, using both solid media and broth, should be obtained to isolate *P. acnes* (routine cultures also are obtained; see 12.10, Postoperative Endophthalmitis). The anaerobic cultures should be incubated in an anaerobic environment as rapidly as possible and allowed to grow for at least 2 weeks.

5. Consider an anterior chamber paracentesis for diagnostic smears and cultures.

6. Consider diagnostic medium-power argon laser treatment to the areas of iris thought to be covered by epithelial downgrowth.

If this workup is negative, no underlying etiology can be elicited, and a trial of steroids reduces the inflammation only transiently, surgical removal of the capsular bag and intraocular lens should be considered in an effort to isolate *P. acnes*.

See 12.1, Anterior Uveitis; 12.3, Posterior Uveitis; 12.10, Postoperative Endophthalmitis; and 12.15, Sympathetic Ophthalmia for more specific information on diagnosis and treatment.

12.12 TRAUMATIC ENDOPHTHALMITIS

This condition constitutes an emergency. If suspected, prompt action is required.

SYMPTOMS AND SIGNS

Same as 12.10, Postoperative Endophthalmitis.

Note: Patients with Bacillus *endophthalmitis may have a high fever, leukocytosis, proptosis, a corneal abscess in the form of a ring, and rapid visual deterioration.*

ORGANISMS

Bacillus species, *S. epidermidis,* gram-negative species, fungi, *Streptococcus* species, others. A mixed flora may be present.

DIFFERENTIAL DIAGNOSIS

• Sterile inflammatory response from a retained intraocular foreign body or blood in the vitreous.

• Sterile inflammation as a result of surgical manipulation.

• Phacoanaphylactic endophthalmitis (A sterile autoimmune inflammatory reaction as a result of exposed lens protein.).

WORKUP

Same as for 12.10, Postoperative Endophthalmitis. An orbital CT scan (axial and coronal views) or ultrasonography also is performed to rule out an intraocular foreign body.

TREATMENT

1. Hospitalization.

2. Management for a ruptured globe or penetrating ocular injury if present (see 3.14, Ruptured Globe and Penetrating Ocular Injury).

3. Topical antibiotics (e.g., fortified tobramycin, q1h, and fortified cefazolin or fortified vancomycin, q1h, alternating every half hour). See Appendix 9, which describes fortified drop preparation.

4. Systemic antibiotics (e.g., ciprofloxacin 400 mg i.v., q12h, and clindamycin 600 mg i.v., q8h).[3]

5. Intravitreal antibiotics (e.g., amikacin, 0.4 mg in 0.1 mL, or ceftriaxone, 2 mg in 0.1 mL, and vancomycin, 1 mg in 0.1 mL, or clindamycin, 1 mg in 0.1 mL). These may be repeated every 48 to 72 hours, as needed.

6. The benefit of pars plana vitrectomy is unknown for this type of endophthalmitis. However, pars plana vitrectomy offers the benefit of reducing infectious load and pro-

viding sufficient material for diagnostic culture and pathologic investigation.

7. If tetanus immunization not up to date, give tetanus toxoid, 0.5 mL intramuscularly.

8. Steroids should *not* be used until fungal organisms are ruled out. If no fungi are isolated, may use prednisolone acetate, 1%, q4h, and subconjunctival dexamethasone, 4 mg. Prednisone, 40 to 80 mg p.o., q.d., is at the discretion of the surgeon. If fungus is isolated, specific antifungal regimens may be used.

Note: Antibiotics are usually withheld until after the vitrectomy is performed unless a prolonged delay until surgery is expected.

FOLLOW-UP

Same as for 12.10, Postoperative Endophthalmitis. The specific antibiotics and the frequency of their administration should be modified in accordance with the patient's response to treatment, as well as the culture and sensitivity results.

---

[3]Drug doses may need to be reduced in children and patients with renal disease. Check gentamicin peak and trough levels one-half hour before and after the fifth dose, and follow the blood urea nitrogen and creatinine levels.

12.13   ENDOGENOUS BACTERIAL ENDOPHTHALMITIS

SYMPTOMS

Decreased vision in an acutely ill (e.g., septic) patient, an immunocompromised host, or an i.v. drug abuser. No history of recent intraocular surgery.

SIGNS

Critical. Vitreous cells and debris, anterior chamber cell and flare, or a hypopyon in a high-risk patient.

Other. Iris microabscess, absent red fundus reflex, retinal inflammatory infiltrates, flame-shaped retinal hemorrhages with or without white centers, corneal edema, eyelid edema, chemosis, conjunctival injection. Panophthalmitis [orbital involvement (proptosis, restricted ocular motility) and endophthalmitis] may develop.

ORGANISMS

Bacillus cereus (especially in i.v. drug abusers), streptococci, *Neisseria meningitidis, S. aureus, H. influenzae,* others.

DIFFERENTIAL DIAGNOSIS

• Endogenous fungal endophthalmitis (May see fluffy, white vitreous opacities. Fungi grow on cultures. See 12.14, *Candida* Retinitis/Uveitis/Endophthalmitis.)

• Retinochoroidal infection (e.g., toxoplasmosis and toxocariasis) (Yellow or white retinochoroidal lesion present.)

• Noninfectious posterior uveitis (e.g., sarcoidosis, pars planitis) (May have a known history of uveitis. Unlikely to get coincidentally the first episode during sepsis.)

- Neoplastic conditions [e.g., large cell lymphoma (usually older than 50 to 55 years), retinoblastoma (usually in the first few years of life)].

WORKUP

1. History: Duration of symptoms? Underlying disease or infections? Intravenous drug abuse? Immunocompromised?

2. Complete ocular examination, including a dilated fundus evaluation.

3. B-scan ultrasonography to determine the extent of posterior segment ocular involvement if it cannot be determined on clinical examination.

4. Complete medical workup by an infectious disease expert.

5. Cultures of blood, urine, and all indwelling catheters and i.v. lines, as well as Gram stain of any discharge. A lumbar puncture is indicated when meningeal signs are present.

6. Vitrectomy with intraocular antibiotics (e.g., amikacin, 0.4 mg in 0.1 mL, or ceftriaxone, 2 mg in 0.1 mL, and vancomycin, 1 mg in 0.1 mL; clindamycin, 1 mg in 0.1 mL, may be used in place of vancomycin): The timing of this procedure is controversial. We perform it as soon as possible. Other physicians initially perform aqueous and vitreous aspirations when the systemic cultures are negative and the organism remains unknown.

TREATMENT

In conjunction with a medical internist.

1. Hospitalize the patient.

2. Broad-spectrum antibiotics are started after appropriate smears and cultures are obtained. Antibiotic choices vary according to the suspected source of septic infection (e.g., gastrointestinal tract, genitourinary tract) and are determined by an infectious disease expert. Dosages recommended for meningitis and severe infections are used.

Note: Intravenous drug abusers are given an aminoglycoside and clindamycin to eradicate Bacillus cereus.

3. Topical cycloplegic (e.g., atropine, 1%, t.i.d.).

4. Topical steroid (e.g., prednisolone acetate, 1%, q1h to q6h, depending on the degree of anterior segment inflammation).

5. Periocular antibiotics (e.g., subconjunctival or subtenon injections) are sometimes used. See Appendix 7 for injection techniques.

6. Intravitreal antibiotics offer higher intraocular concentrations.

7. Vitrectomy offers the benefit of reducing infective load and providing sufficient material for diagnostic culture and pathologic study.

FOLLOW-UP

1. Daily in the hospital.

2. Peak and trough levels for many antibiotic agents are examined every few days. Blood urea nitrogen and creatinine levels are monitored during aminoglycoside therapy. The antibiotic regimen is guided by the culture and sensitivity results, as well as the patient's clinical response to treatment. Intravenous antibiotics are maintained for at least 2 weeks and until the condition has resolved.

12.14 *CANDIDA* RETINITIS/UVEITIS/ENDOPHTHALMITIS

SYMPTOMS

Decreased vision, floaters, pain, often bilateral. Patients typically are i.v. drug abusers, immuno-compromised hosts (e.g., as a result of cancer, immunosuppressive agents, AIDS, long-term antibiotics, or systemic steroids) or possess a long-term indwelling catheter (e.g., for hyperalimentation or hemodialysis).

SIGNS

Critical. Multifocal, yellow–white, fluffy retinal lesions from one to several disc diameters in size. With time, the lesions increase in size, spread into the vitreous, and appear as "cotton balls."

Other. Vitreous cells and haze, vitreous abscesses, retinal hemorrhages with or without pale centers (pale centers indicate Roth spots), aqueous cells and flare, hypopyon. Retinal detachment may develop.

DIFFERENTIAL DIAGNOSIS

The following should be considered in immunocompromised hosts.

• CMV retinitis (Minimal to mild vitreous reaction, more retinal hemorrhage, tends to concentrate along vessels; consider strongly in patients with AIDS. See 13.4, Acquired Immunodeficiency Syndrome.).

• Toxoplasmosis (Yellow–white lesion confined to the retina. An adjacent chorioretinal scar may or may not be present. Vitreous cells and debris are common, but vitreous abscesses or "cotton balls" are not. See 12.5, Toxoplasmosis.).

• Others (e.g., herpes simplex; *Mycobacterium avium-intracellulare*; *Nocardia, Aspergillus,* and *Cryptococcus* species; coccidioidomycosis).

WORKUP

1. History: Medications? Medical problems? Intravenous drug abuse? Other risk factors for AIDS?

2. Search the skin for scars from i.v. drug injection.

3. Complete ocular examination, including a dilated retinal evaluation.

4. Blood, urine, and catheter site (if present) cultures for *Candida* species; these often need to be repeated several times and may be negative despite ocular candidiasis.

5. Diagnostic (and therapeutic) vitrectomy is indicated when a significant amount of vitreous involvement is present. Cultures and smears are taken at the time of vitrectomy to confirm the diagnosis and to evaluate the organisms' sensitivity to antifungal agents. Amphotericin B, 5 μg in 0.1 mL, is injected into the central vitreous cavity at the conclusion of the procedure.

6. Baseline CBC, blood urea nitrogen, creatinine, and liver function tests.

TREATMENT

1. Hospitalize all unreliable patients, systemically ill patients, or those with moderate to severe vitreous involvement.

2. An infectious disease specialist or internist familiar with antifungal therapy should be consulted.

3. Fluconazole, 200 to 400 mg p.o., q.d.

4. In resistant cases, amphotericin B may be administered. For the first few days, amphotericin B, 1 mg i.v., is given five times per day, then larger doses totaling 20 mg/day are administered. Therapy is discontinued when a total dose of 1,000 mg has been given. Patients with endophthalmitis can be given up

to 1 mg/kg/day for several weeks, not to exceed a total dose of 2 g.

5. Topical cycloplegic agent (e.g., atropine, 1%, t.i.d.).

6. See 9.4, Inflammatory Open-Angle Glaucoma, for IOP control. Note, however, that steroids are usually contraindicated in candidiasis.

FOLLOW-UP

1. Patients are seen daily. Visual acuity, IOP, and the degree of anterior chamber and vitreous inflammation are assessed.

2. Serum blood urea nitrogen levels, creatinine levels, and CBC are repeated a few times per week. Liver function tests are repeated periodically. Serum levels of antifungal agents are followed, and dosages are adjusted accordingly.

Note: Systemic antifungal agents may not be necessary if no systemic disease is uncovered.

12.15 SYMPATHETIC OPHTHALMIA

SYMPTOMS

Bilateral eye pain, photophobia, decreased vision (near vision is often affected before distance vision), red eye. A history of penetrating trauma or intraocular surgery to one eye (usually 4 to 8 weeks before, but the range is from 5 days to 66 years, with 90% occurring within 1 year) may be elicited.

SIGNS

Critical. Any inflammation in the uninvolved eye after unilateral ocular trauma is suspect. Bilateral severe anterior chamber reaction with large mutton-fat KP, small depigmented nodules at the level of the retinal pigment epithelium (Dalen–Fuchs nodules), and thickening of the uveal tract. Signs of previous injury or surgery in one eye are usually present, including indications of previous laser therapy or cryotherapy.

Other. Nodular infiltration of the iris, peripheral anterior synechiae, neovascularization of the iris, occlusion and seclusion of the pupil, cataract, exudative retinal detachment, papillitis. The earliest sign may be loss of accommodation or a mild anterior or posterior uveitis in the uninjured eye.

DIFFERENTIAL DIAGNOSIS

• VKH syndrome (Similar signs, but often no history of ocular trauma or surgery. Other symptoms and signs may include headache, nausea, vomiting, fever, malaise, vertigo, bizarre behavior, focal neurologic symptoms, alopecia, vitiligo, or poliosis. Darkly pigmented people, especially Asians, are more commonly affected. See 12.9, Vogt–Koyanagi–Harada Syndrome.).

• Phacoanaphylactic endophthalmitis (Severe anterior chamber reaction from injury to the lens capsule, usually from trauma or surgery. No posterior uveitis is present. Contralateral eye is uninvolved.).

• Sarcoidosis (May cause a granulomatous panuveitis with exudates over retinal veins or white clumps in the anterior vitreous inferiorly. Concomitant pulmonary disease is common. No history of trauma. See 12.6, Sarcoidosis.).

• Syphilis (Granulomatous panuveitis may be accompanied by interstitial keratitis, dilated capillary nests on the iris, or a diffuse pigmentary retinopathy. Positive FTA-ABS. No history of trauma. See 13.5, Acquired Syphilis.).

WORKUP

1. History: Any prior eye surgery or injury? Venereal disease? Difficulty breathing?

2. Complete ophthalmic examination, including a dilated retinal examination.

3. CBC, RPR, FTA-ABS, and ACE level (if sarcoidosis is a serious consideration).

4. Consider a chest radiograph to evaluate for tuberculosis or sarcoidosis.

5. IVFA or B-scan ultrasonography, or both, to help confirm the diagnosis.

TREATMENT

1. Prevention: Enucleation of a blind, traumatized eye before a sympathetic reaction can develop (usually considered within 7 to 14 days of the trauma). If sympathetic ophthalmia develops, enucleation may still be beneficial, regardless of the time since trauma.

   Inflammation is controlled with steroids; the dose depends on the severity of the inflammation. In moderate to severe cases, the following regimen can be used initially. Steroids are tapered slowly as the condition improves.

2. Topical steroids (e.g., prednisolone acetate, 1%, q1–2h).

3. Periocular steroids (e.g., subconjunctival dexamethasone, 4 to 5 mg in 0.5 mL, two to three times per week). See Appendix 7 for the administration technique.

4. Systemic steroids [e.g., prednisone, 60 to 80 mg p.o., q.d., and an antacid or H_2 blocker (e.g., ranitidine, 150 mg p.o., b.i.d.)]. Before using systemic steroids, should consider evaluation of fasting blood sugar, PPD, and chest radiograph.

5. Cycloplegic (e.g., scopolamine, 0.25%, t.i.d.).

6. If steroids are ineffective or contraindicated, an immunosuppressive agent (e.g., methotrexate or cyclosporine) may be tried, usually in conjunction with a medical consultant.

FOLLOW-UP

1. Every 1 to 7 days initially, to monitor the effectiveness of therapy.

2. As the condition improves, the follow-up interval may be extended to every 3 to 4 weeks.

3. IOP must be monitored closely.

4. Steroids should be maintained for 3 to 6 months after all signs of inflammation have resolved. Because of the possibility of recurrence, periodic checkups are important.

CHAPTER 13

GENERAL OPHTHALMIC PROBLEMS

13.1 ACQUIRED CATARACT

SYMPTOMS

Slowly progressive visual loss or blurring, usually over months to years, affecting one or both eyes. Glare, particularly from oncoming headlights while driving at night, and reduced color perception may occur, but not to the same degree of dyschromatopsia as can occur with optic neuropathies. The particular symptoms are based on the location and density of the lens opacity.

SIGNS

Critical. Opacification of the normally clear crystalline lens (see the respective types).

Other. The retina often appears indistinct on funduscopic examination, and the dilated red reflex may be dim on retinoscopy. A direct ophthalmoscope at distances of 3 to 5 feet also may show a decreased red reflex or the hardened nucleus or cortical spokes on retroillumination. The patient may be found to be more myopic than previously noted (so-called "second sight"). A cataract alone does not cause a relative afferent pupillary defect.

ETIOLOGY

• Age-related (Most common).

• Trauma (Ocular or head contusion, electrocution, others.).

• Toxic [Steroids, anticholinesterases, antipsychotics (e.g., phenothiazines), others.].

• Intraocular inflammation (e.g., uveitis).

• Radiation.

• Intraocular tumor (A ciliary body malignant melanoma may produce a sector cortical cataract.).

• Degenerative ocular disease (e.g., retinitis pigmentosa).

• Diabetes (The juvenile form is characterized by white "snowflake" opacities in the anterior and posterior subcapsular locations. It often progresses rapidly. Adults develop age-related cataracts as described previously, but at an earlier age.).

• Hypocalcemia (Small, white, iridescent cortical changes, usually seen in the presence of tetany.).

• Wilson disease [Red–brown pigment deposition in the cortex beneath the anterior capsule (a "sunflower" cataract). Seen with a corneal Kayser–Fleischer ring.].

• Myotonic dystrophy (Multicolored opacities cause a "Christmas-tree cataract" behind the anterior capsule.).

• Others (e.g., Down syndrome, atopic dermatitis).

TYPES

1. Nuclear: Yellow or brown discoloration of the central part of the lens on slit-lamp ex-

amination. Typically blurs distance vision more than near vision.

2. Posterior subcapsular: Opacities appear near the posterior aspect of the lens, often forming a plaque. They are best seen in retroillumination against a red fundus reflex. Glare and difficulty reading are common complaints. May be associated with ocular inflammation, prolonged steroid use, diabetes, trauma, or radiation. Classically occurs in patients younger than 50 years.

3. Cortical: Radial or spokelike opacities in the lens periphery that expand to involve the anterior and posterior lens. Often asymptomatic until the changes develop centrally.

Note: A mature cataract is defined as anterior cortical changes sufficiently dense to obscure totally the view of the posterior lens and posterior segment of the eye.

WORKUP

Determine the etiology, whether the cataract is responsible for the decreased vision, and whether surgical removal would improve vision.

1. History: Medications? Systemic diseases? Trauma? Ocular disease or poor vision in youth or young adulthood (before the cataract)?

2. Complete ocular examination, including distance and near vision, pupillary examination, and refraction. A dilated slit-lamp examination by using both direct and retroillumination techniques is usually required to view the cataract properly. Fundus examination, concentrating on the macula, is essential in ruling out other causes of decreased vision. It is helpful for preoperative planning to note the degree of pupil dilation, density of the cataract, and presence or absence of pseudo-exfoliation syndrome or phacodonesis.

3. B-scan ultrasonography when the fundus is obscured by a dense cataract to rule out posterior segment disease.

4. The potential acuity meter (PAM) or laser interferometry can be used to estimate the visual potential when cataract extraction is being considered in an eye with posterior segment disease.

Note: Laser interferometry and PAM often overestimate the eye's visual potential in the presence of macular holes or macular pigment epithelial detachments. Interferometry also makes an overprediction of results in cases of amblyopia. Near vision is often the most accurate manner of evaluating macular function if the cataract is not too dense. Nonetheless, both laser interferometry and PAM are useful clinical tools.

5. When surgery is planned, keratometry readings and an A-scan ultrasonographic measurement of axial length are required for determining the power of the desired intraocular lens. An evaluation of the corneal endothelium, usually done at the slit lamp but occasionally requiring an endothelial cell count, is also needed.

TREATMENT

1. Cataract surgery may be performed for the following reasons:

   —To improve visual function in patients with symptomatic visual disability.

   —As surgical therapy for ocular disease (e.g., lens-related glaucoma or uveitis).

   —To facilitate management of ocular disease (e.g., to monitor or treat diabetic retinopathy or glaucoma).

2. Correct any refractive error if the patient declines cataract surgery.

3. A trial of mydriasis (e.g., scopolamine, 0.25%, q.d.) may be used successfully in some patients if the patient desires nonsurgical treatment. The benefits of this therapy are only temporary.

FOLLOW-UP

Unless there is a secondary complication from the cataract (e.g., glaucoma; quite rare), a cataract itself does not require urgent action. Patients who decline surgical removal are reexamined yearly, and sooner if there is a symptomatic decrease in visual acuity.

If congenital, see 8.7, Congenital Cataract.

13.2 DIABETES MELLITUS

DIABETIC RETINOPATHY

SIGNS

• Mild nonproliferative diabetic retinopathy (NPDR): Dot-and-blot hemorrhages, microaneurysms, and hard exudates, usually most prominent in the posterior pole. Nearly always bilateral.

• Moderate NPDR: Same findings as mild NPDR, plus cotton-wool spots, venous beading and loops, and moderate capillary nonperfusion [seen on intravenous fluorescein angiography (IVFA)].

• Severe NPDR: Same findings as moderate NPDR, plus four quadrants of intraretinal hemorrhages, or two quadrants of venous beading, or one quadrant of intraretinal microvascular abnormalities.

• Proliferative diabetic retinopathy (PDR): The findings in mild, moderate, or severe NPDR, or a combination of these, are often present plus neovascularization on or within one disc diameter of the optic disc (NVD), neovascularization elsewhere (retina) (NVE), or neovascularization of the iris (NVI). Fibrovascular tissue along the posterior surface of or extending into the vitreous and adherent to the retina, traction retinal detachment, or vitreous hemorrhage also may be present. Usually bilateral, but can be asymmetric. Almost always in the posterior pole.

Note: Macular edema may be present in any of the stages listed.

DIFFERENTIAL DIAGNOSIS

Nonproliferative

• Central retinal vein occlusion (CRVO) (Optic disc swelling is present, veins are more tortuous, hard exudates are usually not found, hemorrhages are more prominent, and CRVO is generally unilateral and of more sudden onset. See 11.7, Central Retinal Vein Occlusion.).

• Branch retinal vein occlusion (BRVO) [The hemorrhages are distributed along the course of a vein, and do not extend across the horizontal raphe (midline). See 11.8, Branch Retinal Vein Occlusion.].

• Ocular ischemic syndrome (The hemorrhages are larger and mostly in the mid-periphery; exudate is absent. See 11.10, Ocular Ischemic Syndrome.).

• Hypertensive retinopathy (The hemorrhages are more commonly flame shaped and rarely abundant, microaneurysms occur less frequently, and the retinal arterioles are narrowed. See 11.9, Hypertensive Retinopathy.).

• Radiation retinopathy (Microaneurysms are rarely present. Follows radiation therapy to the eye or adnexal structures such as the brain, sinus, or nasopharynx, when the eye is irradiated inadvertently. May develop any time after the radiation therapy, but occurs most commonly within a few years. Hold a high suspicion for it even in patients in whom the eye was reportedly shielded. Usually, 3,000 cGy is necessary, but it has been noted to occur with 1,500 cGy.).

Proliferative

• Neovascular complications of BRVO, CRVO, or central retinal artery occlusion (History of one of these events. See previous discussion.).

• Sickle cell retinopathy (Retinal neovascularization occurs peripherally, usually not in the macula. "Sea-fans" of peripheral retinal neovascularization are present. See 11.23, Sickle Cell Disease.).

• Embolization from intravenous (i.v.) drug abuse (e.g., talc retinopathy) (History of i.v. drug abuse, peripheral retinal neovascularization, may see particles of talc in macular vessels.).

• Sarcoidosis [May have uveitis, exudates around veins ("candle-wax drippings") or systemic findings. See 12.6, Sarcoidosis.].

- Ocular ischemic syndrome (Usually accompanied by pain; mild anterior chamber reaction; corneal edema; episcleral vascular congestion; a mid-dilated, poorly reactive pupil; iris neovascularization; and pulsations of the central retinal artery induced by light digital pressure. See 11.10, Ocular Ischemic Syndrome.).

- Radiation retinopathy (See prior discussion.).

WORKUP

1. Examine the iris carefully for neovascularization, preferably before pharmacologic dilation. [Check the angle with gonioscopy, especially if intraocular pressure (IOP) is increased.]

2. Dilated fundus examination by using a 90- or 60-diopter or fundus contact lens with a slit lamp to obtain a stereoscopic view of the posterior pole. Rule out neovascularization and macular edema. Use indirect ophthalmoscopy to examine the retinal periphery.

3. Fasting blood sugar, glycosylated hemoglobin, and, if necessary, a glucose tolerance test if the diagnosis is not established.

4. Check the blood pressure.

5. Consider IVFA to determine areas of perfusion abnormalities, foveal ischemia, microaneurysms, and clinically inapparent neovascularization (especially if considering focal macular laser therapy).

6. Consider blood tests for hyperlipidemia if extensive exudate is present.

TREATMENT

Clinically Signficant Macular Edema

Focal or grid laser treatment should be considered when any of the following forms of macular edema are present (Fig. 13.1):

1. Retinal thickening within 500 μm (one third of disc diameter) of the center of the macula.

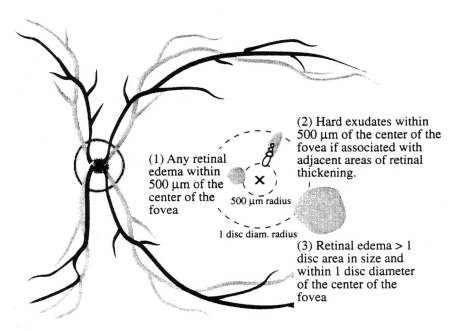

(1) Any retinal edema within 500 μm of the center of the fovea

500 μm radius

1 disc diam. radius

(2) Hard exudates within 500 μm of the center of the fovea if associated with adjacent areas of retinal thickening.

(3) Retinal edema > 1 disc area in size and within 1 disc diameter of the center of the fovea

FIGURE 13.1 Clinically significant macular edema in diabetic retinopathy that warrants grid-pattern photocoagulation.

2. Hard exudates within 500 μm of the center of the macula, if associated with thickening of the adjacent retina.

3. Retinal thickening greater than one disc area in size, part of which is within one disc diameter of the center of the macula.

Note: Patients with enlarged foveal avascular zones on IVFA are treated lightly, away from the regions of foveal ischemia, if they are treated at all. Patients with extensive, frank foveal ischemia are poor candidates for treatment. Younger patients and diet-controlled diabetic patients tend to have a better treatment response.

Proliferative Diabetic Retinopathy

Panretinal laser photocoagulation is indicated for any one of the following high-risk characteristics (Fig. 13.2):

1. NVD greater than one fourth to one third of the disc area in size.

2. Any degree of NVD when associated with preretinal or vitreous hemorrhage.

3. NVE greater than one half of the disc area in size when associated with a preretinal or vitreous hemorrhage.

4. Any NVI.

Note: Some physicians treat NVE or any degree of NVD without preretinal or vitreous hemorrhage, especially in unreliable patients.

Note: If the ocular media are too hazy for an adequate fundus view, yet one of these conditions is met, peripheral retinal cryotherapy may be indicated, if there is no vitreous traction. Pars plana vitrectomy and endolaser therapy with or without lensectomy and posterior chamber intraocular lens is another alternative.

Indications for Vitrectomy

Vitrectomy may be indicated for any one of the following conditions:

1. Dense vitreous hemorrhage causing decreased vision, especially when present for several months.

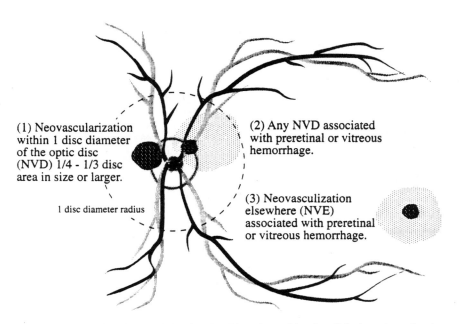

(1) Neovascularization within 1 disc diameter of the optic disc (NVD) 1/4 - 1/3 disc area in size or larger.

1 disc diameter radius

(2) Any NVD associated with preretinal or vitreous hemorrhage.

(3) Neovasculization elsewhere (NVE) associated with preretinal or vitreous hemorrhage.

FIGURE 13.2 High-risk characteristics for visual loss in proliferative diabetic retinopathy that warrant panretinal photocoagulation.

2. Traction retinal detachment involving and progressing within the macula.

3. Macular epiretinal membranes or recent-onset displacement of the macula.

4. Severe retinal neovascularization and fibrous proliferation that are unresponsive to laser photocoagulation.

5. Dense premacular hemorrhage.

Note: Patients with juvenile type 1 diabetes are known to have more aggressive proliferative diabetic retinopathy and therefore may benefit from earlier vitrectomy and laser photocoagulation. B-scan ultrasonography may be required to rule out tractional detachment of the macula in eyes with dense vitreous hemorrhage obscuring a fundus view.

FOLLOW-UP

1. *Diabetes without retinopathy.* Annual dilated examination.

2. *Mild NPDR.* Dilated examination every 6 months.

3. *Moderate to severe NPDR.* Dilated examination every 2 to 4 months.

4. *PDR (not meeting high-risk criteria).* Dilated examination every 1 to 3 months.

See 13.3, Pregnancy for the follow-up of diabetic retinopathy in pregnant women.

Note: The Diabetes Control and Complications Trial showed that intensive control of blood sugar with insulin (in type 1 diabetes) decreases the progression of diabetic retinopathy (as well as nephropathy and neuropathy).[1]

NEUROOPHTHALMIC PROBLEMS
CRANIAL NERVE ABNORMALITIES

An isolated third, fourth, or sixth cranial nerve palsy, often associated with pain in or around the eye, may result from diabetic microvascular disease. Only very rarely are two nerves involved simultaneously. Typically, third nerve in-

[1]*N Engl J Med* 1993;329:977–986.

volvement spares the pupil (i.e., it does not become dilated). A diabetic cranial nerve paralysis usually resolves within 3 months. No treatment is indicated.

ACUTE DISC EDEMA (DIABETIC PAPILLOPATHY)

Benign disc edema may occur in one or both eyes of a diabetic patient, most commonly with mild visual loss. There is no correlation with the severity of diabetic retinopathy. In addition to disc edema, disc hyperemia due to telangiectases of the disc vessels may occur, simulating neovascularization. This entity is more common in patients with juvenile-onset diabetes. No treatment is indicated. Spontaneous resolution usually occurs after 3 to 4 months.

Idiopathic anterior ischemic optic neuropathy also may occur in diabetic patients. Usually it is associated with more dramatic visual loss than in nondiabetic patients (manifested as a decrease in acuity and visual field loss).

GLAUCOMA
PRIMARY OPEN-ANGLE GLAUCOMA

Patients with diabetes are probably at an increased risk for this form of glaucoma. When treating with a topical beta-blocker, additional care must be exercised in monitoring for side effects. Beta-blockers may mask the warning symptoms of hypoglycemia (e.g., sweating, shaking, nightmares, restlessness).

NEOVASCULAR GLAUCOMA

As discussed previously, neovascularization of the iris and glaucoma are complications of diabetes, and panretinal photocoagulation is indicated as soon as possible.

MISCELLANEOUS
REFRACTIVE CHANGES

Acute hyperglycemia may produce a sudden hyperopic or myopic shift, causing bilateral blurred vision. Glasses should not be prescribed until the patient's blood sugar has been stable for several months.

CATARACT

Diabetic patients are at an increased risk of cataract, especially posterior subcapsular cataracts.

MUCORMYCOSIS

A rare, life-threatening orbital infection caused by this ubiquitous fungus can occur in diabetic patients, particularly those with ketoacidosis. Any diabetic or compromised host with the appearance of orbital cellulitis (eyelid edema, proptosis, external ophthalmoplegia, and fever) should be further examined for necrosis of the skin, nasal mucosa, or palate. An emergency computed tomography (CT) scan of the sinuses, orbit, and brain should be performed to aid in diagnosis. A biopsy should be obtained from any necrotic tissue as well as the nasopharynx and paranasal sinuses if this condition is suspected. Treat with liposomal amphotericin B. (See 10.9, Cavernous Sinus and Associated Syndromes.)

13.3 PREGNANCY

ANTERIOR SEGMENT

Changes include a transient loss of accommodation and increased corneal thickness and curvature with secondary change in the corneal refractive index. The change in refraction is probably the result of a shift in fluid or hormonal status and will most likely revert to normal after delivery. Unless the patient is insistent, it is best to defer prescribing new glasses until several weeks postpartum.

In addition, these physiologic corneal changes may hinder contact lens wear. Because corneal sensitivity is known to decrease during pregnancy, possibly increasing the risk of infection, discontinuation of contact lenses is often advisable.

PREECLAMPSIA/ECLAMPSIA

Occurs in 5% of pregnancy and presents after 20 weeks of gestation.

SYMPTOMS

Headaches, blurred or loss of vision, photopsias, diplopia.

SIGNS

Systemic

- Preeclampsia: Hypertension, proteinuria, and peripheral edema.

- Eclampsia: Preeclampsia with seizures.

Ocular. Focal retinal arteriolar spasm and narrowing, peripapillary or focal areas of retinal edema, serous retinal detachments in 1% of preeclamptic and 10% of eclamptic patients, acute nonarteritic ischemic optic neuropathy, and bilateral occipital lobe infarcts (preeclampsia–eclampsia hypertensive posterior encephalopathy syndrome, or PEHPES). Differential diagnosis of PEHPES includes posterior circulation stroke, infectious cerebritis, coagulation disorder causing intracranial venous thrombosis, intracranial hemorrhage, occult tumor with secondary bleed, migraines, atypical seizure, or demyelination.

NATURAL HISTORY

1. Magnetic resonance imaging (MRI) abnormalities resolve 1 to 2 weeks after blood pressure control, at which time complete neurologic recovery can be expected.

2. Serous retinal detachment resolve postpartum with residual pigment epithelial changes.

3. Retinal vascular changes also normalize postpartum.

WORKUP

1. Complete neuroophthalmologic and fundus examinations including pupillary evaluation. Brisk pupils and no relative afferent pupillary defect in a patient with poor vision suggest the possibility of occipital lesions.

2. MRI findings in PEHPES include bilateral occipital lobe lesions involving subcortical white matter with possible extension into the gray–white junction, cortical surface, external capsule, and basal ganglia. MRI abnormalities are identical in obstetric and nonobstetric hypertensive encephalopathy.

3. With a typical presentation, further invasive studies are discouraged.

4. Systemic workup, including blood pressure monitoring and urinalysis, in conjunction with a gynecologic consult.

TREATMENT

1. Control blood pressure and electrolyte imbalances.

2. When possible, prompt delivery would be ideal.

CENTRAL SEROUS CHORIORETINOPATHY

See 11.11, Central Serous Chorioretinopathy.

More frequently (90%) associated with subretinal exudates than the nonpregnant population (less than 20%). The diagnosis is a clinical one, with IVFA being rarely necessary. Observation is the treatment of choice for the vast majority of cases, with most resolving postpartum. A more hyperopic correction may provide temporary visual assistance.

DIABETIC RETINOPATHY

See 13.2, Diabetes Mellitus.

Risk factors for progression of diabetic retinopathy during pregnancy include baseline severity of diabetic retinopathy, duration of diabetes, associated hypertension, elevated glycosylated hemoglobin, and rapid glycemic control. NPDR, PDR, and diabetic macular edema that occur during pregnancy have a high likelihood of postpartum regression. Table 13.1 summarizes recommendations based on the baseline degree of diabetic retinopathy.

PURTSCHER RETINOPATHY

Extensive cotton-wool spots and nerve fiber layer or preretinal hemorrhages in the posterior pole classically occurring in the setting of major trauma. Exact etiology is unknown but may be related to sudden increase in venous pressure, fat or amniotic fluid embolization, or release of inflammatory mediators at the time of labor and delivery. Visible fundus changes resolve in several weeks, but some visual impairment persists in approximately 50% of cases. No treatment has been established.

PITUITARY ADENOMA

Pituitary adenomas may enlarge during pregnancy, producing a visual field disturbance (classically a bitemporal hemianopsia) or headache. Because subclinical pituitary adenomas may produce amenorrhea, women who underwent treatment to induce ovulation should be examined with a high index of suspicion.

A possible cause of pituitary adenoma enlargement during pregnancy is pituitary apoplexy, a potentially life-threatening event. Therefore, any woman with a pituitary adenoma who presents with a headache or a new visual field defect should have an MRI. Peripartum hemorrhage or shock can cause an in-

TABLE 13.1 RECOMMENDATIONS BASED ON THE BASELINE DEGREE OF DIABETIC RETINOPATHY

Baseline Diabetic Retinopathy	Gestational Diabetes	None or Minimal NPDR	Mild to Moderate NPDR	High-Risk NPDR	PDR
Gestational course	No risk of retinopathy	No progression in vast majority. Of those who progress, only a few have visual impairment	Progression in up to 50%. Postpartum regression in many	Progression in up to 50%. Postpartum regression in some	Tends to progress rapidly
Eye examinations	None	First and third trimester	Every trimester	Monthly	Monthly
Treatment	None	None	None, unless high-risk proliferative changes occur	None, unless high-risk proliferative changes occur	Treat PDR with panretinal photocoagulation by the same criteria as defined by the Diabetic Retinopathy Study. Observe diabetic macular edema because of the high rate of spontaneous postpartum regression. Consider cesarean section to prevent vitreous hemorrhage due to Valsalva maneuver used during labor. Not an indication to terminate pregnancy.

NPDR, nonproliferative diabetic retinopathy; PDR, proliferative diabetic retinopathy.

farction of the pituitary gland, leading to hypopituitarism (Sheehan syndrome).

Migraines are usually worse during pregnancy and immediately postpartum.

PSEUDOTUMOR CEREBRI

See 10.15, Pseudotumor Cerebri.

The incidence of pseudotumor cerebri has not been shown to increase during pregnancy. However, management may prove challenging, given that many of the medications used to treat pseudotumor cerebri are contraindicated in pregnant women.

MIGRAINE HEADACHE

See 10.25, Migraine.

MENINGIOMA OF PREGNANCY

Meningiomas may have a very aggressive growth pattern during pregnancy that is difficult to manage. They may regress postpartum but may regrow during subsequent pregnancies.

Note: All pregnant women complaining of a headache should have their blood pressure, visual fields, and fundus checked (particularly looking for papilledema). As mentioned, MRI or lumbar puncture is often required if a hemorrhage or cortical venous thrombosis is suspected.

13.4   ACQUIRED IMMUNODEFICIENCY SYNDROME

RISK GROUPS

The symptoms of acquired immunodeficiency syndrome (AIDS) appear after the human immunodeficiency virus (HIV) has severely depleted the immune system of CD4+ T lymphocytes. Risk groups include homosexual or bisexual men, i.v. drug abusers, hemophiliacs and transfusion recipients, sexual partners of HIV-infected (HIV+) individuals, prostitutes and their sexual partners, and infants born to HIV+ mothers.

LABORATORY TESTING

For initial diagnosis (establishes HIV+ status):

1. Serum enzyme-linked immunosorbent assay (ELISA) for HIV antibody (highly sensitive, less specific).

2. If ELISA is positive, Western blot to confirm (highly specific). If Western blot is positive, patient is considered HIV+.

3. Polymerase chain reaction is available if the preceding two tests are negative in high-risk individuals.

For monitoring the patient's clinical status:

4. CD4+ cell counts.

5. HIV viral titers.

Note: A diagnosis of AIDS is made on the basis of CD4+ counts less than 200 cells/mm³ or the presence of an AIDS-defining illness, in an HIV+ patient.

OCULAR COMPLICATIONS OF AIDS

CORNEA AND EXTERNAL DISEASES

HERPES ZOSTER OPHTHALMICUS

May be the initial clinical manifestation of HIV infection. Herpes zoster ophthalmicus in patients younger than 40 years without known immunocompromise should raise the clinical suspicion for AIDS.

SIGNS

Vesicular lesions of the face in the distribution of the ophthalmic division of the trigeminal nerve. May be associated with almost any ocular abnormality, including keratitis, uveitis, scleritis, and cranial nerve palsies. (See 4.15, Herpes Zoster Virus.)

WORKUP

Complete ophthalmic examination, including dilated fundus examination. An associated late complication of patients with AIDS with herpes zoster ophthalmicus is progressive outer retinal necrosis (PORN), a rapidly progressive retinitis characterized by clear vitreous and sheetlike opacification deep to normal-looking retinal vessels. PORN also may be seen with spontaneous vitreous hemorrhage. This condition frequently leads to bilateral blindness due either to the infection itself or to secondary retinal detachment, making prompt diagnosis and treatment essential. (See 12.8, Acute Retinal Necrosis.)

TREATMENT

See Table 13.2 for treatment details.

1. Nucleoside analog antiviral medications, tailored to the individual patient. The location and extent of the lesions as well as the stage of the HIV infection are all factors that play a role in selecting an appropriate therapy.

2. When intraocular inflammation is present, a topical cycloplegic (e.g., scopolamine, 0.25%, t.i.d.) and a topical steroid (e.g., prednisolone acetate, 1%, q1–2h) are given.

3. Bacitracin ointment to the skin lesions, b.i.d.

4. If associated with PORN, i.v. plus intraocular antivirals may be used.

*Note: Patients should not receive oral steroids because of the risk of further immunosuppression and extension of the infection.

Kaposi Sarcoma

Kaposi sarcoma (KS) of the ocular adnexal tissues occurs in approximately 5% of patients with AIDS. (See 5.12, Conjunctival Tumors.)

SIGNS

Skin lesions are more common than conjunctival lesions. Eyelid lesions are purple–red, nontender nodules and can have associated edema, trichiasis, or entropion formation. Bright red subconjunctival lesions are most commonly located in the inferior cul-de-sac. (These may be mistaken for benign subconjunctival hemorrhage.) Orbital lesions with associated periorbital edema occur rarely.

TREATMENT

1. Vinblastine and vincristine have had some success in causing remission of KS.

2. Local treatment by excision, cryotherapy, or irradiation may be performed for single lesions if systemic chemotherapy is not used or has failed.

TABLE 13.2 HERPES ZOSTER OPHTHALMICUS

Drug	Dosing Information	Toxicities	Contraindications
Acyclovir (e.g., Zovirax)	10 mg/kg i.v., q8h (q12h if creatinine >2.0) ×7–10 days. Consider maintenance with 800 mg p.o., 5×/day to prevent reactivation.	Intravenous: reversible renal and neurologic toxicity	Use with caution in patients with a history of renal impairment.
Famciclovir (e.g., Famvir)	500 mg p.o., q8h. Adjust dosage for creatinine clearance <60 mL/min.	Headache, nausea, diarrhea, dizziness, fatigue	Use with caution in patients with a history of renal impairment.
Valacyclovir HCl (e.g., Valtrex)	1 g p.o., q8h. Adjust dosage for creatinine clearance <60 mL/min.	Headache, nausea, vomiting, diarrhea	See comment.[a]

[a]Comment: In patients with advanced human immunodeficiency virus or acquired immunodeficiency syndrome, thrombotic thrombocytopenic purpura/hemolytic–uremic syndrome has been reported in association with valacyclovir doses of 8 g/day.
i.v., intravenously; p.o., orally.

Note: KS lesions may resolve when patients are given HIV protease inhibitors.

OTHER CORNEA AND EXTERNAL DISEASE

• Molluscum contagiosum: Chronic follicular conjunctivitis, umbilicated eyelid nodules. Few lesions in immunocompetent patients, but multiple and bilateral in patients with AIDS. Treated with excision or cryotherapy. (See 5.2, Chronic Conjunctivitis.)

• Microsporidial keratoconjunctivitis: Chronic superficial punctate keratitis and conjunctival injection not responsive to conservative treatment. Diagnosed with Giemsa stain of corneal scraping. Treated with topical fumagillin or oral itraconazole or both. Epithelial debridement followed by topical antibiotic ointment (e.g., bacitracin, t.i.d.) may be useful for mild cases.

• Bacterial and fungal keratitis: May occur without prior corneal injury. (See 4.12, Fungal Keratitis.) Not more common in patients with AIDS, but more severe presentation.

• Herpes simplex virus keratitis: May be associated with more frequent recurrence and prolonged, peripheral ulceration. (See 4.14, Herpes Simplex Virus.)

• Herpes zoster disciform keratitis: May occur without preceding skin eruption. (See 4.15, Herpes Zoster Virus.)

• Cytomegalovirus (CMV) keratitis: Stellate keratic precipitates are suggestive of concomitant CMV retinitis and CMV keratitis. Treatment for CMV keratitis is not well established.

UVEITIS

• CMV infection.

• Syphilis (see 13.5, Acquired Syphilis).

• Toxoplasmosis.

• Drug-induced uveitis (Several agents used in HIV+ patients may cause uveitis/hypopyon, including rifabutin, cidofovir, and sulfonamides. If rifabutin is the inciting agent, reduce the dose, and add topical steroids to control the uveitis. For all others, stop the inciting agent.).

• Pseudohypopyon secondary to lymphoma.

• HIV infection–associated uveitis [Consider this condition if inflammation is poorly responsive to steroids and no other etiology is present (e.g., drug reaction).].

POSTERIOR SEGMENT DISEASE

NONINFECTIOUS RETINAL MICROVASCULOPATHY ("HIV RETINOPATHY")

Noninfectious retinopathy is the most common ocular manifestation of AIDS. Fifty to 70% of patients with AIDS have this condition. It may be the presenting sign of AIDS.

SYMPTOMS

Usually asymptomatic.

SIGNS

Cotton-wool spots, intraretinal hemorrhages, microaneurysms (resembles diabetic retinopathy, not specific for AIDS). An ischemic maculopathy may occur, causing significant visual loss in 3% of patients.

WORKUP

HIV retinopathy is a marker of low CD4+ counts; thus, the presence of retinal microvasculopathy should prompt a complete slit-lamp and dilated fundus examination looking for concomitant opportunistic infections (e.g., CMV retinitis).

TREATMENT

No specific ocular treatment is available. This condition improves with systemic antiviral treatment for HIV and improving CD4 counts.

CYTOMEGALOVIRUS RETINITIS

The most common ocular opportunistic infection in patients with AIDS (34% prevalence) and the leading cause of AIDS-related blindness. CMV is usually seen in patients with CD4+ counts of 50 cells/mm^3 or less. Because active retinitis may be asymptomatic, dilated fundus examination should be performed at least every 3 months in patients with CD4+ counts of 50 cells/mm^3 or less to rule out opportunistic disease.

SYMPTOMS

Patients may notice a scotoma or decreased vision in one or both eyes. Patients may also experience floaters, but most patients do not have vitreous cells owing to profound immunosuppression. Pain or photophobia is usually not found. Patients often have few to no symptoms, emphasizing the importance of routine examinations.

SIGNS

Critical

• Indolent form: Peripheral granular opacities with occasional hemorrhage.

• Fulminant form: Confluent areas of necrosis with associated hemorrhage, starting along the major retinal vascular arcades. Progressive retinal atrophy may also indicate active CMV.

Other. The eye is typically quiet and white with few to no aqueous or vitreous cells. Retinal pigment epithelial (RPE) atrophy and pigment clumping result once the active process resolves. Rhegmatogenous retinal detachment (RRD) occurs in approximately one third of patients with CMV retinitis. (There is an increased risk of RRD when more than 25% of the retina is affected by retinitis.)

WORKUP

See Table 13.3 for treatment details.

1. History and complete ocular examination, including dilated fundus examination.

TABLE 13.3 CYTOMEGALOVIRUS RETINITIS

Drug	Dosing Information	Toxicities	Contraindications
Ganciclovir (e.g., Cytovene)	i.v. induction: 5 mg/kg i.v. b.i.d. ×2–3 wk i.v. maintenance: 5 mg/kg i.v. q.d., or 6 mg/kg i.v. 5 days/wk	Neutropenia[a], thrombocytopenia, anemia, renal toxicity.	Absolute neutrophil count <500/mm^3 platelets <25,000/mm^3; potentially embryotoxic. Discontinue nursing.
Ganciclovir implant	4.5 mg sustained-release	Well-tolerated[b] device implanted in the anterior vitreous. Lasts 6–10 mo.	Surgical complications occur (e.g., retinal detachment, vitreous hemorrhage).
Foscarnet (e.g., Foscavir)	i.v. induction: 90 mg/kg i.v. b.i.d. ×2 wk i.v. maintenance: 120 mg/kg i.v. q.d.[c] Monitor creatinine/ electrolytes and adjust dosing as needed.	Renal impairment; neutropenia; anemia; electrolyte imbalances.	Use caution with renal impairment or electrolyte imbalances.
Cidofovir, HPMPC (e.g., Vistide)	i.v. induction: 5 mg/kg i.v. weekly ×3 wk i.v. maintenance: 3–5 mg/kg biweekly Intravitreal: 20 mg every 5–6 wk	Dose- and schedule-dependent nephrotoxicity, hypotony (necessitates discontinuation), iritis (steroid responsive).	Intravitreal injection in the fellow eye is contraindicated if permanent hypotony develops in the first (treated) eye.

[a]Concomitant use of granulocyte colony-stimulating factor (G-CSF, also known as Neupogen) can reduce the incidence of neutropenia.
[b]Compared with i.v. ganciclovir. With implant therapy, there is an increased risk of systemic disease (30%) and fellow eye involvement (50%) after 6 months. However, the relapse-free interval is greatly increased.
[c]During induction phase, each dose is delivered in 500 mL of normal saline. During maintenance, 1,000 mL of saline should be used.
b.i.d., twice daily; i.v., intravenous; q.d., daily.

2. Serial fundus photographs are useful to document progression and should be taken at each visit.

3. Refer the patient to an internist for a systemic CMV evaluation and treatment.

TREATMENT

1. Intravenous ganciclovir, cidofovir, and foscarnet are used individually or in combination. The goal of treatment is quiescent retinitis: nonprogressive areas of RPE atrophy with a stable opacified border.

   Note: Ganciclovir can cause myelosuppression.

   Note: If ganciclovir is used to treat CMV in a patient already taking zidovudine for HIV therapy, the dose of zidovudine must be reduced because together they can cause severe myelosuppression.

2. Under the direction of an internist, protease inhibitors are often helpful. Regression of CMV has been documented without anti-CMV therapy in patients taking protease inhibitors.

3. CMV-associated retinal detachments are managed as follows: An RRD that spares the macula may be treated with laser demarcation. Pars plana vitrectomy with silicone oil is indicated for detachments involving the macula.

4. When ganciclovir implants are used, an RRD also may occur as a complication of implantation.

5. The role of oral ganciclovir prophylaxis against CMV is controversial.

FOLLOW-UP

1. Ganciclovir resistance (reflected by positive blood or urine CMV cultures) may occur at any point during treatment.

2. Almost all patients relapse eventually. Because relapse may be difficult to recognize clinically, serial fundus photographs are highly recommended. Relapse is defined as recurrent or new retinitis, movement of opacified border, or expansion of the atrophic zone.

3. Relapse does not necessarily indicate drug resistance. Reinduction with the same medication is the first line of treatment. Subtherapeutic intraocular drug levels may occur in patients on maintenance and allow for relapse.

4. Clinical resistance is defined as persistent or progressive retinitis in spite of induction-level medication for 6 weeks (usually, induction lasts 2 weeks).

5. Laboratory confirmation is possible for ganciclovir resistance (screen for UL97 mutation).

6. If resistance is recognized, a change in therapy is indicated.

7. Cross-resistance may be a problem. Because ganciclovir, foscarnet, and cidofovir are all DNA polymerase inhibitors, viral polymerase mutations may lead to resistance to several drugs in this class. Cross-resistance between ganciclovir and cidofovir is especially common. Ganciclovir–foscarnet cross-resistance is uncommon.

8. Discontinuation of anti-CMV maintenance therapy may be considered in selected patients receiving highly active antiretroviral therapy (HAART; protease inhibitors with other antiretroviral agents), who have CD4+ counts greater than 100 cells/mm^3 and completely quiescent CMV retinitis. In these patients whose immune system can control CMV, stopping maintenance therapy may prevent drug toxicity and forestall development of drug-resistant organisms.

TOXOPLASMOSIS (TOXOPLASMA GONDII)

SYMPTOMS

Decreased vision, floaters, photophobia, pain, red eye.

SIGNS

Retinochoroidal lesions clinically indistinguishable from CMV. Unlike CMV, significant vitreous response is typically present, and patients typically have higher CD4+ counts. Adjacent retinochoroidal scars are usually not observed. The lesions may be single or multifocal, discrete or diffuse, and unilateral or bilateral.

WORKUP

1. Complete ocular examination with special emphasis on the neuroophthalmic aspects.

2. Referral to an internist for a complete medical evaluation, which must include central nervous system (CNS) imaging because of a high association with CNS disease.

3. Toxoplasmosis antibody titers may be unreliable in HIV+ patients.

4. Because many infectious organisms [e.g., CMV, *Toxoplasma,* herpes simplex virus, herpes zoster virus, *Treponema pallidum* (syphilis), *Cryptococcus*] and lymphoma can cause a similar-appearing necrotizing retinitis, diagnostic vitrectomy may be necessary.

TREATMENT

1. Sulfadiazine and pyrimethamine together are the preferred treatment. In severe cases can add clindamycin or atovaquone (e.g., Mepron). Long-term maintenance therapy may be necessary to prevent recurrence.

2. Folinic acid, 5 to 10 mg orally (p.o.), q.d. minimizes pyrimethamine toxicity.

3. For patients who cannot take sulfonamides, clindamycin is substituted (not recommended for maintenance therapy).

4. Topical steroid (e.g., prednisolone acetate, 1%, q1–6h). The dosage depends on the degree of anterior segment inflammation.

5. Topical cycloplegic (e.g., scopolamine, 0.25%, t.i.d.) in the presence of anterior segment inflammation.

6. Systemic steroids are contraindicated for ocular toxoplasmosis in AIDS.

See Table 13.4 for treatment details.

PNEUMOCYSTIS CARINII CHOROIDOPATHY

A rare ocular manifestation of AIDS in patients with widely disseminated *P. carinii* infection.

SYMPTOMS

Mild decrease in visual acuity; may be asymptomatic.

SIGNS

Multifocal, yellow, round, deep choroidal lesions approximately one-half to two disc diam-

TABLE 13.4 TOXOPLASMOSIS *(TOXOPLASMA GONDII)*

Drug	Dosing Information	Toxicities	Contraindications
Sulfadiazine	Loading dose: 2 g p.o. ×1 Maintenance dose: 1 g p.o., q.i.d. for 3–6 wk[a]	Hypersensitivity, crystalluria, hematuria, renal stones, anemia.	Pregnancy, nursing mothers.
Pyrimethamine	Loading dose: 100–200 mg p.o. ×1 Maintenance dose: 25 mg p.o., b.i.d. for 3–6 wk[a] Check complete blood count weekly. Reduce dose if platelet count <100,000/mm³.	Hypersensitivity, megaloblastic anemia, leukopenia, thrombocytopenia.	Use with caution in pregnant and nursing women. Megaloblastic anemia due to folate deficiency.
Clindamycin	300–600 mg p.o., q.i.d. for 3–6 wk[a]	Pseudomembranous colitis, renal and hepatic toxicity.	Use with caution in patients with gastrointestinal, renal, or hepatic disease.

[a]May need chronic maintenance therapy.
p.o., orally; q.i.d., four times daily.

eters in size, located in the posterior pole. Typically, no retinal vascular changes or vitritis. Patients are often very ill.

WORKUP

1. Elicit history of *P. carinii* pneumonia and associated treatment (e.g., aerosolized pentamidine).

2. Complete dilated ocular examination.

3. Refer the patient to an internist for medical evaluation and management consultation.

TREATMENT

In conjunction with an internist or infectious disease specialist, the following treatments may be used.

1. Intravenous trimethoprim/sulfamethoxazole, or

2. Intravenous pentamidine.

   See Table 13.5 for treatment details.

SYPHILIS

Strictly speaking, syphilis is not an opportunistic infection (because it may be found in patients with CD4+ counts greater than 200 cells/mm^3).

Nonetheless, there is an increased incidence of neurosyphilis in the AIDS population. Therefore, lumbar puncture is mandatory in all HIV+ patients with syphilis. In patients with AIDS, the rapid plasma reagin (RPR) may be negative despite active syphilis, but the specific treponemal antibody test [e.g., fluorescent treponemal antibody, absorbed (FTA-ABS), microhemagglutination–*T. pallidum* (MHA-TP)] is usually positive. (See 13.5, Acquired Syphilis.)

Note: Ocular syphilis can mimic CMV retinitis in clinical appearance.

NEURO-OPHTHALMOLOGIC DISEASE

Two to 12% of patients with AIDS may develop neuroophthalmologic abnormalities (e.g., cranial nerve palsies, pupillary abnormalities, brainstem ocular motility defects, ischemic or infectious optic neuropathy, visual field defects, visual hallucinations) resulting from CNS infection (e.g., toxoplasmosis), lymphoma, or primary HIV disease. Steroids are absolutely contraindicated in patients with AIDS with retrobulbar optic neuritis or other optic neuropathies until infection is ruled out. Syphilis, *Cryptococcus*, and herpes zoster virus are the primary causes of infectious retrobulbar optic neuritis.

TABLE 13.5 *PNEUMOCYSTIS CARINII* CHOROIDITIS

Drug	Dosing Information	Toxicities	Contraindications
Trimethoprim (TMP)/ sulfamethoxazole (SMX)	i.v.: 5 mg/kg TMP and 25 mg/kg SMX i.v., q8h for 3 wk	Megaloblastic anemia, leukopenia, thrombocytopenia, Stevens–Johnson syndrome. Discontinue if any skin rashes or toxicities occur—fatalities have been reported.	History of hypersensitivity to related drugs. Megaloblastic anemia due to folate deficiency. Use with caution in and nursing pregnant women.
Pentamidine	4 mg/kg i.v., q.d. infused over 2 h	Leukopenia, hypoglycemia, thrombocytopenia, hypotension, renal failure, hypocalcemia, Stevens–Johnson syndrome.	No absolute contraindications.

i.v., intravenous; q.d., daily.

13.5 ACQUIRED SYPHILIS

SIGNS

Systemic

• Primary: Chancre (ulcerated, painless lesion), regional lymphadenopathy.

• Secondary: Skin or mucous membrane lesions, generalized lymphadenopathy, constitutional symptoms (e.g., sore throat, fever), other, less common but more severe abnormalities, including symptomatic or asymptomatic meningitis.

• Latent: No clinical manifestations.

• Tertiary: Cardiovascular disease (e.g., aortitis), CNS disease (e.g., meningovascular disease, general paresis, tabes dorsalis).

Ocular

• Primary: A chancre may occur on the eyelid or conjunctiva.

• Secondary: Uveitis, optic neuritis, active chorioretinitis, retinitis, retinal vasculitis, conjunctivitis, dacryoadenitis, dacryocystitis, episcleritis, scleritis, monocular interstitial keratitis, others.

• Tertiary: Optic atrophy, old chorioretinitis, interstitial keratitis, chronic iritis, Argyll Robertson pupil (will not react to light, but will accommodate; see 10.3, Argyll Robertson Pupil), in addition to the other signs seen in secondary disease.

Note: Patchy hyperemia of the iris with the development of fleshy, pink nodules near the iris sphincter is pathognomonic of syphilis.

DIFFERENTIAL DIAGNOSIS

See 12.1, Anterior Uveitis, and 12.3, Posterior Uveitis.

WORKUP

See 12.1, Anterior Uveitis, and 12.3, Posterior Uveitis, for a nonspecific uveitis workup.

1. Complete ophthalmic examination, including pupillary evaluation, slit-lamp examination, and dilated fundus examination.

2. Venereal Disease Research Laboratories test (VDRL) or RPR reflects the activity of the disease and is important in monitoring the patient's response to treatment. Used for screening, but many false-negative results can occur in early primary, latent, or late syphilis. Not as specific as FTA-ABS or MHA-TP.

3. FTA-ABS or MHA-TP are very sensitive and specific in all stages of syphilis. Once reactive, these tests do not revert to normal and therefore cannot be used to assess the patient's response to treatment.

4. HIV serology: Should be offered to patients with sexually transmitted diseases.

5. Lumbar puncture: The indications are controversial. We consider lumbar puncture in the following situations:

—Positive FTA-ABS and neurologic or neuroophthalmologic signs, papillitis, active chorioretinitis, or anterior or posterior uveitis.

—Patients who are HIV+ as well as FTA-ABS positive.

—Those for whom treatment has failed.

—Patients to be treated with a nonpenicillin regimen (as a baseline).

—Patients with untreated syphilis of unknown duration or longer than 1 year's duration.

TREATMENT INDICATIONS

1. **FTA-ABS negative:** No treatment indicated. Patient probably does not have syphilis. Consider retesting if clinical circumstances are compelling.

2. **FTA-ABS positive and VDRL negative**

a. If appropriate past treatment cannot be documented, treatment is indicated.

b. If appropriate past treatment can be documented, treatment is not indicated.

3. **FTA-ABS positive and VDRL positive:** A VDRL titer of 1:8 or greater (e.g., 1:64) is expected to decline at least fourfold within 1 year of appropriate treatment, and should revert to negative (or at least to 1:4 or less) within 1 year in primary syphilis, 2 years in secondary syphilis, and 5 years in tertiary syphilis. A VDRL titer of less than 1:8 (e.g., 1:4) often does not decrease fourfold. Therefore, the following recommendations are made:

a. If appropriate past treatment cannot be documented, treatment is indicated.

b. If appropriate past treatment can be documented, and

—If a previous VDRL titer greater than or equal to 4 times the current titer can be documented, no treatment is indicated (unless 5 years have passed and the titer is still greater than 1:4).

—If a previous VDRL titer was at least 1:8 and did not decrease fourfold, treatment is indicated.

—If the previous VDRL titer was less than 1:8, treatment is not indicated, unless the current titer has increased fourfold.

—If a previous VDRL is unavailable, treatment is not required unless treatment was more than 5 years earlier and the VDRL is still greater than 1:4.

*Notes:

1. If active syphilitic signs (e.g., active chorioretinitis, papillitis) are present despite appropriate past treatment (regardless of the VDRL titer), lumbar puncture and treatment may be needed.

2. Patients with concurrent HIV and active syphilis may have negative serologies (FTA-ABS, RPR) because of their immunocompromised state. These patients manifest aggressive, recalcitrant syphilis. They should be treated with neurosyphilis dosages, usually over longer treatment periods. Consultation with an infectious disease specialist is recommended.

TREATMENT

1. Neurosyphilis [positive FTA-ABS in the serum and either cell count greater than 5 white blood cells/mm³, protein greater than 45 mg/dL, or positive cerebrospinal fluid (CSF) VDRL on lumbar puncture]: Intravenous aqueous crystalline penicillin G, 2 to 4 million U, q4h, for 10 to 14 days, followed by benzathine penicillin, 2.4 million U intramuscularly (i.m.), weekly for 3 weeks (1.2 million U in each buttock).

2. Syphilis with abnormal ocular but normal CSF findings: Benzathine penicillin, 2.4 million U i.m., weekly for 3 weeks.

3. If anterior segment inflammation is present, treatment with a cycloplegic (e.g., cyclopentolate, 2%, t.i.d.) and topical steroid (e.g., prednisolone acetate, 1%, q.i.d.) may be beneficial.

*Notes:

1. Treatment for possible chlamydial infection with tetracycline, 250 mg p.o., q.i.d., doxycycline, 100 mg p.o., b.i.d., or erythromycin, 250 mg p.o., q.i.d. for 3 to 6 weeks, is typically indicated.

2. Therapy for penicillin-allergic patients is not well established. Tetracycline, 500 mg p.o., q.i.d., for 30 days, is used by some for both late syphilis and neurosyphilis, but better CSF penetration may be obtained with doxycycline (200 mg p.o., b.i.d., for 30 days) or a third-generation cephalosporin.

FOLLOW-UP

1. **Neurosyphilis:** Repeat lumbar puncture every 6 months for 2 years, less if the cell

count returns to normal sooner. The cell count should decrease to a normal level within this period, and the CSF VDRL titer should decrease fourfold (these changes typically occur within 6 to 12 months). An increased CSF protein decreases more slowly. If these indices do not decrease as expected, retreatment may be indicated.

2. **Other forms of syphilis:** Repeat the VDRL titer at 3 and 6 months after treatment. If a VDRL titer of 1:8 or more does not decline fourfold within 6 months, or if the VDRL titer increases fourfold at any point, or if clinical symptoms or signs of syphilis persist or recur, lumbar puncture and retreatment are indicated. If a pretreatment VDRL titer is less than 1:8, retreatment is indicated only when the titer increases during follow-up or when symptoms or signs of syphilis recur.

See 8.8, Congenital Syphilis, for additional information.

13.6 LYME DISEASE

SYMPTOMS

Decreased vision, double vision, pain, photophobia, facial weakness. Patients may also complain of headache, malaise, fatigue, fever, chills, palpitations, or muscle or joint pains. A history of a tick bite within the previous few months may be elicited.

SIGNS

Ocular. Optic neuritis; vitritis; iritis; stromal keratitis; choroiditis; exudative retinal detachment; third, fourth, or sixth cranial nerve palsy; bilateral optic nerve swelling; conjunctivitis; episcleritis; exposure keratopathy; other rare abnormalities, including orbital inflammatory pseudotumor.

Critical Systemic. One or more flat, erythematous or "bull's-eye" skin lesions, which enlarge in all directions (erythema migrans); unilateral or bilateral facial nerve palsies; arthritis. The skin lesions and arthritis may be transient and migratory. These findings may not be present at the time the ocular signs develop. A high serum antibody titer against the causative agent, *Borrelia burgdorferi,* is often, but not always present.

Other Systemic. Meningitis, peripheral radiculoneuropathy, synovitis, joint effusions, cardiac abnormalities, or a low false-positive FTA-ABS titer, or a combination of these.

DIFFERENTIAL DIAGNOSIS

• Syphilis (High positive FTA-ABS titer may produce a low false-positive antibody titer against *B. burgdorferi*. No history of a tick bite. History of chancre, maculopapular rash on palms and soles, exposure to or risk factors for sexually transmitted disease. May have interstitial keratitis, uveitis, optic neuritis, patchy iris hyperemia, a salt-and-pepper chorioretinitis, or pigmented "bone spicules" on fundus examination. See 13.5, Acquired Syphilis.).

• Others (Rickettsial infections, acute rheumatic fever, juvenile rheumatoid arthritis.).

WORKUP

1. History: Does patient live in endemic area? Prior tick bite, skin rash, Bell palsy, joint or muscle pains, flulike illness? Meningeal symptoms? Prior positive Lyme titer?

2. Complete systemic (especially neurologic) and ocular examinations.

3. Two-step diagnosis with a screening assay and confirmatory Western blot for *B. burgdorferi.*

4. Serum RPR and FTA-ABS.

5. Consider lumbar puncture when meningitis is suspected or neurologic signs or symptoms are present.

TREATMENT

Early Lyme Disease

(Including Lyme-related uveitis, keratitis, or seventh nerve palsy.)

1. Doxycycline, 100 mg p.o., b.i.d., for 10 to 21 days.

2. In children, pregnant women, and those who cannot take doxycycline, substitute amoxicillin, 500 mg p.o., t.i.d.

3. Other alternatives include cefuroxime axetil (e.g., Ceftin) 500 mg p.o., b.i.d., clarithromycin, 500 mg p.o., b.i.d., or azithromycin, 500 mg p.o., q.d.

Patients with Neuroophthalmic Signs or Recurrent or Resistant Infection

1. Ceftriaxone, 2 g i.v., q.d., for 2 to 3 weeks.

2. Alternatively, penicillin G, 20 million units i.v., q.d., for 2 to 3 weeks.

FOLLOW-UP

Every 1 to 3 days until improvement is demonstrated, and then weekly until resolved.

13.7 CHICKEN POX (VARICELLA-ZOSTER VIRUS)

SYMPTOMS

Facial rash, red eye, foreign-body sensation.

SIGNS

Early. Acute conjunctivitis with vesicles or papules at the limbus, on the eyelid, or on the conjunctiva. Pseudodendritic corneal epithelial lesions, stromal keratitis, anterior uveitis, optic neuritis, retinitis, and ophthalmoplegia occur rarely.

Late. (Weeks to months after the outbreak.) Immune stromal or neurotrophic keratitis may occur.

TREATMENT

1. **Conjunctival involvement:** Cool compresses and erythromycin ointment to the eye and periorbital lesions, t.i.d.

2. **Corneal epithelial lesions:** Same as for conjunctival involvement.

3. **Stromal keratitis with uveitis:** Topical steroid (e.g., prednisolone acetate, 1%, q.i.d.), cycloplegic (e.g., scopolamine, 0.25%, b.i.d.), and erythromycin ointment, q.h.s.

4. **Neurotrophic keratitis:** Uncommon; see 4.6, Neurotrophic Keratopathy.

5. **Canalicular obstruction:** Uncommon. Managed by intubation of puncta.

Notes:

1. *Do* not *give aspirin to these children because of the possible risk of Reye syndrome.*

2. *Immunocompromised children with chicken pox may require i.v. acyclovir.*

3. *Varicella-zoster virus vaccination is now available for children and will likely prevent ophthalmic complications of chicken pox in immunocompetent patients if given at least 8 to 12 weeks before exposure.*

FOLLOW-UP

1. Follow up in 1 to 7 days, depending on the severity of ocular disease. Taper the topical steroids slowly.

2. Watch for stromal or neurotrophic keratitis approximately 4 to 6 weeks after the chicken pox resolves. Varicella-zoster virus stromal keratitis can have a chronic course requiring long-term topical steroids with a very gradual taper.

13.8 CONVERGENCE INSUFFICIENCY

SYMPTOMS

Eye discomfort, headache, sleepiness, or blurred vision from reading or doing near work. It is most common in teenagers and young adults, but may be seen in presbyopes.

SIGNS

Critical. An inability to maintain fusion at near as a result of a reduced amplitude of fusional convergence power (see Workup).

Other. A distant near point of convergence, an exophoria greater at near than at distance, and a reduced amplitude of accommodation.

DIFFERENTIAL DIAGNOSIS

Other causes of eyestrain with reading.

• Uncorrected refractive error (especially hyperopia and astigmatism).

• Accommodative insufficiency (AI) [Symptoms develop after 20 to 40 minutes of reading, same age group as convergence insufficiency (CI), but these patients have normal fusional capacities. When a 4-diopter base-in prism is placed in front of the eye while reading, the print is noted to blur in patients with AI, but become clearer in those with CI. Patients with AI usually benefit from reading glasses; those with CI do not.].

ETIOLOGY

• Fatigue or illness.

• Drugs (parasympatholytics).

• Uveitis.

• Adie tonic pupil.

• Glasses inducing a base-out prism effect.

• Postexanthematous encephalitis.

• Traumatic injury.

• Often idiopathic.

WORKUP

1. Manifest (without cycloplegia) refraction.

2. Determine the near point of convergence. Ask the patient to focus on an accommodative target (e.g., the eraser of a pencil) and to inform you when double vision develops as you bring the target toward him or her; a normal near point of convergence is less than 6 to 8 cm.

3. Check for exodeviations or esodeviations at distance and near by using the cover tests (see Appendix 2) or the Maddox rod test. See 10.6, Isolated Fourth Nerve Palsy.

4. Measure the patient's fusional ability at near. Have the patient focus on an accommodative target at his or her reading distance. With a prism bar, slowly increase the amount of base-out prism in front of one eye until the patient notes double vision (the break point), and then slowly reduce the amount of base-out prism until a single image is again noted (the recovery point). A low break point (i.e., 10 to 15 prism diopters) or a low recovery point, or both, are consistent with CI.

5. Place a 4-diopter base-in prism in front of one eye while the patient is reading and determine whether the print becomes clearer or more blurred to rule out AI.

6. Cycloplegic refraction (performed after the previous tests and measurements).

   Note: These tests are performed with the patient's spectacle correction in place (if glasses are worn for near work).

TREATMENT

1. Correct any refractive error (hyperopia should be slightly undercorrected, whereas myopia should be fully corrected).

2. Near-point exercises (e.g., pencil push-ups): The patient is taught to focus on the eraser of

a pencil while slowly moving it from arm's length toward the face. The patient must concentrate on maintaining one image of the eraser. When double vision results, the maneuver is repeated. An attempt is made to draw the pencil in closer each time while maintaining single vision. The exercise is repeated 15 times, 5 times per day.

3. Near-point exercises with base-out prisms (for patients whose near point of convergence is satisfactory or for those who have mastered pencil push-ups without a prism): Pencil push-ups as described previously are performed while the patient additionally holds a 6-diopter base-out prism in front of one eye.

4. Encourage use of good lighting and time for relaxation between periods of concentrated close work.

5. For older patients, or those whose condition shows no improvement despite near-point exercises, reading glasses with base-in prism can be useful.

FOLLOW-UP

This is not an urgent condition. Patients are reexamined in 1 month.

13.9 ACCOMMODATIVE SPASM

SYMPTOMS

Bilateral blurred distance vision or fluctuating vision, headache, and eyestrain while reading. Typically, patients are teenagers who are under stress. Symptoms may occur after prolonged and intense periods of near work.

SIGNS

Critical. Cycloplegic refraction reveals substantially less myopia (or more hyperopia) than was originally found when the refraction was performed without cycloplegia (the manifest refraction). Manifest myopia may be as high as 10 diopters. Spasm of the near reflex is associated with excess accommodation, excess convergence, and miosis.

Other. Abnormally close near point of focus, miosis, a normal amplitude of accommodation that may appear low.

ETIOLOGY

• Inability to relax the ciliary muscles. Accommodative spasm is involuntary and is associated with stressful situations or functional neuroses.

• Fatigue.

• Prolonged reading may also precipitate episodes.

DIFFERENTIAL DIAGNOSIS

• Uncorrected hyperopia (Patients accept plus lenses during the manifest refraction.).

• Other causes of pseudomyopia [Hyperglycemia, medication induced (e.g., sulfa drugs and anticholinesterase medications), forward displacement of the lens.].

• Manifestation of iridocyclitis.

WORKUP

1. Complete ophthalmic examination, including an initial manifest refraction. The manifest refraction may be highly variable, but it is important to determine the least

amount of minus power or the most amount of plus power that provides clear distance vision.

2. Cycloplegic refraction.

TREATMENT

1. True refractive errors should be corrected. If a significant amount of esophoria at near is present, additional plus power (e.g., +2.50 diopters) in reading glasses or bifocal form may be helpful for close work.

2. Gentle counseling of the patient and parents to provide a more relaxed atmosphere and avoid stressful situations is important.

3. Cycloplegics, including atropine, have been used to break the spasm, but are rarely needed except in the most resistant cases.

FOLLOW-UP

Reevaluate in several weeks. The physician should also be available for additional consultative support.

13.10 STEVENS–JOHNSON SYNDROME
(ERYTHEMA MULTIFORME MAJOR)

SYMPTOMS

Acute onset of fever, rash, red eyes, malaise, arthralgias, and respiratory tract symptoms.

SIGNS

Systemic. Classic "target" skin lesions (maculopapules with a red center and a white surround on an erythematous base) concentrated on hands and feet; ulcerative stomatitis; and hemorrhagic lip crusting. The mortality rate is 10% to 33%.

Ocular

• Acute phase: Mucopurulent or pseudomembranous conjunctivitis, episcleritis, iritis.

• Late complications: Conjunctival scarring or symblepharon; trichiasis; eyelid deformities; tear deficiency; corneal neovascularization, ulcer, perforation, or scarring.

ETIOLOGY

May be precipitated by many agents, including:

• Drugs: Including sulfonamides, barbiturates, chlorpropamide, thiazide diuretics, phenytoin, salicylates, allopurinol, chlormezanone, corticosteroids, isoniazid, tetracycline, codeine, aminopenicillins, cancer chemotherapeutic agents.

• Infectious agents: Most commonly *Mycoplasma pneumoniae*, herpes simplex virus, and adenovirus.

• Allergy and autoimmune diseases.

• Radiation therapy.

• Malignancy.

TYPES

1. Erythema multiforme major (Stevens–Johnson syndrome): Immune complex deposition in dermis with subepithelial vesiculobullous reaction of skin and mucous membranes.

2. Erythema multiforme minor: Only skin involvement.

3. Toxic epidermal necrolysis: The most severe form, causing extensive intraepithelial vesiculobullous eruptions and epidermal sloughing. More common in children and immunosuppressed patients.

WORKUP

1. History: Attempt to determine the precipitating factor.

2. Slit-lamp examination, including eyelid eversion with examination of the fornices.

3. Conjunctival or corneal cultures if infection is suspected (see 4.11, Bacterial Keratitis).

4. Consult internal medicine for a systemic workup.

TREATMENT

1. Hospitalization.

2. Remove (e.g., drug) or treat (e.g., infection) the inciting factor.

3. Supportive care is the mainstay of therapy.

Ocular

a. Tear deficiency: Aggressive lubrication with artificial tears (e.g., Refresh Plus or TheraTears drops, q1–2h), ointments, punctal occlusion, moisture chambers, or tarsorrhaphy.

b. Iritis: Topical steroid drops[2] (e.g., prednisolone acetate, 1%, four to eight times per day) and cycloplegic (e.g., atropine, 1%, t.i.d.).

c. Infections: Culture and treat as outlined in 4.11, Bacterial Keratitis.

d. Controversial treatments:

—Topical steroids for ocular surface inflammation.

—Daily pseudomembrane peel and symblepharon lysis with glass rod or moistened cotton swab.

—Systemic or topical vitamin A.

—Intravenous immunoglobulin.

Systemic: Manage by burn unit protocol, including hydration, wound care, and system antibiotics. Medical consultation recommended.

FOLLOW-UP

1. **During hospitalization:** Follow daily, with infection and IOP surveillance.

2. **Outpatient:** Weekly follow-ups initially, watching for long-term ocular complications.

—Steroid and antibiotic treatment are maintained for 48 hours after the eye is healed and are then tapered.

—Artificial tears and lubricating ointment may need to be maintained indefinitely if the conjunctiva has been severely scarred.

3. Possible late surgical interventions.

—Trichiasis: Repeated epilation, electrolysis, cryotherapy, or surgical repair.

—Entropion repair with buccal mucosal grafts.

—Penetrating keratoplasty: Poor prognosis even when combined with limbal stem cell or amniotic membrane transplantation because of underlying deficiencies, such as dry eyes.

—Permanent keratoprosthesis.

[2]Use with caution in the presence of an epithelial defect.

13.11 VITAMIN A DEFICIENCY

See Table 13.6.

SYMPTOMS

Night blindness (earliest and most common manifestation), dry eyes, foreign body sensation, ocular pain, and severe loss of vision.

SIGNS

Bitot spots (triangular perilimbal gray plaques of keratinized conjunctival debris); decreased tear breakup time; bilateral conjunctival and corneal dryness with lack of normal luster; corneal epithelial defects, sterile or infectious

TABLE 13.6 WORLD HEALTH ORGANIZATION CLASSIFICATION OF VITAMIN A DEFICIENCY

XN	Night blindness
X1A	Conjunctival xerosis
X1B	Bitot spot
X2	Corneal xerosis
X3A	Corneal ulceration or keratomalacia with ≤1/3 corneal involvement
X3B	Corneal ulceration or keratomalacia with ≥1/3 corneal involvement
XS	Corneal scar
XF	Xerophthalmia fundus

ulceration, perforation, scarring; keratomalacia (often preceded by a gastrointestinal or respiratory infection); fundus abnormalities (yellow or white peripheral retinal dots representing focal RPE defects).

DIFFERENTIAL DIAGNOSIS

Keratoconjunctivitis sicca (see 4.3, Dry-Eye Syndrome).

ETIOLOGY

• Primary: Dietary deficiency or chronic alcoholism (relatively uncommon in developed countries).

• Secondary: Lipid malabsorption [e.g., cystic fibrosis, chronic pancreatitis, inflammatory bowel disease, postgastrectomy or post-intestinal bypass surgery, chronic liver disease, abetalipoproteinemia (Bassen–Kornzweig syndrome)].

WORKUP

1. History: Malnutrition? Poor or extreme diet? Gastrointestinal or liver disease? Previous surgery? Measles?

2. Complete ophthalmic examination, including careful inspection of eyelid margins and inferior fornices.

3. Serum vitamin A level before treatment is initiated.

4. Consider impression cytology of the conjunctiva, looking for decreased conjunctival goblet cell density.

5. Consider dark-adaptation studies and electroretinogram (may be more sensitive than the serum vitamin A level, which may not decrease until the body's reserves are depleted).

6. Corneal cultures if an infection is suspected (see 4.11, Bacterial Keratitis).

TREATMENT

1. Vitamin A replacement therapy (oral or intramuscular) in the following dosages:

—Adults and children older than 1 year: 200,000 IU, q.d., for 2 days, repeat in 2 weeks, then every 4 to 6 months.

—Pregnant women and children younger than 1 year: 100,000 IU every 4 to 6 months.

—Infants: 50,000 IU prophylactic dose.

2. Intensive ocular lubrication with artificial tears (e.g., Refresh Plus, GenTeal gel, or Celluvisc) every 15 to 60 minutes and artificial tear ointment (e.g., Refresh PM), q.h.s.

3. Treat malnutrition if present.

4. Consider supplementing the patient's diet with zinc.

5. Consider a penetrating keratoplasty or keratoprosthesis for corneal scars in eyes with potentially good vision.

FOLLOW-UP

Determined by the clinical presentation and response to treatment. Some patients need to be hospitalized, whereas others can be followed every few days or weeks. Vitamin A deficiency associated with measles may be especially severe.

13.12 ALBINISM

SYMPTOMS

Decreased vision and photosensitivity.

SIGNS

Best corrected visual acuity of 20/40 to 20/200; high refractive error; strabismus; absence of stereopsis; nystagmus starting at age 2 to 3 months; amblyopia secondary to strabismus or anisometropia; iris transillumination defects; retinal hypopigmentation, especially peripherally, with visible underlying choroidal vasculature; failure of the retinal vessels to wreathe the fovea; foveal aplasia or hypoplasia (the only ocular finding consistently present).

Note: Albinos show an entire range of visual acuities, refractive errors, nystagmus, and amblyopia.

ASSOCIATED DISORDERS

• Hermansky–Pudlak syndrome: An autosomal recessive defect in platelet function leading to easy bruisability and bleeding. More common in patients of Puerto Rican descent.

• Chediak–Higashi syndrome: An autosomal recessive disorder affecting white blood cell function, resulting in an increased susceptibility to infections and a predisposition for a lymphoma-like condition.

TYPES

1. Oculocutaneous albinism: Autosomal recessive, hypopigmentation of hair, skin, and eye.

   —Tyrosinase positive: Varying degree of pigmentation.

   —Tyrosinase negative: No pigmentation.

2. Ocular albinism: Only ocular hypopigmentation is clinically apparent. Usually inherited as X-linked recessive (Nettleship–Falls). Female carriers may have partial iris transillumination and mottled areas of hypopigmentation in peripheral retina.

WORKUP

1. History: Easy bruisability? Frequent nosebleeds? Prolonged bleeding after dental work? Frequent infections?

2. Family history: Puerto Rican heritage?

3. External (including hair and skin color) examination.

4. Complete ocular examination, including slit-lamp and dilated fundus examinations.

5. Before surgery, obtain bleeding time. Platelet aggregation studies and platelet electron microscopy are also indicated if the Hermansky–Pudlak syndrome is suspected.

6. If the Chediak–Higashi syndrome is suspected, check polymorphonuclear leukocyte function.

7. Flash visual evoked potential testing to demonstrate excessive decussation of retinal ganglion cell axons at the chiasm.

TREATMENT

There is currently no effective treatment for albinism, but the following may be helpful:

1. Treating amblyopia may reduce nystagmus.

2. Appropriate refraction and early use of bifocals may be necessary as amplitude of accommodation diminishes.

3. Eye muscle surgery may be considered for patients with significant strabismus or an abnormal head position due to nystagmus. However, albinos with strabismus rarely achieve binocularity after surgical correc-

tion, possibly because of a lack of the necessary neuronal connections.

4. Genetic counseling.

5. Dermatologic consultation.

6. Consult hematology if either Chediak–Higashi syndrome or Hermansky–Pudlak syndrome is suspected. Patients with the Hermansky–Pudlak syndrome may require platelet transfusions before surgery.

13.13 WILSON DISEASE

SYMPTOMS

Ocular complaints are rare. Patients experience symptoms of cirrhosis, renal disease, or motor dysfunction starting before 40 years of age.

SIGNS

Critical. Kayser–Fleischer ring: a 1- to 3-mm, brown, green, or red band that forms in the peripheral Descemet membrane in 95% of patients. It first appears superiorly and eventually forms a ring involving the entire corneal periphery, extending to the limbus without intervening clear cornea. An autosomal recessive defect leads a low serum ceruloplasmin level and resultant elevated serum and urine copper levels.

Other. "Sunflower" cataract due to anterior and posterior subcapsular copper deposition.

DIFFERENTIAL DIAGNOSIS

• Kayser–Fleischer–like ring (Seen in primary biliary cirrhosis, chronic active hepatitis, progressive intrahepatic cholestasis, multiple myeloma. Unlike Wilson disease, these patients have a normal serum ceruloplasmin level and no neurologic symptoms.).

• Arcus senilis (Corneal stromal lipid deposition, initially appears inferiorly and superiorly before extending around the entire periphery. A clear zone of cornea separates the edge of the arcus from the limbus. Check a fasting lipid profile in patients younger than 40 years.).

• Chalcosis (Copper deposition in basement membranes, including Descemet membrane, caused by copper-containing intraocular foreign body. Alloys containing more than 85% copper induce severe inflammation, including retinal toxicity.).

WORKUP

1. Slit-lamp examination: Deposition at the level of Descemet membrane is apparent through a narrow slit beam.

2. Gonioscopy if the Kayser–Fleischer ring is not evident on slit-lamp examination.

3. Serum copper and ceruloplasmin levels.

4. Urine copper level.

5. Serum protein electrophoresis if the ceruloplasmin level is normal.

6. Referral to an internist or neurologist.

TREATMENT

1. Systemic therapy (e.g., D-penicillamine or tetrathiomolybdate) is instituted by an internist or neurologist.

2. The ocular manifestations usually require no specific treatment.

FOLLOW-UP

1. Systemic therapy and complete blood count (CBC) monitoring with an internist or neurologist.

2. Successful treatment should lead to resorption of the corneal copper deposition and clearing of the Kayser–Fleischer ring, although residual corneal changes may remain. This change can be used to monitor treatment response.

3. There are no ocular complications from a Kayser–Fleischer ring.

13.14 SUBLUXED OR DISLOCATED LENS

DEFINITION

• Subluxation: Partial disruption of the zonular fibers; the lens is decentered but remains partially in the pupillary aperture.

• Dislocation: Complete disruption of the zonular fibers; the lens is displaced out of the pupillary aperture.

SYMPTOMS

Decreased vision, double vision that persists when covering one eye (monocular diplopia).

SIGNS

Critical. Decentered or displaced lens, iridodonesis (quivering of the iris), phacodonesis (quivering of the lens).

Other. Marked astigmatism, cataract, angle-closure glaucoma as a result of pupillary block, acquired high myopia, vitreous in the anterior chamber, asymmetry of the anterior chamber depth.

ETIOLOGY

• Trauma [Most common cause. Results in subluxation if more than 25% of the zonular fibers are ruptured. Need to rule out a predisposing condition (see other etiologies). Can be associated with syphilis.].

• Marfan syndrome (Cardiomyopathy, aortic aneurysm, tall stature with long extremities and kyphoscoliosis. Typically, bilateral lens subluxation superiorly and temporally. Patients are at increased risk for a retinal detachment. Often autosomal dominant.).

• Homocystinuria [Frequent mental retardation, skeletal deformities, resembles Marfan syndrome in stature, high incidence of thromboembolic events (particularly with general anesthesia). Patients with a mild clinical course may be undiagnosed before occurrence of lens subluxation. Typically, bilateral lens subluxation inferiorly and nasally. Increased risk of retinal detachment. Autosomal recessive.].

• Weill–Marchesani syndrome [Short fingers and short stature, seizures, microspherophakia (small, round lens), myopia, no mental retardation. Often autosomal recessive. The small lens can dislocate into the anterior chamber, causing reverse pupillary block.].

• Others (Acquired syphilis, congenital ectopia lentis, aniridia, Ehlers–Danlos syndrome, Crouzon disease, hyperlysinemia, sulfite oxidase deficiency, high myopia, chronic inflammations, hypermature cataract, others.).

WORKUP

1. History: Family history of the disorders listed? Trauma? Systemic illness (e.g., syphilis, seizures)?

2. Complete ocular examination: At the slit lamp, note whether the condition is unilateral or bilateral and determine the direction of the displaced lens. Evaluation for subtle phacodonesis by having the patient look back and forth while observing the lens at the slit lamp.

3. Systemic examination: Evaluate stature, extremities, hands, and fingers; often in conjunction with an internist.

4. RPR and FTA-ABS, even if there is a history of trauma.

5. Sodium nitroprusside test or urine chromatography to rule out homocystinuria as needed.

6. Echocardiography to rule out aortic aneurysms associated with Marfan syndrome as needed.

Note: Systemic evaluations of Marfan syndrome and homocystinuria should be performed in conjunction with an internist.

TREATMENT

1. **Lens dislocated into the anterior chamber.**

   —Dilate the pupil, place the patient on his or her back, and replace the lens into the posterior chamber by head manipulation. It may be necessary to indent the cornea after topical anesthesia (e.g., proparacaine) with a Zeiss gonioprism or a cotton swab to reposition the lens. After the lens is repositioned in the posterior chamber, constrict the pupil with chronic pilocarpine, 0.5% to 1%, q.i.d., and perform a peripheral laser iridotomy.

or

—Surgically remove the lens (usually performed if the lens is a cataract, if treatment described previously fails, if the patient experiences recurrent dislocations, or if there are compliance issues with pilocarpine).

2. **Lens dislocated into the vitreous.**

—Lens capsule intact, patient asymptomatic, no signs of inflammation: Observe.

—Lens capsule broken, eye inflamed: Lensectomy either through the pars plana or by using a limbal approach.

3. **Subluxation**

—Asymptomatic: Observe.

—High uncorrectable astigmatism or monocular diplopia: Surgical removal of the lens.

—Symptomatic cataract: Options include surgical removal of the lens, mydriasis (e.g.,

scopolamine, 0.25%, q.d.) and aphakic correction, pupillary constriction (e.g., pilocarpine, 4% gel, q.h.s.) and phakic correction, or a large optical iridectomy (away from the lens).

4. **Pupillary block:** Treatment is identical to that for aphakic pupillary block (see 9.16, Postoperative Glaucoma).

5. **If Marfan syndrome is present:** Refer the patient to a cardiologist for an annual echocardiogram and management of any cardiac-related abnormalities. Prophylactic systemic antibiotics are required if the patient undergoes surgery (or a dental procedure) to prevent endocarditis.

6. **If homocystinuria is present,** refer to an internist. The usual therapy consists of:

—Pyridoxine, 50 to 1,000 mg p.o., q.d.

—Reduce dietary methionine.

—Avoid surgery if possible because of the risk of thromboembolic complications. If surgical intervention is necessary, anticoagulant therapy is indicated.

FOLLOW-UP

Depends on the etiology, degree of subluxation or dislocation, and symptoms.

13.15   HYPOTONY SYNDROME

DEFINITION

Decreased visual function and other ocular symptoms related to low IOP.

SYMPTOMS

May have mild to severe pain. Vision may be reduced. Excessive tearing in patients after glaucoma filtering procedures.

SIGNS

Critical. Low IOP, usually less than 6 mm Hg, but may occur with an IOP as high as 10 mm Hg. Low IOP, even as low as 2 mm Hg, may not cause problems or symptoms.

Other. Corneal edema and folds, corneal decompensation, aqueous cell and flare, shallow or flat anterior chamber, retinal edema, hypotony maculopathy, retinal vascular tortuosity, chorioretinal folds, serous choroidal detachment, suprachoroidal hemorrhage, the appearance of optic disc swelling.

ETIOLOGY

• Postsurgical [Wound leak, overfiltering bleb or glaucoma drainage device, cyclodialysis cleft (disinsertion of the ciliary body from the sclera at the scleral spur), perforation of the sclera from a superior rectus bridle suture or retrobulbar injection, iridocyclitis, retinal or choroidal detachment, others.].

• Posttraumatic (Same causes as postsurgical.).

• Pharmacologic (Usually from a carbonic anhydrase inhibitor in combination with a topical beta-blocker.).

• Systemic (bilateral hypotony) [Conditions that cause blood hypertonicity (e.g., dehydration, uremia, exacerbation of diabetes), myotonic dystrophy, others.].

• Vascular occlusive disease (e.g., ocular ischemic syndrome, giant cell arteritis, central retinal vein or artery occlusion) (Usually a mild hypotony.).

• Uveitis (causing ciliary body shutdown).

WORKUP

1. History: Recent ocular surgery or trauma? Other systemic symptoms (nausea, vomiting, twitching, drowsiness, polyuria)? History of renal disease, diabetes, or myotonic dystrophy? Medications?

2. Complete ocular examination, including a slit-lamp evaluation of surgical or traumatic ocular wounds (check for poor wound apposition), IOP check, gonioscopy of the anterior chamber angle to rule out a cyclodialysis cleft, and indirect ophthalmoscopy to rule out a retinal or choroidal detachment or both and to look for signs of a scleral perforation. High-frequency ultrasonographic biomicroscopy is often useful for identifying cyclodialysis clefts.

3. Seidel test (with and without gentle pressure) to rule out a wound leak (see Appendix 4).

   Note: A wound leak may drain under the conjunctiva, producing a filtering bleb. Seidel test will then be negative.

4. B-scan ultrasonography when the fundus cannot be seen clinically. Consider ultrasonographic biomicroscopy for evaluation of the anterior chamber angle.

5. Blood tests in bilateral cases: Glucose, blood urea nitrogen, and creatinine.

TREATMENT

Repair of the underlying disorder may be needed if symptoms are significant or progressive.

Wound Leak

1. **Large wound leaks:** Suture the wound closed.

2. **Small wound leaks:** Can be sutured closed or can be patched with a pressure dressing and an antibiotic ointment (e.g., erythromycin) for 1 night to allow the wound to close spontaneously. A carbonic anhydrase inhibitor and a nonselective topical beta-blocker (e.g., acetazolamide, 500 mg sequel p.o., and a drop of levobunolol or timolol, 0.5%) are usually given if patching is to be used.

   Note: Occasionally, cyanoacrylate glue is applied to small wound leaks and covered with a bandage contact lens.

3. **Wound leaks under a conjunctival flap** (repaired only if the hypotony is affecting vision or producing a secondary ocular complication such as a flat anterior chamber): Consider cryotherapy or argon laser therapy after painting the conjunctiva with methylene blue or rose bengal, or autologous blood injection.

Cyclodialysis Cleft

Reattach the ciliary body to the sclera by suturing, cryotherapy, laser photocoagulation, or diathermy.

Scleral Perforation

The site may be closed by suturing or cryotherapy.

Iridocyclitis

Topical steroid (e.g., prednisolone acetate, 1%, q1h to q6h) and a topical cycloplegic (e.g., scopolamine, 0.25%, t.i.d.).

Retinal Detachment

Surgical repair.

Choroidal Detachment

See also 11.21, Choroidal Detachment.
    Treated as iridocyclitis. Surgical drainage of the choroidal effusion along with reformation of the eye and anterior chamber is indicated for any of the following:

1. Retinal apposition ("kissing" choroidal detachments).

2. Lens–corneal touch (needs emergency attention).

3. A flat or persistently shallow anterior chamber accompanied by a failing filtering bleb or an inflamed eye.

Pharmacologic

Reduce or discontinue the IOP-reducing medications.

Systemic Disorder

Refer to an internist.

__Note:__ In myotonic dystrophy, the hypotony is rarely severe enough to produce deleterious effects, and treatment of hypotony, from an ocular standpoint, is unnecessary.

FOLLOW-UP

If vision is good, the anterior chamber is well formed, and there is no wound leak, retinal detachment, or kissing choroidal detachments, then the low IOP poses no immediate problem, and treatment and follow-up are not urgent. Fixed retinal folds in the macula may develop from long-standing hypotony.

13.16 BLIND, PAINFUL EYE

A patient with a nonseeing eye and unsalvageable vision may experience mild to severe pain in it for a variety of reasons. The etiology, workup, and treatment are discussed.

CAUSES OF PAIN

• Corneal decompensation (Fluorescein-staining defect on slit-lamp examination.).

• Uveitis (Anterior chamber or vitreal white blood cells. If the cornea is opaque, the cells may not be seen.).

• Extremely high IOP (May result from neovascular glaucoma and angle closure, uveitis, or intraocular tumor–related glaucoma. IOP may be difficult to measure if the corneal surface is irregular.).

WORKUP

1. History: Determine the etiology and duration of the blindness.

2. Ocular examination: Stain the cornea with fluorescein to detect an epithelial defect and measure the IOP. Tono-Pen measurements may be required if the corneal surface is irregular. If the cornea is clear, look for neovascularization of the iris and angle by go-

nioscopy, and inspect the anterior chamber for cells and flare. Attempt a dilated retinal examination to rule out an intraocular tumor.

3. B-scan ultrasonography of the posterior segment is required to rule out an intraocular tumor when the fundus cannot be adequately visualized.

TREATMENT

1. Sterile corneal decompensation (if it appears infected, see 4.11, Bacterial Keratitis).

    —Antibiotic ointment (e.g., erythromycin), cycloplegic (e.g., atropine, 1%), and a pressure patch for 24 to 48 hours.

    —Antibiotic or lubricating ointment (e.g., Refresh PM) q.d. to q.i.d. (after the patch is removed) for weeks to months (or even permanently).

    —Consider teaching the patient to patch his or her own eye nightly.

    —Consider a tarsorrhaphy or Gunderson conjunctival flap in refractory cases.

2. Uveitis

    —Cycloplegic (e.g., atropine, 1%, t.i.d.).

    —Topical steroid (e.g., prednisolone acetate, 1%, q1–6h).

    —Treat uveitis if it is present or if the cornea is opaque and its presence cannot be ruled out.

    —Endophthalmitis should be ruled out if severe uveitis or a hypopyon is present.

3. Markedly increased IOP

    —Topical beta-blocker (e.g., levobunolol or timolol, 0.5%, b.i.d.) with or without an adrenergic agonist compounds (e.g., brimonidine, 0.2%, or apraclonidine, 0.5%, b.i.d. to t.i.d.). Topical carbonic anhydrase inhibitors (e.g., dorzolamide, 2%, or brinzolamide, 1%, t.i.d.) are effective, but their potential systemic side effects may not warrant

their use for pain relief; miotics may increase ocular irritation.

—If the IOP remains markedly increased and is thought to be responsible for the pain, a cyclodestructive procedure (e.g., yttrium–aluminum garnet or diode laser cyclophotocoagulation or cyclocryotherapy) may be attempted. The potential for sympathetic ophthalmia must be considered.

—If pain persists despite the previously described treatment, a retrobulbar alcohol block may be given. This is typically effective for approximately 3 to 6 months. Technique: 2 to 3 mL of lidocaine is administered in the retrobulbar region. The needle is then held in place while the syringe of lidocaine is replaced with a 1-mL syringe containing 95% to 100% alcohol (some physicians use 50% alcohol). The contents of the alcohol syringe are then injected into the retrobulbar space through the needle. The syringes are again switched, so a small amount of lidocaine can rinse out the remaining alcohol. The retrobulbar needle is then withdrawn. Patients are warned that transient eyelid droop or swelling, limitation of eye movement, or anesthesia may result. Retrobulbar chlorpromazine can also be used to control pain in a blind and painful eye. After the eye is prepared, 1 to 4 mL 2% lidocaine hydrochloride (with or without epinephrine 1:100,00) is injected after the retrobulbar needle (25 gauge, 40 mm) is positioned in the retrobulbar space. The syringe is switched and 1 to 2 mL chlorpromazine (25 to 50 mg, using 25 mg/mL) is injected.

4. Cause of pain unknown.

    a. Cycloplegic (e.g., atropine, 1%, t.i.d.).

    b. Topical steroid (e.g., prednisolone acetate, 1%, q1–6h).

5. Enucleation or evisceration: Patients with ocular pain refractory to topical or retrobulbar injections should be considered for enucleation or evisceration of the eye, both

highly effective procedures for symptoms of a blind, painful eye. Enucleation, however, does not relieve facial paresthesias.

6. Monocular patients: All monocular patients should wear protective eye wear (e.g., polycarbonate lenses) at all times to prevent injury to the contralateral eye.

FOLLOW-UP

Depends on the degree of pain and the clinical abnormalities present. Once the pain resolves, patients are reexamined every 6 to 12 months. B-scan ultrasonography should be performed periodically to rule out an intraocular tumor, when the posterior pole cannot be visualized.

BIBLIOGRAPHY

Chen TC, Ahn Yuen SJ, Sangalang MA, et al. Retrobulbar chlorpromazine injections for the management of blind and seeing painful eyes. *J Glaucoma* 2002;11:209–213.

13.17 NEUROFIBROMATOSIS

(VON RECKLINGHAUSEN SYNDROME)

CRITERIA FOR DIAGNOSIS

See Table 13.7.

Note: Lisch nodules are highly sensitive and specific for neurofibromatosis 1 and precede the development of cutaneous neurofibromas. The onset of these iris nodules is at age 5 years or older, and are unusual in neurofibromatosis 2.

SIGNS

Ocular. Glaucoma (a common complication of orbital plexiform neurofibromas), pulsating proptosis (absence of the greater wing of the sphenoid bone with a herniated encephalocele), prominent corneal nerves, retinal astrocytoma, myelinated nerve fibers, combined hamartoma of the retina and RPE, diffuse uveal thickening, choroidal nevus or melanoma.

Systemic. Intracranial astrocytoma (glioma), pituitary adenoma, cranial or spinal nerve schwannoma, mental deficiency, pheochromocytoma, gastrointestinal or genitourinary malignancies (including Wilms tumor).

WORKUP

1. Family history and examination of family members.

2. Complete general and ophthalmic examinations.

3. CBC and electrolytes.

4. MRI of the orbit and brain: Ophthalmic indications include orbital pain, proptosis, optic disc changes, decreased vision, visual field defect.

5. IQ and psychological testing.

6. Electroencephalography.

7. Audiography.

TREATMENT

1. Depends on the findings.

2. Genetic counseling.

3. Psychological support and counseling.

FOLLOW-UP

1. Every 6 to 12 months in the absence of a disorder requiring therapy.

2. Neonates with an eyelid plexiform neurofibroma should be seen more frequently because of a 50% risk of early glaucoma.

TABLE 13.7 CHARACTERISTICS OF NEUROFIBROMATOSIS 1 AND 2

Neurofibromatosis 1	Neurofibromatosis 2
At least two of the following: 1. At least six café-au-lait spots —>5 mm prepubertal *or* —>15 mm postpubertal 2. Neurofibromas —One plexiform neurofibroma *or* —At least two of any other type 3. Intertriginous freckling 4. Optic nerve glioma 5. At least two Lisch nodules (iris hamartomas) 6. Distinctive osseous dysplasia (sphenoid or tibial) 7. Affected first-degree relative	Either A or B: A. Bilateral acoustic nerve masses (by computed tomography or magnetic resonance imaging) *or* B. Affected first-degree relative *and* 1. Unilateral acoustic nerve mass *or* 2. At least two of the following: —neurofibroma —meningioma —glioma —schwannoma —juvenile posterior subcapsular cataract
Inheritance: Autosomal dominant Gene location: Chromosome 17 Frequency: 1:4,000	Autosomal dominant Chromosome 21 1:50,000

13.18 TUBEROUS SCLEROSIS

(BOURNEVILLE SYNDROME)

SIGNS

Ocular. Astrocytic hamartoma of the retina or optic disc (a white, semitransparent, or mulberry-appearing tumor in the superficial retina that may undergo calcification with age; no prominent feeder vessels, no associated retinal detachment).

Critical Systemic. Adenoma sebaceum (yellow–red papules in a butterfly distribution on the upper cheeks, apparent in the prepubertal years), astrocytic hamartomas of the brain with seizures, subnormal intelligence, or mental retardation, or a combination of these.

Other Systemic. Subungual angiofibromas (yellow–red papules around and beneath the nails of the fingers or toes); shagreen patches; ash-leaf sign (depigmented macules on the skin); café-au-lait spots; renal angiomyolipoma; cardiac rhabdomyoma; pleural cysts causing spontaneous pneumothorax; cystic bone lesions; hamartomas of the liver, thyroid, pancreas, or testes.

DIFFERENTIAL DIAGNOSIS

Retinoblastoma. (Flat or elevated white retinal tumor that has prominent feeder vessels; may be bilateral or multifocal or both. Vitreous seeding, retinal detachment, pseudohypopyon, iris neovascularization, or vitreous hemorrhage may be present. No systemic signs, initially.)

INHERITANCE

Autosomal dominant with incomplete penetrance.

WORKUP

1. Family history: Examination of the family members is important.

2. Complete general physical and ophthalmic examinations.

3. CBC, electrolytes.

4. CT scan (axial and coronal views) or MRI of the brain.

5. Electroencephalography.

6. Echocardiography.

7. Chest radiography.

8. Abdominal CT scan.

TREATMENT

1. Retinal astrocytomas usually require no treatment.

2. Genetic counseling.

FOLLOW-UP

Yearly in the absence of a disorder requiring therapy.

13.19   STURGE–WEBER SYNDROME

(ENCEPHALOFACIAL CAVERNOUS HEMANGIOMATOSIS)

SIGNS

Ocular. Diffuse choroidal hemangioma ("tomato catsup" fundus: the lesion obscures all detail of the choroidal vasculature and produces a uniform red fundus background; best appreciated when compared with the other eye), unilateral glaucoma (facial hemangioma of the upper eyelid increases the risk of glaucoma), iris heterochromia, blood in Schlemm canal (seen on gonioscopy), secondary serous retinal detachment, secondary RPE alterations (retinitis pigmentosa–like picture).

Critical Systemic. Port-wine stain or nevus flammeus (congenital facial hemangioma along the first and second divisions of the trigeminal nerve).

Other Systemic. Subnormal intelligence or mental retardation, Jacksonian-type seizures, peripheral arteriovenous communications, facial hemihypertrophy ipsilateral to nevus flammeus, leptomeningeal angiomatosis, cerebral calcifications.

INHERITANCE

Sporadic.

WORKUP

1. Complete general and ophthalmic examinations.

2. CT scan (axial and coronal views) or MRI of the brain.

3. Electroencephalography.

TREATMENT

1. Treat glaucoma if present: First-line drugs are aqueous suppressants (e.g., timolol or levobunolol and/or brimonidine and/or dorzolamide); latanoprost, pilocarpine, and epinephrine compounds are less effective because of high episcleral venous pressure. Surgery (goniotomy or trabeculectomy, or both) is often required at an early stage to control the IOP, with moderate to high suc-

cess. (See 9.1, Primary Open-Angle Glaucoma.)

2. Consider treating serous retinal detachments that threaten or involve the macula. Laser photocoagulation has been used, but the success rate is low. Low-dose external-beam radiation therapy or plaque radiation therapy often resolves the subretinal fluid. Photodynamic therapy with verteporphyrin is also successful for more circumscribed tumors.

3. Anticonvulsants for epilepsy, in concert with neurologist or pediatrician.

4. Tunable dye laser for cutaneous nevus flammeus, in concert with dermatologist.

FOLLOW-UP

1. Every 6 months; watch carefully for glaucoma or a serous retinal detachment.

2. If glaucoma is present, closer follow-up may be required.

3. If skin involvement is only in the mandibular area, the risk of glaucoma is much lower, and the interval for follow-up may be extended to 1 year.

13.20 VON HIPPEL–LINDAU SYNDROME
(RETINOCEREBELLAR CAPILLARY HEMANGIOMATOSIS)

SIGNS

Critical. Retinal capillary hemangioma (small, yellow–red tumor with a tortuous dilated feeder artery and a draining vein), sometimes associated with subretinal exudates, a retinal detachment, or both.

Other. Cerebellar hemangioblastoma, hypernephroma (renal cell carcinoma), pheochromocytoma, renal cysts, pancreatic cysts, epididymal cysts, syringomyelia.

DIFFERENTIAL DIAGNOSIS

• Racemose hemangiomatosis (No definable tumor present; large, dilated, tortuous vessels form arteriovenous communications.).

• Coats disease (Characteristic aneurysmal dilatation of blood vessels is found with prominent subretinal exudate. No identifiable tumor is present.).

• Retinoblastoma (Multiple white rather than pink retinal tumors. Subretinal exudate is rare.).

• Familial exudative vitreoretinopathy (Usually bilateral, temporal, peripheral exudation

with retinal vascular abnormalities, but no tumor.).

INHERITANCE

Autosomal dominant with incomplete penetrance (chromosome 3p).

WORKUP

Indicated when multiple or bilateral retinal capillary hemangiomas are discovered, or when a unilateral retinal capillary hemangioma is found along with characteristic systemic findings or a positive family history.

Note: Some physicians work up all patients with retinal capillary hemangiomas.

1. Family history and examination of family members.

2. Complete general physical and ophthalmic examinations.

3. CBC, electrolytes.

4. MRI of the brain (visualizes the posterior fossa better than CT scan).

5. Urine tests for levels of epinephrine and norepinephrine.

6. Abdominal CT scan.

7. IVFA if treatment of the retinal capillary hemangioma is planned.

TREATMENT

1. Photocoagulation, cryotherapy, or photodynamic therapy with verteporphyrin of a retinal hemangioma is often indicated if it is affecting or threatening vision.

2. Genetic counseling.

3. Systemic therapy, depending on findings.

FOLLOW-UP

Every 3 to 6 months, depending on the retinal condition.

13.21 WYBURN–MASON SYNDROME

(RACEMOSE HEMANGIOMATOSIS)

SIGNS

Ocular. Enormously dilated, tortuous retinal vessels with arteriovenous communications. No distinct mass or subretinal exudate is present. Rarely, proptosis from a racemose hemangioma of the orbit is present.

Systemic. Midbrain racemose hemangiomas, seizures, hemiparesis, mental changes, and ipsilateral pterygoid fossa, mandibular, and maxillary hemangiomas. Intracranial hemorrhage from a midbrain hemangioma can occur.

DIFFERENTIAL DIAGNOSIS

• Retinal capillary hemangioma. (A distinct mass is present, sometimes with subretinal exudate.).

• Coats disease (The vessels are irregularly dilated, and exudative retinal detachment is found.).

INHERITANCE

Sporadic.

WORKUP

1. Complete general and ophthalmic examinations.

2. MRI of the brain.

3. Electroencephalography.

TREATMENT

1. No treatment is required for the retinal lesions. The condition is congenital and does not progress.

2. Warn the patient of the risk of massive hemorrhage with ipsilateral dental and facial surgery.

FOLLOW-UP

Yearly.

13.22 ATAXIA–TELANGIECTASIA

(LOUIS–BAR SYNDROME)

SIGNS

Ocular. Dilated conjunctival vessels, strabismus, impaired convergence, nystagmus, oculomotor apraxia.

Critical Systemic. Cerebellar ataxia that becomes apparent after the child learns to walk; cutaneous telangiectases in a butterfly distribution on the face, on the antecubital and popliteal fossa, behind the ears, or at the base of the neck during the first decade of life. Recurrent sinopulmonary infections as a result of immunoglobulin A deficiency and impaired T-cell function can occur.

Other Systemic. Leukemia or lymphoma (often leading to death in childhood or early adulthood), mental retardation, seborrheic dermatitis, pigmentary changes of the skin, testicular or ovarian atrophy, hypoplastic or atrophic thymus.

INHERITANCE

Autosomal recessive.

WORKUP

1. Family history (examination of the family members often aids in the diagnosis).

2. Complete general and ophthalmic examinations.

3. CBC.

4. Chest radiography.

5. MRI of the brain.

TREATMENT

1. Systemic treatment, depending on findings.

2. Genetic counseling.

FOLLOW-UP

Patients need close medical follow-up. Routine eye examinations should be performed every 1 to 2 years.

CHAPTER 14

GENERAL RADIOLOGY STUDIES IN OPHTHALMOLOGY

14.1 COMPUTED TOMOGRAPHY SCAN

DESCRIPTION

Computed tomography (CT) uses ionizing radiation and computer-assisted formatting to produce multiple cross-sectional planar images. Possible image planes include axial, coronal, reformatted coronal, and reformatted sagittal images. Views that focus primarily on soft tissues or bony structures are available and both should always be reviewed. Slice width for orbital studies is always 3 mm or thinner. Radiodense contrast allows more extensive evaluation of vascular structures and leaks where there is a breakdown of the normal capillary endothelial barrier (as with inflammation).

*Note: Coronal images are obtained by having the patient hyperextend the neck; this should **not** be done if there is any suspicion of neck injury.*

USES IN OPHTHALMOLOGY

1. Locating suspected intraorbital or intraocular metallic foreign bodies. Glass, wood, and plastic are less radiopaque and tend to be more difficult to isolate on CT.

2. Excellent for defining bone lesions such as fractures (orbital wall or optic canal) or bony involvement of a soft tissue mass.

3. Soft tissue windows are good for determining some soft tissue pathologic features such as orbital cellulitis/abscess (loss of radio-

dense margins). May be useful in determining posterior scleral rupture when clinical examination is inconclusive, but B-scan ultrasonography is usually more sensitive.

4. Excellent for diagnosing sinusitis.

5. Excellent for locating intracranial blood or blood in the subarachnoid, subdural, or epidural space in either acute or subacute setting.

6. Excellent for looking for optic canal fractures in cases of suspected traumatic optic neuropathy.

7. Good for evaluation of proptosis and Graves orbitopathy.

8. Less sensitive than magnetic resonance imaging for evaluation of orbital apex and cavernous sinus.

HINTS FOR ORDERING THE STUDY

1. Always order an orbital study (as opposed to looking at the orbits from a head series) when suspecting ocular or orbital pathologic features. Include views of paranasal sinuses and cavernous sinuses.

2. Order both axial and coronal views. If direct coronal views cannot be performed, request finer axial cuts for better coronal reconstructions.

3. When attempting to diagnose traumatic optic neuropathy, request thin (1-mm) cuts of the optic canal.

4. When attempting to localize either ocular or orbital foreign bodies, order 1-mm cuts.

5. Always order contrast with suspected infections or inflammations. Make sure patient is not allergic to iodine or shellfish.

6. In children or noncooperative adults, consider ordering spiral (helical) CT. The entire scan can be performed in 10 to 30 seconds.

7. CT angiography is helpful in diagnosing vascular lesions, including central nervous system (CNS) aneurysms, but requires special hardware and software.

14.2 MAGNETIC RESONANCE IMAGING

DESCRIPTION

1. Magnetic resonance imaging (MRI) uses a large magnetic field to excite protons of water molecules. The energy given off as the protons reequilibrate to their normal state is detected by specialized receivers ("coils"), and that information is reconstructed into a computer image.

2. Obtains multiplanar images without loss of resolution: axial, coronal, sagittal, and so forth.

3. Weighting of the image:

—T_1-weighted images have good anatomic detail, good for intraorbital structures such as optic nerve, extraocular muscles, and orbital veins, but strong fat signal gives poor resolution of lacrimal gland. T_1 weighting gives poor intraorbital contrast (note that subacute blood more than 5 days old appears bright).

—T_2-weighted images give very poor intraocular contrast.

4. Fat suppression (saturation): Very useful in T_1-weighted images. Deletes bright intraconal fat signal from orbit, allowing for better anatomic detail. Essential for all orbital MRIs.

5. Gadolinium-diethylenetriamine pentaacetic acid (Gd-DTPA) is a paramagnetic agent for MRI that distributes in the extracellular space and does not cross the intact blood–brain barrier. Gd-DTPA is best for T_1-weighted fat-suppressed images. The lacrimal gland and extraocular muscles enhance with Gd-DTPA. The optic nerve does *not* normally enhance. Never use gadolinium without also using fat suppression.

6. Interpretation of T_1- and T_2-weighted images:

Image:

a. T_1: Fat looks bright (i.e., high signal intensity); vitreous and intracranial ventricles are dark.

b. T_2: Vitreous is bright, fat is relatively darker.

c. **T_1 with fat suppression:** Vitreous and fat are dark, extraocular muscles are brighter.

d. Most orbital masses are dark on T_1 weighting and become bright with gadolinium. Notable exceptions of processes that appear *bright* on T_1 weighting before gadolinium injection:

—Fat: Lipoma, liposarcoma.

—Mucus: Dermoid cysts, mucocele.

—Melanin: Melanoma.

—Subacute blood: Three to 14 days old.

—Certain fungal pathogens: *Aspergillus.*

e. High flow (arterial blood) creates a dark area on images because the proton has already moved out of the field of view before relaxation occurs. This is seen on MRI as a "flow void" and is helpful in identifying the cavernous sinus (the carotid siphon appears dark).

Radiographic Parameters:

a. T_1: TR (time to repeat) usually less than 1,000 milliseconds (msec) TE (time to echo) usually low (less than 100 msec).

b. T_2: TR usually more than 1,000 msec; TE usually high (more than 100 msec).

USES IN OPHTHALMOLOGY

1. Excellent for defining extent of orbital/CNS masses.

2. Excellent for suspected intracranial lesions affecting neuroophthalmic pathways.

3. Very poor for defining bone or acute blood.

4. Excellent for diagnosing intracranial masses.

5. Useful for characterization of intraocular mass lesion in an eye with opaque media.

6. Excellent for orbital apical/cavernous sinus lesions.

7. For suspected neurogenic tumors (meningioma, glioma), gadolinium is especially helpful in defining extent of lesions.

8. All patients with clinical signs or symptomatic optic neuritis should have *brain* MRI [FLAIR (fluid-attenuated inversion recovery) images are especially useful].

HINTS FOR ORDERING THE STUDY

1. When looking for ocular or unilateral orbital pathologic condition, may request an orbital surface coil; however, for most routine orbital studies, a head coil is indicated to provide bilateral orbital views extending to the optic chiasm.

2. Always request fat suppression and gadolinium enhancement. Orbital studies without these techniques are incomplete and may be misleading.

3. Contraindications to MRI: Cardiac pacemaker, suspected magnetic intraocular/intraorbital foreign bodies, metal surgical clips. Titanium plates or clips are MRI safe.

14.3   MAGNETIC RESONANCE ANGIOGRAPHY

DESCRIPTION

Special application of MRI technology in which the region of interest is imaged repeatedly at short intervals after intravenous injection of paramagnetic agent to evaluate blood flow in the regional vasculature.

USES IN OPHTHALMOLOGY

1. Suspected carotid or ophthalmic artery stenosis/occlusion or dissection.

2. Suspected intracranial and orbital arterial aneurysms (e.g., pupil involving third cranial nerve palsy), arteriovenous malforma-

tions, and acquired arteriovenous communications.

3. Suspected orbital or intracranial vascular mass (hemangioma, varix).

HINTS FOR ORDERING THE STUDY

Cerebral arteriography remains the gold standard for diagnosis of vascular lesions but carries significant morbidity and mortality in certain populations. Currently, the limit of magnetic resonance angiography (MRA) is an aneurysm larger than 2 mm. The sensitivity of MRA is highly dependent on several factors: hardware, software, and the experience of the neuroradiologist.

14.4 MAGNETIC RESONANCE VENOGRAPHY

Magnetic resonance venography (MRV) is helpful in diagnosing venous thrombosis. Used in workup of patient with bilateral disc swelling.

14.5 OPHTHALMIC ULTRASONOGRAPHY

Ophthalmic ultrasonography is a diagnostic imaging technique that uses high-frequency sound waves (10 to 50 MHz) to generate either cross-sectional imaging (B-scan) or amplitude of reflectivity curves (A-scan) of ocular or orbital tissues.

A-SCAN

DESCRIPTION

Uses ultrasound waves to generate linear distance versus amplitude of reflectivity curves of the evaluated ocular and orbital tissues. A-scans are used for measuring and characterizing the composition of tissues based on the reflectivity curves. Not all A-scan instruments are standardized. Standardization means that the linear curve generated by testing the probe against gelatin standard has a defined shape at a particular gain setting of the instrument. Standardization uses an S-shaped curve. Both contact and water-bath techniques may be used.

USES IN OPHTHALMOLOGY

1. Primary use in ophthalmology is measurement of axial length of the globe. This information is critical for intraocular lens (IOL) power calculations for cataract surgery. Axial length information can also be used to identify certain congenital disorders such as microphthalmos, nanophthalmos, and congenital glaucoma.

2. Diagnostic identification of consistency of masses in the globe or orbit with standardized A-scan probe.

3. Specialized A-mode ultrasonography can be used for corneal pachymetry (measurement of corneal thickness).

HINTS FOR ORDERING THE STUDY

1. When used for IOL power calculations, make sure to check both eyes. The two eyes should be within 0.2 mm.

2. Spikes along the baseline should be sharply rising at 90 degrees.

B-MODE

DESCRIPTION

Gives real-time, two-dimensional (cross-sectional) image of the eye posterior to the iris to immediately posterior to the globe. Both contact and water-bath techniques may be used, but the contact method does not visualize the anterior chamber well.

USES IN OPHTHALMOLOGY

1. Define ocular anatomy when media opacities are too great to visualize directly.

2. In setting of trauma, can be used to diagnosis scleral rupture posterior to the muscle in-

sertions or when media opacities prevent direct visualization.

3. Identify intraocular foreign bodies especially if made of metal or glass (spherical objects have a specific echo shadow); wood or vegetable matter has variable echodensity signal; can also give a more precise location if the foreign body is next to the scleral wall.

4. Evaluation of intraocular tumor/mass consistency, retinal detachment, choroidal detachment (serous versus hemorrhagic), and optic disc abnormalities (e.g., optic disc drusen, coloboma).

5. Can be used for lacrimal gland and anterior orbital pathologic conditions, but this has largely been replaced by MRI or CT.

HINTS FOR ORDERING THE STUDY

1. If used in setting of trauma to determine unknown scleral rupture, can be used over closed eyelids with immersion in copious amounts of sterile methylcellulose, such that no pressure is placed on the globe. The gain must be set higher to overcome the sound attenuation of the eyelids. Known ruptured globe is a contraindication to B-scan ultrasonography.

2. When scleral integrity is not in question, B-scan ultrasonography should be performed dynamically. The movement of the globe can help differentiate between different structures, such as with retinal detachment versus posterior vitreous detachment.

3. Dense intraocular calcifications (such as occurs in many eyes with phthisis bulbi) result in images that are of poor quality and usually are uninterpretable.

4. Silicone oil in the vitreous causes distortion of the scanned image, and therefore the study should be performed in an upright position with the patient.

ULTRASONOGRAPHIC BIOMICROSCOPY

DESCRIPTION

Uses very–high-frequency (50 MHz) B-mode ultrasound of the anterior one fifth of the globe to give cross-sections at near-microscopic resolution. Uses a water-bath eyelid speculum with viscous liquid in bowl of the speculum.

USES IN OPHTHALMOLOGY

1. Excellent for defining corneoscleral limbal pathologic conditions, anterior chamber angle, ciliary body, iris pathologic conditions (e.g., ciliary body masses/cysts, plateau iris), and anteriorly located, small foreign bodies.

2. Unexplained unilateral angle narrowing or closure.

3. Suspected cyclodialysis.

HINTS FOR ORDERING THE STUDY

Known ruptured globe is a contraindication to the study.

ORBITAL ULTRASONOGRAPHY/ DOPPLER

DESCRIPTION

Uses B-mode ultrasonography coupled with Doppler technology to visualize flow in the vessels in the orbit.

USES IN OPHTHALMOLOGY

1. Superior ophthalmic vein pathology: High-flow cavernous sinus fistulas, superior ophthalmic vein thrombosis.

2. Orbital varix.

3. Arteriovenous malformations.

14.6 INTRAVENOUS FLUORESCEIN ANGIOGRAPHY

DESCRIPTION

Photographic method of angiography that does not rely on ionizing radiation. After intravenous injection of fluorescein solution (usually in a hand or arm vein), rapid-sequence photography is performed by using a camera with spectrally appropriate excitation and barrier filters. Fluorescein sodium absorbs blue light, with peak absorption and excitation occurring at wavelengths of 465 to 490 nm. Fluorescence then occurs at the yellow-green wavelengths of 520 to 530 nm.

USES IN OPHTHALMOLOGY

1. Used to image retinal, choroidal, optic disc, or iris vasculature, or a combination of these. It is used diagnostically as well as in planning for many retinal laser procedures.

2. Transit times between injection and appearance of dye in the choroid, retinal arteries, and veins also can be used to evaluate flow through the imaged vessels.

3. Suspected retinal hypoxia (capillary nonperfusion) and neovascularization from various conditions (e.g., diabetes, familial exudative vitreoretinopathy).

4. Suspected choroidal neovascularization from various diseases (e.g., age-related macular degeneration, ocular histoplasmosis, conditions associated with angioid streaks).

HINTS FOR ORDERING THE STUDY

1. Side effects of intravenous fluorescein are nausea (less than 10%), vomiting (usually less than 2%), hives, pruritus, vasovagal response. True anaphylaxis is very rare. Extravasation into extracellular space at the injections site can produce local necrosis. Excreted in urine in 24 to 36 hours.

2. Because it is a photographic method, somewhat clear media are required for visualization.

14.7 INDOCYANINE GREEN ANGIOGRAPHY

DESCRIPTION

Photographic method of ocular angiography similar to intravenous fluorescein angiography; indocyanine green angiography (ICG) differs in that fluorescence occurs in the infrared spectrum (835 nm), allowing for penetration through pigment, fluid, and blood. ICG provides better evaluation of the choroidal vasculature. Indocyanine green excitation occurs at 805 nm, with fluorescence at 835 nm.

USES IN OPHTHALMOLOGY

1. Suspected occult choroidal neovascular membranes (CNVMs).

2. Suspected recurrent CNVM after prior treatment.

3. Suspected CNVM with retinal pigment epithelial detachment.

4. Suspected polypoidal choroidal vasculopathy.

HINTS FOR ORDERING THE STUDY

1. Contraindicated in patients with iodine or shellfish allergies.

2. Most common side effect of ICG is a vasovagal response.

3. Metabolized by the liver.

14.8   NUCLEAR MEDICINE

DESCRIPTION

Nuclear medicine imaging uses radioactive contrast (radionuclide) that emits gamma radiation, which is then gathered by a gamma ray detector. The classic types of radionuclide scanning known to ophthalmologists include bone scanning, liver–spleen scanning, and gallium scanning. Radionuclide scintigraphy is rarely, if ever performed for intraocular or orbital disease but is requested occasionally by ophthalmologists to screen for systemic disease that might be associated with ophthalmic findings.

USES IN OPHTHALMOLOGY

1. Scintigraphy (e.g., with technetium-99): Useful for assessing lacrimal drainage physiology. Useful for patients with contradictory or inconsistent irrigation testing.

2. Systemic gallium scan is useful for detecting extraocular sarcoid granulomatous inflammation.

3. Phosphorus-32 test: Not currently used in most countries; provides little, if any useful differential diagnostic information in most patients with suspected choroidal melanoma.

14.9   PLAIN FILMS

DESCRIPTION

Images of radiopaque tissues obtained by exposure of special photographic plates to ionizing radiation. Not used routinely in ophthalmology at present; previously used to diagnose orbital wall fractures, but CT is now the gold standard for diagnosis of this condition.

USES IN OPHTHALMOLOGY

Radiopaque foreign body when CT is unavailable or patient unable to tolerate CT scan. Screening before MRI in patients if occult metallic foreign body is suspected. Plain films should not be used definitively to rule in or out orbital fractures.

14.10   CEREBRAL ARTERIOGRAPHY

DESCRIPTION

This interventional radiologic examination entails intraarterial injection of radiopaque contrast followed by a rapid sequence of x-ray imaging of the region of interest to evaluate the transit of blood through the regional vasculature. Unlike MRA, arteriography also allows the option of simultaneous treatment of lesions by intravascular techniques. It is the gold standard for intracranial aneurysms, but is slowly being replaced in many centers by MRA as resolution improves.

USES IN OPHTHALMOLOGY

1. Suspected arteriovenous malformations, cavernous sinus fistula, and vascular masses (e.g., hemangioma, varix).

2. Diagnosis of carotid cavernous fistulas.

3. Evaluation of ocular ischemic syndrome or amaurosis fugax due to suspected atherosclerotic carotid or ophthalmic artery occlusive disease. Usually carotid Doppler ultrasonography is adequate for diagnosis.

4. Arteriography is contraindicated in cases of suspected carotid artery dissection because the technique may cause extension of the dissection.

14.11 PHOTOGRAPHIC IMAGING STUDIES

DESCRIPTION

Various methods of imaging the appearance of the eyes or selected regions of the eye, using white light or various spectral wavelengths of light.

TYPES OF OPHTHALMIC PHOTOGRAPHIC IMAGING STUDIES

1. Documentary photography: Color pictures of face, external eye, anterior segment, fundus (white light or red-free lighting).

2. Specular microscopy: Contact and noncontact photographic techniques used to image the corneal endothelium. The images can then be used to evaluate the quality of the endothelial cells and determine endothelial cell counts.

14.12 OPTICAL COHERENCE TOMOGRAPHY

DESCRIPTION

Optical coherence tomography (OCT) provides noninvasive, two-dimensional images by measuring optical reflections of light. In this manner, OCT is similar to ultrasonography except that OCT is based on the reflection of light and not sound. The OCT scanner sends low-coherence light (820-nm wavelength) emitted by a superluminescent diode to the tissue to be examined and to a reference beam. The time delays of the light reflections are recorded by an interferometer. Using a reference mirror, these light reflections are then translated into an imaged object with a high resolution of 10 to 20 μm.

USES IN OPHTHALMOLOGY

1. Suspected retinal disease, including macular edema, central serous chorioretinopathy, and age-related macular degeneration.

2. Suspected vitreoretinal interface syndromes, including macular holes and epiretinal membranes.

3. Quantification of the nerve fiber layer thickness for suspected glaucoma.

4. Newer uses will include cross-sectional images and thickness measurement of the cornea.

HINTS FOR ORDERING THE STUDY

Requires patient's ability to fixate, and relatively clear media.

14.13 CONFOCAL SCANNING LASER OPHTHALMOSCOPY

DESCRIPTION

Confocal scanning laser ophthalmoscopy is a noninvasive imaging technique to evaluate the topography of ocular structures. This confocal optical system provides a contour map of the desired structure in the following manner. The system aims to detect light sent to and reflected from a very thin optical plane, the focal plane. Only the light from the focal plane is recorded. By moving the focal plane in incremental units along the intended object, a series of "focal planes" or images may be recorded and combined to create a three-dimensional image. Computer software may dictate the number of images recorded and their recombination to provide analytical data. Heidelberg retinal tomography is one such example.

USES IN OPHTHALMOLOGY

1. Suspected optic nerve disease, including glaucoma and papilledema.

2. Suspected fundus elevations, including macular edema and choroidal nevi.

HINTS FOR ORDERING THE STUDY

1. Requires patient's ability to fixate, and relatively clear media.

2. Because the hallmark of the test is to provide comparative data, subsequent tests in the same patient need accurate alignment in the same focal plane to provide useful information.

14.14 CONFOCAL BIOMICROSCOPY

DESCRIPTION

The confocal microscope optically sections through the cornea in order to nonivasively obtain structural and functional information of the different corneal layers.

USES IN OPHTHALMOLOGY

May be helpful in diagnosing and following eyes with acanthomoeba keratitis, herpetic keratitis, bacterial keratitis, fungal keratitis, and dry eye syndrome.

14.15 DACRYOCYSTOGRAPHY

DESCRIPTION

Special application of plain film radiographs to image the nasolacrimal drainage system after injection of radiopaque contrast into the system.

USES IN OPHTHALMOLOGY

1. Suspected nasolacrimal drainage obstruction.

2. May be used for defining lacrimal drainage system anatomy when cause of obstruction is maldevelopment or tumor, but has no ability to comment on physiology.

14.16 CORNEAL TOPOGRAPHY

DESCRIPTION

Standard keratometry measures central corneal power and the radius of curvature. Corneal topography is performed using a variety of methods, including Placido disc analysis, scanning slit beam and rasterstereography. These techniques project an image onto the cornea to analyze the corneal shape. It can provide information on corneal curvature and regularity. A simulated keratometry reading can be generated.

USES IN OPHTHALMOLOGY

Detecting irregular astigmatism from keratoconus, pellucid marginal degeneration, corneal surgery, corneal trauma, contact lens warpage, corneal dystrophy, postinflammatory or postinfectious etiology. It may be helpful in identifying the cause of decreased vision in patients with no known cause. It can be used before and after refractive surgery.

DILATING DROPS

MYDRIATIC AND CYCLOPLEGIC AGENTS

	Approximate Maximal Effect	Approximate Duration of Action
Mydriatic		
Phenylephrine, 2.5, 10%	20 min	3 h
Cycloplegic/mydriatic		
Tropicamide, 0.5%, 1%	20–30 min	3–6 h
Cyclopentolate, 0.5%, 1%, 2%	20–45 min	24 h
Homatropine, 2%, 5%	20–90 min	2–3 days
Scopolamine, 0.25%	20–45 min	4–7 days
Atropine, 0.5%, 1%, 2%	30–40 min	1–2 wk

The usual regimen for a dilated examination is:

- *Adults:* Phenylephrine, 2.5% and tropicamide, 1%. Repeat these drops in 15–30 min if the eye is not dilated.
- *Children:* Phenylephrine, 2.5%, tropicamide, 1%, and cyclopentolate, 1–2%. Repeat these drops in 25–35 min if the eye is not dilated.
- *Infants:* Phenylephrine, 1% and tropicamide, 0.2%. Homatropine, 2% or cyclopentolate, 0.5% (usually reserved for infants older than 1–2 mo of age) may also be used. The drops can be repeated in 35–45 min if the eye is not dilated.

*Notes

1. Dilating drops are contraindicated in most types of angle-closure glaucoma and in eyes with severely narrow anterior-chamber angles.

2. Dilating drops tend to be less effective at the same concentration in darkly pigmented eyes.

COVER/UNCOVER AND ALTERNATE COVER TESTS

COVER/UNCOVER TEST

Differentiates a phoria (the eyes are straight when fixating on a target, but misaligned when tired or not focusing) from a tropia (the eyes are misaligned at all times).

REQUIREMENTS

Full range of ocular motility, vision adequate to see the target of fixation, foveal fixation in each eye, attention, and patient cooperation. This test should be performed before the alternate cover test.

1. Ask the patient to fixate on an accommodative target at distance (e.g., a letter on the vision chart).

2. Cover one of the patient's eyes while observing the uncovered eye. A refixation movement of the uncovered eye suggests the presence of a tropia.

3. Remove the cover. A phoria is identified by refixation of the eye now being uncovered while the contralateral eye maintains its position and fixation.

4. Repeat the procedure, covering the opposite eye.

   Note: A tropia may be unilateral, the same eye may be always turned in or out, or it may alternate between eyes. In an alternating tropia, the contralateral eye is sometimes deviated after the cover/uncover test.

5. Ask the patient to fixate on an accommodative target at near. Both eyes are tested at near in the manner described previously.

   Note: An esodeviation is detected by a refixation movement temporally (the eye being observed turns away from the nose). An exodeviation is detected by a refixation movement nasally (the eye being observed turns toward the nose). A hyperdeviation is detected by a refixation movement inferiorly.

ALTERNATE COVER TEST (PRISM AND COVER TEST)

Measures the total deviation: phoria combined with tropia.

REQUIREMENTS

Same as for the cover/uncover test.

1. The patient is asked to fixate on an accommodative target at distance.

2. An occluder is held over one eye for a few seconds, and then quickly switched to the other eye. As the occluder alternately covers each eye for a few seconds, the eye being uncovered may be noted to swing into position to refixate on the target. Such eye movement indicates the presence of a deviation.

3. To measure the deviation, prisms are placed in front of one eye until eye movement ceases as the cover is alternated from eye to eye. The base of the prism is placed in the direction of eye movement. The strength of the weakest prism that eliminates eye movement during the alternate cover test is the amount of the deviation.

4. Measurements may be done for any direction of gaze by turning the patient's head away from the target while asking him or her to maintain fixation on it (i.e., right gaze is measured by turning the patient's head toward his or her left shoulder and asking the patient to look at the target).

5. In general, measurements are taken in the straight-ahead position (both at distance and near), in right gaze, left gaze, downgaze (the chin is tilted up while the patient focuses on the target), upgaze (the chin is tilted down while the patient focuses on the target), and with the patient's head tilted toward his or her left shoulder and then toward his or her right shoulder. Measurements are taken both with and without glasses in the straight-ahead position.

AMSLER GRID

Used to test macular function or to detect a central or paracentral scotoma.

1. Have the patient wear his or her glasses and occlude the left eye while an Amsler grid is held approximately 12 inches in front of the right eye (Fig. A.1).

2. The patient is asked what is in the center of the page. Failure to see the central dot may indicate a central scotoma.

3. Have the patient fixate on the central dot (or the center of the page if he or she cannot see the dot), and ask if all four corners of the di-

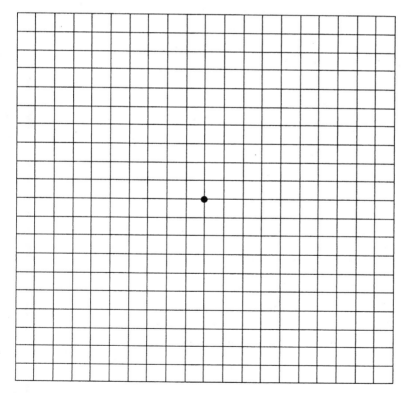

FIGURE A.1   Amsler grid.

agram are visible. Are any of the boxes missing?

4. Again, while staring at the central dot, the patient is asked if all of the lines are straight and continuous or if some are distorted and broken.

5. The patient is asked to outline any missing or distorted areas on the grid with a pencil.

6. Repeat the procedure, covering the right eye and testing the left.

Notes:

1. *It is very important to monitor the patient's eye for movement away from the central dot.*

2. *A red Amsler grid may define more subtle defects.*

SEIDEL TEST TO DETECT A WOUND LEAK

Concentrated fluorescein dye (from a moistened fluorescein strip) is applied directly over the potential site of perforation while observing the site with the slit lamp (by using the white light; Fig. A.2). If a perforation and leak exist, the fluorescein dye is diluted by the aqueous and appears as a green (dilute) stream within the dark orange (concentrated) dye. The stream of aqueous is best seen with the blue light of the slit lamp.

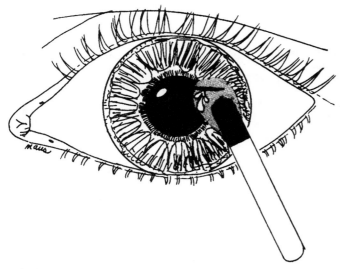

FIGURE A.2   Seidel test.

FORCED-DUCTION TEST AND ACTIVE FORCE GENERATION TEST

FORCED-DUCTION TEST

This test distinguishes restrictive causes of decreased ocular motility from other motility disorders. One technique is the following:

1. Place a drop of topical anesthetic (e.g., proparacaine) into the eye.

2. Place a cotton-tipped applicator soaked with cocaine, 10%, on the muscle to be grasped (i.e., the muscle away from the "paretic" field) for approximately 1 minute.

3. The anesthetized muscle is grasped firmly with toothed forceps (e.g., Graefe fixation forceps), and the eye is rotated in the "paretic" direction (Fig. A.3). If there is resistance to passive rotation of the eye, a restrictive disorder is diagnosed.

ACTIVE FORCE GENERATION TEST

The patient is asked to look in the "paretic" direction while a sterile cotton swab is held just beneath the limbus on that same side. The amount of force generated by the "paretic" muscle is compared with that generated in the normal contralateral eye.

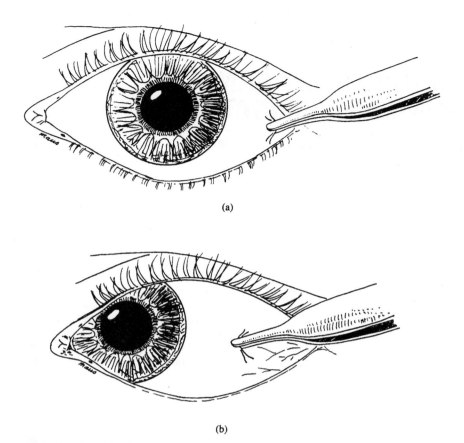

(a)

(b)

FIGURE A.3 Forced ductions. In the case illustrated, the left eye could not look inward. **a:** The lateral rectus muscle is grasped with forceps. **b:** The eye can be moved in the paretic direction (inward in this case) without resistance, ruling out a restrictive muscle condition.

TECHNIQUE FOR DIAGNOSTIC PROBING AND IRRIGATION OF THE LACRIMAL SYSTEM

1. Anesthetize the eye with a drop of topical anesthetic (e.g., proparacaine) and hold a cotton-tipped applicator soaked in the topical anesthetic on the involved punctum for several minutes.

2. Dilate the punctum with a punctum dilator.

3. Gently insert a small Bowman probe into the punctum 2 mm vertically, and then 8 mm horizontally, toward the nose (Fig. A.4). Pull the involved eyelid laterally while slowly moving the probe horizontally to facilitate the procedure and to avoid creating a false passageway.

4. In the presence of an eyelid laceration, a torn canaliculus may be diagnosed by the appearance of the probe in the site of the eyelid laceration.

5. Irrigation of the lacrimal system is performed after removing the probe and inserting an irrigation canula in the same manner in which the probe was inserted. Five to 10 mL of saline is gently pushed into the system. Leakage through a torn eyelid also diagnoses a severed canaliculus. Resistance to injection of the saline, ballooning of the lacrimal sac, or leakage of the saline out of either punctum may be the result of a lacrimal system obstruction. A patent lacrimal system usually drains into the throat quite readily, and the arrival of saline there may be noted by the patient.

*Note: If evaluating solely the patency of the lacrimal system, and not ruling out a laceration, the system can be irrigated as described previously, immediately after punctum dilatation.

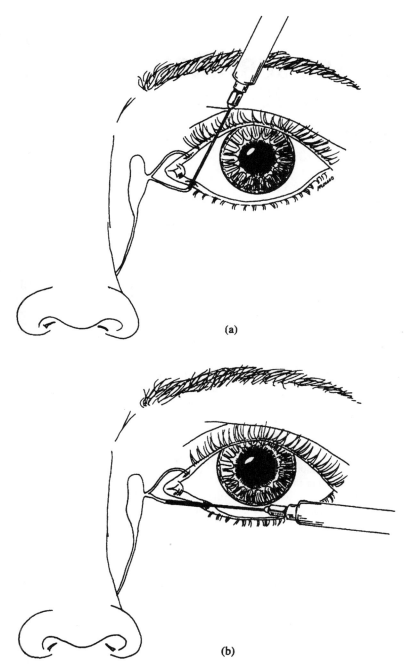

(a)

(b)

FIGURE A.4 Diagnostic probing of the lacrimal system. **a:** After punctum dilatation, the probe or irrigation needle is directed inferiorly for 2 mm. **b:** The instrument is rotated horizontally, and with the eyelid stretched laterally, is inserted toward the nose.

TECHNIQUE FOR SUBTENON AND SUBCONJUNCTIVAL INJECTIONS

TECHNIQUE FOR SUBTENON INJECTION

1. Topical anesthesia is applied to the area to be injected (e.g., topical proparacaine or a cotton-tipped applicator soaked in proparacaine, or both, held on the area for 1 to 2 minutes). If subtenon steroids are to be injected, 0.1 mL of lidocaine may be injected in the same manner as described next, several minutes before the steroids. The inferotemporal quadrant is usually the easiest location for injection.

2. With the aperture of a 25-gauge, ⅝-inch needle facing the sclera, the bulbar conjunctiva is penetrated 2 to 3 mm from the fornix, avoiding the conjunctival blood vessels (Fig. A.5).

3. As the needle is inserted, lateral motions of the needle are made to ensure that the needle has not penetrated the sclera (at which point, lateral motion would be inhibited).

4. The curvature of the eyeball is followed, attempting to place the aperture of the needle near the posterior sclera.

5. When the needle has been pushed in to the hilt, the stopper of the syringe is pulled back to ensure against intravascular penetration.

6. The contents of the syringe are injected, and the needle is removed.

TECHNIQUE FOR SUBCONJUNCTIVAL INJECTION

1. Topical anesthesia is applied as described previously.

2. Forceps are used to tent the conjunctiva, allowing the tip of a 25-gauge, 3/8-inch needle to penetrate the subconjunctival space. The needle is placed several millimeters below the limbus at the 4- or 8-o'clock position, with the aperture facing the sclera and the needle pointed inferiorly toward the fornix (Fig. A.6).

3. When the entire tip of the needle is beneath the conjunctiva, the stopper of the syringe is withdrawn to ensure against intravascular penetration.

4. The contents of the syringe are injected, and the needle is removed.

Note: An eyelid speculum may be helpful in keeping the eyelids open during these procedures.

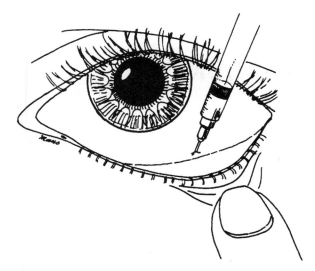

FIGURE A.5 Subtenon injection. The needle is placed 2 to 3 mm from the fornix, through conjunctiva and Tenon capsule. If possible, angle the injection so the syringe does not lie over the cornea.

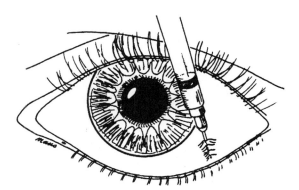

FIGURE A.6 Subconjunctival injection. The tip of the needle is placed into the subconjunctival space.

VITREOUS EXAMINATION FOR CELLS

1. Best performed in a completely darkened room with the patient's pupil widely dilated.

2. Anterior vitreous: Use the high-power magnification of the slit lamp, reduce the beam height to less than the pupil diameter, and narrow the beam width to focus through the pupil. Set the illumination to the brightest setting. Move the slit lamp forward with the joystick, angling the beam of light until the anterior vitreous can be seen posterior to the lens. By moving the joystick, several optical sections can be sampled. Patients are sometimes asked to move their eyes from left to right, facilitating the recognition of vitreous cells as they float by.

3. Middle and posterior vitreous: By using a Hruby (first choice), fundus contact, or 60-diopter lens, the slit beam is initially focused on the disc. The joystick is then used to pull the slit lamp slowly away from the eye, refocusing the light on the posterior vitreous. Again, patients may be asked to look toward their left and right and then to resume primary position to produce movement of cells and to facilitate their recognition.

MAKING FORTIFIED TOPICAL ANTIBIOTICS

FORTIFIED TOBRAMYCIN (OR GENTAMICIN)

With a syringe, inject 2 mL of tobramycin, 40 mg/mL, directly into a 5-mL bottle of tobramycin, 0.3%, ophthalmic solution (e.g., Tobrex). This gives a 7-mL solution of fortified tobramycin (approximately 15 mg/mL). Refrigerate. Expires after 14 days.

FORTIFIED CEFAZOLIN

Add enough sterile water (without preservative) to 500 mg of cefazolin dry powder to form 10 mL of solution. This provides a strength of 50 mg/mL. Refrigerate. Expires after 7 days.

FORTIFIED VANCOMYCIN

Add enough sterile water (without preservative) to 500 mg of vancomycin dry powder to form 10 mL of solution. This provides a strength of 50 mg/mL. To achieve a 25-mg/mL concentration, take 5 mL of 50-mg/mL solution and add 5 mL sterile water. Refrigerate. Expires after 4 days.

FORTIFIED BACITRACIN

Add enough sterile water (without preservative) to 50,000 U bacitracin dry powder to form 5 mL of solution. This provides a strength of 10,000 U/mL. Refrigerate. Expires after 7 days.

TETANUS PROPHYLAXIS

History of Tetanus Immunization (doses)	Clean Minor Wounds		All Other Wounds	
	Tetanus Toxoid	Immune Globulin	Tetanus Toxoid	Immune Globulin
Uncertain	Yes	No	Yes	Yes
0–1	Yes	No	Yes	Yes
2	Yes	No	Yes	No[a]
3 or more	No[b]	No	No[c]	No

Dose of tetanus toxoid is 0.5 mL intramuscularly.
[a]Unless wound is more than 24 h old.
[b]Unless more than 10 years since last dose.
[c]Unless more than 5 years since last dose.

ANGLE CLASSIFICATION

Proper evaluation of the configuration of the anterior chamber requires the use of at least three descriptors: the point at which the iris is adherent to the cornea or uvea, the depth of the anterior chamber, and the curvature of the peripheral iris. The Spaeth grading system of the anterior chamber angle takes into account all three of these attributes, and has proved highly satisfactory.

SPAETH GRADING SYSTEM

See Figure A.7.

IRIS INSERTION

A = *Anterior to Schwalbe line (SL)*

B = *Between SL and scleral spur*

C = *Scleral spur visible* (common in blacks and Asians)

D = *Deep: ciliary body visible* (common in whites)

E = *Extremely deep: greater than 1 mm of ciliary body is visible*

Indentation gonioscopy may be necessary to differentiate false opposition of the iris against structures in the iridocorneal angle (Fig. A.7, letters in parentheses in Examples of Spaeth Grading System) from the true iris insertion (Fig. A.7, letters without parentheses in Examples of Spaeth Grading System).

ANGLE OF ANTERIOR CHAMBER

The angular width that is measured as the angle between a line parallel to the corneal endothelium at Schwalbe's line and a line parallel to the anterior surface of the iris.

CURVATURE OF IRIS

b = bowing anteriorly

p = plateau configuration

f = flat

c = concave posterior bowing

PIGMENTATION OF POSTERIOR TRABECULAR MESHWORK (PTM)

Viewing at 12 o'clock in the angle with mirror at 6 o'clock position, pigmentation graded on a scale of 0 (no PTM pigment seen) to 4+ (intense PTM pigment).

GENERAL GUIDELINES

1. Occludable angles would include the following:

   —Any angle narrower than 10 degrees

   —Any p angle

2. Abnormal iris attachments include:

   —Any A attachment

   —Any B attachment

   —C attachment in certain populations

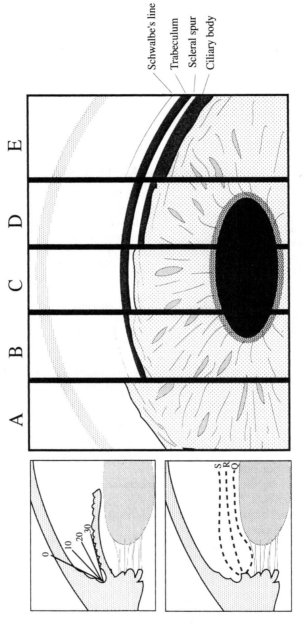

FIGURE A.7 Spaeth classification of the anterior chamber angle.

Schwalbe's line
Trabeculum
Scleral spur
Ciliary body

3. Iris bow greater than 1+ usually indicates pupillary block.

4. Pigmentation greater that 2+ is usually pathologic.

EXAMPLES OF SPAETH GRADING SYSTEM

1. C15b 2+ptm = Open but narrow occludable angle

2. A40f = closed angle

3. (B)D30p 0ptm = open, atypical narrow angle, occludable with dilation

4. D40c 4+ptm = open angle characteristic of patients with myopia or iris pigment dispersion syndrome.

SHAFFER CLASSIFICATION

See Figure A.8.

Grade 0 The angle is closed.

Grade 1 Extremely narrow angle (10 degrees). Only Schwalbe line, and perhaps also the top of the trabecula, can be visualized. Closure is probable.

Grade 2 Moderately narrow angle (20 degrees). Only the trabecula can be seen. Closure is possible.

Grade 3 Moderately open angle (20 to 35 degrees). The scleral spur can be seen. Closure is not possible.

Grade 4 Angle wide open (35 to 45 degrees). The ciliary body can be visualized with ease. Closure is not possible.

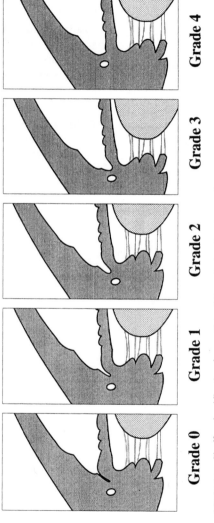

FIGURE A.8 Shaffer classification for grading of the anterior chamber angle.

SELECTED OPHTHALMOLOGY RESOURCES ON THE INTERNET

AMERICAN ACADEMY OF OPHTHALMOLOGY (AAO)

http://www.aao.org
Provides Academy news and services, including annual meeting information, career development assistance, and an online education center.

THE AMERICAN OPHTHALMOLOGICAL SOCIETY (AOS)

http://www.aosonline.org/index.html
Includes a membership directory, annual meeting information, and thesis guidelines and full-text articles and theses for 2001 and 2002.

AMERICAN SOCIETY OF CATARACT AND REFRACTIVE SURGERY/AMERICAN SOCIETY OF OPHTHALMIC ADMINISTRATORS

http://www.ascrs.org/index.html
Presents a variety of professional aids, including links to meeting information, an image library, abstracts for *The Journal of Cataract and Refractive Surgery*, and an online education series.

ASSOCIATION FOR RESEARCH IN VISION AND OPHTHALMOLOGY

http://www.arvo.org/root/index.asp
Provides information on the annual meetings, a career center, and links to the ARVO abstracts.

CENTERS FOR DISEASE CONTROL AND PREVENTION (CDC)

http://www.cdc.gov
Offers full-text access to *Morbidity and Mortality Weekly Report* (*MMWR*); statistical reports; guidelines for prevention and control of disease, injuries, and disabilities; and travelers' health information.

DIGITAL JOURNAL OF OPHTHALMOLOGY

http://www.djo.harvard.edu/
An online journal produced by the Massachusetts Eye and Ear Infirmary. Of particular note are the Grand Rounds case reports.

EYE DISEASE LINKS

http://www.mic.ki.se/Diseases/c11.html
An extensive list developed by Karolinska Institute Library. Arranged by eye disorder, the list includes links to international associations, patient education resources, ophthalmic publications, and drug information.

EYE RESOURCES ON THE INTERNET

http://webeye.ophth.uiowa.edu/
Maintained by the Association of Vision Science Librarians. Includes links to associa-

tions, journals, patient education resources, and support groups.

EYEPALM.COM

http://www.eyepalm.com/
Reviews software programs for personal digital assistants (PDAs) and provides links to vendors.

MEDEM EYE HEALTH

http://www.medem.com/MedLB/bufferpage_aao.cfm
Presents patient education material prepared by the American Academy of Ophthalmology.

NATIONAL ASSOCIATION FOR THE VISUALLY HANDICAPPED

http://www.navh.org
Provides information on various eye diseases for the layman and sells a variety of low-vision aids.

NATIONAL EYE INSTITUTE

http://www.nei.nih.gov
Lists clinical trials, funding information, education programs, and job opportunities. Pho-
tos, images, and video clips are also available as is access to NEIBank, their database of genes and proteins expressed in the eye and visual system.

VISION SCIENCE REFERENCE DATABASE

http://www.bausch.com
Developed by the University of Waterloo Centre for Contact Lens Research and sponsored by Bausch & Lomb, the database includes citations and abstracts to articles from over 40 professional journals, many of them not indexed in PubMed.

WILLS EYE HOSPITAL

http://www.willseye.org
Includes information about the hospital, medical staff, clinical departments, training programs, clinical trials, patient education, and the Charles D. Kelman Medical Library journal holdings.

WILLS EYE HOSPITAL GLAUCOMA FOUNDATION

http://www.wills-glaucoma.org/
Includes resources for both physicians and patients.

LIST OF COMMONLY USED OPHTHALMIC MEDICATIONS

The purpose of this drug glossary is to provide a brief list of common topical ophthalmic medications used in ophthalmology. For more extensive information on the following medications, please consult the *Wills Eye Drug Guide* or a *Physicians' Desk Reference.*

INFECTIOUS DISEASE

Usual dosing: q1–6h, depending on severity

Antibacterial:

Fluoroquinolones	Ciprofloxacin (Ciloxan): solution 0.3%, ointment 0.3%
	Ofloxacin (Ocuflox) solution 0.3%
	Levofloxacin (Quixin) solution 0.5%
	Gatifloxacin (Zymar) solution 0.3%
	Moxifloxacin (Vigamox) solution 0.5%
Aminoglycosides	Tobramycin (solution 3 mg/mL, ointment 3 mg/g)
	Gentamicin (solution 3 mg/mL, ointment 3 mg/g)
Sulfonamides	Sulfisoxazole (solution 4%)
	Sulfacetamide (solution 1%, 10%, 30%; ointment 10%)
Others	Bacitracin ointment 500 units/g
	Polymyxin B Sulfate Powder for solution 500,000 units
	Chloramphenicol (5 mg/mL; ointment 10 mg/g)
	Erythromycin ointment (5 mg/g)
Antifungal	Natamycin (Natacyn) Suspension 5%
	Amphotericin B (Fungizone) Solution 0.1%–0.5%
Antiviral	Vidarabine (Vira-A) Ointment 3.0%
	Trifluridine (Viroptic) solution 1%

GLAUCOMA

ALPHA$_2$-ADRENERGIC AGONISTS

Examples:

- Apraclonidine (Iopidine) solution 0.5%, 1%

- Brimonidine tartrate (Alphagan-P) solution 0.15%

Usual dosing: b.i.d.–t.i.d.

Mechanism: Inhibits aqueous secretion, possible increased uveoscleral outflow

Side effects: Allergy, mydriasis, dry mouth, dry eye, hypotension, lethargy

Contraindications: Monoamine oxidase inhibitor use

BETA-ADRENERGIC ANTAGONISTS

Examples:

- Betaxolol (Betoptic) solution 0.5%

- Carteolol (Ocupress) solution 1%

- Levobetaxolol (Betaxon) solution 0.5%

- Levobunolol (Betagan) solution 0.25%, 0.5%

- Metipranolol (OptiPranolol) solution 0.3%

- Timolol hemihydrate (Betimol) solution 0.25%, 0.5%

- Timolol maleate (Timoptic) solution 0.25%, 0.5%

Usual dosing: b.i.d.

Mechanism: Decreased aqueous humor production

Side effects: Blurred vision, corneal anesthesia, superficial punctate keratopathy, bradycardia/heart block, bronchospasm, fatigue, mood change, impotence, decreases sensitivity to hypoglycemic symptoms in patients with insulin-dependent diabetes, worsening of myasthenia gravis

Contraindications: Asthma, severe chronic obstructive pulmonary disease, bradycardia, heart block, congestive heart failure, myasthenia gravis

CARBONIC ANHYDRASE INHIBITORS

Examples:

- Dorzolamide (Trusopt) solution 2%

- Brinzolamide (Azopt) suspension 1%

Usual dosing: b.i.d.–t.i.d.

Mechanism: Decreased aqueous production in ciliary body

Side effects: Bitter taste, diuresis, fatigue, gastrointestinal upset, Stevens–Johnson syndrome, aplastic anemia

Contraindications: Sulfa allergy, hyponatremia/hypokalemia, renal stones, thiazide diuretics, digitalis use

MIOTICS

Examples:

- Echothiophate iodide (Phospholine Iodide) solution 0.03%–0.25%

- Physostigmine (Isopto Eserine) solution 0.25%, 0.5%, ointment 0.25%

- Demecarium bromide (Humorsol) solution 0.125%, 0.25%

- Acetylcholine (Miochol-E) 1:100 dilution

- Carbachol (Isopto Carbachol) solution 0.75%–3%

- Pilocarpine Hydrochloride (Isopto Carpine) solution 0.25%–8%

- Pilocarpine nitrate (Pilagan) solution 1%–4%

Usual dosing: b.i.d.–q.i.d.

Mechanism: Increased trabecular outflow

Side effects:

—**Direct cholinergic:** Brow ache, breakdown of blood–aqueous barrier, angle closure, decreased night vision, variable myopia, retinal tear/detachment

—**Indirect cholinergic:** Retinal detachment, cataract, myopia, intense miosis, angle closure, increased bleeding postsurgery, punctual stenosis, increased formation of posterior synechiae in chronic uveitis, diarrhea, abdominal cramps, enuresis, increased effect of succinylcholine

Contraindications:

—**Direct cholinergic:** Peripheral retinal disease, central media opacity, uveitis

—**Indirect cholinergic:** Succinylcholine administration, predisposition to retinal tear, anterior subcapsular cataract, ocular surgery, uveitis

PROSTAGLANDINS

Examples:

- Latanoprost (Xalatan) solution 0.005%
- Travoprost (Travatan) solution 0.004%
- Bimatoprost (Lumigan) solution 0.03%
- Unoprostone (Rescula) solution 0.15%

Usual dosing: q.h.s.

Mechanism: Prostaglandin PF agonist, increased uveoscleral outflow

Side effects: Increased melanin pigmentation in iris, blurred vision, eyelid redness, cystoid macular edema, anterior uveitis, upper respiratory tract infection symptoms, backache, chest pain, myalgia

Contraindications: Pregnancy, inflammatory conditions

SYMPATHOMIMETIC

Examples:

- Dipivefrin (Propine) solution 0.1%
- Epinephrine (Epifrin, Glaucon) solution 0.5%, 1%, 2%

Usual dosing: b.i.d.

Mechanism: In ciliary body, variable (beta-adrenergic stimulation increases aqueous production, but alpha-adrenergic stimulation decreases aqueous production); in trabecular meshwork, beta stimulation causes increased trabecular outflow and increased uveoscleral outflow, in total lowering intraocular pressure

Side effects: Cystoid macular edema in aphakia, mydriasis, rebound hyperemia, blurred vision, adrenochrome deposits, allergic blepharoconjunctivitis, tachycardia, hypertension, cardiac disease

Contraindications: Narrow angles, aphakia, pseudophakia, soft lenses, hypertension, cardiac disease

Combination agents:

- Epinephrine/pilocarpine (E-Pilo)
- Timolol/Trusopt (Cosopt)

ANTIINFLAMMATORY

NONSTEROIDAL ANTIINFLAMMATORY AGENTS (NSAIDS)

Examples:

- Diclofenac (Voltaren) solution 0.1%
- Flurbiprofen (Ocufen) solution 0.03%
- Ketorolac (Acular) solution 0.5%
- Suprofen (Profenal) solution 1%

Usual dosing: q.i.d.

MAST CELL INHIBITORS/ ANTIHISTAMINES

Examples:

- Cromolyn sodium (Crolom) solution 4%
- Lodoxamide (Alomide) solution 0.1%
- Nedocromil (Alocril) solution 2%
- Pemirolast (Alamast) solution 0.1%
- Azelastine (Optivar) solution 0.05%
- Emedastine (Emadine) solution 0.05%
- Ketotifen (Zaditor) solution 0.025%
- Levocabastine (Livostin) solution 0.05%
- Olopatadine (Patanol) solution 0.1%

Usual dosing: b.i.d.–q.i.d.

CORTICOSTEROIDS

Examples:

- Dexamethasone acetate suspension 0.1%, ointment 0.05%

- Dexamethasone phosphate solution 0.1%

- Fluorometholone suspension 0.1%, 0.25%; ointment 0.1%

- Loteprednol etabonate 0.2, 0.5%

- Medrysone suspension 1%

- Prednisolone suspension 0.12%, 0.125%, 1%

- Rimexolone suspension 1%

Usual dosing: q1h–q.d., depending on severity

COMBINATION STEROID/ANTIBIOTIC

Examples:

- Dexamethasone acetate/neomycin/polymyxin B (Maxitrol) suspension 0.1%, ointment 0.1%

- Dexamethasone/tobramycin (TobraDex) suspension 0.1%, ointment 0.1%

- Dexamethasone/neomycin (Dexacidin) solution 0.1%, ointment 0.5%

- Fluorometholone/sulfacetamide (FML-S) suspension 0.1%/10%

- Hydrocortisone/neomycin/polymyxin B (Cortimycin, Cortisporin) suspension 1%, ointment

- Hydrocortisone/neomycin/polymyxin B/gramicidin (AK-Spore HC) suspension 1%, ointment

- Prednisolone acetate/sulfacetamide (AK-Cide) suspension 0.1%/10%

- Prednisolone acetate/sulfacetamide (Blephamide) suspension 0.2%/10%, ointment 0.2%/10%

- Prednisolone phosphate/sulfacetamide (Vasocidin) solution 0.23%/10%; ointment 0.5%/10%

Usual dosing: Varies

LUBRICATING

Examples:

- Refresh

- GenTeal

- Tears Naturale

- HypoTears

- TheraTears

CONTRAINDICATIONS AND SIDE EFFECTS

The following is a list of drugs commonly used in ophthalmology, along with some of their contraindications and side effects that have clinical importance. Most of these drugs should not be used in pregnant or breast-feeding women, in infants, in those with significant renal or hepatic disease, or in patients in whom an allergy to the drug is suspected or known (therefore, these contraindications are not listed separately for each drug, and should be investigated further if therapy is desired for a patient who is in one of these circumstances).

Acetazolamide (e.g., Diamox): Contraindicated in patients with sulfa allergy, metabolic acidosis, adrenal insufficiency, and a history of kidney stones (a relative contraindication). Be careful in patients taking another diuretic, a systemic steroid, or digoxin because their potassium level may be reduced to a dangerous level. Side effects: Blood dyscrasias, kidney stones, others.

Acyclovir (e.g., Zovirax): Contraindicated in renal failure, adjust dose for chronic renal insufficiency. Side effects: Gastrointestinal disturbance, rash, renal toxicity.

Aminocaproic acid (e.g., Amicar): Contraindicated in patients with an intravascular clotting disorder. Side effects: Hypotension (particularly postural), nausea, vomiting, others.

Amphotericin B: Highly toxic when used systemically. Side effects: Fever, chills, dyspnea, hypotension, renal failure, electrolyte abnormalities, bone marrow suppression, nausea/vomiting, phlebitis at infusion site.

Apraclonidine (e.g., Iopidine; topical): Contraindicated in patients taking monoamine oxidase inhibitors. Side effects: Allergy, mydriasis, dry mouth, dry eye, hypotension, lethargy.

Atropine (topical): Contraindicated in most angle-closure situations, infants, albinos, and patients with Down syndrome. Use cautiously in pediatric patients because the margin for toxicity is low. Side effects: Urinary retention, tachycardia, delirium, others. *Treatment of anticholinergic (e.g., atropine) overdose* Physostigmine, 1 to 4 mg intravenously (i.v.), repeating 0.5 to 1.0 mg i.v., every 15 minutes until the symptoms improve.

Brimonidine (e.g., Alphagan P; topical): See Apraclonidine.

Brinzolamide (e.g., Azopt; topical): See Acetazolamide.

Carbachol (topical): See Pilocarpine.

Carbogen (95% O_2, 5% CO_2): Contraindicated in patients with pulmonary disease or an electrolyte disorder.

Clindamycin: Side effects: Pseudomembranous colitis, others.

Cocaine (topical): Contraindicated with compromised cardiovascular or cerebrovascular status.

Cyclopentolate (topical): See Atropine.

Dipivefrin (e.g., Propine; topical): See Epinephrine.

Dorzolamide (e.g., Trusopt; topical): See Acetazolamide.

Doxycycline: See Tetracycline.

Echothiophate iodide (e.g., Phospholine iodide; topical): See Pilocarpine. Patients (or parents) are told that succinylcholine should never be given for general anesthesia (the combination of the two drugs can be lethal). *Treatment of anticholinesterase overdose* Atropine, 2 mg i.v., every 5 minutes until relief of symptoms, or pralidoxime, 25 mg/kg i.v., in 500 mL of 5% D_5W over 2 hours (do not use in overdose of neostigmine and physostigmine).

Epinephrine (topical): Contraindicated in patients with severe cardiovascular disease. Side effects: Macular edema in aphakic patients, conjunctival reaction, precipitation of narrow-angle glaucoma, others. Allergic conjunctivitis is common.

Fluorometholone (topical): See Prednisolone acetate.

Gentamicin side effects: Nephrotoxicity, ototoxicity, neuromuscular blockade (myasthenia-like syndrome), others.

Homatropine (topical): See Atropine.

Isosorbide: See Mannitol.

Itraconazole (e.g., Sporanox): See Ketoconazole. Less hepatotoxic than ketoconazole.

Ketoconazole: Contraindicated with certain medications metabolized by the hepatic cytochrome P-450 system, including terfenadine, astemizole, cisapride, triazolam. Side effects: Gastrointestinal distress, rash, pruritus, peripheral edema, hepatotoxicity (monitor liver function tests, discontinue if anorexia, nausea/vomiting, or signs of jaundice occur).

Latanoprost (e.g., Xalatan; topical): Increased melanin pigmentation in iris, blurred vision, eyelid redness; cystoid macular edema and anterior uveitis have been reported, systemic upper respiratory infection symptoms, backache, chest pain, myalgia. Contraindicated in pregnancy.

Levobunolol (e.g., Betagan; topical): See Timolol.

Mannitol: Contraindicated in patients with hypotension, cardiovascular compromise, or concomitant administration of another osmotic agent. Side effects: Congestive heart failure, subarachnoid or subdural hemorrhage, mental confusion, others.

Methazolamide (e.g., Neptazane): See Acetazolamide.

Natamycin (topical): Side effects: Mild conjunctival irritation, corneal epithelial toxicity, allergy.

Neomycin (topical): Side effects: Superficial punctate keratitis and allergic conjunctivitis are common.

Phenylephrine (e.g., Neo-Synephrine; topical): Contraindicated in patients with significant cardiac disease, sympathetic denervation (i.e., those taking monoamine oxidase inhibitors and diabetic patients with neuropathy), most angle-closure glaucomas, and in the presence of occludable anterior chamber angles.

Physostigmine (e.g., Eserine; topical): Miotic agent. Contraindicated with succinylcholine. See Echothiophate iodide and Pilocarpine.

Pilocarpine (topical): Side effects: Exacerbates iritis, can precipitate or exacerbate angle-closure glaucoma when used in high concentrations (usually 4% to 6% or greater), retinal detachment (with especially high concentrations, or other strong miotic agents such as echothiophate), brow ache, others.

Prednisolone acetate (topical): Often contraindicated in patients with herpes simplex or fungal keratitis. Side effects: Increased intraocular pressure, cataract, increased susceptibility to infectious organisms, others.

Prednisone: Contraindicated in patients with peptic ulcer disease, tuberculosis, active infection, psychosis, or pregnancy. Workup includes complete blood count, glucose tolerance test, pregnancy test, purified protein derivative, anergy panel, chest radiograph, stool guaiac test. Side effects: Hyperglycemia, hypokalemia, hypertension, peptic ulcer, increased intraocular pressure, cataract, pseudotumor cerebri, mental status changes, aseptic necrosis of bone, osteoporosis, decreased wound healing, growth suppression in children, fluid retention, others.

Proparacaine (topical): Side effects: Corneal epithelial erosions and ulcers with repeated and prolonged use.

Pyridostigmine (e.g., Mestinon): Contraindicated in patients with urinary or intestinal obstruction; use with caution in asthmatics. Side effects: Gastrointestinal distress, rash, muscle cramps. Overdose may lead to cholinergic crisis.

Scopolamine (topical): See Atropine.

Steroids: See Prednisone.

Sulfacetamide (topical): Side effects: Stevens–Johnson syndrome, bone marrow suppression, others.

Sulfadiazine: See Sulfacetamide.

Tetracycline: Contraindicated in children younger than 8 years (tooth discoloration). Side effects: Gastrointestinal upset, pseudotumor cerebri, hepatotoxicity, skin sensitivity to sunlight (patients are told on starting the drug to avoid sunlight if possible), others.

Timolol (e.g., Timoptic; topical): Contraindicated in patients with asthma or other breathing problems, bradycardia (the patient's pulse is checked before administering a beta-blocker), arrhythmias, congestive heart failure, hypotension, others.

Tobramycin: See Gentamicin.

Tropicamide (topical): See Atropine.

Valacyclovir (e.g., Valtrex): Associated with thrombotic thrombocytopenic purpura/hemolytic–uremic syndrome in immunocompromised patients. See also Acyclovir.

Vancomycin: Side effects: Nephrotoxicity, ototoxicity, others.

GENERAL GLOSSARY

Accommodation: Adjustment in convexity of the natural lens of the eye to maintain a focused image on the retina at near.

Amaurosis fugax: Fleeting, partial or total blindness of vision; may be associated with visible emboli in retinal vessels.

Amblyopia: Defective vision without identifiable organic cause; a unilateral or bilateral reduction of best-corrected central visual acuity in absence of visible organic lesion corresponding to the degree of visual loss.

Anisocoria: Unequal size in the diameter of two pupils.

Anisometropia: Inequality in refractive power between two eyes.

Anterior chamber: Space in the eye bordered anteriorly by cornea and posteriorly by the iris and pupil; it is filled with aqueous.

Applanation tonometer: Instrument to measure intraocular pressure.

Astigmatism: The refracting power of the eye is not the same in all meridians (e.g., more hyperopic vertically than horizontally).

Bell phenomenon: Reflexive upturning of the eye with active lid closure.

Bulbar conjunctiva: Freely movable tissue that forms most superficial covering of the globe from limbus to fornices.

Buphthalmos: Meaning "ox eye"; distention of globe in response to elevated intraocular pressure; seen in patients with congenital glaucoma.

Chemosis: Edema or swelling of the bulbar conjunctiva.

Choroid: Middle pigmented vascular coat of the posterior five-sixths of the eyeball continuous with the iris in front; it lies between sclera externally and retina internally.

Choroiditis: Inflammation of the choroid.

Ciliary body: Specialized structure of eye connecting anterior part of choroid to circumference of iris composed of ciliary muscle and process.

Coloboma: Congenital absence of any eye structure.

Conjunctiva: Transparent membrane covering anterior portion of sclera.

Conjunctivitis: Inflammation of conjunctiva.

Cornea: Transparent anterior portion of the eye contiguous with the sclera.

Cotton-wool spot: A superficial retinal infarction appearing as a fluffy white lesion, sometimes obscuring retinal vessels.

Crowding phenomenon: Individual letters can be read better than a whole line; most commonly seen in amblyopic patients.

Cyclodialysis: Separation of the ciliary body from the sclera.

Cycloplegic: Drug that causes paralysis of ciliary muscle causing paralysis of accommodation.

Dacryoadenitis: Inflammation of the lacrimal gland.

Dacryocystitis: Inflammation of the lacrimal sac.

Descemet membrane: An inner (posterior) corneal layer.

Diplopia: Double vision.

Ectopia lentis: Dislocated lens.

Ectropion iridis (ectropion uveae): Eversion of the iris at pupillary rim such that pigmented posterior aspect of the iris is visualized.

Enophthalmos: An abnormal retraction of the globe within bony orbit.

Enucleation: Removal of the eyeball from orbit.

Episclera: Loose connective tissue between conjunctiva and sclera.

Episcleritis: Inflammation of external surface of the sclera (beneath the bulbar conjunctiva).

Esophoria: The eyes are aligned during binocular vision, but have a latent tendency to cross (e.g., while not focusing).

Esotropia: The eye is deviated so that the cornea is rotated nasally and the fovea temporally; nonfixating eye is turned inward ("cross-eyed").

Exenteration: Removal of the eye and orbital contents.

Exophoria: The eyes are aligned during binocular vision, but have a latent tendency to turn away from one another.

Exophthalmos: An abnormal protrusion of the globe from the bony orbit.

Exotropia: The eye is deviated so that the cornea is rotated temporally and the fovea nasally; nonfixating eye is turned outward ("wall-eyed").

Flare: Increased protein in the anterior chamber fluid, permitting visualization of the slit-lamp beam.

Floaters: Visual perception of dots or spots which may seem to "swim" or shift location when the position of gaze is shifted.

Fluorescein: An orange substance that forms a green fluorescent solution when viewed with a cobalt blue light.

Fluorescein angiography: A diagnostic test using intravenously injected fluorescein to highlight vascular abnormalities in the eye, most commonly in the fundus.

Fovea: An area of the retina corresponding to central vision, approximately 1.5 mm in diameter, located temporal and slightly inferior to the center of the optic disc.

Foveola: The center of the fovea, 0.5 mm in diameter.

Ghost vessels: Corneal stromal blood vessels containing no blood.

Gonioscopy: Examination of anterior chamber angle structures of eye, including trabecular meshwork.

Guttata (corneal): Droplet-like excrescences on the posterior surface of Descemet membrane.

Hard exudates: Deep retinal lipid, often glistening yellow in appearance.

Hering law of motor correspondence: Equal and simultaneous innervation flows to synergistic muscles concerned with the desired direction of gaze.

Heterochromia: Difference in coloration, especially between the two irides.

Hyperopia: Farsightedness; caused by an eye too short or refractive power such that light rays focus beyond the retina.

Hyphema: Blood in the anterior chamber; when layering or clotting of the blood is present, the term *hyphema* is used; when only suspended red blood cells are present, the term *microhyphema* is used.

Hypopyon: Layering of white blood cells inferiorly in the anterior chamber.

Hypotony: Abnormally low intraocular pressure, usually below 6 mm Hg.

Indirect ophthalmoscopy: The use of a relatively large lens located between the patient and the observer, in combination with a light source, to view the fundus.

Intraretinal microvascular abnormalities: Dilated, often telangiectatic, retinal capillaries that act as shunts between arterioles and venules.

Iris: Anterior pigmented portion of the vascular coat of the globe found posterior to the cornea and anterior to the lens; its middle opening forms the pupil.

Iritis (anterior uveitis, iridocyclitis, cyclitis): Inflammation of the iris, ciliary body, or both.

Keratitis: Inflammation of the cornea.

Keratoconus: Conelike protrusion of the cornea.

Keratic precipitates: Cellular aggregates that form on the corneal endothelium, often inferiorly, in a base-down triangular pattern.

Krukenberg spindle: Narrow, vertically oriented band of pigment located along the central corneal endothelium developing in pigment dispersion syndrome.

LASEK (laser assisted subepithelial keratectomy): Type of refractive surgery.

LASIK (laser in-situ keratomileusis): Type of refractive surgery in which an excimer laser is used to reshape the corneal stromal bed beneath a corneal flap created by a microkeratome or femtosecond laser.

Leukocoria: A grossly visible white pupil.

Macula: An area three to four disc diameters in size centered at the posterior part of the retina.

Meibomian glands: Sebaceous glands lying in grooves on inner surface eyelids, with ducts opening on the free margins of the lids.

Meibomianitis: Inflamed, inspissated oil glands along the eyelid margins, reflecting inflammation of the meibomian glands.

Metamorphopsia: Abnormal visual perception causing objects to appear distorted or variable in size/shape.

Microkeratome: Suction ring with moving blade used to create partial-thickness corneal flap for LASIK refractive surgery.

Microphthalmia: A congenitally small, disorganized eye.

Micropsia: Abnormal visual perception causing objects to appear smaller than normal.

Miosis: Constriction of the pupil.

Mydriasis: Dilatation of the pupil.

Myopia: Nearsightedness; light rays come to focus before reaching the retina.

Nanophthalmos: A congenitally small but otherwise normal eye.

Neovascularization: Growth of new blood vessels.

Nystagmus: Involuntary repetitive tremors of the eyes.

Orbit: Bony socket containing globe and surrounding contents.

Ophthalmoplegia (internal): Paralysis of the pupil.

Ophthalmoplegia (external): Paralysis of the extraocular muscles.

Optic neuritis: Inflammation of the optic nerve.

Ora serrata: The most peripheral portion of the retina.

Oscillopsia: The perception that the environment is moving back and forth.

Palpebral conjunctiva: The most superficial covering of the underside of the eyelids from the fornices to the eyelid margins.

Papilledema: Edema of the optic disc produced by increased intracranial pressure.

Papillitis: Inflammation of the most anterior portion of the optic disc.

Peripapillary: Surrounding the optic disc.

Peripheral anterior synechiae: Adhesions between the peripheral iris and anterior chamber angle or peripheral cornea.

Peripheral iridectomy: Removal of a portion of the peripheral iris.

Phakomatosis: A group of several heritable disorders characterized by systemic and ocular findings.

Phoria: A latent deviation that is controlled by fusional mechanism so that under normal binocular vision the eyes remain aligned.

Photophobia: Ocular pain on exposure to light.

Photopsia: A sensation of instantaneous flashes of light; most commonly indicative of retinal traction.

Photorefractive keratectomy (PRK): A laser surgery to correct refractive errors.

Phototherapeutic keratectomy (PTK): Type of surgery in which an excimer laser is used to ablate anterior corneal opacities or abnormalities.

Polycoria: Presence of many openings in the iris.

Posterior synechiae: Adhesions between the iris and the anterior lens capsule, most commonly at the pupillary border.

Proptosis: Forward protrusion of the globe from the bony orbit.

Pseudohypopon: A layered collection of non-inflammatory cells in the anterior chamber, usually associated with neoplastic conditions.

Ptosis (blepharoptosis): Drooping of the upper eyelid.

Punctum: The opening of the tear drainage system in the eyelid margin.

Pupillary block: Aqueous humor is prevented from flowing from the posterior chamber into the anterior chamber between the iris and lens.

Radial keratotomy (RK): A surgical technique in which radial incisions are made into the superficial cornea in an effort to change the corneal curvature and therefore the patient's refractive error.

Relative afferent pupillary defect: A decreased pupillary constriction to light in one eye compared with the other eye, using the swinging-flashlight test.

Retina: Thin, transparent membrane lying between the vitreous and sclera extending from the ora serrata to the optic nerve, often referred to as the "film of the camera."

Retinitis: Inflammation of the retina.

Retinoscopy: A technique by which the reflex from a streak of light shined on the retina is used to estimate the refractive error of the eye.

Rhegmatogenous retinal detachment: Detachment of the retina as a result of a retinal break (hole).

Sclera: Tough, white, opaque outer coat of the globe continuous with cornea anteriorly.

Scleral depression: A technique by which indentation of the peripheral retina is combined with indirect ophthalmoscopy to view the peripheral retina.

Scleritis: Inflammation of the sclera.

Scotoma: An area of loss of sensitivity in the visual field.

Sherrington law of reciprocal innervation: Increased innervation and contraction of a given extraocular muscle are accompanied by a reciprocal decrease in innervation and contraction of its agonist.

Staphyloma: An outpouching of the sclera that involves the uvea.

Strabismus: Ocular misalignment.

Tarsorrhaphy: Suturing of the upper and lower eyelids together, either partially or completely.

Trabeculectomy: A surgical technique to improve aqueous outflow in patients with glaucoma.

Tropia: Manifest deviation that exceeds the control of the fusional mechanism so that eyes are not aligned.

Vitreous humour: Clear, gelatinous fluid filling the portion of the globe between the lens, ciliary body, and retina.

Vitritis: Inflammation of the vitreous.

SUBJECT INDEX

Page numbers followed by an *f* indicate figures; page numbers followed by a *t* indicate tables.

A

A-scan ultrasonography, 363

Abetalipoproteinemia
CPEO *vs.*, 219
hereditary
retinitis pigmentosa and, 279

Abrasion(s)
corneal, 17–18

Acanthamoeba, 58–59

Accommodation
defined, 398

Accommodative spasm, 343–344

Acetazolamide
contraindications and side effects of, 395

Acquired cataract, 322–323

Acquired immunodeficiency syndrome (AIDS), 331–337,
332t, 334t, 336t, 337t
CMV retinopathy in, 333–335, 334f
CMV-related, 333
cornea diseases due to, 332t, 331–333
herpes zoster disciform keratitis in, 333
herpes zoster ophthalmicus in, 331–332, 332t
HSV keratitis in, 333
Kaposi sarcoma in, 332–333
keratitis in, 333
microsporidial keratoconjunctivitis in, 333
molluscum contagiosum in, 333
neuro-ophthalmologic disease in, 337
noninfectious retinopathy in, 333
ocular complications of, 331–337
posterior segment disease in, 333–337, 334f, 336f, 337f
risk groups for, 331
toxoplasmosis in, 335–336, 336f
uveitis in, 333

Acquired syphilis, 338–340. *See also* Syphilis, acquired

Active force generation test, 376

Acute angle-closure glaucoma, 179–183
anterior uveitis *vs.*, 290
causes of, 179–180
differential diagnosis of, 180
glaucomatocyclitic crisis *vs.*, 186
inflammatory open-angle glaucoma *vs.*, 171
malignant glaucoma *vs.*, 193, 193t
phacolytic glaucoma *vs.*, 177
primary

neovascular glaucoma *vs.*, 187–188
signs of, 179
symptoms of, 179
treatment of, 181–183
workup for, 180–181

Acute conjunctivitis, 89–93, 90f

Acute disc edema
diabetes mellitus and, 327

Acute posterior multifocal placoid pigment epitheliopathy
(AMPPE)
posterior uveitis due to, 299
VKH syndrome *vs.*, 311

Acute retinal necrosis
posterior uveitis due to, 299

Acute retinal necrosis (ARN), 308–310, 309t
Behçet disease *vs.*, 308
causes of, 308
differential diagnosis of, 309, 309t
follow-up care, 310
signs of, 308
symptoms of, 308
treatment of, 309–310
workup for, 309

Acute zonal occult outer retinopathy
posterior uveitis due to, 299

Acyclovir
contraindications and side effects of, 395

Adenoma(s)
pituitary
during pregnancy, 329, 331

Adie tonic pupil, 203

Adolescent(s)
pseudotumor cerebri in, 226

Age
as factor in degenerative retinoschisis, 251–252

Age-related macular degeneration (ARMD)
chloroquine/hydroxychloroquine toxicity *vs.*, 287
cone dystrophies *vs.*, 283
exudative, 264–265
vitreous hemorrhage due to, 276
malignant melanoma of choroid *vs.*, 288–289
nonexudative, 263–264
vitreous hemorrhage due to, 276

AIDS. *See* Acquired immunodeficiency syndrome
(AIDS)

Convergence spasm
  isolated sixth nerve palsy *vs.*, 209
Cornea, 40–88
  defined, 398
  disorders of
    acanthamoeba, 58–59
    aphakic bullous keratopathy, 81–82
    band keratopathy, 51–52
    contact lens—related induced giant papillary
      conjunctivitis, 73
    contact lens—related problems, 69–72
    crystals
      differential diagnosis of, 6
    dellen, 77
    differential diagnosis of, 6–8
    dry-eye syndrome, 43–45
    dystrophies, 79–81
    edema
      differential diagnosis of, 6–7
    Fuchs endothelial dystrophy, 80–81
    graft rejection, 82–83
    herpes zoster virus, 63–65
    HSV, 59–63
    keratitis
      bacterial, 52–56
      fungal, 57–58
      interstitial, 66–67
    keratoconus, 78–79
    keratopathy
      aphakic bullous, 81–82
      exposure, 46–47
      filamentary, 45–46
      pseudophakic bullous, 81–82
    neurotrophic keratopathy, 47–48
    ocular vaccinia, 86–88
    peripheral corneal thinning/ulceration, 74–77
    phlyctenulosis, 68–69
    pterygium/pinguecula, 50–51
    refractive surgery complications of, 83–86
    staphylococcal hypersensitivity, 67–68
    superficial punctate keratitis, 40–42
    superficial vascular invasion of
      differential diagnosis of, 7
    thermal/ultraviolet keratopathy, 48–49
    Thygeson superficial punctate keratopathy, 49–50
  epithelium of
    whorl-like opacity in
      differential diagnosis of, 8
  foreign bodies of, 18–19
  nerves of
    enlarged
      differential diagnosis of, 7
  ossification of
    in infancy
      differential diagnosis of, 7
  recurrent corneal erosion of, 42–43
Cornea diseases
  AIDS-related, 331–333, 332t
Corneal abrasion, 17–18
Corneal erosion
  recurrent, 42–43

Corneal laceration, 35
Corneal topography, 369
Cortical blindness, 237
  nonphysiologic visual loss *vs.*, 238
Corticosteroid(s), 393–394
Cotton-wool spot
  defined, 398
Cotton-wool spots
  differential diagnosis of, 8–9
Cover/uncover test, 371
CPA masses
  isolated seventh nerve palsy due to, 211
CPEO. *See* Chronic progressive external ophthalmoplegia
  (CPEO)
Crabs, 93
Cranial nerve abnormalities
  diabetes mellitus and, 327
Cranial nerve palsy
  orbital disease *vs.*, 126
Crossed eyes
  in children
    differential diagnosis of, 1
Crowding phenomenon
  defined, 398
CRVO. *See* Central retinal vein occlusion (CRVO)
CT. *See* Computed tomography (CT)
Cyanoacrylate
  eye injury due to, 16
Cyclodialysis
  defined, 398
Cyclopentolate
  contraindications and side effects of, 395
Cycloplegic
  defined, 398
Cyst(s)
  dermoid
    orbital tumors in children due to, 133–134
  epidermoid
    orbital tumors in children due to, 133–134
Cystoid macular edema, 270–271
Cytomegalovirus (CMV)
  AIDS-related, 333
  posterior uveitis due to, 298
Cytomegalovirus (CMV) retinopathy
  AIDS-related, 333–335, 334f

D

Dacryoadenitis
  acute infectious, 119–121
  chronic, 139–140
  defined, 398
Dacryocystitis, 117–119
  defined, 399
Dacryocystography, 368
Decreased vision
  differential diagnosis of, 1
  normal fundus in presence of decreased vision
    differential diagnosis of, 9
Degenerative ocular disease
  cataract due to, 322
Dellen, 77

diabetes mellitus and, 327
eyelid
　differential diagnosis of, 8
macular
　cystoid, 270–271
Embolic retinopathy
　sickle cell disease *vs.*, 278
Embolus
　differential diagnosis of, 9
Embryotoxon
　posterior, 159
Encephalofacial cavernous hemangiomatosis, 356–357
Endogenous bacterial endophthalmitis, 317–318
Endogenous endophthalmitis
　posterior uveitis due to, 298–299
Endophthalmitis
　bacterial
　　endogenous, 317–318
　blebitis *vs.*, 197
　endogenous
　　posterior uveitis due to, 298–299
　infectious
　　anterior uveitis *vs.*, 291
　　lens-particle glaucoma *vs.*, 178–179
　phacoanaphylactic
　　lens-particle glaucoma *vs.*, 179
　phacolytic glaucoma *vs.*, 177
　postoperative, 312–314 (*See also* Postoperative
　　endophthalmitis)
　traumatic, 316–317
Enophthalmos
　defined, 399
　of fellow eye
　　orbital disease *vs.*, 126
Entropion, 113
Enucleation
　defined, 399
Epibulbar osseous choristoma, 108
Epidermoid cysts
　orbital tumors in children due to, 133–134
Epinephrine
　contraindications and side effects of, 396
Epiretinal membrane, 273
Episclera
　defined, 399
Episcleral vessels
　dilated
　　differential diagnosis of, 7
Episcleritis, 99–100
　blebitis *vs.*, 197
　defined, 399
Eserine
　contraindications and side effects of, 396
Esodeviations
　in children, 144–146
　　differential diagnosis of, 144
　　follow-up care, 146
　　signs of, 144
　　treatment of, 146
　　types of, 144–145
　　workup for, 145–146

Esophoria
　defined, 399
Esotropia
　defined, 399
　in children
　　types of, 144–145
Exenteration
　defined, 399
Exfoliative glaucoma, 176–177
　defined, 176
　differential diagnosis of, 176
　follow-up care, 177
　pigment dispersion/pigmentary glaucoma *vs.*,
　　174
　signs of, 176
　symptoms of, 176
　treatment of, 176
　workup for, 176
Exodeviations
　in children, 147–148
　　differential diagnosis of, 147
　　signs of, 147
　　treatment of, 148
　　types of, 147
　　workup for, 147–148
Exophoria
　defined, 399
Exophthalmos
　defined, 399
Exotropia(s)
　defined, 399
　in children
　　types of, 147
Exposure
　keratopathy, 46–47
Exudate(s)
　hard
　　defined, 399
　macular
　　differential diagnosis of, 9
Exudative ARMD, 264–265
Eye disease
　Internet links on, 389
Eye drops
　for toxic conjunctivitis, 95
Eye(s)
　blind, painful, 352–354
　bulging (*See* Orbital disease)
　Internet resources on, 389–390
　itchy
　　differential diagnosis of, 4
　jumping
　　differential diagnosis of, 3
　red
　　differential diagnosis of, 4–5
Eyelash loss
　differential diagnosis of, 2
Eyelid disorders
　acute infectious dacryoadenitis, 119–121
　blepharospasm, 115–116
　canaliculitis, 116–117

postoperative glaucoma and, 191–192, 193t
Hypocalcemia
 cataract due to, 322
Hypopyon
 defined, 399
 differential diagnosis of, 6
Hypopyon uveitis
 HLA B27—associated uveitis *vs.*, 302
Hypotony
 defined, 399
 differential diagnosis of, 12
Hypotony syndrome, 350–352
 causes of, 351
 defined, 350
 follow-up care, 352
 signs of, 350–351
 symptoms of, 350
 treatment of, 351–352
 workup for, 351

I

ICG. *See* Indocyanine green (ICG) angiography
Idiopathic intracranial hypertension, 225–226. *See also*
  Pseudotumor cerebri
Indirect ophthalmoscopy
 defined, 399
Indocyanine green (ICG) angiography, 365
Infant(s)
 blind, 161–163 (*See* Blind infant)
 nystagmus in
  differential diagnosis of, 12
 ossification of cornea in
  differential diagnosis of, 7
Infectious disease
 drugs for, 391
Infectious endophthalmitis
 anterior uveitis *vs.*, 291
 lens-particle glaucoma *vs.*, 178–179
Infectious keratouveitis
 anterior uveitis *vs.*, 291
Inflammation
 intraocular
  cataract due to, 322
Inflammatory glaucoma
 neovascular glaucoma *vs.*, 187
 open-angle, 171–172
  acute angle-closure glaucoma *vs.*, 180
  causes of, 172
  differential diagnosis of, 171–172
  glaucomatocyclitic crisis *vs.*, 186
  pigment dispersion/pigmentary glaucoma *vs.*, 174–175
  signs of, 171
  symptoms of, 171
  treatment of, 172
  workup for, 172
 phacolytic glaucoma *vs.*, 177
Inflammatory optic neuritis
 arteritic ischemic optic neuropathy *vs.*, 227
Injection(s)
 subconjunctival
  technique for, 380, 381f

subtenon
 technique for, 380, 381f
INO. *See* Internuclear ophthalmoplegia (INO)
Intermediate uveitis, 296–297
Intermittent intraocular hemorrhage
 amaurosis fugax *vs.*, 234
Internet
 ophthalmology resources on, 389–390
Internuclear ophthalmoplegia (INO), 220–221
 causes of, 220–221
 differential diagnosis of, 220
 follow-up care, 221
 isolated third nerve palsy *vs.*, 204
 signs of, 220
 symptoms of, 220
 treatment of, 221
 workup for, 221
Interstitial keratitis, 66–67
 congenital syphilis and, 152
Intracavernous aneurysm
 cavernous sinus syndrome due to, 214
Intracranial mass compressing afferent visual pathway
 optic neuritis *vs.*, 222
Intraepithelial neoplasia
 conjunctival, 107
Intraocular foreign bodies, 37–38
 retained
  posterior uveitis *vs.*, 297
Intraocular hemorrhage
 intermittent
  amaurosis fugax *vs.*, 234
Intraocular inflammation
 cataract due to, 322
Intraocular pressure
 decreased
  differential diagnosis of, 10
 differential diagnosis of, 10
 increase in
  acute
   differential diagnosis of, 10
  chronic
   differential diagnosis of, 10
Intraocular tumor
 cataract due to, 322
 glaucoma secondary to
  phacolytic glaucoma *vs.*, 177
 vitreous hemorrhage due to, 276
Intraorbital foreign body, 32–33
Intraretinal microvascular abnormalities
 defined, 399–400
Intravenous fluorescein angiography (IVFA), 365
Iridectomy
 peripheral
  defined, 400
Iridocorneal endothelial syndrome, 189–190
 defined, 189
 differential diagnosis of, 189–190
 follow-up care, 190
 signs of, 189
 symptoms of, 189
 treatment of, 190

Large cell lymphoma
posterior uveitis *vs.*, 297
LASEK (laser-assisted subepithelial keratectomy)
defined, 400
Laser in-situ keratomileusis (LASIK)
defined, 400
Laser-assisted subepithelial keratectomy (LASEK)
defined, 400
LASIK (laser in-situ keratomileusis)
defined, 400
Latanoprost
contraindications and side effects of, 396
Leber's congenital amaurosis
nystagmus due to, 232
Leber's optic neuropathy, 230
optic neuritis *vs.*, 222
papilledema *vs.*, 224
Lens
differential diagnosis of, 10–11
dislocated, 349–350
differential diagnosis of, 10
subluxed, 349–350
Lens particles
iridescent
differential diagnosis of, 10
Lens-induced uveitis
anterior uveitis due to, 291
Lens-particle glaucoma, 178–179
defined, 178
differential diagnosis of, 178–179
follow-up care, 179
phacolytic glaucoma *vs.*, 177
signs of, 178
symptoms of, 178
treatment of, 179
Lenticonus
anterior, 159
differential diagnosis of, 10–11
posterior, 159
Lesion(s)
amelanotic
conjunctival, 106
eyelid
differential diagnosis of, 8
macular
bull's-eye
differential diagnosis of, 8
melanotic
conjunctival, 108–109
orbital
cavernous sinus syndrome *vs.*, 213–214
differential diagnosis of, 12
peripheral
isolated seventh nerve palsy due to, 211
Leukemia
orbital tumors in children due to, 134
posterior uveitis *vs.*, 298
Leukocoria
in children, 141–142
causes of, 141–142
defined, 141, 400

follow-up care, 142
in children
differential diagnosis of, 12
treatment of, 142
workup for, 142
Levator muscle dehiscence
myasthenia gravis *vs.*, 217
Levobunolol
contraindications and side effects of, 396
Lice, 93
Light
flashes of
differential diagnosis of, 3
Light sensitivity
differential diagnosis of, 4
Limbal dermoid
conjunctival, 106
Louis-Bar syndrome, 359
Lowe syndrome
congenital cataracts in children due to, 151
congenital glaucoma in children due to, 157
Lubricating medications, 394
Lyme disease, 340–341
anterior uveitis due to, 291
differential diagnosis of, 340
follow-up care, 341
isolated seventh nerve palsy due to, 211
posterior uveitis due to, 300
signs of, 340
symptoms of, 340
treatment of, 341
workup for, 340
Lymphangioma
conjunctival, 107
orbital tumors in children due to, 134
Lymphoid tumors
conjunctival, 108
orbital tumors in adults due to, 137
Lymphoma
large cell
posterior uveitis *vs.*, 297
malignant melanoma of choroid *vs.*, 289

M
Macula
defined, 400
Macular degeneration
age-related [*See* Age-related macular degeneration
(ARMD)]
Macular edema
cystoid, 270–271
Macular exudates
differential diagnosis of, 9
Macular hole, 271–272
Macular lesions
bull's-eye
differential diagnosis of, 8
Maculopathy
chloroquine/hydroxychloroquine
Stargardt disease *vs.*, 285
Magnetic resonance angiography (MRA), 362

Opacity(ies)
  vitreous
    differential diagnosis of, 13
Open-angle glaucoma
  inflammatory, 171–172 (*See also* Inflammatory
    glaucoma, open-angle)
  secondary
    primary open-angle glaucoma *vs.*, 164–165
Ophthalmia
  sympathetic, 320–321
    VKH syndrome *vs.*, 311
Ophthalmia neonatorum, 154–156
  causes of, 154
  differential diagnosis of, 154
  follow-up care, 157
  signs of, 154
  treatment of, 155–156
  workup for, 154–155
Ophthalmic medications
  commonly used, 391–394
  contraindications and side effects of, 395–397
Ophthalmic problems
  general, 322–359 [*See also* specific problem, e.g.,
    Cataract(s)]
Ophthalmic ultrasonography, 363–364
Ophthalmology resources
  on Internet, 389–390
Ophthalmopathy
  Graves
    papilledema *vs.*, 224
Ophthalmoplegia
  external
    defined, 400
  internal
    defined, 400
  internuclear, 220–221
    isolated third nerve palsy *vs.*, 204
Ophthalmoscopy
  confocal scanning laser, 368
  indirect
    defined, 399
Opsoclonus
  nystagmus *vs.*, 231, 233
Optic atrophy
  congenital syphilis and, 152
  hereditary
    complicated, 231
  primary open-angle glaucoma *vs.*, 165
Optic disc
  atrophy of
    differential diagnosis of, 11
  infiltration of
    papilledema *vs.*, 224
  swelling of
    differential diagnosis of, 11
Optic disc vasculitis
  papilledema *vs.*, 224
Optic nerve
  lesions of
    differential diagnosis of, 11–12
  melanocytoma of

    malignant melanoma of choroid *vs.*, 289
Optic nerve defects
  congenital
    primary open-angle glaucoma *vs.*, 165
Optic nerve drusen
  primary open-angle glaucoma *vs.*, 165
Optic nerve glioma
  orbital tumors in children due to, 134
Optic nerve sheath meningioma
  orbital tumors in adults due to, 137
Optic nerve tumors
  compressive
    arteritic ischemic optic neuropathy *vs.*, 227
  orbital
    papilledema *vs.*, 224
Optic neuritis, 221–223
  causes of, 222
  defined, 400
  differential diagnosis of, 221–222
  follow-up care, 223
  inflammatory
    arteritic ischemic optic neuropathy *vs.*,
      227
  retrobulbar
    nonphysiologic visual loss *vs.*, 238
  signs of, 221
  symptoms of, 221
  treatment of, 222–223
  workup for, 222
Optic neuropathy
  arteritic ischemic, 227–228
  compressive, 230
  cone dystrophies *vs.*, 283
  dominant, 230–231
  hypertensive
    papilledema *vs.*, 224
  ischemic
    nonarteritic, 228–229 (*See also* Nonarteritic ischemic
      optic neuropathy)
    optic neuritis *vs.*, 221
    papilledema *vs.*, 224
  Leber's, 230
    optic neuritis *vs.*, 222
  optic neuritis *vs.*, 221
  radiation, 231
  toxic, 229–230
    optic neuritis *vs.*, 222
Optic pit, 262–263
  differential diagnosis of, 262
  follow-up care, 263
  signs of, 262
  symptoms of, 262
  treatment of, 263
  workup for, 262–263
Optical coherence tomography (OCT), 367
Optociliary shunt vessels
  differential diagnosis of, 11
  on disc
    differential diagnosis of, 9
Ora serrata
  defined, 400

Orbit, 126–140
  cellulitis of, 131–133
  dacryoadenitis of
    chronic, 139–140
  defined, 400
  disease of, 126–128 (*See also* Orbital disease)
  inflammatory disease of
    pseudotumor, 130–131
  lacrimal gland mass of, 139–140
  thyroid-related disease of, 128–130 (*See also* Thyroid-related orbitopathy)
  tumors of
    in children, 133–136 (*See also* Orbital tumors, in children)
Orbital blow-out fracture, 28–29
Orbital cellulitis, 131–133
  causes of, 131
  follow-up care, 133
  orbital disease due to, 127
  organisms in, 131–132
  signs of, 131
  symptoms of, 131
  treatment of, 132–133
  workup for, 132
Orbital disease, 126–128
  causes of, 126–127
  defined, 401
  differential diagnosis of, 11–12, 126
  internuclear ophthalmoplegia *vs.*, 220
  signs of, 126
  symptoms of, 126
  workup for, 127–128
Orbital fracture
  isolated fourth nerve palsy *vs.*, 207
Orbital inflammatory disease
  isolated fourth nerve palsy *vs.*, 207
  isolated sixth nerve palsy *vs.*, 209
  myasthenia gravis *vs.*, 217
Orbital inflammatory pseudotumor, 130–131
  causes of, 130
  follow-up care, 131
  isolated third nerve palsy *vs.*, 204
  orbital disease due to, 127
  signs of, 130
  symptoms of, 130
  treatment of, 131
  workup for, 130–131
Orbital lesions
  cavernous sinus syndrome *vs.*, 213–214
  differential diagnosis of, 12
Orbital optic nerve tumors
  papilledema *vs.*, 224
Orbital trauma
  isolated sixth nerve palsy *vs.*, 209
Orbital tumor compressing optic nerve
  optic neuritis *vs.*, 222
Orbital tumor(s)
  in adults, 136–138, 136t
    causes of, 136–137
    follow-up care, 138
    signs of, 136, 136t

  symptoms of, 136
  treatment of, 138
  workup for, 137–138
  in children, 133–136, 133t
    causes of, 133–135
    signs of, 133, 133t
    treatment of, 135–136
    workup for, 135
  orbital disease due to, 127
Orbital vasculitis
  orbital disease due to, 127
Orbitopathy
  thyroid-related, 128–130 (*See also* Thyroid-related orbitopathy)
Organic amblyopia, 149
Oscillopsia
  defined, 400
  differential diagnosis of, 3
Osteoma
  choroidal
    malignant melanoma of choroid *vs.*, 289
Otitis
  isolated seventh nerve palsy due to, 211

P
Pain
  differential diagnosis of, 4
Painful eyes
  blind, 352–354
Palpebral conjunctiva
  defined, 400
Palsy(ies)
  cranial nerve
    orbital disease *vs.*, 126
  double-elevator, 148
  progressive supranuclear
    cavernous sinus syndrome *vs.*, 214
Pannus
  differential diagnosis of, 7
Panuveitis
  posterior uveitis due to, 299
Papilla(ae)
  conjunctival
    differential diagnosis of, 7
Papilledema, 223–225
  acute
    optic neuritis *vs.*, 222
  amaurosis fugax *vs.*, 234
  causes of, 224–225
  defined, 223, 400
  diabetic
    central retinal vein occlusion *vs.*, 256
  differential diagnosis of, 224
  signs of, 223–224
  symptoms of, 223
  treatment of, 225
  workup for, 225
Papillitis
  defined, 400
  diabetic
    papilledema *vs.*, 224

papilledema *vs.*, 224
Papilloma(s)
 conjunctival, 107
Parinaud oculoglandular conjunctivitis, 96
Parinaud syndrome
 isolated third nerve palsy *vs.*, 204
 thyroid-related orbitopathy *vs.*, 128–129
Parotid neoplasm
 isolated seventh nerve palsy due to, 211
Paroxysmal hemicrania
 chronic
  cluster headache *vs.*, 244
Pars planitis, 296–297
 posterior uveitis due to, 298
PAS
 acute angle-closure glaucoma *vs.*, 180
Pediatrics. *See* Children
Pediculosis, 93
Pemphigoid
 ocular cicatricial, 104–105
Peripapillary
 defined, 400
Peripheral anterior synechiae
 defined, 400
Peripheral corneal thinning/ulceration, 74–77
Peripheral field
 constriction of
  differential diagnosis of, 13
Peripheral iridectomy
 defined, 400
Peripheral lesions
 isolated seventh nerve palsy due to, 211
Periphlebitis
 differential diagnosis of, 9
 posterior uveitis due to, 299
Persistent hyperplastic primary vitreous (PHPV)
 congenital cataracts in children due to, 150–151
 leukocoria due to, 141
Peter's anomaly, 159
Phacoanaphylactic endophthalmitis
 lens-particle glaucoma *vs.*, 179
Phacolytic glaucoma, 177–178
 defined, 177
 differential diagnosis of, 177
 signs of, 177
 symptoms of, 177
 treatment of, 178
 workup for, 177–178
Phacomorphic glaucoma
 lens-particle glaucoma *vs.*, 179
Phakomatosis
 defined, 400
Phenothiazine
 toxicity
  retinitis pigmentosa *vs.*, 279
Phenothiazine toxicity, 286–287
 chlorpromazine, 287
 thioridazine, 286–287
Phenylephrine
 contraindications and side effects of, 396
Phlyctenulosis, 68–69

Phoria
 defined, 401
Phospholine iodide
 contraindications and side effects of, 396
Photographic imaging studies, 367
Photophobia
 defined, 401
 differential diagnosis of, 4
Photopsia
 defined, 401
Photorefractive keratectomy (PRK)
 defined, 401
Phototherapeutic keratectomy (PTK)
 defined, 401
PHPV. *See* Persistent hyperplastic primary vitreous (PHPV)
Physiologic optic nerve cupping
 primary open-angle glaucoma *vs.*, 164
Physostigmine
 contraindications and side effects of, 396
Pigment dispersion/pigmentary glaucoma, 174–175
 defined, 174
 differential diagnosis of, 174–175
 follow-up care, 175
 signs of, 174
 symptoms of, 174
 treatment of, 175
 workup for, 175
Pigmentary glaucoma
 acute angle-closure glaucoma *vs.*, 180
 glaucomatocyclitic crisis *vs.*, 186
 inflammatory open-angle glaucoma *vs.*, 171
Pigmented paravenous retinochoroidal atrophy
 retinitis pigmentosa *vs.*, 280
Pilocarpine
 contraindications and side effects of, 396
Pituitary adenoma
 during pregnancy, 329, 331
Pituitary apoplexy
 cavernous sinus syndrome due to, 214
Plain films, 366
Plateau iris, 184–185
Plateau iris configuration, 184
Plateau iris syndrome, 184
Plexiform neurofibroma
 orbital tumors in children due to, 134–135
Pneumocystis carinii pneumonia
 AIDS-related, 336–337, 337f
Pneumonia(s)
 Pneumocystis carinii
  AIDS-related, 336–337, 337f
Polycoria
 defined, 401
Posner-Schlossman syndrome. *See* Acute angle-closure glaucoma
Posterior embryotoxon, 159
Posterior polymorphous dystrophy
 iridocorneal endothelial syndrome *vs.*, 190
Posterior scleritis
 malignant melanoma of choroid *vs.*, 289
 posterior uveitis *vs.*, 298

posterior uveitis after, 298
retrobulbar hemorrhage, 29–30, 31f
ruptured globe, 35–36
vitreous hemorrhage due to, 276
Traumatic endophthalmitis, 316–317
Traumatic glaucoma
acute angle-closure glaucoma *vs.*, 180
Trichiasis, 113–114
Tropia
defined, 401
Tropicamide
contraindications and side effects of, 397
Tuberculosis
anterior uveitis due to, 292
posterior uveitis due to, 300
toxoplasmosis *vs.*, 303
Tuberous sclerosis, 355–356
Tumor(s)
anterior uveitis *vs.*, 291
chiasmal
nonphysiologic visual loss *vs.*, 238
conjunctival, 106–109
eyelid
malignant, 124–125
intraocular
cataract due to, 322
glaucoma secondary to phacolytic glaucoma *vs.*, 177
vitreous hemorrhage due to, 276
lacrimal gland
orbital disease due to, 127
lymphoid
conjunctival, 108
orbital tumors in adults due to, 137
optic nerve
compressive
arteritis ischemic optic neuropathy *vs.*, 227
orbital
papilledema *vs.*, 224
orbital
compressing optic nerve
optic neuritis *vs.*, 222
in adults, 136–138 (*See also* Orbital tumors, in adults)
in children, 133–136 (*See also* Orbital tumors, in children)
orbital disease due to, 127
skull base
cavernous sinus syndrome *vs.*, 214
within cavernous sinus
cavernous sinus syndrome due to, 214

U

Ulceration
peripheral corneal thinning, 74–77
Ultrasonography
A-scan, 363
B-mode, 363–364
Doppler orbital, 364
ophthalmic, 363–364
Uveitis, 290–321
acute retinal necrosis, 308–310, 309t
AIDS-related, 333

anterior, 290–295
blebitis *vs.*, 197
causes of, 291–292
congenital syphilis and, 152
differential diagnosis of, 290–291
epidemiology of, 292t
follow-up care, 295
signs of, 290
symptoms of, 290
systems review in, 293t
treatment of, 293–295
workup for, 292–293, 292t–294t
Behçet disease, 307–308
Candida retinitis/uveitis/endophthalmitis, 319–320
drug-induced
anterior uveitis *vs.*, 290
endophthalmitis
endogenous bacterial, 317–318
postoperative, 312–314
traumatic, 316–317
HLA B26—associated
Behçet disease *vs.*, 307–308
HLA B27—associated, 302
hypopyon
HLA B27—associated uveitis *vs.*, 302
intermediate, 296–297
lens-induced
anterior uveitis due to, 291
papilledema *vs.*, 224
posterior, 297–301
causes of, 298–301
differential diagnosis of, 297–298
signs of, 297
symptoms of, 297
with spillover into anterior chamber
anterior uveitis *vs.*, 290
workup for, 301
postoperative
chronic, 315–316
postoperative glaucoma and, 191–192
prior
iridocorneal endothelial syndrome *vs.*, 190
sarcoidosis, 305–307
sympathetic ophthalmia, 320–321
toxoplasmosis, 303–305
Vogt-Koyanagi-Harada syndrome, 310–312, 311t
Uveitis-glaucoma-hyphema (UGH) syndrome
anterior uveitis due to, 291

V

Vaccinia
ocular, 86–88 (*See also* Ocular vaccinia)
Valacyclovir
contraindications and side effects of, 397
Vancomycin
contraindications and side effects of, 397
fortified
making of, 383
Varicella-zoster virus, 341
Varix
orbital disease due to, 127